CONTEMPORARY ASPECTS OF ENDOCRINOLOGY

Edited by **Evanthia Diamanti-Kandarakis**

Contemporary Aspects of Endocrinology
Edited by Evanthia Diamanti-Kandarakisca

Published by InTech

Janeza Trdine 9, 51000 Rijeka, Croatia

Publishing Process Manager Petra Nenadic

Technical Editor Teodora Smiljanic

Cover Designer InTech Design Team

Additional hard copies can be obtained from orders@intechopen.com

Contemporary Aspects of Endocrinology, Edited by Evanthia Diamanti-Kandarakis
p. cm.
978-953-307-357-6

For EU product safety concerns:
IN TECH d.o.o., Prolaz Marije Krucifikse Kozulić 3, 51000 Rijeka, Croatia,
info@intechopen.com or visit our website at intechopen.com.

Meet the editor

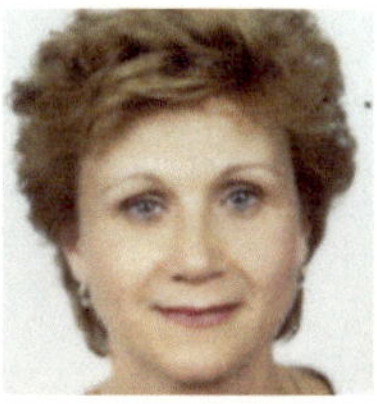

Dr Evanthia Diamanti-Kandarakis is professor of Internal Medicine, Endocrinology and Metabolism in addition to holding the position of Chairman of the Third Department of Medicine, Medical School University of Athens. She received her MD from Medical School of Athens and her PhD in experimental Endocrinology on the effects of androgens in hypophysectomised rats, from the same University. Dr Diamanti-Kandarakis completed her initial training in internal medicine in England before continuing in the United States. For the past 15 years, her research interests have been focused on clinical, molecular and environmental aspects of metabolic and hormonal abnormalities in Polycystic ovarian syndrome. This work has generated more than 120 publications and more than 3,500 citations. Dr Diamanti-Kandarakis has been invited by the international academic community as a speaker and has given more than 100 lectures, in Europe, Asia, Africa, North and South America.

Contents

Preface

Comprehending endocrine disorders requires a combination of basic knowledge on molecular biology and genetics as well as a good grasp of the clinical aspects. Given the recent advances in these fields, an overview of the latest trends and developments affecting endocrinology is provided.

As one of the most up to date publications on this specialist field, this book is the result of a collaboration between a number of leading researchers and practitioners in the field who are recognized for their work over the years in the field of endocrinology. The book provides and indepth analysis across a range of topics focused on hormonal and metabolic disorders.

The book aims to provide a basic as well as advanced recent trends in endocrine disorders in addition to an analytical focus on those topics less well-studied. Readers will find a large spectrum of endocrinopathise from thyroid carcinogenesis and pituitary adenomas to adrenal tumors and metabolic bone disease. Emphasis has also been focused on more specific issues not yet fully elucidated (e.g. the molecular pathways involved in thyrotropin beta gene regulation or monogenic phosphate balance disorders).

We hope that the scope of this book is not only to answer questions but mainly to stimulate new questions.In sharing the knowledge, of the eminent scientists and clinicians in this book with a broad spectrum of readers,it will spark new interest in the expanding spectrum of endocrine disorders.

The book is organized into the following sections:

I. INTRODUCTION TO ENDOCRINOLOGY including the chapter « The power of an evolutionary perspective in studies of endocrinology» by Dr. Zhang Yaping et al.; a review focused on recent advances in the understanding of the evolution of hormone signalling pathways.

II. PITUITARY ADENOMAS including the following chapters:

- «The Genetics of Pituitary Adenomas» by Dr. Fedele Monica et al.; a review on pituitary adenomas covering a wide spectrum from pituitary tumorigenesis to sporadic and familiar pituitary adenomas.

- «Acromegaly and Gigantism» by Dr. Akin Fulya et al.; authors attempt to provide data concerning the history, epidemiology, etiology, pathophysiology, clinical features, diagnosis and treatment of acromegaly.

- «Effects of Growth hormone (GH) over-expression on signaling cascades involved in promotion of cell proliferation and survival» by Dr. González Lorena et al.; authors analyze the effects of long term exposure to growth hormone (GH) at the molecular level in the liver.

III. THE THYROID GLAND including the following chapters:

- «Negative regulation of the thyrotropin beta gene by T3» by Dr. Sasaki Shigekazu et al.; an up-to-date review focused on the molecular mechanisms of negative regulation of the TSH beta gene by T3.

- «Clinical management of thyroid nodules in the areas of various iodine supply» by Prof. Słowińska-Klencka Dorota et al.; a review is focused on the clinical management of thyroid nodules in areas of different iodine status (high, sufficient or inadequate iodine supply).

- «Clinical Workup of Nodular and Mass Lesions of the Endocrine Organs» by Dr. Lin Xiaoqi et al.; a review focused on the application of FNA biopsy for thyroid and parathyroid lessions.

- «Molecular biology of thyroid cancer» by Prof. Viglietto Giuseppe et al.; a revision on thyroid tumorigenesis covering a wide literature spectrum from epidemiology and risk factors of thyroid cancer to the mechanisms and molecular pathways that underlie onset and progression of these neoplasms.

- «Diagnosis and differential diagnosis of medullary thyroid cancer» by Dr. Faggiano Antongiulio et al.; a review focused on the pathogenesis, diagnosis and therapeutic approach of medullary thyroid cancer.

- «Molecular Diagnostics in Treatment of Medullary Thyroid Carcinoma» by Prof. Pützer Brigitte et al.; a review focused on new perspectives in the molecular diagnostic approach of patients with medullary thyroid cancer.

- «Medullary thyroid carcinoma associated with RET mutations located in exon» by Dr. Peppa Melpomeni et al.; a chapter focused on the genetic analysis of the RET protooncogene -apart from the known somatic mutations in exons 10, 11, 13-16, authors analyze another " non classical" exon mutation in exon 8.

- «Status for congenital hypothyroidism at advanced ages» by Dr. Ari Yuca Sevil; a review focused on the multi-systemic abnormalities provoked by congenital hypothyroidism later in life.

IV. ADRENAL GLANDS including the following chapters:

- «Adrenal incidentaloma and adrenocortical carcinoma» by Dr. Sasaki Shigekazu et al.; an up-to-date review focused on the molecular mechanisms of negative regulation of the TSH beta gene by T3.

- «Adrenal Cortex Tumors and Hyperplasias» by Prof. Pignatelli Duarte; a thorough revision on adrenal cortex tumors and hyperplasias.

- «Autoimmunity to steroid-producing cells» by Dr. Falorni Alberto et al; a review of the genetic basis of adrenal autoimmunity.

- «Exrretion of Steroid Hormones in Rodent: An overview on species differences for new biomedical animal research models» by Dr. Busso Juan Manuel et al.; a review analyzing the routes of gonadal and adrenocortical steroid excretion based on data derived from wild , laboratory and farm rodents.

V. METABOLIC BONE DISEASE including the following chapters:

- «New trends in Calcium and Phosphorus metabolism. Hypoparathyroidism» by Dr. Puig-Domingo Manuel et al.; a review specialized on the regulation of the metabolism of calcium and phosphorus and their integrated pathways to maintain their levels within physiological limits.

- «Monogenic phosphate balance disorders» by Dr. Raeder et al.; a review focused on phosphate disorders- diagnosis and treatment.

- «Pseudohypoparathyroidism in Children» Dr. Nwosu Benjamin; a review focused on pseudohypoparathyroidism's diagnosis , treatment and management in children.

- «Retinoids and Bone» by Prof. Lerner Ulf et al.; a review on the impact of Vitamin A on bone remodeling, skeletal mass and osteoclast differentiation.

We have learned that there is an endocrinology of elation and despair, a chemistry of mystical insight, and, in relation to the autonomic nervous system, a meteorology and even... an astro-physics of changing moods. - Aldous (Leonard) Huxley, *Literature and Science (1963)*

Prof. Dr. Evanthia Diamanti-Kandarakis
University of Athens Medical School, Sotiria Hospital, Athens,
Greece

Part 1

Introduction to Endocrinology

1

The Power of an Evolutionary Perspective in Studies of Endocrinology

Jing He[1], David M. Irwin[1,2] and Ya-Ping Zhang[1,3]
[1]*State Key Laboratory of Genetic Resource and Evolution, Kunming Institute of Zoology, Chinese Academy of Sciences*
[2]*Department of Laboratory Medicine and Pathobiology and Banting and Best Diabetes Centre, University of Toronto*
[3]*Laboratory for Conservation and Utilization of Bioresource, Yunnan University*
[1,3]*China*
[2]*Canada*

1. Introduction

Much of our understanding of the molecular basis of endocrinology has been the product of highly productive studies that have focused on specific molecules (e.g., hormones) and their specific immediate interacting partners. However, biomolecules are not isolated particles, but instead they are elements of highly integrated interaction networks, and specific interactions among them drive virtually all cellular functions and underlie phenotypic complexity and diversity. Many hormones, and their specific receptors and other interacting proteins, are known to be evolutionarily related, which raises intriguing questions concerning how specificity originated within these systems.

Our previous studies have illustrated that biochemical entities are developmentally and evolutionarily fluid, with capabilities to be altered both in composition and behavior. Gene birth and death are widespread phenomena in genome evolution and accounts for the great diversity of gene families involved in endocrinology. While concordance of evolutionary histories both in pattern and process of hormones, receptors and interacting proteins might be expected for integrated systems, studies have shown that the evolutionary history of receptors need not mirror that of their ligands. Simultaneous emergence, or loss, of multiple interacting partners by multiple gene duplication or gene loss is unlikely in evolution. Gene duplication is essential in the development of complex endocrinology. It is creative in producing elements that allow evolutionary tinkering and thus plays a major role in gene co-option (i.e., recruitment for novel functions) facilitating the evolution of greater biological complexity. Alternatively, if an interacting partner is lost, the retained partner may either be subsequently lost or, more interestingly, serve as raw material in evolution and become recruited into a new interaction yielding a new function. Thus, a stepwise process of elaboration through mutation and optimization ensues, adapting genes (and their encoded proteins) into the physiology of an organism.

Here we review several recent advances in our understanding of the evolution of hormone signalling pathways that illustrate the power of an evolutionary perspective. Among our examples are the motilin and ghrelin signalling pathways where we have demonstrated that both the hormones (motilin and ghrelin) and their specific receptors descended from common ancestors through independent gene duplications. The motilin receptor originated well before the evolution of the hormone, and the motilin-motilin receptor specificity has arisen, as the result of ligand-receptor coevolution, after the hormone gene duplicated. Similarly, motilin and its specific receptor gene specifically lost on the rodent lineage followed a stepwise process. Once one of the interacting partners is lost, the retained partner may subsequently be lost, or serve as raw material in evolution and become recruited into a new function.

Given the evolutionary dynamics of the genome and the plasticity of biomolecule networks, an evolutionary perspective is necessary to understand many aspects of the molecular basis of endocrinology. An integrated evolutionary comparative strategy helps enhance our understanding of the assemblage of the complex endocrine systems, provide important clues in interaction capacity exploration, and identify the main diversification events of the endocrine systems and potential cross-talk between them through evolutionary related interacting proteins. In addition, knowledge of how elements of the endocrine systems that underlie cellular functions are evolutionarily and developmentally interact, help not only in choosing appropriate species to examine function, but also provide genetic makers to probe the emergence of specific traits and characteristics, uncovering the genetic basis that underlie the morphological and behavior changes, and thus enhance our understanding of how organisms adapt to changing environments.

2. The molecular basis of endocrine systems

Endocrinology is the branch of biology that focuses on regulatory systems involving a group of specialized chemical substances called hormones that travel though blood. New developments in endocrinology have been dominated by progress in molecular genetics. Although these investigations often relate to rare single gene disorders, they have resulted in major advances in our understanding of the cellular mechanisms of hormone action (Cegla, Tan and Bloom 2010; Hodson et al. 2010; Peter and Vallo 1998). Most endocrinology studies are medically orientated, and thus anthropocentric, with little or no comparative or evolutionary perspective, and therefore provide few insights into our comprehension of the enigmatic origin and diversification of these systems (Markov et al. 2008).

Much of our understanding of the molecular basis of endocrinology has come from highly productive studies that have focused on specific molecules and their immediate interacting partners, in fact, hormonal systems are a central part. Indeed the specificity of each hormone ligand and receptor pair is maintained in divergent species (Moyle et al. 1994), while biochemical entities are developmentally and evolutionarily fluid, with a much wider range of capabilities for alteration in both composition and behavior (Avise and Ayala 2007; Wilkins 2007). Thus intriguing questions concerning how the diversity and specificity occur within these systems remain to be answered.

Genomes are documents of life history, and their structures continually change throughout evolution. Humans represent only a leaf on the tree of life. The anthropocentrism view of evolution, where humans are the pinnacle of gradually developed complexity, is a one-sided and incorrect view (Markov et al. 2008). In the light of evolution, an approach that considers each taxa equally, adopts a comparative strategy, integrates information from diverse organisms and various scientific approaches, helps enhance our understanding of the assemblage of the complex endocrine systems and the main events that have prompted their diversification, and yields better insight into their biological functions and potential cross-talk between them through evolutionary related interacting proteins.

3. Evolutionary mechanisms for the diversification of endocrine systems

Genomes are the entirety of organisms' hereditary information, and encode all the information necessary to give rise to biomolecular products. The structure and content of genomes do not remain static, and continually change through evolutionary time. Major evolutionary mechanisms that have been instrumental in shaping the genome include gene duplication, gene loss and evolutionary shift.

3.1 Gene duplication

As genome size increases, gene content tends to increase, although at a disproportionately lower rate in eukaryotes compared to non-eukaryotes (Gregory 2005; Hou and Lin 2009; Konstantinidis and Tiedje 2004; Lynch and Conery 2003). The gene number increases with genome size, and morphological complexity is mostly generated by expanding the sizes of gene families rather than due to a growth of the number of unique gene types, hence multicellular organisms employ large sets of similar gene products while exhibiting extraordinary biodiversity. The elements of endocrine systems often group into families (e.g., hormones and their specific receptors), whose members have diverged to various extents in regulation and function (Danks et al. 2011; Hoffmann and Opazo 2011; Irwin 2010; Kim et al. 2011; Sundström, Dreborg and Larhammar 2010).

Gene duplication is the most important mechanism for generating new genes and new biochemical processes and has facilitated the evolution of biodiversity and complexity (Li 2006; Ohno 1970). The most obvious contribution is supplying the raw genetic material for the various evolutionary forces (e.g., mutation, genetic drift and natural selection) to act upon, which lead to specialized or new gene functions (Zhang 2003). Without gene duplication, the capability and plasticity of organisms in adapting to changing environments would be severely limited. Gene duplication can also contribute to species divergence (Ting et al. 2004) along with the origin of species-specific features (Zhang et al. 2002). Duplication may involve part of gene, a single gene, part of a chromosome, an entire chromosome, or the whole genome. The first four scenarios are also known as regional duplications, because they do not result in a doubling of the entire genome. Hereinafter, the role of whole genome duplication and regional duplication will be discussed respectively.

3.1.1 Whole genome duplication

Genome duplication is often considered to be more important than regional duplication in evolution, as it allows for the duplication of the entire regulatory systems. Regional duplications, on the other hand, generally allow for part of a regulatory system to be duplicated, which may lead to imbalances that may disrupt normal function. The significance of whole genome duplication has been highlighted by the studies of invertebrate chordates and the base of vertebrate evolution (Garcia-Fernández and Holland 1994), as well as fish diversification (Dehal and Boore 2005; Jaillon et al. 2004). Genome duplication facilitated the appearance and diversification of complex features, such as the endocrine system (Holland et al. 2008). The amphioxus genome exhibits considerable synteny with the human genome, but lacks the whole-genome duplications characteristic of vertebrates (Dehal and Boore 2005). Holland et al. (2008) examined the existence of endocrine components based on the amphioxus genome, and reasoned that ancestral chordate only possess a basic set of endocrine functions. Hereby a fully functional endocrine system must have arisen after the divergence of cephalochordate, which was driven in all probability by subsequent genome duplications.

3.1.2 Regional duplication

While whole genome duplication events are not uncommon, nevertheless they only infrequently contribute to the evolution of well-developed bisexual organisms, as they likely disrupt the mechanism of sex determination and would be quickly eliminated (Li 1997). Regional duplications make up the gap, providing new genetic material for local elaboration and optimization, and fuel the evolution of lineage-specific variability (Li 1997; Ohno 1970). Whole genome duplications and small-scale duplications have very different consequences. Selective retention of different duplicates, and enrichment of signaling proteins and transcription factors, have been observed in yeast, plants, early vertebrate and fish following whole genome duplications (Conant 2010; Gout, Duret and Kahn 2009; Huminiecki and Heldin 2010; Kassahn et al. 2009; Manning and Scheeff 2010). This indicates that the individual duplication of signaling proteins and transcriptional regulators may be deleterious, since interactions between them are relatively transient and subtle, requiring a dosage balance from the whole genome duplication to survive. It is reasonably to expect that, simultaneous duplications of ligands and downstream signaling genes are required to allow the expansion of the complex endocrine systems. As it is, only part of the regulatory system has been duplicated in regional duplication, then, what are the evolutionary consequences of such an imbalanced outcome?

3.2 Gene loss

Studies on genome evolution have focused on the creation of new genes, including changes in regulatory mechanisms, and often neglect the role of selective gene loss in shaping these genomes. Gene loss or pseudogenization is a widespread phenomenon in genome evolution (Wang, Grus and Zhang 2006). The differential fixation of mutational gene loss after genome duplication illustrates the power of these types of events (Semyonov et al. 2008; van Hoek and Hogeweg 2009). Within gene families gene turnover, caused by differential gene gain and loss, leads to diverse patterns of gene distributions on different lineages, and contributes significantly to the evolution of biodiversity and may be the basis for reproductive isolation and speciation in geographically isolated populations (Gagneux and Varki 2001; Gout, Duret and Kahn 2009; Hahn, Demuth and Han 2007; Kettler et al. 2007; Powell et al. 2008). Sometimes, the ubiquitous, and near-stochastic, gene loss process can lead to the loss of single copy genes. By taking advantages of the availability of large amounts of vertebrate genomic information, it has been shown that many important human endocrine genes have been found to be missing or inactivated in other vertebrates, and vice versa (He et al. 2010; Irwin 2010; Pitel et al. 2010). In the same way, evolutionary comparisons among different taxa can help identify novel elements of endocrine systems that are not possessed by model animals. Endocrine entities are not isolated particles, but are elements of highly integrated interaction networks, and play their role through specific interactions (Carroll, Bridgham and Thornton 2008). As a random process, the simultaneous loss of multiple interacting partners is unlikely, despite the intimate association between them. Gene loss, a dramatic genetic event, leads to the immediate loss of specific interactions, and probably affects interaction turnover as greatly as gene duplication. If a signaling protein is lost, then what are the evolutionary consequences for the retained partners?

3.3 Evolutionary shift

Genes are not only duplicated and lost, there are many genes which have been conserved and are unambiguous orthologues in a wide variety of taxonomic species, but evolutionary shifts occur frequently and orthologues genes can have distinct functions in different taxa (Macqueen et al. 2010; Zhou et al. 2008). Species adapt to diverse ecosystems and environments, and have differing genetic backgrounds. As selective constraints vary, it impacts the pattern of gene evolution, and changes in selection can yield changes in function (Irwin 2001). In some cases, positive selection appears to underlie the evolutionary shift (Wallis 2001; Liu et al. 2001); while in others, inefficient purifying selection and increased genetic drift, associated with a reduction in effective population size, are the cause (Macqueen et al. 2010).

The genetic network of the endocrine systems are developmentally and evolutionarily fictile, the elemental composition is prone to be altered via gene gain and loss, and its physiological properties frequently change through mutations in endocrine gene coding sequences and/or regulatory systems, and turnover of interacting biomolecules. Using a comparative strategy, integrating information on species phylogenetic relationships, gene evolutionary history, gene sequences and functional properties such as expression, interaction and physiological data, should enhance our understanding of how they evolved and yield better insight into their biological functions. The large amounts of accumulating genetic information is a powerful resource for addressing these questions.

4. Case studies for evolutionary endocrinology: Lessons from the motilin/ghrelin hormone family and their receptors

4.1 Gene duplication plays a major role in gene co-option

4.1.1 Ghrelin and motilin

Ghrelin and motilin represent a novel gastrointestinal hormone family in mammals (Inui 2001). Not only are ghrelin and motilin structurally related, but, the sequence and overall structure of their precursor genes show considerable similarity (Fig. 1).

Ghrelin is derived by posttranslational cleavage from its precursor preproghrelin (GHRL), and is a circulating peptide hormone that is secreted mainly by the stomach and acts upon the hypothalamus and hindbrain (Nakazato et al. 2001; Kojima and Kangawa 2005). Growth hormone secretagogue receptor (GHSR) is the specific receptor for ghrelin and a G protein-coupled receptor, and upon stimulation releases growth hormone (GH) from the pituitary (Howard et al. 1996; Kojima et al. 1999; Sun, Ahmed and Smith 2003). Evidence from mammals suggests that ghrelin also acts to stimulate gastric motility, increase appetite and food intake, and induce a positive energy balance leading to body weight gain (Murray et al. 2003; Peeters 2005). Prepromotilin (MLN) is posttranslationaly processed to yield a secreted peptide that is then cleaved at a paired basic amino acid site and gives rise to motilin (Poitras 1993). Motilin primarily acts to increase gastrointestinal motility by activating neural pathways or via the direct stimulation of smooth muscles. In human and dog it has been suggested that motilin has a physiological role in the regulation of a motor pattern

typical for the fasted state (Poitras 1993). It is of interest to note that motilin also has a weak GH-releasing effect (Samson et al. 1984). GPR38, an orphan G protein coupled receptor, was identified as the motilin receptor, MLNR, through a remarkable process of reverse pharmacology (Feighner et al 1999). GHSR and MLNR, whose sequences are very similar, are members of the β-group of rhodopsin-like receptor family (Holst et al. 2004).
Despite the very close resemblance of the hormones and receptors, to date there is no evidence for any cross-reactivity between the ligands, which corresponds to the fact that the pharmacophore of the peptides are quite different (Peeters 2005). Octanoylation of serine[3] is a unique and crucially important feature of ghrelin and studies have demonstrated that without the octanoyl group the potency of GHRL is dramatically decreased (Peeters 2005; Kaiya et al. 2001).

4.1.2 Evolution of the motilin/ghrelin hormone gene family

Genes for ghrelin have been cloned from a number of vertebrate species. Using bioinformatic methods, we have identified additional ghrelin gene sequences from diverse mammalian species and a frog *Xenopus tropicalis* (Table 1). Motilin genes have only been identified and characterized in mammals and birds, even after the use of bioinformatic approaches (Table 2). Ghrelin and motilin genes are both single copy genes in all of the species studied, and reside in conserved gene neighborhoods respectively, strongly supporting their orthology. The amino acid sequences of ghrelin are well conserved among species, especially in the N terminal region, and the same principle holds for motilin (Table 1-2). Interestingly, when the comparative genomic analysis was conducted between human and other vertebrates (chicken, *X. tropicalis*, medaka, tetraodon, and zebrafish) aimed at the GHRL and MLN neighborhood regions, it was revealed that homologs of the human GHRL and MLN flanking genes, which are located on different chromosomes in amniotes, were found to reside on the same chromosome near the GHRL locus in medaka, tetraodon, zebrafish, and *X. tropicalis*. This observation suggests that there was a duplication of the GHRL gene yielding MLN on the amniote lineage however there was no overlap in the genomic neighborhoods for GHRL and MLN. We could not identify any sequences similar to ghrelin and/or motilin genes in the recently released lamprey and deuterostome draft genomes. GHRL sequences from fish and amphibians posses only a single putative endoproteinase recognition site C-terminal to the signal peptidase cleavage site, thus can produce only a single posttranslational-processed peptide, ghrelin. In contrast, GHRL of amniotes (reptiles, birds, and mammals) possess three putative endoproteinase recognition sites, potentially giving rise to a second posttranslational-processed peptide, a 24-residue ghrelin-associated peptide (Fig. 1). The second peptide has recently been identified to be obestatin in mammals (Zhang et al. 2005). All MLNs, which are only found in reptiles, birds and mammals, possess three putative endoproteinase recognition sites, thus potentially give rise to two posttranslational-processed peptides, motilin and a 17-residue peptide in a position homologous to obestatin (Fig 1). Phylogenetic analysis revealed that bullfrog GHRL groups with amniote MLN rather than amnitote GHRL, although the bootstrap support for this conclusion is low (Fig. 2).
Based on the distribution of GHRL and MLN genes in the species studied, comparative genomics analysis between human and other vertebrates, and endoproteinase cleavage sites distribution in GHRL/MLN genes, we surmise that MLN was generated by a gene duplication on the early amniote lineage as illustrated in figure 2 (He et al. 2011). Other potential evolutionary scenarios (e.g., duplication prior to the fish-tetrapod divergence) require a larger number of gene deletion events along with parallel gain or loss of endopeptidease cleavage sites, and thus are less parsimonious.

Species	Ghrelin sequence	Obestatin homolog sequence
Homo sapiens	GSSFLSPEHQRVQQRKESKKPP AKLQP	FNAPFDVGIKLSGVQYQQHS QALG
Pan troglodytes	GSSFLSPEHQRVQQRKESKKPP AKLQP	FNAPFDVGIKLSGVQYQQHS QALG
Pongo pygmaeus	GSSFLSPEHQRVQQRKESKKPP AKLQP	FNAPFDVGIKLSGVQYQQHS QALG
Hylobates lar	GSSFLSPEHQRVQQRKESKKPP AKLQP	FNAPFDVGIKLSGVQYQQHS QALG
Macaca fuscata	GSSFLSPEHQRAQQRKESKKPP AKLQP	FNAPFDVGIKLSGVQYQQHS QALG
Papio hamadryas	GSSFLSPEHQRAQQRKESKKPP AKLQP	FNAPFDVGIKLSGVQYQQHS QALG
Saimiri sciureus	GSSFLSPEHQRIQQRKESKKPPA KLQP	FNAPFDVGIKLSGVQYQQHS QALG
Macaca mulatta	GSSFLSPEHQRAQQRKESKKPP AKLQP	FNAPFDVGIKLSGVQYQQHS QALG
Otolemur garnettii	GSSFLSPDHQKIQQRKESKKPPA KLQP	FNSPLDVGIKLSGAQYQQHS QALG
Cebus paella	GSSFLSPEHQRMQQRKESKKPP AKLQS	FNVPFDVGIKLSGVQYQQHS QALG
Aotus trivirgatus	GSSFLSPEHQRIQQRKESKKPPA KLQP	FNAPFDVGIKLSGIQYQQHSQ ALG
Mesocricetus auratus	GSSFLSPEHQKAQQRKESKKPQ AKLQP	FNAPFDVGIKLSGAQYQQHG RALG
Mus musculus	GSSFLSPEHQKAQQRKESKKPP AKLQP	FNAPFDVGIKLSGAQYQQHG RALG
Rattus norvegicus	GSSFLSPEHQKAQQRKESKKPP AKLQP	FNAPFDVGIKLSGAQYQQHG RALG
Meriones unguiculatus	GSSFLSPEHQKTQQRKESKKPP AKLQP	FNAPFDVGIKLSGAQYQQHG RALG
Oryctolagus cuniculus	GSSFLSPEHQKAQQRKDAKKPP ARLQP	
Felis catus	GSSFLSPEHQKVQQRKESKKPP AKLQP	FNAPFDVGIKLSGAQYHQHG QALG
Canis familiaris	GSSFLSPEHQKLQQRKESKKPP AKLQP	FNAPFDVGIKLSGPQYHQHG QALG
Equus caballus	GSSFLSPEHHKVQHRKESKKPP AKLKP	FNAPFDVGIKLSGAQYHQHS QALG
Rangifer tarandus	GSSFLSPEHQKLQRKEPKKPSGR LKP	FNAPFDIGIKLSGAQSLQHGQ TLG
Capra hircus	GSSFLSPEHQKLQRKEPKKPSGR LKP	FNAPFNIGIKLSGAQSLQHGQ TLG
Ovis aries	GSSFLSPEHQKLQRKEPKKPSGR LKP	FNAPFNIGIKLSGAQSLQHGQ TLG
Bos taurus	GSSFLSPEHQKLQRKEAKKPSG	FNAPFNIGIKLAGAQSLQHG

Species	Ghrelin sequence	Obestatin homolog sequence
	RLKP	QTLG
Bubalus bubalis	GSSFLSPEHQKLQRKEPKKPSGRLKP	FNAPFNIGIKLSGAQSLQHGQTLG
Ailuropoda melanoleuca	GSSFLSPEHQKVQRKESKKPPAKLQP	FNAPFDVGIKLSGAQYQEHGQALG
Sus scrofa	GSSFLSPEHQKVQQRKESKKPAAKLKP	FNAPCDVGIKLSGAQSDQHGQPLG
Kogia breviceps	GSSFLSPEHQKLQRKEAKKPSGRLKP	
Myotis lucifugus	GSSFLSPEHQKAQQRKESKKPPAKLQP	FNAPFDVGIKLSGAQSHWHGQALG
Erinaceus europaeus	GSSFLSPEHQKGQQRKEPKKPPGKVQP	FSAPFDVGLRLSGAQYEQHGEALR
Dasypus novemcinctus	GSSFLSPEHQKTQLRKEFKKPATKLQP	FNAPFDVGIKLSGAQYQQHGRSLG
Echinops telfairi	GSSFLSPGHPKVQPQRKESKTPAGKLQA	FNVPFDIGIKVSVAQYGEHGRALD
Loxodonta africana	GSSFLSPKNQKLQQRKESKKPPAKLQP	
Monodelphis domestica	GSSFLSPEHPKTQRKETKKPSVKLQP	FNAPFDIGIKVAEAQYQQYGHALE
Gallus gallus	GSSFLSPTYKNIQQQKDTRKPTARLH	FNVPFEIGVKITEREYQEYGQALE
Meleagris gallopavo	GSSFLSPAYKNIQQQKDTRKPTARLHP	FNVPFEIGVKITEREYQEYGQALE
Anas platyrhynchos	GSSFLSPEFKKIQQQNDPTKTTAKIH	FHVPFEIGVKITEEEYQEYGQTLE
Anser sp.	GSSFLSPEFKKIQQQNDPAKATAKIH	FNVPFEIGVKITEEEYQEYGQTLE
Dromaius novaehollandiae	GSSFLSPDYKKIQQRKDPRKPTTKLH	FNVPFEIGVKITEEQYQEYGQMLE
Trachemys scripta elegans	GSSFLSPEYQNTQQRKDPKKHTKLN	LNVPFEIGVKITEDQYQEYGQVLE
Rana catesbeiana	GLTFLSPADMQKIAERQSQNKLRHGNMN	
Rana esculenta	GLTFLSPADMRKIAERQSQNKLRHGNMN	
Danio rerio	GTSFLSPTQKPQGRRPPRVG	
Carassius auratus	GTSFLSPAQKPQGRRPPRMG	
Ictalurus punctatus	GSSFLSPTQKPQNRGDRKPPRVG	
Oreochromis mossambicus	GSSFLSPSQKPQNKVKSSRIG	

Species	Ghrelin sequence	Obestatin homolog sequence
Oreochromis niloticus	GSSFLSPSQKPQNKVKSSRIG	
Oncorhynchus mykiss	GSSFLSPSQKPQGKGKPPRVG	
Acanthopagrus schlegelii	GSSFLSPSQKPQNRGKSSRVG	
Anguilla japonica	GSSFLSPSQRPQGKDKKPPRVG	

Table 1. Bioactive peptide sequences from diverse vertebrata ghrelin gene.

Species	Motilin sequence
Homo sapiens	FVPIFTYGELQRMQEKERNKGQ
Pan troglodytes	FVPIFTYGELQRMQEKERNKGQ
Macaca mulatta	FVPIFTYGELQRMQEKERSKGQ
Cavia porcellus	FVPIFTYSELRRTQEREQNKRL
Oryctolagus cuniculus	FVPIFTYSELQRMQERERNRGH
Felis catus	FVPIFTHSELQRIREKERNKGQ
Canis familiaris	FVPIFTHSELQKIREKERNKGQ
Ovis aries	FVPIFTYGEVQRMQEKERYKGQ
Bos taurus	FVPIFTYGEVRRMQEKERYKGQ
Sus scrofa	FVPSFTYGELQRMQEKERNKGQ
Equus caballus	FVPIFTYSELQRMQEKERNRGQ
Myotis lucifugus	FVPIFTHSELQRMQEKERNKEQ
Dasypus novemcinctus	FVPIFTYSELQRMQEKEWNKGQ
Loxodonta africana	FVPIFTYSEIRRMQERERNNGQ
Monodelphis domestica	FVPIFTYSDVQRMQEKERNKGQ
Ornithorhynchus anatinus	FIPIFTHSDVQRMQERERNKGQ
Gallus gallus	FVPFFTQSDIQKMQEKERNKGQ

Table 2. Bioactive peptide sequences from diverse vertebrata motlin gene.

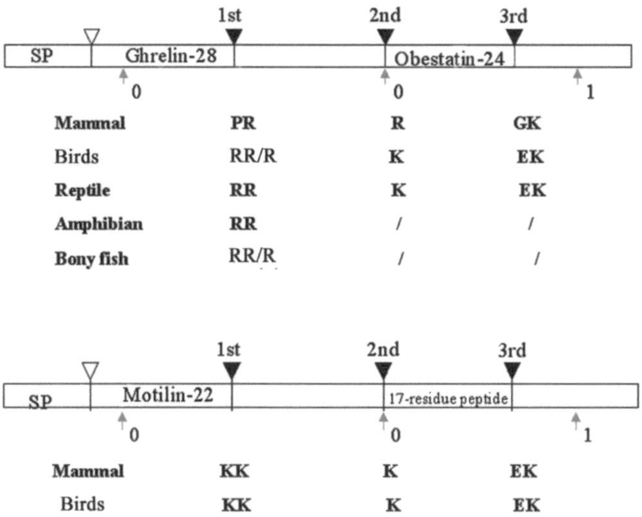

Fig. 1. Schematic representation of ghrelin and motilin preproproteins. The preproproteins of ghrelin and motilin are represented by boxes divided into protein domains, proportional to their length. The open and filled triangles indicate the locations of cleavage sites used by signal peptidase and proprotein convertase, respectively. The sequences of the putative endoproteinase cleavage sites of various vertebrate classes are shown bellow. Alternative processing sites in birds and bony fish are indicated, "↑" denotes intron position with intron phase shown beside the arrow. SP, signal peptide. "/", lack of putative endoproteinase recognition sites.

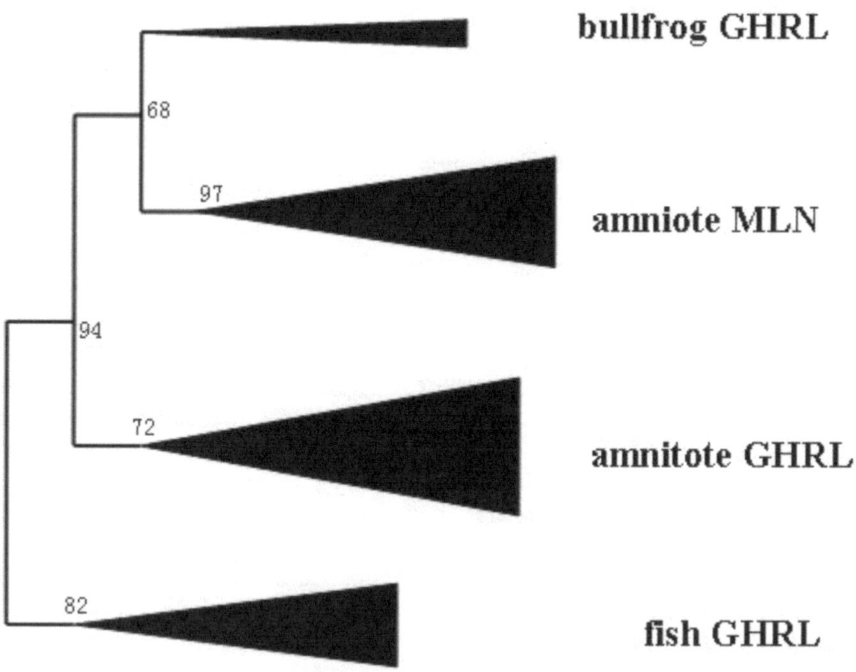

Fig. 2. Schematic representation of the motilin/ghrelin gene family phylogenetic relationships. Bootstrap percentages are shown on interior branches. GHRL, preproghrelin. MLN, prepromotilin.

4.1.3 Evolution of ghrelin and motilin receptors

Only a small number of Ghrelin and motilin receptor genes are known and most of these are from mammals, with ortholog from only two species of fish having previously being characterized (Palyha et al. 2000; Chan and Cheng 2004). Our bioinformatic searches of diverse vertebrate genomes resulted in the identification of a great number of potential receptors. The orthology of the different receptors was established using analysis of synteny of the genes. In combination with phylogenetic reconstruction, the monophyly of each receptor type was established, and no more than one copy of each type of receptor was identified in any of the studied species. GHSR and MLNR are more closely related to each other than they are to any other characterized receptor, and the gene duplication that generated them happened more than 450 million years ago, before the divergence of ray-finned fish and tetrapods (He et al. 2011). Through comparative and evolutionary analyses, we found a new type of receptor in fish, which does not have an ortholog in any non-fish vertebrate. The function of this new receptor is unknown. The sequence of this new receptor has some peculiarities, such as possessing long extracellular loops 2 and 3, which are about 100 residues longer than the analogous loops in GHSR and MLNR (He et al. 2011). Residues at both ends of these loops have been shown to be functionally important for hormone binding and action in homologous receptors; however, the function of these residues in the loops of these novel receptors is not clear (Matsuura, Dong and Miller 2002).

Studies have shown that the GHSR orthologs in fish can be activated by growth hormone secretagogues (GHSs), while MLNR orthologs in fish failed to be activated by GHSs or mammalian motilin (Palyha et al. 2000). The identification of the ancient binding state of MLNR prior to the emergence of motilin has proven challenging, however it is reasonable to speculate that GHSR and MLNR experienced functional diversification shortly after their duplication, and the ancient MLNR did not have either ghrelin or motilin binding properties. Evolutionary studies suggest MLNR experienced an episode of rapid evolution on the branch leading to amniotes, which was driven by positive selection, and accumulated amino acid changes in ligand binding cleft. This time period of rapid evolution coincides with the date of the GHRL/ MLN gene duplication event, thus it is reasonable to speculate, that the burst of rapid evolution in MLNR was a consequence of coevolution with its new ligand, and that motilin binding specificity of MLNR only evolved as a result of ligand-receptor coevolution after the motilin gene diverged from the ghrelin gene on the amniote lineage. In contrast, GHSR has evolved under a constant selective constraint throughout vertebrates, with the ghrelin/GHSR system being maintained and functionally conserved from fish to mammals (He et al. 2011).

4.1.4 Gene duplication and gene co-option

The motilin/ghrelin hormone and their receptors were produced by independent duplication events that occurred at different points in time. The discordance of the evolutionary histories for the hormones and receptors indicate that the intimate interacting partners of an endocrine system can be produced by individual duplications, the composition and functions of each part of the endocrine network do not remain static, and that parts of a system can be co-opted for novelties, and that these processes often involve gene duplication and subsequent divergence. Structural and evolutionary relatedness allows promiscuous interaction properties, which can serve as the starting point for accommodation. Divergence of function in different species is accomplished by hormone/receptor coevolution to improve binding affinity and/or specificity. A major role for gene co-option, involving gene duplication and divergence, should be recognized that creates potential elements which selection can act upon within a biological network to evolve new functions (He et al. 2011; True and Carroll 2002). The growth of gene families allows for more flexible gene expression and/or the evolution of new biochemical specificities (Rubenstein 1990; Sharman and Holland 1996), thus facilitating the evolution of greater biological complexity (Duboule and Wilkins1998).

4.2 Loss of the motilin and its specific receptor genes in rodents

The evolution of motilin and its specific receptor in rodents provides an illustration of the consequences of gene loss. Motilin is a 22-amino acid peptide synthesized by endocrine cells of the duodeno-jejunal mucosa and has a profound stimulatory effect on gastrointestinal contractility (Poitras and Peeters 2008), indicating that motilin and its specific receptor serve as potent active prokinetic drug target candidates. However, the clinical development of potential therapies is limited as both the mouse and rat, the most frequently used laboratory animals, are natural knockouts for the motilin and its specific receptor, that is these animal lack these genes and functional targets (He et al. 2010). These observations raise a number of intriguing questions - how can these animals survive without motilin? How were the genes lost? Did any other endocrine system compensate? What does this mean for our understanding of the human hormones? While we can't answer all of these questions, our studies revealed that the motilin receptor was pseudogenized specifically on the rodent lineage, while the motilin gene exhibited diverse evolutionary consequences in different rodent species (He et al. 2010). Once an interacting partner is lost, retained partners may be lost, as demonstrated by the independent loss of MLN in mice, rats and in the guinea pig, or serve as raw material in evolution, as suggested by the retention of MLN in the kangaroo rat. Genomic sequence information suggest, that in the the monophyletic Dipodomyinae subfamily, the MLN gene is intact and is under sustained evolutionary constraint, suggesting it has been recruited into a novel function, a function distinct from traditional motilin signaling (our unpublished observations). Intriguingly, studies have suggested that, after the break down of the MLN signaling pathway, the ghrelin signaling pathway was recruited to compensate for this loss in the rat (Dass et al. 2003; Depoortere et al. 2003). Given the ubiquity and its stochastic nature, the simultaneous loss of a hormone and its specific receptor is unlikely. As a dramatic genetic change, a gene loss leads to an immediate loss of specific interactions. The functional redundancy among gene family members could allow a compromise for the deleterious gene loss. Existing genes can be modified, or recruited, into new interactions that yield new functions through mutation and optimization (Jacob 1977; Khersonsky, Roodveldt and Tawfik 2006; Tokuriki and Tawfik 2009). Motilin is not a unique case. As similar events have occurred to leptin, an important adipose derived hormone (Brennan and Mantzoros 2006; Zhang et al. 1994), which does not exist in the chicken, and likely other birds, while a functional leptin receptor has conserved in these species (Horev et al. 2000; Ohkubo, Tanaka and Nakashima 2000; Pitel et al. 2010). It is possible that the lineage specific losses of motilin and leptin during evolution contributed to the evolution of novel metabolic regulatory mechanisms in these species.

4.3 Evolutionary shifts in existing genes

The proglucagon gene illustrates some of these issues. The vertebrate proglucagon gene encodes three glucagonlike sequences (glucagon, glucagon-like peptide-1 [GLP-1], and glucagon-like peptide-2 [GLP-2]) that play distinct roles in mammalian metabolic regulation

(Drucker 2001; Drucker 2002; Jiang and Zhang 2003; Kieffer and Habener 1999). Glucagon, produced by the A cells of the pancreatic islets, counteracts insulin's effect on blood glucose level depression (Jiang and Zhang 2003). GLP-1 functions as an incretin hormone in mammals, potentiating insulin release, and thus regulating glucose metabolism (Drucker 2001, 2002). In contrast, glucagon and GLP-1 have similar physiological functions in fish, and resemble that of mammalian glucagon (Duguay and Mommsen 1994; Plisetskaya and Mommsen 1996). The receptors for glucagon, GLP-1, and GLP-2 have emerged before the divergence of fish and mammals; however, the GLP-1 class of receptors has specifically been lost in fish, and accordingly the incretin action of GLP-1. A fish specific duplication produced a second glucagon receptor-like gene on the ancestral fish lineage. The new glucagon receptor-like gene shifted its binding specificity from glucagon to GLP-1 ensues, meanwhile maintained the ancestral downstream signaling. Thus through receptor loss and gain, existing hormone was recruited into new roles, and undoubtedly enabled evolutionary divergence (Irwin and Wong 2005).

While ghrelin and its specific receptor (GHSR) genes has been maintained and functionally conserved from fish to mammals, there are some significant differences in the function of the ghrelin/GHSR system in birds compared to other vertebrates (Richards 2010). Some of the actions of ghrelin are conserved in birds (e.g., GH release), while others, such as the effect of ghrelin on food intake, are opposite to those found in mammals and other vertebrate species (Hiroyuki et al. 2007; Kaiya et al. 2009; Kaiya et al. 2008). Besides ghrelin, the ghrelin gene has the potential to encode another peptide hormone——obstatin (Zhang et al. 2005). We observed episodic evolution for both the ghrelin and motilin genes during primitive placental mammal evolution, the period when a functional obestatin hormone might have originated (He, Irwin and Zhang 2010). It is possible that some of the lineage-specific physiological adaptations are due to the episodic evolution of the motilin and ghrelin genes.

Gene duplication, pseudonization, and the gain and loss of interactions through mutations in existing genes are major evolutionary processes shaping the specific interaction among biomolecules (Berg, Lässig and Wagner 2004; Wagner 2001; Wagner 2003; He et al. 2010). Thus, once a mutation arises, a stepwise process of elaboration and optimization ensues, which gradually integrates and orders mutations into a coherent pattern. Given the evolutionary dynamics of the genome and the plasticity of biomolecular networks, an evolutionary perspective is necessary to understand many aspects of the molecular basis of endocrinology.

5. Conclusion

Biological evolution is the process of generating biodiversity. Different phenotype corresponds to a given genomic control. New genes, new interactions, and new biochemical processes are essential for the molecular basis of the evolution of biodiversity and complexity. Genetic networks of endocrine systems are developmentally and evolutionarily fictile, elemental compositions within them are prone to be altered through gene gain and loss, and its physiological properties frequently change with mutations in gene coding sequences and/or regulatory systems, and turnover of interacting biomolecules.

The endocrine system consists of several glands in different parts of the body, which secrete hormones directly into the blood. Hormones usually have many different functions and modes of action; one hormone may play roles in different target organs, and conversely, target organs are affected by more than one hormone. Although quite irregular, there are still some formulas that can be followed. Structural and evolutionary relatedness generate promiscuous interaction properties, and provide important clues to interaction capacity exploration. Tracing the origin and studying the molecular evolution of endocrine systems should help us comprehend the main events that have prompted the diversification of these systems. In the light of evolution, through a comparative strategy, integrating information from diverse species helps to enhance our understanding of the assemblage of complex endocrine systems, identifying novel components of endocrine systems, and potential cross-talk between them through evolutionarily related interacting proteins. In addition, knowledge of how elements that underlie cellular functions are evolutionarily and developmentally interact, not only helps in choosing appropriate species to examine function, but also provide genetic makers to probe the evolution of specific traits and characteristics, disclosing the genetic basis that underlie the morphological and behavior changes, and thus helping enhance our understanding of how changing environments led to biochemical adjustments.

6. Acknowledgments

This work was supported by grants from the National Basic Research Program of China (973 Program, 2007CB411600), the National Natural Science Foundation of China (30621092, 30623007), and Bureau of Science and Technology of Yunnan Province (O803481101).

7. References

Avise JC, Ayala FJ. From the Academy: Colloquium Perspective: In the light of evolution I: Adaptation and complex design. Proc Natl Acad Sci USA. 2007 104 Suppl 1:8563-8566.

Berg J, Lässig M, Wagner A. Structure and evolution of protein interaction networks: a statistical model for link dynamics and gene duplications. BMC Evol Biol. 2004 4:51.

Brennan AM, Mantzoros CS. Drug Insight: the role of leptin in human physiology and pathophysiology--emerging clinical applications. Nat Clin Pract Endocrinol Metab. 2006 2:318-327.

Carroll SM, Bridgham JT, Thornton JW Evolution of hormone signaling in elasmobranchs by exploitation of promiscuous receptors. Mol Biol Evol. 2008 25:2643–2652.

Cegla J, Tan TM, Bloom SR. Gut-brain cross-talk in appetite regulation. Curr Opin Clin Nutr Metab Care. 2010 13:588-593.

Chan CB, Cheng CH. Identification and functional characterization of two alternatively spliced growth hormone secretagogue receptor transcripts from the pituitary of black seabream Acanthopagrus schlegeli. Mol Cell Endocrinol. 2004 214:81-95.

Conant GC. Rapid reorganization of the transcriptional regulatory network after genome duplication in yeast. Proc Biol Sci. 2010 277:869-876.

Danks JA, D'Souza DG, Gunn HJ, Milley KM, Richardson SJ. Evolution of the parathyroid hormone family and skeletal formation pathways. Gen Comp Endocrinol. 2011 170:79-91.

Dass NB, Munonyara M, Bassil AK, Hervieu GJ, Osbourne S, Corcoran S, Morgan M, Sanger GJ. Growth hormone secretagogue receptors in rat and human gastrointestinal tract and the effects of ghrelin. Neuroscience 120:443–453.

Dehal P, Boore JL. Two rounds of whole genome duplication in the ancestral vertebrate. PLoS Biol. 2005 3:e314.

Depoortere I, De Winter B, Thijs T, De Man J, Pelckman P, Peeters T 2003 Comparison of the prokinetic effects of ghrelin, GHRP-6 and motilin in rats in vivo and in vitro. Gastroenterology 124:580.

Drucker DJ. Biological actions and therapeutic potential of the glucagon-like peptides. Gastroenterology 2002 122:531–544.

Drucker DJ. The glucagon-like peptides. Endocrinology 2001 142:521–527

Duboule D and Wilkins A S. The evolution of 'bricolage'. Trends Genet. 1998 14:54–59.

Duguay SJ, Mommsen TP. Molecular aspects of pancreatic peptides. In: Fish physiology, vol. 13 (Hoar WS and Randall DJ, eds). Academic Press, San Diego. 1994 225–271.

Feighner SD, Tan CP, McKee KK, et al. Receptor for motilin identified in the human gastrointestinal system. Science 1999 284:2184-2188.

Gagneux P, Varki A. Genetic differences between humans and great apes. Mol Phylogenet Evol. 2001 18:2–13.

Garcia-Fernández J, Holland PW. Archetypal organization of the amphioxus Hox gene cluster. Nature 1994 370:563–566.

Gout JF, Duret L, Kahn D. Differential Retention of Metabolic Genes Following Whole-Genome Duplication. Mol Biol Evol. 2009 265:1067-1072.

Gregory TR. Synergy between sequence and size in large-scale genomics. Nature Rev Genet. 2005 6:699–708.

Hahn MW, Demuth JP, Han SG. Accelerated rate of gene gain and loss in primates. Genetics 2007 177:1941-1949.

He J, Irwin DM, Chen R, Zhang YP. Stepwise loss of motilin and its specific receptor genes in rodents. J Mol Endocrinol. 2010 44:37-44.

He J, Irwin DM, Zhang YP. Motilin and ghrelin gene experienced episodic evolution during primitive placental mammal evolution. Sci China Life Sci. 2010 53:677-682.

He J, Irwin DM, Zhang YP. Gene duplication plays a major role in gene co-option: Studies into the evolution of the motilin/ghrelin family and their receptors. Chinese Science Bulletin. 2011 56: 2690-2697.

Hiroyuki Kaiya, Veerle M Darras, Kenji Kangawa. Ghrelin in Birds: Its Structure, Distribution and Function. Journal of Poultry Science 2007 44:1–18.

Hodson DJ, Molino F, Fontanaud P, Bonnefont X, Mollard P. Investigating and modelling pituitary endocrine network function. J Neuroendocrinol. 2010 22:1217-1225.

Hoffmann FG, Opazo JC. Evolution of the relaxin/insulin-like gene family in placental mammals: implications for its early evolution. J Mol Evol. 2011 72:72-79.

Holland LZ, Albalat R, Azumi K, et al. The amphioxus genome illuminates vertebrate origins and cephalochordate biology. Genome Res. 2008 18:1100-1111.

Holst B, Holliday ND, Bach A, Elling CE, Cox HM, Schwartz TW. Common structural basis for constitutive activity of the ghrelin receptor family. J Biol Chem. 2004 279:53806-53817.

Horev G, Einat P, Aharoni T, Eshdat Y, Friedman-Einat M. Molecular cloning and properties of the chicken leptin-receptor (CLEPR) gene. Mol Cell Endocrinol. 2000 162:95-106.

Hou Y, Lin S. Distinct gene number-genome size relationships for eukaryotes and non-eukaryotes: gene content estimation for dinoflagellate genomes. PLoS One. 2009 4:e6978.

Howard AD, Feighner SD, Cully DF, et al. A Receptor in Pituitary and Hypothalamus That Functions in Growth Hormone Release. Science 1996 273:974-977.

Huminiecki L, Heldin C-H: 2R and modeling of vertebrate signal transduction engine. BMC Biol 2010 8:146.

Inui A. Ghrelin: an orexigenic and somatotrophic signal from stomach. Nat. Rev. Neurosci. 2001 2:551-560.

Irwin DM, Wong K. Evolution of new hormone function: loss and gain of a receptor. J Hered. 2005 96:205-11.

Irwin DM. Evolution of genes for incretin hormones and their receptors. Vitam Horm. 2010 84:1-20.

Irwin DM. Molecular evolution of proglucagon. Regul Pept. 2001 98:1-12

Jacob F. Evolution and tinkering. Science 1977, 196: 1161–1166.

Jaillon O, Aury J, Brunet F, et al., Genome duplication in the teleost fish Tetraodon nigroviridis reveals the early vertebrate proto-karyotype. Nature 2004 431:946–957.

Jiang G, Zhang BB. Glucagon and regulation of glucose metabolism. Am J Physiol. 2003 284:E671–E678.

Kaiya H, Furuse M, Miyazato M, Kangawa K. Current knowledge of the roles of ghrelin in regulating food intake and energy balance in birds. Gen Comp Endocrinol. 2009 163:33-38.

Kaiya H, Kojima M, Hosoda H, et al. Bullfrog ghrelin is modified by n-octanoic acid at its third threonine residue. J Biol Chem. 2001 276:40441-40448.

Kaiya H, Miyazato M, Kangawa K, Peter RE, Unniappan S. Ghrelin: a multifunctional hormone in non-mammalian vertebrates. Comp Biochem Physiol A Mol Integr Physiol. 2008 149:109-128.

Kassahn KS, Dang VT, Wilkins SJ, Perkins AC, Ragan MA. Evolution of gene function and regulatory control after whole-genome duplication: comparative analyses in vertebrates. Genome Res. 2009 19:1404-1418.

Kettler GC, Martiny AC, Huang K, et al. Patterns and implications of gene gain and loss in the evolution of Prochlorococcus. PLoS Genet. 2007 312:e231.

Khersonsky O, Roodveldt C, Tawfik DS. Enzyme promiscuity: evolutionary and mechanistic aspects. Curr Opin Chem Biol. 2006 10:498-508.

Kieffer TJ, Habener JF. The glucagon-like peptides. Endocr Rev. 1999 20:876–913.

Kim DK, Cho EB, Moon MJ, Park S, Hwang JI, Kah O, Sower SA, Vaudry H, Seong JY. Revisiting the evolution of gonadotropin-releasing hormones and their receptors in vertebrates: secrets hidden in genomes. Gen Comp Endocrinol. 2011 170:68-78.

Kojima M, Hosoda H, Date Y, Nakazato M, Matsuo H, Kangawa K. Ghrelin is a growth-hormone-releasing acylated peptide from stomach. Nature 1999 402:656-60.

Kojima M, Kangawa K. Ghrelin: structure and function. Physiol Rev. 2005 85:495-52.

Konstantinidis KT, Tiedje JM. Trends between gene content and genome size in prokaryotic species with larger genomes. Proc Natl Acad Sci USA. 2004 101:3160–3165.

Li WH. Molecular Evolution. Sinauer Associates, Sunderland, 1997.

Liu JC, Makova KD, Adkins RM, Gibson S, Li WH. Episodic evolution of growth hormone in primates and emergence of the species specificity of human growth hormone receptor. Mol Biol Evol. 2001 18:945-953.

Lynch M, Conery JS. The origins of genome complexity. Science 2003 302:1401–1404.

Macqueen DJ, Delbridge ML, Manthri S, Johnston IA. A newly classified vertebrate calpain protease, directly ancestral to CAPN1 and 2, episodically evolved a restricted physiological function in placental mammals. Mol Biol Evol. 2010 27:1886-1902.

Manning G, Scheeff E. How the vertebrates were made: selective pruning of a double-duplicated genome. BMC Biol. 2010 8:144.

Markov GV, Paris M, Bertrand S, Laudet V. The evolution of the ligand/receptor couple: a long road from comparative endocrinology to comparative genomics. Mol Cell Endocrinol. 2008 293:5-16.

Matsuura B, Dong M and Miller LJ. Differential determinants for peptide and non-peptidyl ligand binding to the motilin receptor. Critical role of second extracellular loop for peptide binding and action. J Biol Chem. 2002 277:9834-9839.

Moyle WR, Campbell RK, Myers RV, Bernard MP, Han Y, Wang X. Co-evolution of ligand-receptor pairs. Nature 1994 368:251-255.

Murray C D, Kamm M A, Bloom S R, et al. Ghrelin for the gastroenterologist: history and potential. Gastroenterology 2003 125:1492-1502.

Nakazato M, Murakami N, Date Y, Kojima M, Matsuo H, Kangawa K, Matsukura S. A role for ghrelin in the central regulation of feeding. Nature 2001 409:194-198.

Ohkubo T, Tanaka M, Nakashima K. Structure and tissue distribution of chicken leptin receptor (cOb-R) mRNA. Biochim Biophys Acta. 2000 1491:303-308.

Ohno S. Evolution by gene duplication. Springer-Verlag. Berlin, 1970.

Palyha OC, Feighner SD, Tan CP, et al. Ligand activation domain of human orphan growth hormone (GH) secretagogue receptor (GHS-R) conserved from Pufferfish to humans. Mol Endocrinol. 2000 14:160-169.

Peeters T L. Ghrelin: a new player in the control of gastrointestinal functions. Gut 2005 54:1638-649.

Peter EC, Vallo T. Recent advances Advances in endocrinology. Arch Dis Child. 1998 78:278-284.

Pitel F, Faraut T, Bruneau G, Monget P. Is there a leptin gene in the chicken genome? Lessons from phylogenetics, bioinformatics and genomics. Gen Comp Endocrinol. 2010 167:1-5.

Plisetskaya EM, Mommsen TP. Glucagon and glucagon-like peptides in fishes. Int Rev Cytol, 1996 168:187–257.

Poitras P, Peeters TL. Motilin. Current Opinion in Endocrinology, Diabetes and Obesity 2008 15:54–57.

Poitras P: Motilin. In: Gut Peptides: Biochemistry and Physiology. Edited by Walsh JH, Dockaray GJ. Raven Press. New York, 1993. 261–303.

Powell AJ, Conant GC, Brown DE, Carbone I, Dean RA. Altered patterns of gene duplication and differential gene gain and loss in fungal pathogens. BMC Genomics. 2008 9:147.

Richards MP, McMurtry JP. The avian proghrelin system. Int J Pept. 2010. pii: 749401.

Rubenstein PA. The functional importance of multiple actin isoforms. Bioessays 1990 12:309-315.

Samson WK, Lumpkin MD, Nilaver G, McCann SM. Motilin: a novel growth hormone releasing agent. Brain Res Bull. 1984 12:57-62.

Semyonov J, Park JI, Chang CL, Hsu SY. GPCR genes are preferentially retained after whole genome duplication. PLoS One. 2008 3:e1903.

Sharman A C and Holland P W H. Conservation duplication and divergence of developmental genes during chordate evolution. Netherlands Journal of Zoology 1996 46:47-67.

Sun Y, Ahmed S, Smith RG. Deletion of ghrelin impairs neither growth nor appetite. Mol Cell Biol. 2003 23:7973-7981.

Sundström G, Dreborg S, Larhammar D. Concomitant duplications of opioid peptide and receptor genes before the origin of jawed vertebrates. PLoS One. 2010 5:e10512.

Ting CT, Tsaur SC, Sun S, Browne WE, Chen YC, Patel NH, Wu CI. Gene duplication and speciation in Drosophila: evidence from the Odysseus locus. Proc Natl Acad Sci USA. 2004 101:12232-12235.

Tokuriki N, Tawfik DS. Protein dynamism and evolvability. Science 2009 324:203-207.

True JR, Carroll SB. Gene co-option in physiological and morphological evolution. Annu Rev Cell Dev Biol. 2002 18:53-80.

van Hoek MJ, Hogeweg P. Metabolic adaptation after whole genome duplication. Mol Biol Evol. 2009 26:2441-2453.

Wagner A. How the global structure of protein interaction networks evolves. Proc Biol Sci. 2003 270:457-466.

Wagner A. The yeast protein interaction network evolves rapidly and contains few redundant duplicate genes. Mol Biol Evol. 2001 18:1283-1292.

Wallis M. Episodic evolution of protein hormones in mammals. J Mol Evol. 2001 53:10-18.

Wang X, Grus WE, Zhang J. Gene losses during human origins. PLoS Biology. 2006 4:e52.

Wilkins AS. Between "design" and "bricolage": genetic networks, levels of selection, and adaptive evolution. Proc Natl Acad Sci USA. 2007 104 Suppl 1:8590-8596.

Zhang J, Zhang YP, Rosenberg HF. Adaptive evolution of a duplicated pancreatic ribonuclease gene in a leaf-eating monkey. Nat Genet. 2002 30:411–415.

Zhang J. Evolution by gene duplication: an update. Trends in Ecology & Evolution 2003 18:292-298.

Zhang JV, Ren PG, Avsian-Kretchmer O, et al. Obestatin, a peptide encoded by the ghrelin gene, opposes ghrelin's effects on food intake. Science 2005 310:996-999.

Zhang Y, Proenca R, Maffei M, Barone M, Leopold L, Friedman JM. Positional cloning of the mouse obese gene and its human homologue. Nature 1994 372:425-32.

Zhou XR, Wang YZ, Smith JF, Chen R. Altered expression patterns of TCP and MYB genes relating to the floral developmental transition from initial zygomorphy to actinomorphy in Bournea (Gesneriaceae). New Phytol. 2008 178:532-543.

Part 2

Pituitary Adenomas

2

The Genetics of Pituitary Adenomas

Monica Fedele, Giovanna Maria Pierantoni and Alfredo Fusco
Istituto di Endocrinologia e Oncologia Sperimentale (IEOS) del CNR, and Dipartimento di Biologia e Patologia Cellulare e Molecolare, Università di Napoli Federico II
Italy

1. Introduction

Cancer is considered a disease of the genome since the development of the vast majority of the human neoplasias is due to the accumulation of gene mutations. Indeed, the vast majority of tumours occur due to a considerable number of mutations that human cells accumulate during lifetime. Approximately 380 genes, representing about 1% of all human genes, have been implicated *via* mutation in tumorigenesis (Futreal et al., 2004). Most (90%), of these mutations are somatic, whereas germline mutations are a minority (20%). Some mutations may be both somatic and germline (10%) (Futreal et al., 2004).

Pituitary adenomas (PA) are one of the most frequent intracranial tumours with a prevalence of clinically-apparent tumours close to one in 1,000 of the general population and are the third most common intracranial tumour type after meningiomas and gliomas (Scheithauer et al., 2006). The majority of pituitary adenomas are sporadic and only a small subset (5% of all pituitary tumours) are familial, and often occur as component of familial endocrine-related tumour syndromes. Despite their benign nature, PA can cause significant morbidity because of hormonal hyper-secretion, or compressive effects to surrounding tissues. For example, GH-producing adenomas are associated with a GH excess that leads to gigantism or acromegaly, depending on whether the excessive GH occurs prior or not to epiphyseal-plate closure, respectively. In addition, if the pituitary mass overgrows, it can impinge upon the optic chiasm interfering with vision or generally results in headache due to the increased pressure on the surrounding brain structures.

Therefore, molecular understanding of pituitary adenoma formation is essential for the development of medical therapies and the treatment of post-operative recurrences.

2. The pituitary gland

The pituitary gland, also known as hypophysis, is one of the most important glands of the mammalian endocrine system. Through its secreted hormones, it controls the growth and activity of other glands: the thyroid, the adrenals, the gonads, the liver, the adipose tissue and the mammary glands (Fig. 1). The pituitary does not act independently, but it is under the continuous control of the nervous system through the hypothalamus. A wide range of external stimuli, including supply of nutrients, the ambient temperature, the exercise, and physical or psycological stress, causes secretion of hypothalamic hormones. As a response to hypothalamic control, the pituitary secretes the hypophyseal hormones, which maintain crucial homeostatic functions, including metabolism, growth, and reproduction. Apart from the hypothalamic inputs, pituitary hormone secretion is also regulated by feedback effects of the circulating hormones, as well as the autocrine and paracrine secretions of the pituitary cells (Bilezikjian et al., 2004; Mechenthaler, 2008) (Fig. 1).

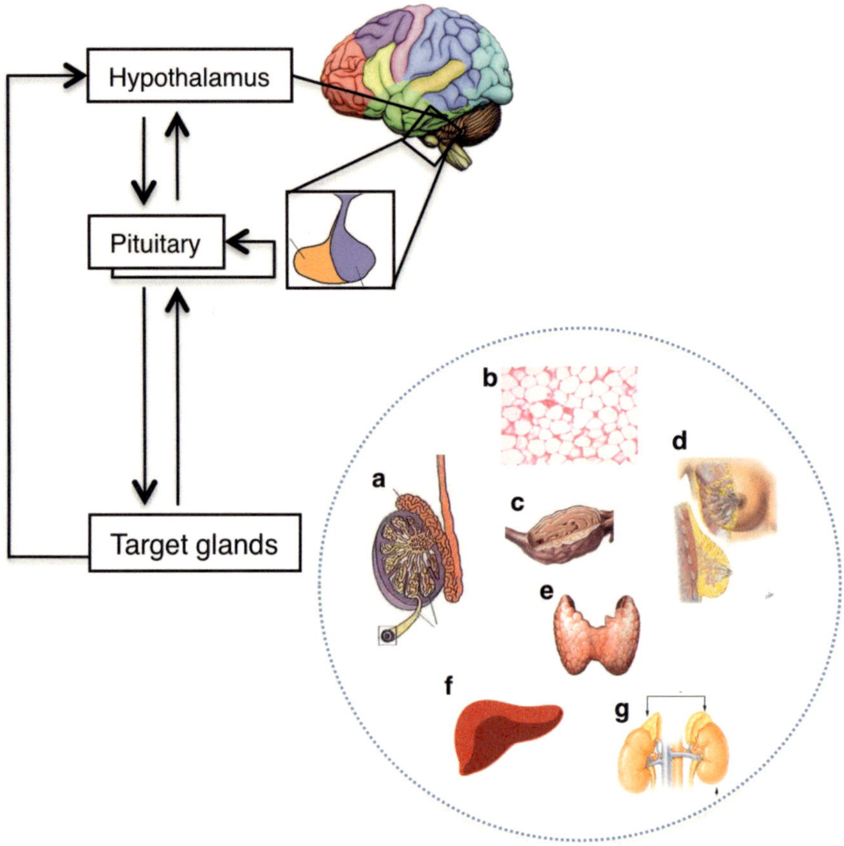

Fig. 1. Schematic representation of the hypothalamic-pituitary axis. Hypothalamic hormones, through the portal system, directly target anterior pituitary cell surface receptors that elicit positive or negative signals mediating pituitary hormone gene transcription and secretion. Pituitary hormones exert negative feedback on hypothalamus. Intrapituitary cytokines and growth factors regulate pituitary cell function by paracrine and autocrine control. Peripheral hormones from pituitary target glands exert negative feedback on respective pituitary hormone synthesis and secretion as well as on hypothalamic releasing factors. a, testis; b, adipose tissue; c, ovary; d, mammary gland; e, thyroid; f, liver; g, adrenal glands (arrows).

The human hypophysis is composed of the neurohypophysis (or posterior lobe) and the adenohypophysis (or anterior lobe). The posterior lobe consists of cells secreting antidiuretic (ADH) or vasopressin and oxytocin, whereas the anterior lobe is composed of five distinct cell types (Table 1). Approximately 50% of all anterior lobe cells are growth hormone (GH)-secreting cells, also known as somatotrophs (Hearney & Melmed, 2004). GH has a crucial role in controlling body growth and metabolism, by acting either directly on multiple tissues or indirectly, via the hepatic production of insulin-like growth factors (mainly IGF-1) (Brook & Marshall, 2001). Prolactin (PRL)-secreting cells, also known as lactotrophs, in men and nulliparous women may account for approximately 10% of the anterior pituitary cells, whereas in multiparous women their number can be up to three times higher (Heaney & Melmed, 2004). PRL inhibits the function of the gonads and stimulates breast enlargement and milk production during pregnancy. GH- and PRL-secreting cells derive from progenitor mammosomatotrophs, which are bi-hormonal cells that can differentiate into either somatotrophs or lactotrophs depending on the needs of each phase the body is in (i.e. growth, or pregnancy and lactation) (Asa & Ezzat, 2002). Adrenocorticotrophin (ACTH)-secreting cells, also known as corticotrophs, account for approximately 10-20% of all anterior lobe cells (Heaney & Melmed, 2004). ACTH stimulates the secretion of glucocorticoid hormone (cortisol) from the adrenal gland cortex, while cortisol, in turn, concerts metabolic and anti-inflammatory effects (Goodman, 2003). Apart from ACTH, corticotrophs secrete endorphins, γ-lipotrophins and other pro-opiomelanocortin derivatives.

Follicle stimulating hormone (FSH) and luteinizing hormone (LH)-secreting cells, or gonadotroph cells, account for roughly equal numbers as corticotrophs (Heaney & Melmed, 2004). These hormones regulate the sex steroid hormone production in the gonads, as well as the development and maturation of the germ cells. Lastly, a small percentage of thyrotroph cells (5%) secrete the thyroid stimulating hormone (TSH) (Heaney & Melmed, 2004). TSH is the stimulus for thyroid hormone (T3/T4) production from the thyroid gland. Thyroid hormone mainly controls GH synthesis and secretion, metabolism and thermogenesis, as well as foetal skeletal maturation, and central nervous system development and maturation (Goodman, 2003).

Pituitary cells	Secreting hormone	Target tissue
Corticotrophs	Adrenocorticotropic hormone (ACTH)	Adrenal gland
Gonadotrophs	Follicle-stimulating hormone (FSH) and luteinizing hormone (LH)	Ovary, Testis
Somatotrophs	Growth hormone (GH)	Liver, adipose tissue
Lactotrophs	Prolactin	Ovary, mammary gland
Thyrotrophs	Thyroid-stimulating hormone (TSH)	Thyroid gland

Table 1. Anterior pituitary cell functions

3. Origin and development of pituitary adenomas

Pituitary tumours are believed to develop by monoclonal expansion of a single neoplastic cell, due to an acquired intrinsic primary cell defect (genetic or epigenetic) that confers growth advantage (Asa & Ezzat, 2002). Indeed, early molecular studies of pituitary tumours, employing X-chromosome inactivation as a means of determining clonality, show that, in most cases, these tumours are monoclonal in origin, suggesting an intrinsic discrete genetic/molecular defect driving the transforming event and perhaps other ones driving progression (Fig. 2). However, these tumours do not follow the sequential classic paradigm apparent in multiple other tumour types, that is, initiation/transformation, hyperplasia, benign adenoma, invasive/aggressive adenoma and, ultimately, carcinoma. Conversely, they can arise from a hyper-plastic pituitary tissue, in which there are a number of different clones each with variable potential to develop into a discrete tumour. Consistent with this hypothesis is the finding of different patterns of genetic alterations in recurrent/re-grown tumours compared to primary PA from the same patient (Clayton et al., 2000). Therefore, alongside the monoclonal hypothesis, more recently the polyclonal hypothesis has been proposed. According to it PA originate from the expansion of a single clone coming from a polyclonal hyper-plastic tissue. The initiating stimulus, which might include pituitary-specific oncogenes, intra-pituitary growth factors, or hypothalamic releasing hormones, would result in hyperplasia of specific cell subtypes in the pituitary giving rise to a number of different clones each one with variable potential to develop into a discrete tumour (Clayton & Farrell, 2004) (Fig. 2).

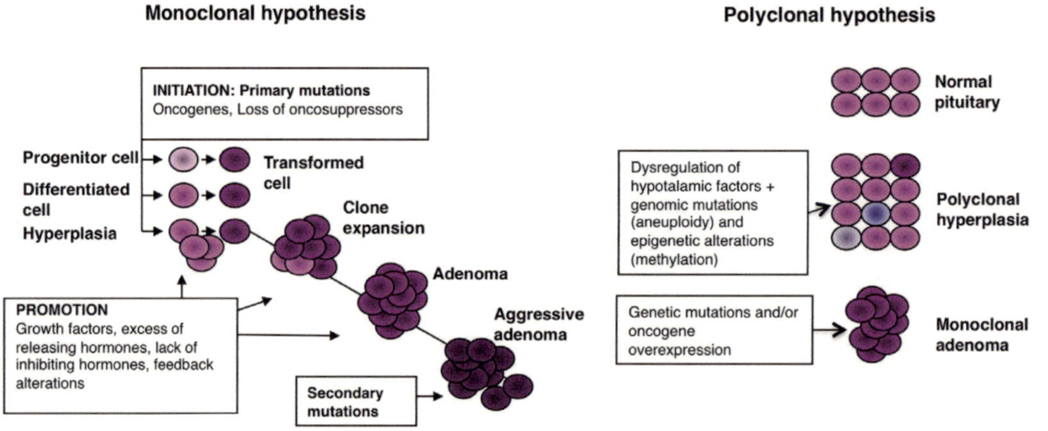

Fig. 2. Schematic representation of the two models of PA genesis (monoclonal and polyclonal hypotheses)

Pituitary tumours are in most of the cases benign and can grow both slowly and expansively. However, although defined as benign, nearly 50% of PA invade surrounding tissues, but invasiveness rate differs between various PA types (Brook & Marshall, 2001; Saeger et al., 2007), and mitotic activity is low even in aggressive PA, in contrast to tumours arising from more rapidly replicating tissues (Melmed, 2003). Very rarely PA become metastatic, and are then referred as pituitary carcinomas. Their incidence has been suggested to be 0.2% of symptomatic pituitary tumours (Pernicone et al., 1997), with almost equal frequency in both sexes (DeLellis et al., 2004; Kaltsas et al., 2005). Most are ACTH- or PRL-secreting tumours (Saeger et al., 2007). The time interval between initial adenoma diagnosis and carcinoma development may vary greatly, depending on the tumour subtype, with a mean of seven years (Pernicone et al., 1997; Sidibe, 2007). The reason of the unique feature of PA to rarely progress to carcinomas has been recently attributed to "premature" senescence-associated molecular pathways activated in PA (Chesnokova & Melmed, 2010). Premature senescence is a mechanism of irreversible cell cycle arrest and constitutes a strong anti-proliferative response, which can be triggered by DNA damage, chromosomal instability and aneuploidy, loss of tumour suppressive signalling or oncogene activation (Sharpless & Depinho, 2004). It occurs in benign or early stage tumours, but not in the advanced ones, as a mean to buffer the cell from pro-proliferative signals (Michaloglou et al., 2005, as cited in Chesnokova & Melmed, 2010), and functions to protect against oncogenic transformation, thereby suppressing unscheduled proliferation of damaged and early transformed cells.

4. Classification and pathogenesis of sporadic pituitary adenomas

Sporadic PA account for 10-15% of diagnosed brain tumours and although some differences in their frequencies exist, each of the five hormone-secreting cell types within the gland can give rise to an adenoma (Table 2) (Asa & Ezzat, 2002; Melmed, 2003). Apart from these adenomas, which are easily diagnosed upon the appearance of the clinical symptomatology consequent to the specific hormone hyper-secreted, micro-adenomas, known as "incidentalomas", are present in 10% of the general population and are encountered inadvertently by MRI (Melmed & Kleinberg, 2008). Micro-adenomas are intra-sellar and generally less than 10 mm in widest diameter. Macro-adenomas, mainly including non functioning pituitary adenomas (NFPA), are greater than 10 mm and usually impinge upon adjacent sellar structures determining mass effects, including pituitary failure, blindness, headache and various CNS disorders. Immunocytochemistry detects pituitary cell gene products and allows classification of pituitary tumours based on their function (Table 2). With the only exception of the glycoprotein α-subunit (α-GSU), immunohistochemical positivity of more than 5% of cells in the tumour usually reflects peripheral circulating hormone levels (Melmed & Kleinberg, 2008).

Adenoma type	Incidence	Principal hormone immunoreactivity	Clinical manifestation
Prolactinoma	29%	Prolactin	Hypogonadism, galactorrhea
NFPA (gonadotroph and null-cell adenoma)	27%	FSH/LH/α-GSU	Mass effects
Somatotropinoma	15%	GH	Gigantism or acromegaly
Adrenocorticotropinoma	10%	ACTH	Cushing's disease
Mixed GH/PRL cell adenoma	5%	GH/prolactin	Hypogonadism, acromegaly, galactorrhea
Mammosomatotroph cell adenoma	1%	GH/prolactin	Hypogonadism, acromegaly, galactorrhea
Thyrotroph cell adenoma	0,9%	TSH	Hypothyroidism

Table 2. Clinical and pathological characteristics of pituitary adenomas (adapted from Melmed & Kleinberg, 2008)

A considerable literature details the pathogenic changes occurring in sporadic tumours. However, in marked contrast to most other tumour types, there are few reports that describe genetic mutations (either activating oncogenes or inactivating tumour suppressor genes) that "drive" the inappropriate proliferation of pituitary cells. More often, altered control of gene expression, which results in either over-expression or down-regulation of certain proteins, is involved in PA pathogenesis. These proteins include hormones, growth factors, their receptors, the associated signal transduction pathways, cell-cycle regulators and factors involved in chromosomal instability.

4.1 Gain-of-function mutations

Oncogenes commonly mutated in the majority of human tumours are very rarely involved in pituitary tumorigenesis. Indeed, apart from *GNAS* and *HMGA2* genes that are mutated in a considerable percentage of GH-secreting adenomas and prolactinomas, respectively, few gain-of-function mutations have been reported in PA.

4.1.1 GNAS

Activating *gsp* mutation is present in up to 40% of human GH-secreting adenomas (Lyons et al., 1990). They consist in somatic heterozygous point mutations of the G protein α-subunit ($G_s\alpha$) gene (*GNAS*) involving either arginine 201 (replaced with cysteine or histidine) or glutamine 227 (replaced with arginine or leucine) that constitutively activate the $G_s\alpha$ protein (Vallar et al., 1987). Similar early post-zygotic somatic mutations in codon 201 of the $G_s\alpha$ were identified in tissues derived from patients with McCune-Albright syndrome (MAS), which includes GH-secreting pituitary adenomas (Weinstein et al., 1991). Interestingly, only in the pituitary the $G_s\alpha$ expression is mono-allelic - subject to imprinting - and is derived from the maternal allele (Hayward et al., 2001). When expressed in cell lines, mutant $G_s\alpha$ showed a 30-fold decrease in the rate of α subunit-mediated hydrolysis of GTP to GDP, a mechanism required to turn-off its activation (Landis et al., 1989). The resulting G protein activation increases cyclic adenosine mono-phosphate (cAMP) levels and activates protein kinase A (PKA), which in turn phosphorylates the cAMP response element-binding protein (CREB) and leads to sustained constitutive GH secretion and cell proliferation.
The *gsp* mutations have been identified also in NFPAs and ACTH-secreting adenomas (<10%), but quite rarely and not in all the studies (Melmed & Kleinberg; Lania et al., 2003).

4.1.2 GNAI2

Activating *gip* mutations, involving the *GNAI2* gene that encodes a G protein subunit involved in the inhibition of adenylyl ciclase and calcium influx, have been observed in a subset of NFPAs (Williamson et al., 1994). The mutation, observed in 3 out of 22 samples (13%), consists in an aminoacid substitution that replaces Gln 205 (corresponding to Gln 227 of $G_s\alpha$) with Arg, which causes activation of Ras (Edamatsu et al., 1998). Interestingly, two tumours with *gip* mutations also harboured *gsp* mutations, suggesting the possibility of multiple hits in a stepwise pathogenesis of pituitary neoplasia (Williamson et al., 1994).

4.1.3 RAS

The family of RAS genes encodes a 21-kD monomeric GDP/GTP binding protein mainly involved in the transduction of growth factor signalling. These genes may acquire mitogenic properties by point mutations that increase the affinity for GTP in the GTP-binding domain (codons 12 and 13) or prevent GTP-ase activity (codon 61). These mutations are present with high frequency in human neoplasias but are very rare in pituitary tumours (Karga et al., 1992; Cai et al., 1994; Pei et al., 1994, as cited in Lania et al., 2003). Indeed, a Gly12 to Val substitution has been observed in one aggressive prolactinoma resistant to dopaminergic inhibition that eventually was lethal. RAS mutations have been also described in metastases of three pituitary carcinomas, but not in the primitive tumours (Lania et al., 2003). Therefore, the rare RAS mutations in pituitary tumours are associated with malignant features, likely representing a late event in pituitary tumorigenesis.

4.1.4 PKCα

The Ca^{2+}/calmodulin and phospholipid-dependent protein kinase C (PKC) is a large ubiquitous kinase family that participates in growth factor- and hormone-mediated signalling and cell proliferation. Point mutations in the gene encoding the PKCα isoform, replacing Gly294 with Asp - a strategic region of PKC containing the calcium-binding site - have been observed in four invasive pituitary tumours (Alvaro et al., 1993), causing its over-expression with respect to normal pituitary. These findings were not confirmed by subsequent studies (Schiemann et al., 1997), but ectopic expression of a mutant form of PKCα originally found in human tumours leads to aberrant sub-cellular translocation of the enzyme, together with effects on growth control (Alvaro et al., 1997).

4.1.5 FGFR4

The normal pituitary and pituitary tumours produce a wide number of substances with secretory, differentiating, and proliferative potentials and express specific receptors (Lania et al., 2003). The aberrant expression of an N-terminally truncated fibroblast growth factor (FGF) receptor-4, containing the third Ig-like domain, the trans-membrane region and the kinase domain, that is constitutively phosphorylated and causes transformation *in vitro* and *in vivo,* has been reported in about 40% of pituitary adenomas, composed of the various hormone-secreting cell types, but not in normal pituitary. Consistently, the expression of this truncated receptor in lactotroph pituitary cells of transgenic mice results in the development of PA (Ezzat et al., 2002).

4.1.6 HMGA2

The HMGA2 protein belongs to the High Mobility Group A (HMGA) family, also including HMGA1, composed of small, non-histone, chromatin-associated proteins that alter the architecture of chromatin and facilitate the assembly of multi-protein complexes of transcriptional factors (Thanos & Maniatis, 1995). These functions have important rebounds in a wide spectrum of biological processes, ranging from embryonic development, cell differentiation and transformation, cell cycle progression, apoptosis, senescence, DNA repair, up to different aspects of cell physiopathology, including body growth, cardiogenesis, self-renewal of neural stem cells, inflammation and cancer (Hock et al., 2007; Fedele et al., 2010).
The *HMGA2* gene is over-expressed in human prolactinomas (Finelli et al., 2002). Its over-expression is associated, in most of the prolactin-secreting adenomas analised, with gain of chromosome 12 (trisomy/tetrasomy), the most frequent cytogenetic alteration in these tumours, and amplification of the *HMGA2* locus (region 12q13-15) or structural rearrangements of chromosome 12 (Finelli et al., 2002).
HMGA2 over-expression was also found in 12 out of 18 NFPA, which rarely harbour trisomy 12 but, differently from what occurs in prolactinomas, HMGA2 up-regulation was associated with amplification and/or rearrangement of the *HMGA2 locus* in only two cases (Pierantoni et al., 2005).

It is noteworthy that animal models clearly identified a critical role for *HMGA* genes in pituitary tumorigenesis since, as more deeply described below, transgenic mice over-expressing either the *Hmga1* or the *Hmga2* genes develop mixed prolactin/GH-secreting adenomas with a high penetrance (Fedele et al., 2002; 2005).

4.2 Loss-of-function mutations

Aberrant pituitary cell proliferation may result from the inactivation of either common tumour suppressor genes (TSGs) or specific inhibitors of pituitary cell function and growth. Unlike oncogenes that drive neoplastic transformation also when mutated in heterozygosity, TSGs are usually recessive and the inactivation of both alleles is required to cause the loss of anti-tumoral action.

Even though the key role of some TSGs ($p27^{kip1}$, RB) in pituitary tumorigenesis has been clearly demonstrated in mice (Fero et al., 1996; Jacks et al., 1992, as cited in Fedele & Fusco, 2010), they are not or very rarely mutated in human PA.

Low expression levels of $p27^{Kip1}$ protein have been found in ACTH-secreting adenomas, recurrent PA, and pituitary carcinomas by immunohistochemistry. However, as it occurs in other human neoplasias, no changes in $p27^{kip1}$ mRNA levels were observed, suggesting the involvement of post-translational mechanisms accounting for the impairment of $p27^{kip1}$ protein stabilization in these tumours (Dahia et al., 1998).

Recently, reduced $p27^{kip1}$ protein levels were found in a NFPA harbouring a novel mutation of DKC1, encoding for dyskerin, a pseudouridine synthase that modifies rRNA and regulates telomerase activity. This mutation, consisting in a specific aminoacid substitution (S485G), significantly alters DKC1 stability/pseudouridylation activity (Bellodi et al., 2010). However, the link between DKC1 mutation and $p27^{kip1}$ expression is not clear yet.

Loss of heterozygosity (LOH) on chromosome 13q14, where *RB* is located, is a relatively frequent event. In particular, deletion of one *RB* allele is observed in most highly invasive or malignant pituitary tumours and their metastases. The retained allele is not mutated but, as better described below, it is frequently hyper-methylated (Pei et al., 1995; Simpson et al., 1999; 2000, as cited in Lania et al., 2003). However, the presence of cases of LOH at 13q14 in PA in the absence of mutation or hyper-methylation of the *RB* allele may suggest the involvement in PA of another still unknown TSG located in the same chromosomal region (Bates et al., 1997, as cited in Vandeva et al., 2010).

MEN1 gene mutations, responsible for the MEN-1 syndrome (fully described in paragraph 5.1), are uncommon in sporadic PA (~3%), even in the presence of LOH of 11q13 (Melmed & Kleinberg). Indeed, just four cases have been described: in one NFPA, in one ACTH-secreting adenoma (Zhuang et al., 1997), in one prolactinoma (Wembin et al., 1999) and in one TSH-secreting adenoma (Schmidt et al., 1999), suggesting, also in this case, the presence of another adenoma-relevant TSG on chromosome 11.

More recently, the aryl hydrocarbon receptor interacting protein (*AIP)* gene, also located on chromosome 11q13 and responsible for familial isolated pituitary adenomas (fully described in paragraph 5.4), has been found to be mutated in about 3% of sporadic GH-secreting adenoma (Occhi et al., 2010). The AIP protein is a co-chaperone and though to be important in keeping proteins and protein complexes in functional formation. It interacts with several protein partners, including hydrocarbon receptor, phosphodiesterases, survivin, G proteins and RET, and currently it is uncertain which of them plays a key role in pituitary tumorigenesis. The AIP mutation types identified in sporadic PA include nonsense, splice

site substitutions, missense, frameshift and in-frame deletions. Some of them have been only identified in sporadic PA, whereas some others have been identified in both familial and sporadic cases (Ozfirat & Korbonits, 2010).
Interestingly, no mutations in the *TP53* gene have been found in PA, even though they have been detected in more than 50% of all human cancers, including tumours of the central nervous system (Lania et al., 2003). Since *TP53* mutations are associated with tumour progression, this result appears consistent with the intrinsic nature of pituitary tumour evolution, which rarely progress to carcinoma.

Pituitary tumour type	Mutated gene	Incidence
GH-secreting NFPA/ACTH-secreting	*GNAS*	40% <10%
NFPA	*GNAI2*	13%
Pituitary carcinomas/invasive prolactinomas	*RAS*	rare
Invasive NFPA	*PKCα*	rare
All types	*FGFR4*	~40%
Prolactinomas NFPA	*HMGA2*	~80% ~10%
NFPA, ACTH-secreting, prolactinoma, TSH-secreting	*MEN1*	~3%
GH-secreting	*AIP*	~3%
NFPA	*DKC1*	rare

Table 3. Summary of gene mutations and their incidence in sporadic pituitary adenomas.

4.3 Gene over-expression

To identify novel factors involved in pituitary tumour pathogenesis, several studies have been focused on differences in gene expression between PA and normal pituitary tissue. Indeed, more frequently than gene mutations, alterations of gene expression have been reported in human PA. They include both gene over-expression and down-regulation, the latter being mainly associated with epigenetic gene silencing.

4.3.1 Cyclins

Cell cycle dysregulation is the main pathogenetic event in the development of pituitary tumors. In fact, it has been estimated that more than 80% of human pituitary tumours display alterations at least in one of the regulators of the G1/S transition of the cell cycle (Malumbres & Barbacid, 2001, as cited in Fedele & Fusco, 2010). In particular, over-expression of different cyclins has been reported in various functioning and non functioning PA.
Cyclin E expression is increased in ACTH adenomas compared to normal pituitary tissue (Jordan et al., 2000, as cited by Fedele & Fusco, 2010), likely related to the low levels of nuclear $p27^{kip1}$ in these tumours (Musat et al., 2010).
Cyclin D1, as well as cyclin D3, is over-expressed in aggressive NFPA (Jordan et al., 2000, Turner et al., 2000, Saeger et al., 2001, Simpson et al., 2001, as cited in Fedele & Fusco, 2010). One of the possible mechanisms responsible of such over-expression could be the activation of the Wnt-β-catenin pathway that targets cyclin D1. Indeed, transfecting GH3 pituitary cells

with Wnt inhibitory factor-1 (WIF1) decreased cell proliferation and colony formation, suggesting an involvement of Wnt pathway in pituitary tumorigenesis (Elston et al., as cited in Musat et al., 2010). Moreover, cyclin D1 gene allelic imbalance has been described in about 25% of analysed adenomas (Hibberts et al.,1999, as cited in Fedele & Fusco, 2010).
B-type cyclins have recently been found over-expressed in many human pituitary adenomas, with prevalence in prolactinomas (Wierinckx et al., 2007; De Martino et al., 2009).

4.3.2 PTTG

Pituitary tumour transforming gene (PTTG) was isolated from experimental pituitary tumours by mRNA differential display PCR between rat pituitary tumor cells and normal pituitary tissue (Pei & Melmed, 1997). Subsequent experiments showed its abundant expression in nearly all pituitary tumour types, especially prolactinomas, but not in normal pituitary (Zhang et al., 1999).
PTTG codes for securin that interacts and inhibits the proteolitic protein separase, which degrades the cohesin complex involved in holding together replicated paired sister chromatids during metaphase, leading, when over-expressed, to cell aneuploidy, which is frequently observed in PA (Uhlmann et al., 1999; Zou et al., 1999, as cyted by Fedele & Fusco, 2010). In addition, PTTG also induces FGF production and angiogenesis and is up-regulated by oestrogen (Melmed & Kleinberg, 2008) and modulates the G1/S phase transition by interacting with Sp1 and regulating the transcriptional activity of the cyclin D3 promoter (Tong et al., 2007, as cyted by Fedele & Fusco, 2010). Interestingly, PTTG is regulated by CDK1-mediated phosphorylation suggesting a link between the control of the cell cycle by CDKs and securin function (Holt et al., 2008, as cyted by Fedele & Fusco, 2010).
Finally, PTTG has been implicated in the premature senescence that typically characterizes PA and that is responsible for the benign nature of this tumour (see paragraph 3). Indeed, both PTTG deletion and over-expression cause extensive pituitary cell aneuploidy, which causes intracellular p53 accumulation and p21 induction, resulting in senescence (Chesnokova & Melmed, 2010). Therefore, high PTTG levels in PA may initially mediate excessive proliferation, and lead to defective DNA replication and aneuploidy. Activation of pituitary DNA damage pathways triggers p21, a barrier to tumour growth, which in turn may restrain further growth and malignant transformation (Chesnokova & Melmed, 2010).

4.3.3 HMGA1 and HMGA2

Both *HMGA1* and *HMGA2* genes are over-expressed in different subtypes of PA, with the highest levels in prolactin- and/or GH-secreting tumours, compared to normal pituitary (De Martino et al., 2009). In addition, HMGA1 expression is significantly higher in invasive adenomas or macro-adenomas than in non-invasive adenomas or micro-adenomas and shows the highest level in grade IV, more aggressive pituitary adenomas, than in grades I, II and III (Wang et al., 2010). However, while HMGA2 over-expression is associated to gene amplification (see paragraph 4.1.6), HMGA1 over-expression does not appear to depend upon cytogenetic alterations involving the 6p21 chromosomal region, where the *HMGA1* gene is located (Fedele et al., 2010).
Studies in mice over-expressing either *Hmga1* or *Hmga2* gene under the transcriptional control of the cytomegalovirus promoter, clearly demonstrated the causal role of both these genes in pituitary tumorigenesis. Indeed, both these transgenic mouse models, with different incidence and latency period, develop mixed GH/PRL-secreting PA (Fedele et al.,

2002; 2005). The mechanism by which HMGA proteins induce the onset of PA mainly involves the interaction with pRB, which causes the displacement of HDAC1 from the pRB/E2F1 complex, and the resulting enhancement of E2F1 activity (Fedele et al., 2006). The crucial role of the HMGA-mediated E2F1 activation in pituitary tumorigenesis was confirmed by crossing Hmga2-overexpressing with E2f1-knockout mice, which resulted in the suppression of pituitary tumorigenesis in double mutant mice (Fedele et al., 2006). The analysis of the expression profile of pituitary adenomas developed by Hmga transgenic mice in comparison with normal pituitary from wild-type mice led to the identification of other genes potentially down-stream in the molecular pathway leading to PA onset in Hmga transgenic mice (De Martino et al., 2007; 2009). Among these genes, *Mia/Cd-rap*, coding for a secreted product of malignant melanoma cells, and *Ccnb2*, encoding the cyclin B2, which plays an important role in cell cycle progression, are directly regulated, by the HMGA proteins at transcriptional level (De Martino et al., 2007; 2009). Consistent with these data, the *MIA* gene, which is down-regulated by HMGA proteins, is down-regulated in human prolactinomas compared to normal pituitary (Evans et al., 2008), and the *CCNB2* gene, which is up-regulated by HMGAs, is over-expressed in PA *versus* normal pituitary, in statistically significant association with *HMGA* expression (De Martino et al., 2009).

4.3.4 Galectin 3

Recent evidences suggest that galectin-3 (Gal-3), a member of a phylogenetically conserved family of lectins sharing a consensus sequence of about 130 amino acids and a carbohydrate-recognition domain responsible for β-galactosides binding, plays an important role in pituitary progression (Righi et al., 2010). Gal-3, encoded by the *LGALS3* gene on chromosome 14q21-22, is ubiquitously expressed mainly in the cytosol, but it can easily traverse the intracellular and plasma membranes. Extracellular Gal-3 mediates cell migration, cell adhesion, and cell-to-cell interactions, whereas intracellular Gal-3 inhibits apoptosis and is up-regulated during neoplastic progression and metastasis in several human cancer (Righi et al., 2010). In different studies, Gal-3 expression was reported in folliculo-stellate cells and in normal and neoplastic pituitary prolactin- and ACTH-secreting cells, with a significantly higher presence in carcinomas *versus* adenomas (Riss et al., 2003; Ruebel et al., 2006, as cited in Righi et al., 2010). Indeed, down-regulation of Gal-3 , by RNA interference induced a significant decrease in cell proliferation and an important increase in apoptosis of pituitary HP75 cells (Riss et al., 2003, as cited in Righi et al., 2010), indicating a causal role of Gal-3 expression in pituitary tumorigenesis.

Recent studies suggest that the consequences of Gal-3 over-expression in pituitary carcinoma development could be related to changes in the expression levels of cell cycle targets of the Wnt/β-catenin signalling pathway, such as cyclin D1 and the proto-oncogene c-myc (Kim et al., 1999; Lin et al., 2000; Shimura et al., 2004, as cited in Righi et al., 2010).

4.4 Gene down-regulation and epigenetic gene silencing

For many of the genes whose expression is lost or drastically reduced in PA *versus* normal pituitary, the epigenetic gene silencing is the common mechanism .

The term epigenetic refers to a process that heritably influences the expression of a gene without genetic change to the underlying DNA sequence itself (Jaenish & Bird, 2003). The silencing of TSGs, through or associated with CpG island methylation, is recognized as a major mechanism of gene inactivation that frequently coexists with genetic lesions in most cancers studied to date (Esteller, 2007). It has been proposed that methylation silences gene expression by hindering the access of transcription factors to their binding sites. Additionally, it is proposed that silencing might be achieved by methyl-binding proteins that recruit chromatin-modifying factors that compact and inactivate the chromatin (Tateno et al., 2010). The epigenetic events involved in pituitary tumorigenesis that lead to down-regulation of gene and/or protein expression are mainly due to promoter hyper-methylation and/or microRNA (miRNA)-dependent impairment of protein translation.

In the following subsections we will describe the main genes down-regulated by promoter methylation in PA compared to normal pituitary tissue.

4.4.1 Cell cycle inhibitors

The retinoblastoma (pRB) family members are the main inhibitors of cell cycle progression from G1 to S phase. Even though heterozygous pRb-knockout mice develop PA, no mutations at the *RB* gene have been so far found in human pituitary tumours. However, lack of expression of pRB has been found in a small number of pituitary tumours where the promoter region of *RB* is hyper-methylated (Simpson et al., 2000).

Hyper-methylation of the promoter region also accounts for the loss of $p16^{INK4}$ protein expression, which is relatively frequent in PA (Simpson et al., 1999). *RB* and $p16^{INK4a}$ methylations tended to be mutually exclusive (Yoshino et al., 2007).

As for pRB and $p16^{INK4a}$, down-regulation of $p21^{Cip1}$ and $p27^{kip1}$ in pituitary adenomas may also be due to epigenetic modifications, including DNA and/or histone methylation (Yoshino et al., 2007, Zhu et al., 2008).

4.4.2 Hypotalamic hormone receptors

Somatostatin (SS) and dopamine (DA) are among the key regulators of hormone secretion by the anterior pituitary gland. SS mediates its inhibitory activity on pituitary hormone secretion via specific seven trans-membrane G-protein coupled SS receptors (sst). Human adult pituitary tissue expresses sst1, sst2, sst3 and sst5. Similarly, DA action is mediated by five receptors, named D1, D2, D3, D4 and D5, being D2 the only one highly expressed in pituitary cells (lactotroph and non-lactotroph). DA and SS receptors can form heterodimers that may have influence on ligand binding, signalling and internalization of the respective receptors (Hofland et al., 2010).

The expression of sst subtypes in human PA is different in comparison with pituitary and from tumour to tumour. GH-secreting adenomas display a predominant expression of sst2 and sst5, whereas a subset of GH-secreting adenomas expresses sst1 and sst3 as well. In prolactinomas, sst1 and sst5 are the predominantly expressed ssts, whereas sst2 is expressed at a detectable level in only a minority of them. ACTH-secreting adenomas express sst5 at highest level, and most of them co-express sst2 at low level. Silent corticotroph adenomas display considerable higher sst1 and sst2, but lower sst5 expression, compared with ACTH-secreting PA. NFPA mainly express sst3 and to a lesser degree sst2. In TSH-secreting PA, sst2 is mainly expressed, with co-expression of sst3 and sst5 in a subset. Finally, two novel truncated isoforms of sst5 (sst5MD5 and sst5MD4) with five and four trans-membrane domains, respectively, have been identified in PA. In particular, sst5MD4 was found in 85% of GH-secreting adenomas and its expression was negatively associated with the inhibitory effect of octreotide on circulating GH levels *in vivo* (Hofland et al., 2010).

The differential expression of specific sst subtypes in PA may be caused by epigenetic events. Indeed, it has been recently identified an upstream promoter of the human somatostatin receptor, hSSTR2, which is controlled by epigenetic modifications, including DNA methylation and histone acetylation (Torrisani et al., 2008).

As far as DA receptor expression, mainly D2 has been demonstrated in the majority of PA, although expression levels may vary among adenomas. Interestingly, the loss of D2 expression correlates with increased CpG island-associated methylation and enrichment for histone H3K27me3. Conversely, D2 expression is associated to enrichment for H3K9Ac and barely detectable H3K27me3 (Al-Azzawi et al., 2011).

Therefore, a combined treatment with epigenetic drugs and DA agonists for the medical management of different pituitary tumour subtypes, resistant to conventional therapies, could be envisaged.

4.4.3 GADD45γ

One of the growth inhibitory genes whose expression is lost in the majority of human PA is *GADD45γ*, a p53-regulated gene involved in inhibition of cell growth. Indeed, it was found abundantly expressed in normal pituitary and strongly down-regulated in different PA subtypes. Moreover, suppression of cell proliferation was observed when GADD45γ was expressed in pituitary cell lines (as reviewed by Zhang et al., 2010), suggesting a causal role of its loss in pituitary tumorigenesis. The loss of GADD45γ expression in pituitary tumour cells has been associated with methylation of the *GADD45γ* CpG island, frequently (58%) reported in PA not expressing the *GADD45γ* gene (Bahar et al., 2004).

4.4.4 MEG3

The *Maternally Expressed Gene 3 (MEG3)*, a large maternal imprinted non-coding RNA gene located on chromosome 14q32, is highly expressed in the pituitary but specifically absent in gonadotroph-derived NFPA (Zhang et al., 2010). No gene deletion or mutation at the *MEG3* gene was found in such tumours, but increased DNA methylation in promoter and enhancer regions, responsible for loss of MEG3 expression, was identified in tumours in comparison with normal pituitary (Zhao et al., 2005).

MEG3 is able to suppress proliferation of different types of human tumour cells due to its ability to act up-stream of two well known TSGs, such as p53 and pRB. Indeed, MEG3 stimulates p53-mediated transcriptional activation of specific targets, such as GDF15, a TGF-β family member with an anti-proliferative activity, and leads to the accumulation of p53 protein levels. However, it can also suppress cell proliferation in the absence of p53 through a pRB-dependent mechanism (Zhou et al., 2007, as cited in Zhang et al., 2010).

4.4.5 ZAC1

The zinc-finger protein ZAC1 is a transcription factor and co-regulator that plays a key role in pituitary development, maturation and tumorigenesis. Indeed, it lies downstream to the mitogenic MAPK and survival PI3K pathways, and its target genes control cell proliferation and hormone synthesis of pituitary cells (Theodoropoulou et al., 2010). As co-regulator, ZAC1 is involved in the activation of different members of the nuclear receptor and p53 family (Huang & Stallcup, 2000; Huang et al., 2001, as cited in Theodoropoulou et al., 2010), which are key regulators of cell growth, differentiation, homeostasis and development. In particular, through activation of p53, ZAC1 induces the cell-cycle inhibitor $p21^{Cip1}$ causing

growth arrest. Moreover, ZAC1 can also directly bind to the proximal promoter of p21^{Cip1} and confer trans-activation to the GC-rich Sp1-responsive elements (Huang et al., 2007, as cited in Theodoropoulou et al., 2010).
ZAC1 is highly expressed in all types of hormone-producing pituitary cells (Pagotto et al., 2000, as cited in Theodoropoulou et al., 2010). The chromosomal region where it maps (6q24-25) is frequently deleted in solid tumours, and LOH at least at one informative marker has been reported in 50% of pituitary adenomas analysed, but no mutations in the ZAC1 coding region have been found (Pagotto et al. 2000, as cited in Theodoropoulou et al., 2010). However, ZAC1 mRNA and protein levels were found reduced in all types of PA, especially in null cell NFPA, where ZAC1 expression may be completely absent, suggesting a putative role of ZAC1 in pituitary differentiation, since null cell adenomas are thought to be de-differentiated tumours (Theodoropoulou et al., 2010).
It is likely that the loss of ZAC1 expression may be due to an aberrant methylation of a 5'-CpG island in the *ZAC1/LOT1* gene, since it has been reported that this region is differentially methylated in ovarian and breast cancer compared to normal tissues (Abdollahi et al., 2003). Moreover, histone deacetylation, elicited by a mechanism up-stream of the *LOT1* gene, has been suggested as an additional epigenetic modification that controls ZAC1 expression (Abdollahi et al., 2003).

4.5 microRNA expression in pituitary adenomas

MicroRNAs (miRNAs/miRs) are a huge class of non-coding small RNAs that post-transcriptionally regulate gene expression by targeting the 3' un-translated mRNA regions. miRNAs control a wide range of biological functions, including cell proliferation, differentiation, apoptosis and metabolism, and are involved in human pathology, including cancer (Bartel, 2004). Indeed, it has been suggested that some miRNAs might have oncogenic or tumour suppressor functions, playing key roles in tumorigenesis (Croce, 2009).
In PA of different histotypes, a significant down-regulation of miR-15a and miR-16-1, that inversely correlates with tumour diameter and directly correlates with the secretion of the anti-neoplastic cytokine p43, has been shown in comparison with normal pituitary (Bottoni et al., 2005).
The analysis of the differential expression profile of PA of specific histotypes in comparison with normal pituitary, has identified several other miRNAs potentially involved in pituitary tumorigenesis (Bottoni et al., 2007; Amaral et al., 2009; Mao et al., 2010). In ACTH-secreting adenomas six more miRNAs (miR-145, miR-21, miR-141, let-7a, miR-150 and miR-143), other than miR-15a and miR-16, have been shown to be down-regulated (Amaral et al., 2009). In GH-secreting adenomas 52 miRNAs have been reported to be differentially expressed (23 up-regulated and 29 down-regulated). Nine of them are differentially expressed between micro- and macro-adenomas (Mao et al., 2010). Also in NFPAs, six miRNA, including miR-140, miR-99b, miR-99a, miR-30c, miR-30b and miR-138-2, (the first five up-regulated and the last one down-regulated) are differentially expressed in macro- *versus* micro-adenomas (Bottoni et al., 2007).
Interestingly, most of the identified miRNAs differentially expressed in PA *versus* normal pituitary tissue are involved in cell growth, apoptosis, cell proliferation and tumour development. In particular, miR-126 and miR-381, both down-regulated in somatotropinomas, target PTTG (Mao et al., 2010). Furthermore, recent studies have demonstrated that the down-regulation of five miRNAs (let-7, miR-15, miR-16, miR-26 and

miR-196a-2), able to target the HMGA proteins, plays a key role in pituitary tumorigenesis (De Martino et al., 2009b; Kaddar et al., 2009; Quian et al., 2009; Palmieri et al., manuscript in preparation, as cited in Fedele et al., 2010).
Therefore, an innovative therapeutic approach for PA could be the use of miRNAs able to target proteins playing key role in pituitary tumorigenesis and whose expression is down-regulated in PA. Indeed, such approach has been suggested for PA resistant to classical PA therapies, in which the resistance to SS and DA agonists is associated to different miRNA expression (Bottoni et al., 2007; Mao et al., 2010).

5. Familial pituitary adenomas

The vast majority of pituitary adenomas occur spontaneously, which means that they are not inherited, while familial pituitary tumours account for approximately 5% of all pituitary adenomas (Marx & Simonds, 2005). These tumours arise as a component of endocrine-related tumour syndromes, namely Multiple Endocrine Neoplasia type I (MEN1), Multiple Endocrine Neoplasia type IV (MEN4) and Carney complex (CNC), or, if the condition seems to affect only the pituitary gland, as Familial Isolated Pituitary Adenomas (FIPA).
Different gene mutations have been identified in patients affected by familial pituitary adenomas. In highly penetrant conditions, affected individuals manifest the disease phenotype at a considerably younger age (on average 4 years) than their sporadic counterparts; this is due to the shorter time elapse before a "second hit" occurs in a predisposed tissue that already harbours a germline genetic defect. On the contrary, low-penetrance alleles may be more common in the general population, since the presence of a predisposing allele does not necessarily cause a disease-associated phenotype, or it may be associated with age-related penetrance and gender-specific risks (Fearon, 1997; Nagy et al., 2004).

5.1 Multiple Endocrine Neoplasia type I (MEN1)

MEN1 is an inherited autosomal dominant disorder that causes tumours in various endocrine glands (Brandi et al., 2001). MEN1 is sometimes called multiple endocrine adenomatosis or Wermer's syndrome, after one of the first doctor recognised and described it. MEN1 is rare, occurring in about one in 30,000 people. The disorder affects both sexes equally and shows no geographical, racial, or ethnic preferences (Teh et al., 1998).
The gene causing MEN1, identified in 1997, was located on chromosome 11q13, and consists of 10 exons that encode a 610-amino acid protein referred to as Menin (Teh et al., 2005). Menin is predominantly a nuclear protein that has roles in transcriptional regulation, genome stability, cell division and proliferation (Marx & Simonds, 2005). Thus, in transcriptional regulation, Menin interacts with the activating protein-1 (AP-1) transcription factors JunD and C-Jun, and members of the NF-kB family transcriptional regulators, to repress transcriptional activation; members of the Smad family, to inhibit the transforming growth factor-β (TGF-β) and the bone morphogenetic protein-2 (BMP-2) signalling pathways. A wider role in transcription regulation has also been suggested, as Menin has been shown to be an integral component of histone methyltransferase complexes (Agarval et al., 2004).
MEN1 tumours frequently have LOH of the *MEN1* locus, which is consistent with a tumour suppressor role of MEN1. Also mutations of the *MEN1* gene have been identified, and, to

date, about 1300 mutations have been reported: approximately 23% are nonsense mutations, around 41% are frameshift deletions or insertions, 6% are in-frame deletions or insertions, 9% are splice-site mutations, 20% are missense mutations, and 1% are whole or particular gene deletions. The majority (>70%) of these mutations are predicted to lead to truncated forms of Menin disrupting the interactions of Menin with other proteins and altering critical events in cell cycle regulation and proliferation. However, a comparison of the clinical features in patients and their families with the same mutations reveals an absence of phenotype–genotype correlations (Lemos & Thakker, 2008).

In patients with MEN1, several endocrine glands form tumours and become hormonally overactive (Brandi et al., 2001). In MEN1, the overactive glands most often include the parathyroid glands, the pancreas and the pituitary. The parathyroids are the endocrine glands earliest and most often affected by MEN1. In MEN1 patients, all four parathyroid glands tend to be overactive, causing hyperparathyroidism. The parathyroid glands form tumours that release too much PTH, leading to hyper-calcemia. People with MEN1 have about a 20 to 60 percent chance of developing gastrinomas. Gastrin is a hormone that stimulates secretion of gastric acid (HCl) by the parietal cells of the stomach and aids in gastric motility. The pituitary gland develops a tumour in about one in four people with MEN1. This tumour most often releases too much prolactin, developing a prolactinoma. High prolactin levels can cause excessive production of breast milk or interfere with fertility in women or with sex drive and fertility in men. Other pituitary tumour types in MEN1 can be NFPA or GH-secreting adenoma.

5.2 The novel Multiple Endocrine Neoplasia type IV (MEN4) syndrome

Recently, it has been recognized a new rare type MEN1-like syndrome named Multiple Endocrine Neoplasia type 4 (MEN4) caused by mutation of *CDKN1B* (Pellegata et al., 2006). This gene, which maps at 12p13 locus, codes for the 196 amino acid cyclin-dependent kinase inhibitor $p27^{kip1}$. CDKN1B/$p27^{Kip1}$ protein plays an important role in the cell cycle regulation, through the binding and inhibition of cyclin/CDK complexes during the cellular G1 to S phase transition (Sherr & Roberts, 1999); thus, CDKN1B/$p27^{Kip1}$ participates in determining several cell fate decisions, including proliferation, differentiation, apoptosis, cell density, and even cell migration (Besson et al., 2004; Chu et al., 2008). The *CDKN1B* changes so far identified in MEN4 patients either affect the localization, the stability or the protein binding abilities of $p27^{kip1}$. Interestingly, it has been shown that *CDKN1B* is a transcriptional gene target of Menin (Karnik et al., 2005). These findings point to a critical role for p27-mediated cell cycle regulation in neuroendocrine cell homeostasis.

Six germline mutations have been identified so far. Two of them determine a truncated protein with an aberrant cytoplasmic localization. Other two mutations are located in $p27^{kip1}$ region involved in the binding to Grb2 or CDK2. Another one is in the $p27^{kip1}$ regulatory region at -7 position of the Kozak sequence, and is associated with reduction in $p27^{kip1}$ protein levels. Lastly, a mutation at stop codon to Q, coding for an aberrant longer $p27^{kip1}$ including 60 aa more in comparison with the wild-type protein, has been recently identified (Molatore & Pellegata, 2010). Bi-allelic inactivation of *CDKN1B* is an exceedingly rare condition in human tumours, which usually exhibit hemizygous loss of the locus. Therefore, the finding that tumours in *CDKN1B* mutation carriers show loss of heterozygosity or lack of $p27^{kip1}$ expression suggests that $p27^{kip1}$ may behave as a 'canonical' tumour suppressor in neuroendocrine cells.

The phenotypic features associated with MEN4 are still undefined due to the small number of patients reported so far. It is worth noting that these families do not exhibit significant phenotypic differences when compared to *MEN1* mutation-positive families (Bassett et al., 1998).

5.3 Carney complex (CNC)

Carney complex is a hereditary condition. It is associated with spotty skin pigmentation, myxomas (benign or non cancerous connective tissue tumours), and benign or cancerous tumours of the endocrine glands such as the adrenal (Cushing's syndrome), thyroid and pituitary gland (GH-secreting tumours). Although people with Carney complex have an increased risk of cancer, most tumours are benign.

About 60% of people with Carney complex have a mutation in the *CNC1* locus, which maps on chromosome 17q24 (Stratakis et al., 1996). This locus was found to harbour the predisposing gene protein kinase A type I-alpha regulatory subunit (PRKAR1A), encoding a serine/threonine protein kinase A (PKA) regulatory subunit that is the main mediator in cAMP signalling. The function of PRKAR1A is to bind cAMP and regulate the function of the catalytic subunits of the protein kinase A (PKA) holoenzyme. Inactivating *PRKAR1A* mutations have been identified in up to 60% of CNC patients meeting the diagnostic criteria (Kirschner et al., 2000). Almost all 40 distinct germline *PRKAR1A* mutations reported so far lead to mRNA instability, abnormal PRKAR1A and increased PKA activity with elevated cAMP levels in the affected tissues (Groussin et al., 2002), leading to typical manifestations of CNC. However, it is likely that other genes may be associated with Carney complex. Indeed, many of CNC tumours show amplification or deletion of the 2p16 region (the *CNC2* locus) (Matyakhina et al., 2003).

Carney complex follows an autosomal dominant inheritance pattern, in which a mutation happens in only one copy of the gene. It is estimated that between 50% and 70% of cases of Carney complex are familial, while the remaining 30% to 50% of cases result from new mutations.

5.4 Familial Isolated Pituitary Adenomas (FIPA)

Recently, a distinct clinical entity, namely Familial Isolated Pituitary Adenomas (FIPA), has been reported. It characterizes families with isolated pituitary adenomas outside the clinical and genetic contexts of MEN1 and CNC (Daly et al., 2005).

The pituitary tumour types occurring in these families are most commonly GH-secreting adenomas (causing acromegaly or acromegalic gigantism), prolactinomas or NFPA, very rarely ACTH-secreting adenomas (causing Cushing's disease) or TSH-secreting adenomas (Daly et al., 2006). The disease most often starts in adulthood, very rarely in childhood.

The gene responsible for this familial disease has been identified in only 20% of the families. It is called Aryl hydrocarbon receptor (AHR) Interacting Protein, in short AIP, which is part of AHR pathway (Daly et al., 2007). AIP gene is located on chromosome 11q13, and its product is a member of the immonophilin family of proteins with three tetraicopeptide repeats, the TPR domains, that act as scaffolds for the assembly of different multi-protein complexes. AHR is a ligand-inducible transcription factor that mediates the cellular response to xenobiotic compounds. Upon ligand binding, AHR is activated by a conformation change that exposes a nuclear localization signal: the receptor translocates to the nucleus, where it binds to aryl hydrocarbon receptor nuclear translocator. The

heterodimer binds to the xenobiotic response element and regulates gene expression. Loss of heterozygosity of *AIP* gene has been found in tumours of FIPA patients. According to the Knudson two-hit hypothesis, the first hit is due to an inherited germline mutation of one allele and the second hit is a somatic deletion of the other allele (Knudson, 2001).
Almost 50 different germline AIP mutations have been demonstrated in the setting of FIPA. Most of them are present in the TPR domain. Other nonsense and missense mutations all along the coding sequence have been described (Beckers & Daly, 2007). The appearance of PA occurs earlier in the patients carrying AIP mutations with respect to the AIP negative patients.
In FIPA families with normal AIP, a linkage with loci 2p16, 3q28, 4q32.3–4q33, 8q12.1, 19q13.4, and 21q22.1 has been shown, suggesting that mutations in several other genes may be involved in the development of FIPA syndrome (Toledo et al., 2010).

Adenoma type	Incidence	Mutated gene	Syndrome
GH-secreting PRL-secreting NFPA	10% 30% 5%	*MEN1*	Multiple endocrine neoplasia type 1 (MEN1)
To be defined	To be defined	*CDKN1B*	Multiple endocrine neoplasia type IV (MEN4)
GH secreting GH-PRL secreting	15% 70%	*PRKAR1A* *CNC2 locus*	Carney complex (CNC)
GH-secreting PRL-secreting NFPA	30% 40% 13%	*AIP*	FIPA

Table 4. Familial pituitary adenomas.

6. Conclusions

Based on all the events associated with the pathogenesis of PA, the sequence of genetic alterations likely begins, at least for GH-secreting adenomas, with an aberrant cAMP signalling that causes polyclonal hyperplasia and/or initial adenoma formation (as evidenced by GNAS and PRKAR1A involvement). Then, for all subtypes, growth of a monoclonal pituitary tumour is initiated and/or assisted by cell-cycle dysregulation and aneuploidy. Menin down-regulation, methylation of certain target genes, aneuploidy and/or disruption of genomic integrity in a greater scale lead to a well-growing pituitary adenoma, but still responsive to medical and/or surgical treatment (depending on the type). Finally, E2F1 activation, cell cycle dysregulation, PTTG over-expression and/or additional growth factor up-regulation and increased angiogenesis lead to aggressive tumours. However, mitotic activity is low even in aggressive PA, in contrast to tumours arising from more rapidly replicating tissues, and pituitary tumours rarely progress to carcinoma (Chesnokova & Melmed, 2010).
Indeed, induction of premature senescence in PA, which is triggered in response to aneuploidy, restrains further growth and malignant transformation but allows the cells to remain viable and perform their physiological functions.
Anyway, further studies are required to better understand all the genetic and epigenetic alterations accounting for the development of PA and the sequence with which they occur.

7. References

Abdollahi, A., Pisarcik, D., Roberts, D., Weinstein, J., Cairns, P. & Hamilton, T.C. (2003). LOT1 (PLAGL1/ZAC1), the candidate tumor suppressor gene at chromosome 6q24-25, is epigenetically regulated in cancer. *The Journal of Biological Chemistry,* Vol.278, No.8, pp.6041-6049, ISSN 0021-9258

Agarwal, S.K., Lee Burns, A., Sukhodolets, K.E., Kennedy, P.A., Obungu, V.H., Hickman, A.B., Mullendore, M.E., Whitten, I., Skarulis, M.C., Simonds, W.F., Mateo, C., Crabtree, J.S., Scacheri, P.C., Ji, Y., Novotny, E.A., Garrett-Beal, L., Ward, J.M., Libutti, S.K., Richard, A.H, Cerrato, A., Parisi, M.J., Santa Anna-A, S., Oliver, B., Chandrasekharappa, S.C., Collins, F.S., Spiegel, A.M. & Marx, S.J. (2004). Molecular pathology of the MEN1 gene. *Annals of the New York Academy of Sciences,* Vol.1014, pp.189-198, ISSN 1749-6632

Al-Azzawi, H., Yacqub-Usman, K., Richardson, A., Hofland, L.J., Clayton, R.N. & Farrell, W.E. (2011). Reversal of endogenous dopamine receptor silencing in pituitary cells augments receptor-mediated apoptosis. *Endocrinology,* Vol.152, No.2, pp.364-373, ISSN 0013-7227

Alvaro, V., Lévy, L., Dubray, C., Roche, A., Peillon, F., Quérat, B. & Joubert D. (1993). Invasive human pituitary tumors express a point-mutated alpha-protein kinase-C. *The Journal of Clinical Endocrinology and Metabolism,* Vol.77, No.5, pp.1125-1129, ISSN 0021-972X

Alvaro, V., Prévostel, C., Joubert, D., Slosberg, E. & Weinstein, B.I. (1997). Ectopic expression of a mutant form of PKCalpha originally found in human tumors: aberrant subcellular translocation and effects on growth control. *Oncogene,* Vol.14, No.6, pp.677-685, ISSN 0950-9232

Amaral, F.C., Torres, N., Saggioro, F., Neder, L., Machado, H.R., Silva, W.A. Jr, Moreira, A.C. & Castro, M. (2009). MicroRNAs differentially expressed in ACTH-secreting pituitary tumors. *The Journal of Clinical Endocrinology and Metabolism,* Vol.94, No.1, pp.320-323, ISSN 0021-972X

Asa, S.L. & Ezzat, S. (2002). The pathogenesis of pituitary tumours. *Nature Reviews Cancer,* Vol.2, No.11, pp.836-849, ISSN 1474-1768

Bahar, A., Bicknell, J.E., Simpson, D.J., Clayton, R.N. & Farrell, W.E. (2004). Loss of expression of the growth inhibitory gene GADD45gamma, in human pituitary adenomas, is associated with CpG island methylation. *Oncogene,* Vol.23, No.4, pp.936-944, ISSN 0950-9232

Bartel, D. P. (2004). MicroRNAs: genomics, biogenesis, mechanism and function. *Cell,* Vol.116, No.2, pp.281–297, ISSN 0092-8674

Bassett, J.H., Forbes, S.A., Pannett, A.A., Lloyd, S.E., Christie, P.T., Wooding, C., Harding, B., Besser, G.M., Edwards, C.R., Monson, J.P., Sampson, J., Wass, J.A., Wheeler, M.H. & Thakker, R.V. (1998). Characterization of mutations in patients with multiple endocrine neoplasia type 1. *The American Journal of Human Genetics,* Vol.62, No.2, pp.232-244, ISSN 1552-4825

Beckers, A. & Daly, A.F. (2007). The clinical, pathological, and genetic features of familial isolated pituitary adenomas. *European Journal of Endocrinology,* Vol. 157, No. 4, pp. 371-382, ISSN 0804-4643

Bellodi, C., Krasnykh, O., Haynes, N., Theodoropoulou, M., Peng, G., Montanaro, L.& Ruggero, D. (2010). Loss of function of the tumor suppressor DKC1 perturbs p27 translation control and contributes to pituitary tumorigenesis. *Cancer Research*, Vol.70, No.14, pp.6026-6035, ISSN 0008-5472

Bilezikjian, L.M., Blount, A.L., Leal, A.M., Donaldson, C.J., Fischer, W.H. & Vale, W.W. (2004). Autocrine/paracrine regulation of pituitary function by activin, inhibin and follistatin. *Molecular and Cellular Endocrinology*, Vol.225, No.1-2, pp.29-36, ISSN 0303-7207

Bottoni, A., Piccin, D., Tagliati, F., Luchin, A., Zatelli, M.C. & degli Uberti, E.C. (2005). miR-15a and miR-16-1 down-regulation in pituitary adenomas. *Journal of Cellular Physiology*, Vol.204, No.1, pp.280-285, ISSN 0021-9541

Bottoni, A., Zatelli, M.C., Ferracin, M., Tagliati, F., Piccin, D., Vignali, C., Calin, G.A., Negrini, M., Croce, C.M. & Degli Uberti, E.C. (2007). Identification of differentially expressed microRNAs by microarray: a possible role for microRNA genes in pituitary adenomas. *Journal of Cellular Physiology*. Vol.210, No.2, pp.370-377, ISSN 0021-9541

Brandi, M.L., Gagel, R.F., Angeli, A., Bilezikian, J.P., Beck-Peccoz, P., Bordi, C., Conte-Devolx, B., Falchetti, A., Gheri, R.G., Libroia, A., Lips, C.J., Lombardi, G., Mannelli, M., Pacini, F., Ponder, B.A., Raue, F., Skogseid, B., Tamburrano, G., Thakker, R.V., Thompson, N.W., Tomassetti, P., Tonelli, F., Wells, S.A.Jr & Marx, S.J. (2001). Guidelines for diagnosis and therapy of MEN type 1 and type 2. *The Journal of Clinical Endocrinology and Metabolism*, Vol.86, No.12, pp.5658-5671, ISSN 0021-972X

Brook, C.G.D. & Marshall, N.J. (2001). *Essential Endocrinology* (4th edition), Blackwell Science, ISBN 9780632056156-0632056150, Oxford, England

Chesnokova, V. & Melmed, S. (2010). Pituitary senescence: the evolving role of Pttg. *Molecular and Cellular Endocrinology*, Vol.326, No.1-2, pp.55-59, ISSN 0303-7207

Clayton, R.N., Pfeifer, M., Atkinson, A.B., Belchetz, P., Wass, J.A., Kyrodimou, E., Vanderpump, M., Simpson, D., Bicknell, J. & Farrell, W.E. (2000). Different patterns of allelic loss (loss of heterozygosity) in recurrent human pituitary tumors provide evidence for multiclonal origins. *Clinical Cancer Research*, Vol.6, No.10, pp.3973-3982, ISSN 1078-0432

Clayton, R.N. & Farrell, W.E. (2004). Pituitary tumour clonality revisited. *Frontiers of Hormone Research*, Vol.32, pp.186-204, ISSN 1662-3762

Croce, C.M. (2009). Causes and consequences of microRNA dysregulation in cancer. *Nature Reviews. Genetics*, Vol.10, No.10, pp.704-714, ISSN 1471-0056

Dahia, P.L., Aguiar, R.C., Honegger, J., Fahlbush, R., Jordan, S., Lowe, D.G., Lu, X., Clayton, R.N., Besser, G.M. & Grossman, A.B. (1998). Mutation and expression analysis of the p27/kip1 gene in corticotrophin-secreting tumours. *Oncogene*, Vol.16, No.1, pp.69-76, ISSN 0950-9232

Daly, A.F., Jaffrain-Rea, M.L. & Beckers, A. (2005). Clinical and genetic features of familial pituitary adenomas. *Hormone and metabolic research*, Vol.37, No.6, pp.347-354, ISSN 0018-5043

Daly, A.F., Jaffrain-Rea, M.L., Ciccarelli, A., Valdes-Socin, H., Rohmer, V., Tamburrano, G., Borson-Chazot, C., Estour, B., Ciccarelli, E., Brue, T., Ferolla, P., Emy, P., Colao, A., De Menis, E., Lecomte, P., Penfornis, F., Delemer, B., Bertherat, J., Wemeau, J.L., De Herder, W., Archambeaud, F., Stevenaert, A., Calender, A., Murat, A., Cavagnini, F. & Beckers, A. (2006). Clinical characterization of familial isolated pituitary adenomas. *The Journal of Clinical Endocrinology and Metabolism*, Vol.91, No.9, pp. 3316-3323, ISSN 0952-5041

Daly, A.F., Vanbellinghen, J.F., Khoo, S.K., Jaffrain-Rea, M.L., Naves, L.A., Guitelman, M.A., Murat, A., Emy, P., Gimenez-Roqueplo, A.P., Tamburrano, G., Raverot, G., Barlier, A., De Herder, W., Penfornis, A., Ciccarelli, E., Estour, B., Lecomte, P., Gatta, B., Chabre, O., Sabate, M.I., Bertagna, X., Garcia Basavilbaso, N., Stalldecker, G., Colao, A., Ferolla, P., Wemeau, J.L., Caron, P., Sadoul, J.L., Oneto, A., Archambeaud, F., Calender, A., Sinilnikova, O., Montanana, C.F., Cavagnini, F., Hana, V., Solano, A., Delettieres, D., Luccio-Camelo, D.C., Basso, A., Rohmer, V., Brue, T., Bours, V., Teh, B.T. & Beckers, A. (2007). Aryl hydrocarbon receptor-interacting protein gene mutations in familial isolated pituitary adenomas: analysis in 73 families. *The Journal of Clinical Endocrinology and Metabolism*, Vol.92, No.5, pp.1891-1896, ISSN 0952-5041

De Lellis, R.A., Lloyd, R.V., Heitz, P.U. & Eng, C. (Eds) (2004). *Pathology and genetics of tumours of endocrine organs*, IARC Press, ISBN 9789283224167-9283224167, Lyon, France

De Martino, I., Visone, R., Palmieri, D., Cappabianca, P., Chieffi, P., Forzati, F., Barbieri, A., Kruhoffer, M., Lombardi, G., Fusco, A. & Fedele M. (2007). The Mia/Cd-rap gene expression is downregulated by the high-mobility group A proteins in mouse pituitary adenomas. *Endocrine Related Cancer*, Vol.14, No.3, pp.875-886, ISSN 1351-0088

De Martino, I., Visone, R., Wierinckx, A., Palmieri, D., Ferraro, A., Cappabianca, P., Chiappetta, G., Forzati, F., Lombardi, G., Colao, A., Trouillas, J., Fedele, M. & Fusco A. (2009). HMGA proteins up-regulate CCNB2 gene in mouse and human pituitary adenomas. *Cancer Research*, Vol.69, No.5, pp.1844-1850, ISSN 0008-5472

Edamatsu, H., Kaziro, Y. & Itoh, H. (1998). Expression of an oncogenic mutant G alpha i2 activates Ras in Rat-1 fibroblast cells. *FEBS Letters*, Vol.440, No.1-2, pp.231-234, ISSN 0014-5793

Esteller, M. (2007). Cancer epigenomics: DNA methylomes and histone-modification maps. *Nature Reviews Genetics*, Vol.8, No.4, pp.286-298, ISSN 1471-0056

Evans, C.O., Moreno, C.S., Zhan, X., McCabe, M.T., Vertino, P.M., Desiderio, D.M. & Oyesiku, N.M. (2008). Molecular pathogenesis of human prolactinomas identified by gene expression profiling, RT-qPCR, and proteomic analyses. *Pituitary*, Vol.11, No.3, pp.231-245, ISSN 1386-341X

Ezzat, S., Zheng, L., Zhu, X.F., Wu, G.E. & Asa, S.L. (2002). Targeted expression of a human pituitary tumor-derived isoform of FGF receptor-4 recapitulates pituitary tumorigenesis. *The Journal of Clinical Investigation*, Vol.109, No.1, pp.69-78, ISSN 0021-9738

Fearon, E.R. (1997). Human cancer syndromes: clues to the origin and nature of cancer. *Science*, Vol.278, No.5340, pp.1043-1050, ISSN 0193-4511

Fedele, M., Battista, S., Kenyon, L., Baldassarre, G., Fidanza, V., Klein-Szanto, A.J., Parlow, A.F., Visone, R., Pierantoni, G.M., Outwater, E., Santoro, M., Croce, C.M. & Fusco, A. (2002). Overexpression of the HMGA2 gene in transgenic mice leads to the onset of pituitary adenomas. *Oncogene*, Vol.21, No.20, pp.3190-3198, ISSN 0950-9232

Fedele, M., Pentimalli, F., Baldassarre, G., Battista, S., Klein-Szanto, A.J., Kenyon, L., Visone, R., De Martino, I., Ciarmiello, A., Arra, C., Viglietto, G., Croce, C.M. & Fusco A. (2005). Transgenic mice overexpressing the wild-type form of the HMGA1 gene develop mixed growth hormone/prolactin cell pituitary adenomas and natural killer cell lymphomas. *Oncogene*, Vol.24, No.21, pp.3427-3435, ISSN 0950-9232

Fedele, M., Visone, R., De Martino, I., Troncone, G., Palmieri, D., Battista, S., Ciarmiello, A., Pallante, P., Arra, C., Melillo, R.M., Helin, K., Croce, C.M. & Fusco A. (2006). HMGA2 induces pituitary tumorigenesis by enhancing E2F1 activity. *Cancer Cell*, Vol.9, No.6, pp.459-471, ISSN 1535-6108

Fedele, M. & Fusco, A. (2010). Role of the high mobility group A proteins in the regulation of pituitary cell cycle. *The Journal of Molecular Endocrinolology*, Vol.44, No.6, pp.309-318, ISSN 0952-5041

Fedele, M., Palmieri, D. & Fusco, A. (2010). HMGA2: A pituitary tumour subtype-specific oncogene? *Molecular and Cellular Endocrinology*, Vol.326, No.1-2, pp.19-24, ISSN 0303-7207

Finelli, P., Pierantoni, G.M., Giardino, D., Losa, M., Rodeschini, O., Fedele, M., Valtorta, E., Mortini, P., Croce, C.M., Larizza, L. & Fusco, A. (2002). The High Mobility Group A2 gene is amplified and overexpressed in human prolactinomas. *Cancer Research*, Vol.62, No.8, pp.2398-2405, ISSN 0008-5472

Futreal, P.A., Coin, L., Marshall, M., Down, T., Hubbard, T., Wooster, R., Rahman, N. & Stratton, M.R. (2004). A census of human cancer genes. *Nature Reviews Cancer*, Vol.4, No.3, pp.177-183, ISSN 1474-1768

Goodman, H.M. (2003). Basic Medical Endocrinology (3th edition), Academic Press, ISBN 9780122904219- 0122904214, Amsterdam, Netherlands

Groussin, L., Kirschner, L.S., Vincent-Dejean, C., Perlemoine, K., Jullian, E., Delemer, B., Zacharieva, S., Pignatelli, D., Carney, J.A., Luton, J.P., Bertagna, X., Stratakis, C.A. & Bertherat, J. (2002). Molecular analysis of the cyclic AMP-dependent protein kinase A (PKA) regulatory subunit 1A (PRKAR1A) gene in patients with Carney complex and primary pigmented nodular adrenocortical disease (PPNAD) reveals novel mutations and clues for pathophysiology: augmented PKA signaling is associated with adrenal tumorigenesis in PPNAD. *The American Journal of Human Genetics*, Vol.71, No.6, pp.1433-1442, ISSN 1552-4825

Guru, S.C., Manickam, P., Crabtree, J.S., Olufemi, S.E., Agarwal, S.K., & Debelenko LV. (1998). Identification and characterization of the multiple endocrine neoplasia type 1 (MEN1) gene. *Journal of Internal Medicine*, Vol.243, No.6, pp.433-439, ISSN 1365-2796

Hayward, B.E., Barlier, A., Korbonits, M., Grossman, A.B., Jacquet, P., Enjalbert, A. & Bonthron, D.T. (2001). Imprinting of the G(s)alpha gene GNAS1 in the pathogenesis of acromegaly. *The Journal of Clinical Investigation*, Vol.107, No.6, pp. R31-36, ISSN 0021-972X

Heaney, A.P. & Melmed, S. (2004). Molecular targets in pituitary tumours. *Nature Reviews. Cancer*, Vol.4, No.4, pp.285-295, ISSN 1474-1768

Hock, R., Furusawa, T., Ueda, T. & Bustin, M. (2007). HMG chromosomal proteins in development and disease. *Trends in Cell Biology*, Vol.17, No.2, pp.72-79, ISSN 0962-8924

Hofland, L.J., Feelders, R.A., de Herder, W.W. & Lamberts, S.W. (2010). Pituitary tumours: the sst/D2 receptors as molecular targets. *Molecular and Cellular Endocrinology*, Vol.326, No.1-2, pp.89-98, ISSN 0303-7207

Jaenisch, R. & Bird, A. (2003). Epigenetic regulation of gene expression: how the genome integrates intrinsic and environmental signals. *Nature Genetics*, Vol.33, pp.245-254, ISSN 1061-4036

Kaltsas, G.A., Nomikos, P., Kontogeorgos, G., Buchfelder, M. & Grossman, A.B. (2005). Clinical review: Diagnosis and management of pituitary carcinomas. *The Journal of Clinical Endocrinology and Metabolism*, Vol.90, No.5, pp. 3089-3099, ISSN 1945-7197

Karnik, S.K., Hughes, C.M., Gu, X., Rozenblatt-Rosen, O., McLean, G.W., Xiong, Y., Meyerson, M., & Kim, S.K. (2005). Menin regulates pancreatic islet growth by promoting histone methylation and expression of genes encoding p27Kip1 and p18INK4c. *The Proceedings of the National Academy of Sciences U S A* , Vol.102, No.41, pp.14659-14664, ISSN 0027-8424

Kirschner, L.S., Carney, J.A., Pack, S.D., Taymans, S.E., Giatzakis, C., Cho, Y.S., Cho-Chung, Y.S. & Stratakis, C.A. (2000). Mutations of the gene encoding the protein kinase A type I-alpha regulatory subunit in patients with the Carney Complex. *Nature Genetics*, Vol.26, No.1, pp.89-92, ISSN 1061-4036

Knudson, A.G. (2001). Two genetic hits (more or less) to cancer, *Nature Reviews Cancer*, Vol.1, No.2, pp.157-162, ISSN 1474-1768

Landis, C.A., Masters, S.B., Spada, A., Pace, A.M., Bourne, H.R. & Vallar, L. (1989). GTPase inhibiting mutations activate the alpha chain of Gs and stimulate adenylyl cyclase in human pituitary tumours. *Nature*, Vol.340, No.6236, pp.692-696, ISSN 0028-0836

Lania, A., Mantovani, G. & Spada, A. (2003), Genetics of pituitary tumors: Focus on G-protein mutations. Experimental Biology and Medicine (Maywood). Vol.228, No.9, pp.1004-1017, ISSN 1351-0088

Lemos, M.C. & Thakker, R.V. (2008). Multiple endocrine neoplasia type 1 (MEN1): analysis of 1336 mutations reported in the first decade following identification of the gene. *Human Mutation*, Vol.29, No.1, pp.22-32, ISSN 1059-7794

Lyons, J., Landis, C.A., Harsh, G., Vallar, L., Grünewald, K., Feichtinger, H., Duh, Q.Y., Clark, O.H., Kawasaki, E., Bourne, H.R., et al. (1990). Two G protein oncogenes in human endocrine tumors. *Science*, Vol.249, No.4969, pp.655-659, ISSN 0193-4511

Mao, Z.G., He, D.S., Zhou, J., Yao, B., Xiao, W.W., Chen, C.H., Zhu, Y.H. & Wang, H.J. (2010). Differential expression of microRNAs in GH-secreting pituitary adenomas. *Diagnostic Pathology*, Vol.5, No.1, pp.79-87, ISSN 1746-1596

Marx, S.J. & Simonds, W.F. (2005). Hereditary hormone excess: genes, molecular pathways, and syndromes. *Endocrine Reviews*, Vol.26, No.5, pp.615-661, ISSN 0163-769X.

Matyakhina, L., Pack, S., Kirschner, L..S., Pak, E., Mannan, P., Jaikumar, J., Taymans, S.E., Sandrini, F., Carney, J.A., & Stratakis, C.A. (2003). Chromosome 2 (2p16) abnormalities in Carney complex tumours. *Journal of Medical Genetics*, Vol.40, No.4, pp.268-277, ISSN 0022-2593

Mechenthaler, I. (2008). Galanin and the neuroendocrine axes. *Cellular and Molecular Life Science*, Vol.65, No.12, pp. 1826-1835, ISSN 1420-682X

Melmed, S. (2003). Mechanisms for pituitary tumorigenesis: the plastic pituitary. *The Journal of Clinical Investigation*, Vol.112, No.11, pp.1603-1618, ISSN 0021-9738

Melmed, S. & Kleinberg, D. (2008). Anterior Pituitary, In: *Williams Textbook of Endocrinology*, H.M., Kronenberg, S. Melmed, K.S. Polonsky, P.R. Larsen (Eds.), 155-261, Sounders Elsevier, ISBN 978-1-4160-2911-3, Canada

Molatore, S. & Pellegata, N.S. (2010). The MENX syndrome and p27: relationships with multiple endocrine neoplasia. *Progress in Brain Research*, Vol.182, pp.295-320, ISSN 0079-6123

Muşat, M., Morris, D.G., Korbonits, M. & Grossman, A.B. (2010). Cyclins and their related proteins in pituitary tumourigenesis. *Molecular and Cellular Endocrinolology*, Vol.326, No.1-2, pp.25-29, ISSN 0303-7207

Nagy, R., Sweet, K. & Eng, C. (2004). Highly penetrant hereditary cancer syndromes. *Oncogene,* Vol.23, No.38, pp.6445-6470, ISSN 0950-9232

Occhi, G., Trivellin, G., Ceccato, F., De Lazzari, P., Giorgi, G., Demattè, S., Grimaldi, F., Castello, R., Davì, M.V., Arnaldi, G., Salviati, L., Opocher, G., Mantero, F. & Scaroni, C. (2010). Prevalence of AIP mutations in a large series of sporadic Italian acromegalic patients and evaluation of CDKN1B status in acromegalic patients with multiple endocrine neoplasia. *European Journal of Endocrinology,* Vol.163, No.3, pp.369-376, ISSN 0804-4643

Ozfirat, Z. & Korbonits, M. (2010). AIP gene and familial isolated pituitary adenomas. *Molecular and Cellular Endocrinology,* Vol.326, No.1-2, pp.71-79, ISSN 0303-7207

Pei, L. & Melmed, S. (1997). Isolation and characterization of a pituitary tumor-transforming gene (PTTG). *Molecular Endocrinology,* Vol.11, No.4, pp.433-441, ISSN 0888-8809

Pellegata, N.S., Quintanilla-Martinez, L., Siggelkow, H., Samson, E., Bink, K., Hofler, H., Fend, F., Graw, J. & Atkinson, M.J. (2006). Germline mutations in p27Kip1 cause a multiple endocrine neoplasia syndrome in rats and humans, *Proc Natl Acad Sci U S A,* Vol.103, No.42, pp.15558-15563, ISSN 0027-8424

Pernicone, P.J., Scheithauer, B.W., Sebo, T.J., Kovacs, K.T., Horvath, E., Young, W.F. Jr, Lloyd, R.V., Davis, D.H., Guthrie, B.L. & Schoene, W.C. (1997). Pituitary carcinoma: a clinicopathologic study of 15 cases. *Cancer,* Vol.79, No.4, pp.804-812, ISSN 1097-0142

Pierantoni, G.M., Finelli, P., Valtorta, E., Giardino, D., Rodeschini, O., Esposito, F., Losa, M., Fusco, A. & Larizza, L. (2005). High-mobility group A2 gene expression is frequently induced in non-functioning pituitary adenomas (NFPAs), even in the absence of chromosome 12 polysomy. *Endocrine Related Cancer,* Vol.12, No.4, pp.867-874, ISSN 1351-0088

Righi, A., Jin, L., Zhang, S., Stilling, G., Scheithauer, B.W., Kovacs, K. & Lloyd, R.V. (2010). Identification and consequences of galectin-3 expression in pituitary tumors. *Molecular and Cellular Endocrinology,* Vol.326, No.1-2, pp.8-14, ISSN 0303-7207

Saeger, W., Lüdecke, D.K., Buchfelder, M., Fahlbusch, R., Quabbe, H.J. & Petersenn, S. (2007). Pathohistological classification of pituitary tumors: 10 years of experience with the German Pituitary Tumor Registry. *European Journal of Endocrinology,* Vol.156, No.2 pp.203-216, ISSN 0804-4643

Schiemann, U., Assert, R., Moskopp, D., Gellner, R., Hengst, K., Gullotta, F., Domschke, W. & Pfeiffer, A. (1997). Analysis of a protein kinase C-alpha mutation in human pituitary tumours. *Journal of Endocrinology,* Vol.153, No.1, pp.131-137, ISSN 0022-0795

Sharpless, N.E. & DePinho, R.A. (2004). Telomeres, stem cells, senescence, and cancer. *The Journal of Clinical Investigation,* Vol.113, No.2, pp.160-168, ISSN 0021-9738

Scheithauer, B.W., Gaffey, T.A., Lloyd, R.V., Sebo, T.J., Kovacs, K.T., Horvath, E., Yapicier, O., Young, W.F. Jr, Meyer, F.B., Kuroki, T., Riehle, D.L., Laws, E.R. Jr. (2006). Pathobiology of pituitary adenomas and carcinomas. *Neurosurgery,* Vol.59, No.2, pp.341-353, ISSN 1528-8285

Schmidt, M.C., Henke, R.T., Stang, A.P., Meyer-Puttlitz, B., Stoffel-Wagner, B., Schramm, J. & Von Deimling, A. (1999). Analysis of the *MEN1* gene in sporadic pituitary adenomas. *Journal of Pathology,* Vol.188, pp.168–173, ISSN 0022-3417

Sherr, C.J. & Roberts, J.M. (1999). CDK inhibitors: positive and negative regulators of G1-phase progression. *Genes Development,* Vol.13, No.12, pp.1501-1512, ISSN 0890-9369

Sidibé, E.H. (2007). Pituitary carcinoma. Anatomic and clinical features of cases reported in literature. *Neurochirurgie*, Vol.53, No.4, pp.284-288, ISSN 0028-3770

Simpson, D.J., Bicknell, J.E., McNicol, A.M., Clayton, R.N. & Farrell, W.E. (1999). Hypermethylation of the p16/CDKN2A/MTSI gene and loss of protein expression is associated with nonfunctional pituitary adenomas but not somatotrophinomas. *Genes Chromosomes Cancer,* Vol.24, No.4, pp.328-336, ISSN 1045-2257

Simpson, D.J., Hibberts, N.A., McNicol, A.M., Clayton, R.N. & Farrell, W.E. (2000). Loss of pRb expression in pituitary adenomas is associated with methylation of the RB1 CpG island. *Cancer Research*, Vol.60, No.5, pp.1211-1216, ISSN 0008-5472

Stratakis, C.A., Carney, J.A., Lin, J.P., Papanicolaou, D.A., Karl, M., Kastner, D.L., Pras, E. & Chrousos, G.P. (1996). Carney complex, a familial multiple neoplasia and lentiginosis syndrome. Analysis of 11 kindreds and linkage to the short arm of chromosome 2. *The Journal of Clinical Investigation, Vol.* 97, No. 3, pp. 699-705, ISSN 0021-9738

Tateno, T., Zhu, X., Asa, S.L. & Ezzat, S. (2010). Chromatin remodeling and histone modifications in pituitary tumors. *Molecular and Cellular Endocrinology,* Vol.326, No.1-2, pp.66-70, ISSN 0303-7207

Teh, B.T., Cardinal, J., Shepherd, J, Hayward, N.K., Weber, G., Cameron, D, & Larsson, C. (1995). Genetic mapping of the multiple endocrine neoplasia type 1 locus at 11q13. *Journal of Internal Medicine,* Vol.238, No.3, pp.249-253, ISSN 1365-2796

Teh, B.T., Kytola, S., Farnebo, F., Bergman, L., Wong, F.K., Weber, G., Hayward, N., Larsson, C., Skogseid, B., Beckers, A., Phelan, C., Edwards, M., Epstein, M., Alford, F., Hurley, D., Grimmond, S., Silins, G., Walters, M., Stewart, C., Cardinal, J., Khodaei, S., Parente, F., Tranebjaerg, L., Jorde, R. & Salmela, P. (1998). Mutation analysis of the MEN1 gene in multiple endocrine neoplasia type 1, familial acromegaly and familial isolated hyperparathyroidism. *The Journal of Clinical Endocrinology and Metabolism,* Vol.83, No.8, pp.2621-2626, ISSN 1945-7197

Thanos, D. & Maniatis, T. (1995). Virus induction of human IFN beta gene expression requires the assembly of an enhanceosome. *Cell,* Vol.83, No.7, pp.1091-1100, ISSN 0092-8674

Theodoropoulou, M., Stalla, G.K. & Spengler, D. (2010). ZAC1 target genes and pituitary tumorigenesis. *Molecular and Cellular Endocrinology,* Vol.326, No.1-2, pp.60-65, ISSN 0303-7207

Toledo, R.A., Lourenço, D.M. Jr, & Toledo, S.P. (2010). Familial isolated pituitary adenoma: evidence for genetic heterogeneity. *Frontiers of Hormone Research,* Vol.38, pp.77-86, ISSN 0301-3073

Torrisani, J., Hanoun, N., Laurell, H., Lopez, F., Maoret, J.J., Souque, A., Susini, C., Cordelier, P. & Buscail, L. (2008). Identification of an upstream promoter of the human somatostatin receptor, hSSTR2, which is controlled by epigenetic modifications. *Endocrinology,* Vol.149, No.6, pp.3137-3147, ISSN 0013-7227

Vallar, L., Spada, A. & Giannattasio, G. (1987). Altered Gs and adenylate cyclase activity in human GH-secreting pituitary adenomas. *Nature,* Vol.330, No.6148, pp.566-568, ISSN 0028-0836

Vandeva, S., Jaffrain-Rea, M.L., Daly, A.F., Tichomirowa, M., Zacharieva, S. & Beckers, A. (2010). The genetics of pituitary adenomas. *Best Practice and Research. Clinical Endocrinology and Metabolism,* Vol.24, No.3, pp.461-476, ISSN 1521-690X

Wang, E.L., Qian, Z.R., Rahman, M.M., Yoshimoto, K., Yamada, S., Kudo, E. & Sano, T. (2010). Increased expression of HMGA1 correlates with tumour invasiveness and proliferation in human pituitary adenomas. *Histopathology*, Vol.56, No.4, pp.501-509, ISSN 0309-0167

Weinstein, L.S., Shenker. A., Gejman. P.V., Merino. M.J., Friedman. E. & Spiegel, A.M. (1991). Activating mutations of the stimulatory G protein in the McCune-Albright syndrome. *The New England Journal of Medicine*, Vol.325, No.24, pp.1688-1695, ISSN 0028-4793

Wenbin, C., Asai, A., Teramoto, A., Sanno, N. & Kirino, T. (1999). Mutations of the MEN1 tumor suppressor gene in sporadic pituitary tumors. *Cancer Letters*, Vol.142, No.1, pp.43-47, ISSN 0304-3835

Wierinckx, A., Auger, C., Devauchelle, P., Reynaud, A., Chevallier, P., Jan, M., Perrin, G., Fèvre-Montange, M., Rey, C., Figarella-Branger, D., Raverot, G., Belin, M.F., Lachuer, J. & Trouillas J. (2007). A diagnostic marker set for invasion, proliferation, and aggressiveness of prolactin pituitary tumors. *Endocrine Related Cancer*, Vol.14, No.3, pp.887-900, ISSN 1351-0088

Williamson, E.A., Daniels, M., Foster, S., Kelly, W.F., Kendall-Taylor, P. & Harris, P.E. (1994). Gs alpha and Gi2 alpha mutations in clinically non-functioning pituitary tumours. *Clinical Endocrinology*, Vol.41, No.6, pp.815-820, ISSN 0300-0664

Yoshino, A., Katayama, Y., Ogino, A., Watanabe, T., Yachi, K., Ohta, T., Komine, C., Yokoyama, T. & Fukushima, T. (2007). Promoter hypermethylation profile of cell cycle regulator genes in pituitary adenomas. *Journal of Neuro-oncology*, Vol.83, No.2, pp.153-162, ISSN 0167-594X

Zhang, X., Horwitz, G.A., Heaney, A.P., Nakashima, M., Prezant, T.R., Bronstein, M.D. & Melmed S. (1999). Pituitary tumor transforming gene (PTTG) expression in pituitary adenomas. *The Journal of Clinical Endocrinology and Metabolism*, Vol.84, No.2, pp.761-767, ISSN 1945-7197

Zhang, X., Sun, H., Danila, D.C., Johnson, S.R., Zhou, Y., Swearingen, B. & Klibanski, A. (2002). Loss of expression of GADD45 gamma, a growth inhibitory gene, in human pituitary adenomas: implications for tumorigenesis. *The Journal of Clinical Endocrinology and Metabolism*, Vol.87, No.3, pp.1262-1267, ISSN 0021-972X

Zhang, X., Zhou, Y. & Klibanski, A. (2010). Isolation and characterization of novel pituitary tumor related genes: a cDNA representational difference approach. *Molecular and Cellular Endocrinology*, Vol.326, No.1-2, pp.40-47, ISSN 0303-7207

Zhao, J., Dahle, D., Zhou, Y., Zhang, X. & Klibanski, A. (2005). Hypermethylation of the promoter region is associated with the loss of MEG3 gene expression in human pituitary tumors. *The Journal of Clinical Endocrinology and Metabolism*, Vol.90, No.4, pp.2179-2186, ISSN 0021-972X

Zhu, X., Mao, X., Hurren, R., Schimmer, A.D., Ezzat, S. & Asa, S.L. (2008). Deoxyribonucleic acid methyltransferase 3B promotes epigenetic silencing through histone 3 chromatin modifications in pituitary cells. *The Journal of Clinical Endocrinology and Metabolism*, Vol.93, No.9, pp.3610-3617, ISSN 0021-972X

Zhuang, Z., Ezzat, S.Z,. Vortmeyer, A.O., Weil, R., Oldfield, E.H., Park, W.S., Pack, S., Huang, S., Agarwal, S.K., Guru, S.C., Manickam, P., Debelenko, L.V., Kester, M.B., Olufemi, S.E., Heppner, C., Crabtree, J.S., Burns, A.L., Spiegel, A.M., Marx, S.J., Chandrasekharappa, S.C., Collins, F.S., Emmert-Buck, M.R., Liotta, L.A., Asa, S.L. & Lubensky, I.A. (1997). Mutations of the MEN1 tumor suppressor gene in pituitary tumors. *Cancer Research*, Vol.57, No.24, pp.5446-5451, ISSN 0008-5472

3

Acromegaly and Gigantism

Fulya Akin and Emrah Yerlikaya
Pamukkale University, Faculty Of Medicine
Division of Endocrinology and Metabolism
Turkey

1. Introduction

Human growth hormone (GH), a single-chain peptide of 191 amino acids, was isolated from somatotroph cells of the anterior pituitary gland in 1956 and first used therapeutically for treatment of pituitary dwarfism in 1958 (Raben, 1958). Pituitary dwarfism is the classic form of growth hormone deficiency during childhood. Gigantism refers to any standing height more than 2 standard deviations above the mean for the person's sex, age, and Tanner stage. Abnormally high linear growth due to excessive action of insulin-like growth factor-I (IGF-I)/GH causes gigantism while the epiphyseal growth plates are open during childhood, as puberty occurs it is followed by progressive acromegalic changes leading to a picture of a giant with acromegalic features - acromegalic gigantism. When onset disease is after epiphyseal closure, only acromegaly results.

Acromegaly, a somatic growth and proportion disorder first described by Marie in 1886 (Marie, 1886). Elevated levels of growth hormone and IGF-1 are the hallmarks of this syndrome (Melmed, et al., 1983). When Marie first desribed this syndrome at his patients, pitutiary overgrowth is the cause or reflection of the visceromegaly at these patients. İn 1909, Harvey Cushing reported the remission of clinical symptoms of acromegaly after partial hypophysectomy, thus indicating the etiology of the disease and its potential treatment as well (Cushing, 1909).

2. Epidemiology

It is a rare condition with a prevalence less than or equal to 70 cases per million and annual incidence of 3 to 4 cases per million (Alexander et al., 1980; Ritchie et al., 1990). Acromegaly occurs with equal frequency in males and females. The mean age at diagnosis is 40-45 years.

3. Pathology, etiology, pathophysiology

GH also called somatotropin is main regulator of normal growth. Its actions responsible for the catching up of normal adult height. The GH gene is located on chromosome 17 (Chen et al., 1989). There are at least three monomeric forms of GH-the predominant physiologic 22 kd form, a less abundant 20 kd form, and a third incompletely characterized form (Lin et al., 1992). The principal GH form in the pituitary is a 191 amino acid, single-chain, 22 kDa protein (22K). It is the product coded for by the GH-N gene (N for normal) and has also been termed GH-N (Parks, 1989). A second product arising from the same gene is the 20,000 dalton GH variant (20K) (Lewis et al., 1978). This protein is identical to 22K, except for an internal 15 amino acid deletion (residues 32-46). 20K GH is the result of an alternatively spliced GH pre-mRNA where part of exon 3 is spliced out (DeNoto et al., 1981). İmportance of this heterogenicty is unknown. Both forms of hormone are secreted and have similar growth promoting activity, although metabolic effects of the 20K form are reduced. 20K has decreased insulin-like and perhaps slightly decreased diabetogenic activity compared to 22K (Baumann et al., 1994).

Once secreted from the pituitary, a substantial proportion of GH circulates bound to GH-binding protein (GHBP) (Baumann et al., 1986; Herington et al., 1986; Leung et al., 1987). There are two forms of GHBP, a low-affinity variety and a high-affinity form. GHBP comprises the extracellular domain of the GH receptor (Leung et al., 1987) which is located in peripheral tissues and mediates the effects of GH on target organs. The GH binding protein and GH receptor are products of the same gene. GHBP is produced by proteolytic cleavage of the receptor at the outer surface of target cells (Harrison et al., 1995). GH binding protein prolongs its half-life and regulates changes in free hormone concentration. Free portion can cross capillary membranes and perform its actions.

GH elicits intracellular signaling though a peripheral receptor and initiates a phosphorylation cascade involving the JAK/STAT (Janus kinase/signal transducers and activators of transcription) pathway (Carter-Su et al., 1996). Liver contains most abundant receptors for GH. When GH receptor activated this causes rapid JAK2 tyrosine kinase activation, leading to phosphorylation of intracellular signaling molecule including the STATs. Phosphorylated STAT proteins are directly translocated to the cell nucleus, where they elicit GH-specific target gene expression by binding to nuclear DNA (Xu et al., 1996).

Growth hormone induces hepatic production of IGF-I responsible of many of its growth-promoting effects. Local production of IGF-I acting either in a paracrine or autocrine manner also has important biological effects, predominant of which is stimulating cell proliferation and inhibiting apoptosis (Le Roith et al., 2001).

Secretion of GH from the pituitary is pulsatile. An average half-life is 10-20 minutes, it is metabolized through the kidneys, liver, or target tissues (Casanueva, 1992). In children and young adults, maximal GH secretion occurs within 1 hour after the onset of deep sleep (stage III or IV) (Finkelstein et al., 1972; Mendelson, 1982; Takahashi et al., 1968). Two hypothalamic hormones regulate GH secretion; Growth hormone releasing hormone (GHRH) provides the primary drive for GH synthesis and secretion by inducing GH gene transcription and hormone release and does not induce other anterior pituitary hormones (Barinaga et al., 1983; Thorner et al., 1984). GHRH is needed for normal pulsatile GH secretion (Painson et al., 1991; Wehrenberg et al., 1982]. SRIF powerfully antagonizes the mitogenic effect of GHRH on somatotrophs, but does not inhibit GH synthesis (Billestrup et al., 1986), suppresses GH secretion mainly by high-affinity binding to $SSTR_2$ and $SSTR_5$ receptor subtypes expressed on somatotrophs (Shimon, 1997). It is thought to be interaction between these two hypothalamic hormone plays a role in pulsatile GH secretion.

Ghrelin is another peptide of a primarily gastric origin, although ghrelin mRNA had been found in the hypothalamus playing a role in secretion of GH (Mozid et al., 2003). Synthetic analogues of ghrelin (GHS) had been produced as early as 25 years ago. Acute administration of GHS produces an immediate and massive release of GH. Co-administration of GHS and GH-RH results in powerful GH rise that is greater than the effect of either peptide administered alone (Bowers et al., 1991). GHS potentiate GH release in response to a maximum stimulating dose of exogenous GHRH (Penalva et al., 1993) and after a saturating dose of GHRH, although subsequent GHRH administration is ineffective, GHS remain fully effective (Jaffe et al., 1993).

Stressful changes in the internal and external environments can produce brief episodes of hormone secretion. Hypoglycemia leads to acute GH secretion, which is the basis for the insulin-induced hypoglycemia test, a gold standard evaluation of pituitary function (Gharib et al., 2003). In man, hyperglycemia causes transient GH suppression for 1 to 3 hours, followed by GH rise 3 to 5 hours after oral glucose administration (Roth et al., 1963). Elevation of free fatty acid levels is a strong inhibitor of GH release in normal humans (Imaki et al., 1985).

Secretory episodes are induced by an increase in certain amino acids, particularly arginine and leucine. Neuropeptides, neurotransmitters, and opiates acts on the hypothalamus by affecting GHRH and SRIF release. Three hours after acute glucocorticoid administration, GH levels rise and remain elevated for 2 hours. Glucocorticoids administered to normal subjects dose-dependently inhibit GHRH-simulated GH secretion, similar to that seen in Cushing's syndrome (Casanueva et al., 1990). While acute glucocorticoid administration stimulates GH secretion, chronic steroid treatment inhibits GH.

Activation of the gonadal system during puberty is accompanied by increased GH and IGF-1 concentrations (Veldhuis et al., 2006; Giordano et al., 2005). Estrogen stimulates GH secretory rates, and testosterone increases GH secretory mass per pulse, with resultant IGF-I induction (Giustina & Veldhuis, 1998).

Chronic malnutrition and prolonged fasting are associated with elevated GH pulse frequency and amplitude (Ho et al., 1988). The maximal GH levels occur within minutes of the onset of slow wave sleep (Holl et al., 1991). Emotional deprivation is associated with suppressed GH secretion and attenuated GH responses to provocative stimuli occur in endogenous depression (Sachar et al., 1972). Exercise and physical stress, including trauma, hypovolemic shock, sepsis increase GH levels (Vigas et al., 1977).

Thyroid disorders also affect GH secretion. Some studies have reported several alterations of the GH/IGF axis and their binding proteins in hypothyroidism. The main alterations reported in untreated adult hypothyroid patients have been low serum concentrations of IGF-1 and IGFBP-3 that increase significantly with restoration of euthyroidism (Miell et al., 1993; Valcavi et al., 1987).

In hypothyroidism, GH pulsatility is decreased and GH responses to a number of secretagogues are attenuated (Valcavi et al., 1992). Fasting serum IGF-1 levels were found significantly lower in the subclinical hypothyroid and with levothyroxine treatment IGF-1 concentrations were significantly increased in subclinical hypothyroid subjects (Akin et al., 2008). Also in hyperthroidism GH responses to GHRH was found to be decreased whereas serum IGF-1 levels were increased (Valcavi et al., 1993). It could be expected to be decreased due to decreased pituitary GH contents as a result of permanent somatotrophic cell stimulation. At another study, hyperthyroid men is marked by a higher frequency of spontaneous GH secretory bursts, a higher rate of maximal GH secretion attained per burst, and a larger mass of GH released per burst (Iranmanesh et al., 1990). Effects of hyperthyroidism on GH/IGF-1 axis are still contraversial. GH–IGF axis was not affected in patients with subclinical hyperthyroidism (Akin et al., 2009).

GHRH have other actions which serve to feed back for GH secretory axis. GHRH stimulates SRIF secretion and inhibits further GHRH secretion in vitro (Aguila et al., 1985). SRIF inhibits its own secretion in vitro (Peterfreund & Vale, 1984). GH and IGF-I feed back to modulate the GH axis at several levels. IGF-I acts directly on the pituitary to inhibit basal and GHRH-induced GH secretion and also to suppress GH gene expression (Berelowitz et al., 1981; Ceda et al., 1987; Ceda et al., 1985, Yamashita& Melmed, 1986; Yamashita et al., 1986). IGF-I also seems to have a direct hypothalamic effect, increasing SRIF secretion (Berelowitz et al., 1981).

A benign somatotroph adenoma of the pituitary is the most common cause of acromegaly. Whether intracellular defects or excessive trophic influences from outside causes pitutiary tumor need to be discussed. Growth hormone-releasing hormone has trophic activity in the human pituitary (Thorner et al., 1982) and in addition to a case report of diffuse somatotroph hyperplasia in a patient with a growth hormone-releasing hormone-producing bronchial carcinoid (Ezzat et al., 1994). There are several cases of true somatotroph adenoma formation in patients with growth hormone-releasing hormone-producing hypothalamic gangliocytomas (Asa et al., 1984; Bevan et al., 1989). The clonality of a cellular expansion is a secure archaeologic tool capable of distinguishing an irreversible and potentially inexorably progressive process induced by an intracellular insult or insults from a relatively excessive but possibly reversible or self-limiting trophic response to stromal or microenvironmental signals (Levy, 2000; Levy, 2001). The finding of monoclonality in pituitary adenomas is thought to be an evidence for the neoplastic origin of these lesions. Proto-oncogene activation is also a critical prerequisite for pituitary tumor formation.

Pituitary carcinomas are another exceedingly rare cause of acromegaly. Infrequently acromegaly occurs as a result of a hypothalamic tumor secreting GHRH, ectopic secretion of GHRH from a peripheral neuroendocrine tumour (Thorner et al., 1984) or from excessive hypothalamic GHRH secretion (Asa et al., 1984).

Several genetic disorders including multiple endocrine neoplasia type 1 (MEN1) syndrome, McCune Albright syndrome, familial acromegaly and Carney's syndrome are also characterized with growth hormone excess. Postzygotic GNAS mutations result in a mosaic pattern of organ specificity with clinical features of McCune-Albright syndrome (OMIM 174800), including pigmented skin lesions and polyostotic fibrous dysplasia, and endocrine dysfunction including precocious puberty, thyrotoxicosis, and GH and ACTH hypersecretion (Weinstein, 1991).

4. Clinical features of acromegaly

The clinical features of acromegaly are depend on high serum concentrations of both GH and IGF-I (Melmed, 2006). The effect of hypersomatotropism on tissue growth and metabolic function evolves slowly. 10 or more years may elapse from disease onset until diagnosis of the disease (Colao et al., 2004).

Disease can be manifested also with signs and symptoms of pitutiary mass. Any pituitary adenoma can cause headaches commonly retro-orbital. Another common symptom caused by the size and location of the tumor is decreased vision. This usually presents as temporal visual field defects. It is caused by the tumor growing upward out of the sella and pressing on the optic chiasm. Other findings include diplopia, ptosis, opthalmoplegia as a result of extension into the cavernous sinus and compression of the cranial nerves. Sudden loss of vision secondary to apoplexy within the pituitary adenoma may ocur. Aggressive tumors can invade the roof of the palate and cause nasopharyngeal obstruction, infection and CSF leakage. Parinaud syndrome is caused by ectopic pinealomas most often accompanied with paralysis of upward conjugate gaze. As pituitary tumors grow, they compress the pituitary gland, pituitary stalk and hypothalamus and interfere with normal pituitary hormone production. This reslts in partial or complete anterior pituitary hormone deficiency. Hypothyroidism syptoms, failure to lactate, decreased libido, infertility or oligo/amenorrhoea, sense of not well being are common symptoms of hypopitutiarism. Stalk compression leads to hyperprolactinemia. GH-secreting pituitary adenomas may also cosecrete prolactin.

All patients with acromegaly have acral and soft tissue overgrowth, although the extent of the overgrowth varies. Soft tissue findings are macroglossia, large fleshy lips and nose, deepening of the voice, paresthesias of the hands , thickened skin, skin tags, coarsened body hair. Skin tags are common and may be markers for the adenomatous colonic polyps (Leavitt et al., 1983). These soft tissue changes may be attributed to glycosaminoglycan deposition and increased connective tissue collagen production (Verde et al., 1986). Hair growth increases and some women have hirsutism 56 percent in one series (Kaltsas et al., 1999). Acromegalic patients may have a greater incidence of neuropathies because of compression of nerves by adjacent fibrous tissue and endoneural fibrous proliferation. The size and function of sebaceous and sweat glands increase complain of excessive perspiration and body odor. The heart, liver, kidneys, spleen, thyroid, parathyroid glands, and pancreas are larger than normal.

Thyroid dysfunction in acromegaly may be caused by diffuse or nodular toxic or nontoxic goiter or Graves' disease, especially because IGF-I is a major determinant of thyroid cell growth (Kasagi, et al., 1999). As it can be a part of a MEN1 syndrome, hypercalcemia can also be seen.

In the absence of GH there is severe atrophy of the epiphyseal plates, which become narrow as proliferation of cartilage progenitor cells slows markedly.

Conversely, after GH is given to a hypopituitary subject, resumption of cellular proliferation causes columns of chondrocytes to elongate and epiphyseal plates to widen. Synovial tissue and cartilage enlarge, causing hypertrophic arthropathy of the knees, ankles, hips, spine and other joints (Biermasz et al., 2005). Local periarticular fibrous tissue thickening can cause joint stiffening, deformities, and nerve entrapment. Chondrocyte proliferation with increased joint space, ulcerations and fissures of weight-bearing cartilage areas, often accompanied by new bone formation. Chronic osteoarthritis causes narrowed and deformed joint space, osteophyte formation, subchondral cysts, and lax periarticular ligaments with ossification (Dons et al., 1988; 75 Lieberman et al., 1992). When excess GH secretion begins before the epiphyses of the long bones are fused, linear growth does increase; the result is pituitary gigantism. Skeletal overgrowth owing to periosteal new bone formation in response to IGF-1 (McCarthy, et al., 1989). Subtle skeletal and acral overgrowth and soft tissue enlargement causes increased shoe and ring size. Mandibular overgrowth with prognathism, maxillary widening, teeth separation, jaw malocclusion other skeletal manifestations of the acromegaly. Prognathism, thick lips, macroglossia, and hypertrophied nasal structures can obstruct airways (Rosenow et al., 1996; Grunstein et al., 1994). This result in obstructive sleep apnea syndrome. Sleep apnea may also be central in origin and associated with higher GH and IGF-I levels (Grunstein et al., 1994).

Untreated acromegaly results in premature mortality, most commonly from cardiovascular disease (Ritchie et al., 1990; Wright et al., 1970; Etxabe et al., 1993; Rajasoorya et al., 1994; Orme et al., 1998). Asymmetric septal hypertrophy, left ventricular hypertrophy, cardiomegaly and cardiac failure develop; effective treatment reducing growth hormone and IGF-1 serum levels improves cardiac function (Colao et al., 1999). Heart failure occurs in

3 to 10 percent of patients (Damjanovic et al., 2002; Bihan et al., 2004). An increased prevalence of valvular heart disease has also been reported. Arterial blood pressure (systolic and diastolic) is higher with loss of normal daily circadian variability (Terzolo et al., 1999). Hypertension was reported in approximately one third of patients who had acromegaly (Pietrobelli et al., 2001; Minniti et al., 1998). Insulin resistance and diabetes mellitus occur as a result of direct anti-insulin effects of GH (Coculescu et al., 2007; Kasayama et al., 2000).

Several benign and malignant neoplasms, especially in the gastrointestinal tract, have been reported in association with acromegaly (Cheung et al., 1997; Ron et al., 1991), particularly colorectal tubular adenomas and carcinoma (Jenkins et al., 2001; Jenkins, 2006). It is related to disease activity with patients with elevated serum growth hormone and IGF-I levels being particularly prone to developing colonic adenomas (Jenkins et al., 2000). A compelling cause-and-effect relationship of acromegaly with cancer has not been established (Delhougne et al., 1995; Ladas et al., 1994). A recent controlled study in 161 patients revealed no increase in polyp incidence in acromegaly (Renehan et al., 2000). Analysis of nine retrospective reports (1956-1998) encompassing 21,470 person-years at risk, yielded no significant increased cancer incidence (Melmed et al., 2001).

Whether patients with acromegaly are also prone to other malignancies remains controversial. Certainly there is epidemiological evidence in the general population that serum IGF-I levels in the upper part of the normal range are associated with an increased risk of breast and prostate cancer and some reviews have shown the former to be increased in acromegaly (Renehan et al., 2004; Nabarro, 1987).

5. Molecular pathogenesis of acromegaly

GH elicits intracellular signaling though a peripheral receptor and initiates a phosphorylation cascade involving the JAK/STAT (Janus kinase/signal transducers and activators of transcription) pathway (Carter-Su et al., 1996). The STAT proteins become phosphorylated and translocate into the cell nucleus. Transcription of target proteins, such as IGF-I evoke pleiotropic cell responses including IGF1 synthesis, glucose metabolism, cell proliferation, and cytoskeletal changes.

STAT5b is the key intracellular molecule required for GH mediation of postnatal growth, adipose tissue function, and sexual dimorphism of hepatic gene expression (Lanning et al., 2006). In humans, STAT mutations result in relative GH insensitivity and growth retardation (Kofoed , 2003).

6. Diagnosis

Normal GH production from the pituitary gland is pulsatile with the maximal production occurring at night. Even though episodic basal growth hormone secretion patterns are sustained in acromegaly, diurnal variation and the sleep-related growth hormone rise are lost (Barkan et al., 1989). Most values of GH fall in the range of 0.1–0.2 μg/L in normal subjects. However there are six to ten secretory bursts during the day when GH reaches values of 5–30 μg/L, which may overlap with values seen in acromegalic patients. Therefore the only value of a random GH measurement is that of excluding acromegaly if it is undetectable . Unlike the largely undetectable nadir GH levels in normal subjects, those with acromegaly sampled over 24 hours contain detectable levels of GH (>2 μg/L) Elevated integrated growth hormone levels during 24-hour sampling of less than 2.5 mug/L

effectively exclude acromegaly (Duncan et al., 1999). The optimal way to assess the overall daily GH production is to obtain a mean GH over 24 h by frequent GH sampling. However, this method is inconvenient both for the patient and the clinician (Cordero et al., 2008).
The current international consensus for the diagnosis of acromegaly (Giustina et al., 2000) recommends a nadir GH of more than 1 µg/L during an OGTT for diagnosis in conjunction with clinical suspicion and high IGF-1 levels. Using more sensitive newer assays, the GH cut-off may be even lower (Freda et al., 2003). There is a need to verify the current guidelines and propose lowering the current cut off for GH nadir (Costas et al., 2002; Serri et al., 2004). The standard OGTT consists of the administration of 75 g of glucose with GH measurements at various time points for up to 120 min. Normal subjects demonstrate a suppression of GH concentration to 2 µg/L or less throughout the 2 hours of testing (Chapman et al., 1994; Hattori et al., 1990). Acromegalic subjects often gives response paradoxically higher GH levels. Clinicians should be aware that the OGTT's usefulness is limited in high catabolic states, such as stress, hepatic and renal failure, diabetes mellitus, obesity, pregnancy, patients on estrogen replacement or in tall adolescents in whom GH values may be falsely elevated (Duncan et al., 1999; Melmed et al., 2006).
Serum sex and age-matched elevated IGF-1 levels are highly specific for acromegaly in the nonpregnant adult and correlate with clinical disease activity (Clemmons et al., 1979). IGF-1 is an ideal screening test as it has a long half life of 18–20 h and the levels remain stable throughout the day (Giustina et al., 2000). Furthermore IGF-1 correlates with mean GH levels (Barkan et al., 1988) and with clinical features of acromegaly (Clemmons et al., 1979). Even several months after treatment when growth hormone levels are controlled, IGF-1 serum levels may remain persistently high (Drange et al., 1999). Multiple physiologic factors affect IGF-1 levels and need to be taken into account when interpreting the data. IGF-1 is affected by age and gender (Ghigo et al., 1996) with approximately 14% decrease per decade during adult life (Brabant et al., 2003). Again a uniform standard for age range had not been established (Pokrajac et al., 2007) where serum samples with GH and IGF-1 levels close to the current Cortina consensus (Giustina et al., 2000) cutoffs were distributed to different centers to evaluate variability in assay performance. Other problems include the assay susceptibility to interference from binding proteins and the tendency of IGF-1 to plateau at mean GH levels above approximately 20 µg/L (Barkan et al., 1988). The use of exogenous estrogen, malnutrition, liver and renal failure decrease IGF-1 levels (Ho et al., 1922; Freda et al., 2003; Ho et al., 2003). On the other hand, normal pregnancy and adolescence are associated with elevated IGF-1 levels (Duncan et al., 1999).
IGFBP-3 levels are also elevated. However, considerable overlap of these values with those in normal persons, thereby limiting the utility of this measurement.
Magnetic resonance imaging (MRI) of the pituitary gland is the preferred imaging modality for diagnosis in acromegaly. An MRI provides the best assessment of tumor size, location, extent, and relationship to important surrounding structures and is essential for the neurosurgeon to adequately plan surgery and to monitor treatment. If an MRI is not available, a computed tomography (CT) study directed at the pituitary region may be done.
Ectopic GHRH producing tumors may arise from bronchial and pancreatic neuroendocrine tumors, pheochromocytomas, pulmonary endocrine carcinomas, or rarely thymic carcinod (Vieira et al., 2007; Sugihara et al., 2007; Fainstein et al., 2007; Nasr et al.,2006; Bolanowski et al., 2006; Jansson et al., 1998). The measurement of plasma GHRH concentrations can be very helpful in identifying an ectopic source of GHRH in these particular cases. Total body scintigraphy with radiolabled somatostatin should be performed to localize the tumor and

to demonstrate somatostatin receptor expression by the tumor which may respond favorably to somatostatin analogue therapy (Kwekkeboom et al., 1993; Drange et al., 1998).

7. Differential diagnosis

Exclusion of an abnormality of the somatotrophic axis in a young patient with acromegaloid features should lead the differential diagnosis towards diagnoses such as pachydermoperiostosis (Hambrick et al., 1996; Rimoin, 1965; Harbison et al., 1971) or insulin mediated pseudoacromegaly, a disorder associated with severe insulin resistance (Flier et al., 1993). These nadir entities must be considered at differential diagnosis of acromegaly.

8. Treatment

Treatment should aim at managing the tumor mass and GH hypersecretion to prevent morbidity and increased mortality while preserving normal pituitary function. Complete surgical removal of GH-secreting tumors results in hormonal control of acromegaly and improvement of soft tissue changes. After successful resection, growth hormone levels return to normal within 1 hour, and metabolic dysfunction and soft-tissue swelling quickly resolve. In patients with intrasellar microadenomas, surgical removal provides biochemical control with normalization of IGF-I in 75–95% of patients (De et al., 2003; Ludecke et al., 2006; Nomikos et al., 2005; Kaltsas et al., 2001; Shimon et al., 2001; Beauregard et al., 2003).

Transsphenoidal microsurgical adenomectomy approach is used most commonly and, in the hands of experienced neurosurgeons, cures the majority of patients who are harboring a well-circumscribed microadenoma and who have serum GH levels less than 40 μg/L (Gittoes et al., 1999; Shimon et al., 2001; Kreutzer et al., 2001). Control rates are lower in patients with noninvasive macroadenomas but even in these cases surgical removal provides biochemical biochemical control with normalization of IGF-I in 40–68% of patients (De et al., 2003; Ludecke et al., 2006; Nomikos et al., 2005; Kaltsas et al., 2001; Shimon et al., 2001; Beauregard et al., 2003). The success of surgery depends on the skill and experience of the surgeon in resecting the entire tumor without damaging normal anterior pituitary tissue. Craniotomy is very rarely indicated in patients with acromegaly.

Post-transsphenoidal surgical mortality is rare and most side effects are transient. Permanent diabetes insipidus, cerebrospinal fluid leak, hemorrhage, and meningitis develop in up to 5% and their frequency correlates with tumor size, invasiveness, and neurosurgical experience (Gittoes et al., 1999). In experienced hands, other complications of transsphenoidal surgery are rare including transient oculomotor palsies, deterioration of vision, carotid artery injury and epistaxis (occurring in less than 1% of patients) (Ludecke & Abbe , 2006; Nomikos et al., 2005).

Dopamine agonists (DAs), somatostatin receptor ligands (SRLs), and a GH receptor antagonist (GHRA) are the drugs classes available for the treatment of acromegaly. SRLs are the first-choice pharmacotherapy for treating patients who have acromegaly. Two formulas are available for treatment of acromegaly octreotide and lanreotide. Somatotroph and thyrotroph cells express mainly two of five SRIF receptors, SSTR2 and SSTR5 that mediate growth hormone and TSH secretion (Shimon & Melmed, 1998; Weckbecker et al., 2003).

Octreotide is a short-acting somatostatin analogue that binds mainly to SSTR2 and to a lesser extent to SSTR5 (Lamberts, 1988). Lanreotid also acts in a same way. Octreotide also exhibits some SST3 affinity (Patel, 1999). Sandostatin LAR (octreotide acetate) is a long-acting somatostatin analogue (Flogstad et al., 1995; Lancranjan et al., 1999) requiring monthly injections. Starting dose is 20-mg monthly increasing up to 40 mg depending on clinical and biochemical responses. Depot preparation of lanreotide delivered as an aqueous, small-volume mixture (60, 90, or 120 mg) in prefilled syringes for deep subcutaneous administration every 28 days (Biermasz et al., 2005).

Most studies assessing SRLs efficacy in acromegaly define disease control by mean fasting random serum GH levels less than 2.5 µg/L or normalization of age- and gender-matched IGF-1 plasma levels .Treatment with depot form of lanreotide (60 mg every 21 or 28 days) reduced GH less than 2.5 µg/L in 76% of patients (Attanasio et al.,2003; Ambrosio et al., 2002). In another study, monthly injections sandostatin for 9 years reduced integrated serum GH levels to less than 2 µg/L in more than 75% of patients (Cozzi et al., 2006). More than 70% of patients experience improved general well-being, and soft tissue swelling dissipates within several days of treatment (Ezzat, et al., 1992). Headache, a common symptom in acromegaly, usually resolves within minutes of injection (Pascual et al., 1991) reflecting a specific central analgesic effect.

Joint function and crepitus improve, ultrasound shows evidence of bone or cartilage repair, and after several months, sleep apnea improves (Colao et al., 2004). Asymptomatic patients experience a significant decrease of blood pressure, heart rate, and left ventricular (LV) wall thickness (Colao et al., 2000).

SRLs are effective also in reducing tumor size. Significant tumor size decrease has been reported in 52% of patients on primary therapy (Bevan et al., 2005). A critical analysis of 14 studies reported that 37% of patients treated primarily by SRL experience significant tumor shrinkage (Melmed et al., 2005).

In vivo octreoscan imaging visualizing SRIF receptors demonstrates that GH responsiveness directly correlates with the abundance of pituitary receptors, and patients resistant to octreotide do not have visible receptor binding sites (Ur et al., 1992). Efficacy of octreotide action is determined by frequency of drug administration, total daily dose, tumor size, densely granulated tumors (Bhayana et al., 2005) and pretreatment GH levels.

The use of SRLs is most appropriate; as first-line therapy when there is a low probability of a surgical cure (Melmed et al., 2005; Cozzi et al., 2006; Maiza et al., 2007; Mercado et al., 2007; Colao, et al., 2006) after surgery has failed to achieve biochemical control, before surgery to improve severe comorbidities that prevent or could complicate immediate surgery (Carlsen et al., 2008) to provide disease control, or partial control in the time between administration of radiation therapy and the onset of maximum benefit attained from radiation therapy (Melmed et al., 2009). Gastrointestinal symptoms including nausea, mild malabsorption, flatulence, diarrhea or constipation are common mild side effects of SRLs. Multiple small gallstones and gallbladder sludge may occur, occasionally result in cholecystitis. Abnormal glucose metabolism is described with the use of SRLs, as activation of SST2 and SST5 in the pancreatic insulin-secreting beta cells likely inhibits insulin secretion and counter-regulatory hormones, such as glucagon. Mild hyperglycemia and, rarely hypoglycemia (Bruttomesso et al., 2001) manifest mostly in patients who have pre-existing glucose abnormalities. Octreotide can interact with several drugs including cyclosporine. Absorption of oral hypoglycemic agents, β-blockers, calcium channel blockers can be change and dosage titration should be made slowly with SRL at patients using these agents. Asymptomatic sinus bradycardia can also be seen with these drugs.

Only cabergoline has any efficacy in acromegaly, and this is limited monotherapy effective in less than 10% of patients (Bevan et al., 1992; Colao et al., 1997; Abs et al., 1998; Cozzi et al., 1998). Patients with hyperprolactinemia and minimal GH elevation might benefit most from dopamine agonist treatment. Main usages of DAs are; when the patient prefers oral medication, after surgery in selected patients, such as those with markedly elevated prolactin and/or modestly elevated GH and IGF-I levels (Melmed et al., 2009) as additive therapy to SRL therapy in patients partially responsive to a maximum SRL dose (Wagenaar et al., 1990; Sadoul et al., 1992; Cremonini et al., 1992; Marzullo et al., 1999; Cozzi et al., 2004; Selvarajah et al., 2005). Side effects of DAs include gastrointestinal discomfort, transient nausea and vomiting, nasal congestion, dizziness, postural hypotension, headache, and mood disorders (Colao et al., 1997). It is known that increased incidence of valvular heart disease with high doses of carbegoline.

GH action through the surface membrane GH receptor is mediated by ligand-induced receptor signaling. The postreceptor GH signal is not elicited if the receptor is bound by pegvisomant, a GH-receptor antagonist, which blocks subsequent IGF-I generation (Trainer, et al., 2000). Daily pegvisomant (20 mg) given for 12 weeks, normalized IGF-1 levels in 82% of patients who had acromegaly (Kopchick et al., 2002). The indications for its use are; in patients that have persistently elevated IGF-I levels despite maximal therapy with other treatment modalities, possibly as monotherapy or in combination with a SRL in other patients (Melmed et al., 2009).

Because elevated hepatic transaminases have been reported (Biering et al., 2006) liver enzymes should be measured every 6 months. Serum GH levels are increased as much as 76% over baseline levels and persistent tumor growth is reported (Trainer et al., 2000) even though, in most cases, GH-secreting adenoma volumes do not change (Van der Lely et al.,2001; Barkan et al., 2005). Current recommendations are to perform a pituitary MRI every 6 months in all patients (Melmed et al., 2006).

Primary or adjuvant radiation of GH-secreting tumors may be achieved by conventional external deep X-ray therapy, proton beam, or gamma knife radiation surgery. It is usually reserved for patients who have postoperative persistent or recurrent tumors that are resistant or intolerant to medical treatment may benefit from radiotherapy.After conventional radiation (up to 5000 rads divided in 180-rad fractions over 6 weeks), tumors cease growing and shrink in most of patients (Biermasz et al., 2000). Conventional radiotherapy (conformal fractionated radiotherapy) can lower GH levels and normalize IGF-I in over 60% of patients, but maximum response is achieved 10–15 yr after radiotherapy is administered (Barrande et al., 2000; Jenkins et al., 2006; Minniti et al., 2005).

Stereotactic radiosurgery using gamma knife delivers a single tumor-focused radiation fraction. Five-year remission rates with gamma knife radiotherapy in patients with acromegaly (after surgical debulking) range from 29 to 60% (Attanasio et al., 2003; Castinetti et al., 2005; Jezkova et al., 2006; Pollock et al., 2007). After 10 years, about half of all patients receiving radiation therapy have signs of pituitary trophic hormone disruption, and this prevalence increases annually thereafter. Side effects of conventional radiation including hair loss, cranial nerve palsies, tumor necrosis with hemorrhage, and loss of vision or pituitary apoplexy (both rare) have been documented in up to 2% of patients (Van der Lely, 1997). Lethargy, impaired memory, brain tumors at irradiation site and personality changes can also occur.

9. Posttreatment follow-up

GH and IGF-I should be measured to assess the biochemical response to any medical treatment. OGTT and IGF-1 measurement wit clinical examination should be performed at 3–6 months after surgery, and 3-4 months period thereafter. If patient receivig pegvisomant,

monitoring should be made with only IGF-1. OGTT is not helpful in monitoring therapeutic responses while patients are receiving SRL therapy (Arafat et al., 2008; Carmichael et al., 2009). Biochemical control is generally defined as a normal IGF-I for age and gender and age less than 1.0 ng/ml during an OGTT. After biochemical control is achieved, follow up of patients can be made semiannually. With usage of more sensitive GH level less than 0.4 ng/ml thought to be consistent with remission. Pituitary MRI shhuld be performed annually, especially at patients having residual tumor and medical treatment.
Colonoscopy should be performed at three- to four-year intervals in patients over 50 years old and in those with more than three skin tags for early detection and treatment of premalignant colonic polyps (Melmed, 2002). At follow up patients should be evaluated periodically for cardiovascular, skletal, dental problems.

10. Future prospects of acromegaly

Bogazzi et al. (Bogazzi et al., 2004) reported that thiazolidinedione treatment might slow down the growth of well-established GH-secreting tumors and might effectively reduce the GH hypersecretion. In a study, rosiglitazone, used at maximum approved dosage, did not reduce plasma GH and IGF-1 levels in patients with acromegaly (Bastemir et al., 2007).
In recent years, molecular studies investigated the possible association of gene polymorphisms and susceptibility to diseases. Recently, a polymorphism in the promotor region of the IGF-I gene which is associated with IGF-I serum levels, birthweight and body height in adults has been identified (Vaessen et al., 2001; Rietveld et al., 2004). 194 bp allele (20 CA repeats) of the IGF-I promoter have higher circulating IGF-I levels than others. The patients with 194 bp genotype are the resistant patients with active disease and they required high dose medication responsible from resistance to drugs (Akin et al., 2010). The angiotensinojen MT and AT1R CC1166 genotype carriers may have more risk than other genotypes in the development of hypertension in acromegaly (Turgut , et al., 2011).

11. References

Abs, R; Verhelst, J; Maiter, D; Van Acker, K; Nobels, F; Coolens, JL; Mahler, C; Beckers, A. (1998). Cabergoline in the treatment of acromegaly: a study in 64 patients. J Clin Endocrinol Metab. 83:374–378.

Aguila, MC; McCann, SM. (1985). Stimulation of somatostatin-release in vitro by synthetic growth hormone-releasing factor by a nondopaminergic mechanism. Endocrinology. 117:762-765.

Akin, F; Bastemır, M; Yaylalı, GF, Alkıs E; Kaptanoglu, B. (2008). GH/IGF-1 axis in patients with subclinical hypothyroidism. Clinical Endocrinology. 68: 1009–1010.

Akin, F; Yaylali, GF; Turgut, S; Kaptanoglu, B. (2009). Growth hormone/insulin-like growth factor axis in patients with subclinical thyroid dysfunction. Growth Hormone & IGF Research 19(3):252-5.

Akin, F; Turgut, S; Cirak, B; Kursunluoglu, R. (2010). IGF(CA)19 and IGFBP-3-202A/C gene polymorphism in patients with acromegaly. Growth Hormone & IGF Research. 20:399–403.

Alexander, L; Appleton, D; Hall, R. (1980). Epidemiology of acromegaly in the Newcastle region. Clin Endocrinol (Oxf). 12. (1): 71-79.

Ambrosio, MR; Franceschetti, P; Bondanelli, M. (2002). Efficacy and safety of the new 60-mg formulation of the long-acting somatostatin analog lanreotide in the treatment of acromegaly. Metabolism. 51. (3): 387-393.

Arafat, AM; Mohlig, M; Weickert, MO; Perschel, FH; Purschwitz, J; Spranger, J; Strasburger, CJ; Schofl, C; Pfeiffer, AF. (2008). Growth hormone response during oral glucose tolerance test: the impact of assay method on the estimation of reference values in patients with acromegaly and in healthy controls, and the role of gender, age, and body mass index. J Clin Endocrinol Metab. 93:1254–1262.

Asa, SL; Scheithauer, BW; Bilbao, JM.(1984). A case for hypothalamic acromegaly: a clinicopathological study of six patients with hypothalamic gangliocytomas producing growth hormone-releasing hormone. J Clin Endocrinol Metab. 58:796–803.

Attanasio, R; Baldelli, R; Pivonello, R. (2003). Lanreotide 60 mg, a new long-acting formulation: effectiveness in the chronic treatment of acromegaly. J Clin Endocrinol Metab. 88. (11): 5258-5265.

Attanasio, R; Epaminonda, P; Motti, E; Giugni, E; Ventrella, L; Cozzi, R; Farabola, M; Loli, P; Beck-Peccoz, P; Arosio, M. (2003). Gamma-knife radiosurgery in acromegaly: a 4-year follow-up study. J Clin Endocrinol Metab. 88:3105–3112

Barinaga, M; Yamonoto, G; Rivier, C. (1983). Transcriptional regulation of growth hormone gene expression by growth hormone releasing factor. Nature. 306:84-85.

Barkan, AL; Beitins, IZ; Kelch, RP. (1988). Plasma insulin-like growth factor-I/somatomedin-C in acromegaly: correlation with the degree of growth hormone hypersecretion. Clin Endocrinol Metab. 67(1):69–73.

Barkan, AL; Burman, P; Clemmons, DR. (2005). Glucose homeostasis and safety in patients with acromegaly converted from long-acting octreotide to pegvisomant. J Clin Endocrinol Metab. 90. (10): 5684-5691.

Barkan, AL; Stred, SE; Reno, K. (1989). Increased growth hormone pulse frequency in acromegaly. J Clin Endocrinol Metab. 69:1225-1233.

Barrande, G; Pittino-Lungo, M; Coste, J; Ponvert, D; Bertagna, X; Luton, JP; Bertherat, J. (2000). Hormonal and metabolic effects of radiotherapy in acromegaly: long-term results in 128 patients followed in a single center. J Clin Endocrinol Metab. 85:3779–3785.

Bastemir, M; Akin, F; Yaylali, GF. (2007). The PPAR-gamma activator rosiglitazone fails to lower plasma growth hormone and insulin-like growth factor-1 levels in patients with acromegaly. Neuroendocrinology. 86(2):119-23.

Baumann, G; Shaw, M; Amburn, K; Jan, T; Davila, N; Mercado, M; Stolar, M; MacCART, J. (1994). Nucl Med Biol. 21;309-379.

Baumann, G; Stolar, MW; Amburn, K. (1986). A specific growth hormone-binding protein in human plasma: Initial characterization. J Clin Endocrinol Metab. 62:134-141.

Beauregard, C; Truong, U; Hardy, J; Serri, O. (2003).Long-term outcome and mortality after transsphenoidal adenomectomy for acromegaly. Clin Endocrinol (Oxf). 58:86–91.

Bevan, JS; Asa, SL; Rossi, ML; Esiri, MM; Adams, CB; Burke, CW. (1989). Intrasellar gangliocytoma containing gastrin and growth hormone-releasing hormone associated with a growth hormone secreting pituitary adenoma. Clin Endocrinol (Oxf). 30:213–234.

Bevan, JS; Webster, J; Burke, CW; Scanlon, MF. (1992). Dopamine agonists and pituitary tumor shrinkage. Endocr Rev. 13:220–240.

Bevan, JS. (2005). Clinical review: The antitumoral effects of somatostatin analog therapy in acromegaly. J Clin Endocrinol Metab. 90:1856-1863.

Berelowitz, M; Szabo, M; Frohman, LA. (1981). Somatomedin C mediates growth hormone negative feedback by effects on both the hypothalamus and the pituitary. Science. 212:1279-1281.

Bhayana, S; Booth, GL; Asa, SL. The implication of somatotroph adenoma phenotype to somatostatin analog responsiveness in acromegaly. (2005). J Clin Endocrinol Metab. 90:6290-6295.

Biering, H; Saller, B; Bauditz, J. (2006). Elevated transaminases during medical treatment of acromegaly: a review of the German pegvisomant surveillance experience and a report of a patient with histologically proven chronic mild active hepatitis. Eur J Endocrinol. 154:213-220.

Biermasz, NR; Van Dulken, H; Roelfsema, F. (2000). Long term followup results of postoperative in 36 patients with acromegaly. J Clin Endocrinol Metab. 85:2476-2482.

Biermasz, NR; Pereira, AM; Smit, JW; Romijn, JA; Roelfsema, F. (2005). Morbidity after long-term remission for acromegaly: persisting joint-related complaints cause reduced quality of life. J Clin Endocrinol Metab. 90(5):2731-9.

Biermasz, NR; Romijn, JA; Pereira, AM. (2005). Current pharmacotherapy for acromegaly: a review. Expert Opin Pharmaco ther. 6. (14): 2393-2405.

Bihan, H; Espinosa, C; Valdes-Socin, H; Salenave, S; Young, J; Levasseur, S; Assayag, P; Beckers, A; Chanson, P. (2004). Long-term outcome of patients with acromegaly and congestive heart failure. J Clin Endocrinol Metab. 89(11):5308-13.

Billestrup, N; Swanson, LW; Vale, W. (1986) Growth hormone releasing factor stimulates proliferation of somatotrophs in vitro. Proc Natl Acad Sci U S A ;83. 6854-6857.

Bogazzi, F; Ultimieri, F; Raggi, F; Russo, D; Vanacore, R; Guida, C; Viacava, P; Cecchetti, D; Acerbi, G; Brogioni, S; Cosci, C; Gasperi, M; Bartalena, L; Martino, E. (2004). PPAR-gamma inhibits GH synthesis and secretion and increases apoptosis of pituitary GH-secreting adenomas. Eur J Endocrinol. 150: 863–875.

Bolanowski, M; Kos-Kudła, B; Rzeszutko, M; Marciniak, M; Zatońska, K. (2006). Five year remission of GHRH secreting bronchial neuroendocrine tumor with symptoms of acromegaly. Utility of chromogranin A in the monitoring of the disease. Endokrynol Pol. 57(1):32–6.

Bowers, CY; Sartor, AO; Reynolds, GA. (1991). On the actions of the growth hormone releasing hexapeptide, GHRP. Endocrinology. 128. 2027-2035.

Brabant, G; von zur Mühlen, A; Wüster, C; Ranke, MB; Kratzsch, J; Kiess, W. (2003). Serum insulin-like growth factor I reference values for an automated chemiluminescence immunoassay system: results from a multicenter study. Horm Res. 60(2):53–60.

Bruttomesso, D; Fongher, C; Silvestri, B. (2001). Combination of continuous subcutaneous infusion of insulin and octreotide in Type 1 diabetic patients. Diabetes Res Clin Pract. 51. (2): 97-105.

Carlsen, SM; Lund-Johansen, M; Schreiner, T; Aanderud, S; Johannesen, O; Svartberg, J; Cooper, JG; Hald, JK; Fougner, SL; Bollerslev, J. (2008). Preoperative octreotide treatment in newly diagnosed acromegalic patients with macroadenomas increases cure short-term postoperative rates:a prospective, randomized trial. J Clin Endocrinol Metab. 93:2984–2990.

Carmichael, JD; Bonert, VS; Mirocha, JM; Melmed, S. (2009). The utility of oral glucose tolerance testing for diagnosis and assessment of treatment outcomes in 166 patients with acromegaly J Clin Endocrinol Metab. 94:523–527.

Carter-Su, C; Schwartz J; Smit LS. (1996). Molecular mechanism of growth hormone action. Annu Rev Physiol. 58:187-207.

Casanueva, FF; Burguera, B; Muruais, C; Dieguez, C. (1990). Acute administration of corticoids: a new and peculiar stimulus of growth hormone secretion in man. J Clin Endocrinol Metab 70:234-237.

Casanueva; FF. (1992). Physiology of growth hormone secretion and action. Endocrinol Metab Clin North Am. 21:483-515.

Castinetti, F; Taieb, D; Kuhn, JM; Chanson, P; Tamura, M; Jaquet, P; Conte-Devolx, B; Regis, J; Dufour, H; Brue, T. (2005). Outcome of gamma knife radio-surgery in 82 patients with acromegaly: correlation with initial hypersecretion. J Clin Endocrinol Metab. 2005;90:4483–4488.

Ceda, GP; Hoffman, AR; Silverberg, GD. (1985). Regulation of growth hormone release from cultured human pituitary adenomas by somatomedins and insulin. J Clin Endocrinol Metab. 60:1204-1209.

Ceda, GP; Davies, RG; Rosenfeld, RG. (1987). The growth hormone (GH)-releasing hormone (GHRH)-GH-somatomedin axis: Evidence for rapid inhibition of GHRH-elicited GH release by insulin-like growth factors I and II. Endocrinology. 120:1658-1662.

Chapman, IM; Hartman, ML; Straume, M. (1994). Enhanced sensitivity growth hormone (GH) chemiluminescence assay reveals lower postglucose nadir GH concentrations in men than women. J Clin Endocrinol Metab. 78:1312.

Chen, EY; Yu-Cheng, L; Smith, DH. (1989). The human growth hormone locus: Nucleotide sequence, biology, and evolution. Genomics. 4:479-497.

Cheung, NW; Boyages SC. (1997). Increased incidence of neoplasia in females with acromegaly. Clin Endocrinol (Oxf). 47:323-327.

Clemmons ,DR; Van Wyk JJ; Ridgway E. (1979). Evaluation of acromegaly by radioimmunoassay of somatomedin C. N Engl J Med. 301:1138-1142.

Coculescu, M; Niculescu, D; Lichiardopol, R. (2007). Insulin resistance and insulin secretion in non-diabetic acromegalic patients. Exp Clin Endocrinol Diabetes. 115.(5):308-316.

Colao, A; Ferone, D; Marzullo, P; Di Sarno, A; Cerbone, G; Sarnacchiaro, F; Cirillo, S; Merola, B; Lombardi, G. (1997). Effect of different dopaminergic agents in the treatment of acromegaly. J Clin Endocrinol Metab. 82:518–523.

Colao, A; Cuocolo, A; Marzullo, P. Effects of 1-year treatment with octreotide on cardiac performance in patients with acromegaly. (1999). J Clin Endocrinol Metab. 84:17-23.

Colao, A; Marzullo, P; Ferone, D. (2000). Cardiovascular effects of depot long-acting somatostatin analog Sandostatin LAR in acromegaly. J Clin Endocrinol Metab. 85:3132-3140.

Colao, A; Ferone, D; Marzullo, P; Lombardi, G. (2004). Systemic complications of acromegaly: epidemiology, pathogenesis, and management. Endocr Rev. 25(1):102-52.

Colao, A; Pivonello, R; Auriemma, RS; Briganti, F; Galdiero, M; Tortora, F; Caranci, F; Cirillo, S; Lombardi, G. (2006). Predictors of tumor shrinkage after primary therapy with somatostatin analogs in acromegaly: a prospective study in 99 patients. J Clin Endocrinol Metab. 91:2112–2118.

Cordero, RA; Barkan, AL. (2008). Current diagnosis of acromegaly. Rev Endocr Metab Disord. 9:13–19 .

Costas, ACF; Rossi, A; Martinelli, CE, Jr; Machado, HR; Moreira, AC. (2002). Assessment of disease activity in treated acromegalic patients using a sensitive GH assay: should we achieve strict normal GH levels for a biochemical cure. J Clin Endocrinol Metab. 87(7):3142–7.

Cozzi, R; Attanasio, R; Barausse, M; Dallabonzana, D; Orlandi, P; Da Re, N; Branca, V; Oppizzi, G; Gelli, D. (1998). Cabergoline in acromegaly: a renewed role for dopamine agonist treatment? Eur J Endocrinol. 139:516–521.

Cozzi, R; Attanasio, R; Lodrini, S; Lasio, G. (2004). Cabergoline addition to depot somatostatin analogues in resistant acromegalic patients: efficacy and lack of predictive value of prolactin status. Clin Endocrinol (Oxf). 61:209–215.

Cozzi, R; Montini, M; Attanasio, R; Albizzi, M; Lasio, G; Lodrini, S; Doneda, P; Cortesi, L; Pagani G. (2006). Primary treatment of acromegaly with octreotide LAR: a long-term (up to nine years) prospective study of its efficacy in the control of disease activity and tumor shrinkage. J Clin Endocrinol Metab.91:1397–1403.

Cremonini, N; Graziano, E; Chiarini, V; Sforza, A; Zampa, GA. (1992). Atypical McCune-Albright syndrome associated with growth hormone-prolactin pituitary adenoma: natural history, long-term follow-up, and SMS 201–995—bromocriptine combined treatment results. J Clin Endocrinol Metab. 75:1166–1169.

Cushing, H. (1909). Partial hypophysectomy for acromegaly. Ann Surg. 50:1002–1017.

Damjanovic, SS; Neskovic, AN; Petakov, MS; Popovic, V; Vujisic, B; Petrovic, M; Nikolic-Djurovic, M; Simic, M; Pekic, S; Marinkovic, J. (2002). High output heart failure in patients with newly diagnosed acromegaly. Am J Med. 112(8):610-6.

De, P; Rees, DA; Davies, N; John, R; Neal, J; Mills, RG; Vafidis, J; Davies, JS; Scanlon, MF. (2003). Transsphenoidal surgery for acromegaly in Wales: results based on stringent criteria of remission. J Clin Endocrinol Metab. 88:3567– 3572.

Delhougne, B; Deneux, C; Abs, R. (1995). The prevalence of colonic polyps in acromegaly: a colonoscopic and pathological study in 103 patients. J Clin Endocrinol Metab. 80:3223-3226.

DeNoto, FM; Moore, DD; Goodman, HM. (1981). Human growth hormone DNA sequence and mRNA structure: possible alternative splicing. Nucl Acids Res. 9:3719-3730.

Dons, RF; Roseelet, P; Pastakia, B. (1988). Arthropathy in acromegalic patients before and after treatment: A long-term follow-up study. Clin Endocrinol. 28:515-524.

Drange, MR; Melmed, S. (1998). Long-acting lanreotide induces clinical and biochemical remission of acromegaly caused by disseminated growth hormone releasing hormone-secreting carcinoid. J Clin Endocrinol Metab. 83:3104–9.

Drange, MR; Melmed, S. (1999). IGFs in the evaluation of acromegaly. In Rosenfeld RG, Roberts CT (eds): Contemporary Endocrinology. The IFG System: Molecular Biology, Physiology, and Clinical Applications. Totowa, NJ: Humana Press, pp 699-720.

Duncan, E; Wass, JA. (1999). Investigation protocol: acromegaly and its investigation. Clin Endocrinol (Oxf). 50(3):285–293.

Etxabe, J; Gaztambide, S; Latorre, P; et al. (1993). Acromegaly: An epidemiologic study. J Endocrinol Invest. 16:181–187.

Ezzat, S; Snyder, PJ; Young, WF. (1992). Octreotide treatment of acromegaly. A randomized, multicenter study. Ann Intern Med. 117:711-718.

Ezzat, S; Asa, SL; Stefaneanu, L. (1994). Somatotroph hyperplasia without pituitary adenoma associated with a long standing growth hormone-releasing hormone-producing bronchial carcinoid. J Clin Endocrinol Metab. 78:555–560.

Fainstein, Day P; Frohman, L; Garcia, Rivello H; Reubi, JC; Sevlever, G; Glerean, M. (2007). Ectopic growth hormone-releasing hormone secretion by a metastatic bronchial carcinoid tumor: a case with a non hypophysial intracranial tumor that shrank during long acting octreotide treatment. Pituitary. 10:311–19.

Finkelstein, JW; Boyar, RM; Roffwarg, HP. (1972). Age-related change in the twenty-four hour spontaneous secretion of growth hormone. J Clin Endocrinol Metab 35:665-670.

Flier, JS; Moller, DE; Moses, AC; O'Rahilly, S; Chaiken, RL; Grigorescu, F; Elahi, D; Kahn, BB; Weinreb JE; Eastman R. (1993). Insulin-mediated pseudoacromegaly: clinical and biochemical characterization of a syndrome of selective insulin resistance. J Clin Endocrinol Metab. 76:1533–1541.

Flogstad, AK; Halse, J; Haldorsen, T. (1995). Sandostatin LAR in acromegalic patients: A dose-range study. J Clin Endocrinol Metab. 80:3601-3607.

Freda, PU. (2003). Pitfalls in the biochemical assessment of acromegaly. Pituitary. 6(3):135–40.

Freda, PU; Reyes, CM; Nuruzzaman, AT. (2003). Basal and glucose-suppressed GH levels less than 1 µg/L in newly diagnosed acromegaly. Pituitary. 6:175-180.

Gharib, H; Cook, DM; Saenger, PH. (2003). American Association of Clinical Endocrinologists medical guidelines for clinical practice for growth hormone use in adults and children. Endocr Pract. 9:64-76.

Ghigo, E; Aimaretti, G; Gianotti, L; Bellone, J; Arvat, E; Camanni, F. (1996). New approach to the diagnosis of growth hormone deficiency in adults. Eur J Endocrinol. 134(3):352–6.

Giordano, R; Lanfranco, F; Bo, M. (2005). Somatopause reflects age-related changes in the neural control of GH/IGF-I axis. J Endocrinol Invest. 28:94-98.

Gittoes, NJ; Sheppard, MC; Johnson, AP. (1999). Outcome of surgery for acromegaly the experience of a dedicated pituitary surgeon. QJM. 92. (12): 741-745.

Giustina, A; Veldhuis, JD. (1998). Pathophysiology of the neuroregulation of growth hormone secretion in experimental animals and the human. Endocr Rev. 19:717-797.

Giustina, A; Barkan, A; Casanueva, FF; Cavagnini, F; Frohman, L; Ho, K; et al. (2000). Criteria for cure of acromegaly: a consensus statement. J Clin Endocrinol Metab. 85(2):526–9.

Greenman, Y; Melmed S. (1994). Expression of three somatostatin receptor subtypes in pituitary adenomas: Evidence for preferential SSTR5 expression in the mammosomatotroph lineage. J Clin Endocrinol Metab. 79:724-729.

Grunstein, RR; Ho, KK; Sullivan CE. (1994).Effect of octreotide, a somatostatin analog, on sleep apnea in patients with acromegaly. Ann Intern Med. 121:478-483.

Hambrick, GW, Jr; Carter, DM. Pachydermoperiostosis. (1966). Touraine-Solente-Gole syndrome. Arch Dermatol. 94:594–60.

Harbison, JB; Nice, CM, Jr. (1971). Familial pachydermoperiostosis presenting as an acromegaly-like syndrome. Am J

Harrison, SM; Barnard, R; Ho, KY; Rajkovic, I; Waters, MJ. (1995). Control of growth hormone (GH) binding protein release from human hepatoma cells expressing full-length GH receptor. Endocrinology. 136;651-659.

Hattori, N; Shimatsu, A; Kato, Y. (1990). Growth hormone responses to oral glucose loading measured by highly sensitive enzyme immunoassay in normal subjects and patients with glucose intolerance and acromegaly. J Clin Endocrinol Metab. 70:771.

Herington, AC; Ymer, S; Stevenson, J. (1986). Identification and characterization of specific binding proteins for growth hormone in normal human sera. J Clin Invest. 77:1817-1823.

Ho, KK; O'Sullivan, AJ; Wolthers, T; Leung, KC. (2003). Metabolic effects of estrogens: impact of the route of administration. Ann Endocrinol (Paris). 64(2):170–7.

Ho, KY; Veldhuis, JD; Johnson, ML. (1988). Fasting enhances growth hormone secretion and amplifies the complex rhythms of growth hormone secretion in man. J Clin Invest. 81:968-975.

Ho, PJ; Friberg RD; Barkan AL. (1992). Regulation of pulsatile growth hormone secretion by fasting in normal subjects and patients with acromegaly. J Clin Endocrinol Metab. 75(3):812–9.

Holl, RW; Hartman, ML; Veldhuis, JD. (1991). Thirty-second sampling of plasma growth hormone in man: correlation with sleep stages. J Clin Endocrinol Metab. 72: 854-861.

Imaki, T; Shibasaki, T; Shizume, K. (1985). The effect of free fatty acids on growth hormone (GH) releasing hormone-mediated GH secretion in man. J Clin Endocrinol Metab. 60:290-293.

Iranmanesh, A; Lizaralde, G; Johnson, ML; Veldhuis, JD. (1990). Nature of Altered Growth Hormone Secretion in Hyperthyroidism. J Clin Endocrinol Metab. 72 (1): 108-115.

Jaffe, CA; Friberg, RD; Barkan, AL. (1993). Suppression of growth hormone (GH) secretion by a selective GH-releasing hormone (GHRH) antagonist. Direct evidence for involvement of endogenous GHRH in the generation of GH pulses. J Clin Invest. 92:695-701.

Jenkins, PJ; Frajese, V; Jones, AM; Camacho-Hubner, C; Lowe, DG; Fairclough, PD; Chew, SL; Grossmann, AB; Monson, J & Besser, GM. (2000). IGF-I and the development of colorectal neoplasia in acromegaly. Journal of Clinical Endocrinology and Metabolism. 85:3218-3221.

Jenkins, PJ; Besser, M. (2001). Clinical perspective: acromegaly and cancer: a problem. Journal of Clinical Endocrinology and Metabolism. 86(7), 2935-2941.

Jenkins, PJ. (2006). Cancers associated with acromegaly. Neuroendocrinology. 83(3-4), 218-223.

Jenkins, PJ; Bates, P; Carson, MN; Stewart, PM; Wass, JA. (2006). Conventional pituitary irradiation is effective in lowering serum growth hormone and insulin- like growth factor-I in patients with acromegaly. J Clin Endocrinol Metab. 91:1239–1245.

Jezkova, J; Marek, J; Hana, V; Krsek, M; Weiss, V; Vladyka, V; Lisak, R; Vymazal, J; Pecen, L . (2006). Gamma knife radiosurgery for acromegaly—long-term experience. Clin Endocrinol (Oxf). 64:588–595.

Jansson, JO; Svensson, J; Bengtsson, BA; Frohman, LA; Ahlman, H; Wängberg, B. (1998). Acromegaly and Cushing's syndrome due to ectopic production of GHRH and ACTH by a thymic carcinoid tumour: in vitro responses to GHRH and GHRP-6. Clin Endocrinol. 48:243–50.

Kaltsas, GA; Mukherjee, JJ; Jenkins, PJ. (1999). Menstrual irregularity in women with acromegaly. J Clin Endocrinol Metab. 84:2731.

Kaltsas, GA; Isidori, AM; Florakis, D; Trainer, PJ; Camacho-Hubner, C; Afshar, F; Sabin, I; Jenkins, JP; Chew, SL; Monson, JP; Besser, GM; Grossman, AB. (2001). Predictors of the outcome of surgical treatment in acromegaly and the value of the mean growth hormone day curve in assessing postoperative disease activity. J Clin Endocrinol Metab. 86:1645–1652.

Kasagi, K; Shimatsu, A; Miyamoto, S. (1999). Goiter associated with acromegaly: sonographic and scintigraphic findings of the thyroid gland. Thyroid. 9:791-796.

Kasayama, S; Otsuki, M; Takagi, M. (2000). Impaired beta-cell function in the presence of reduced insulin sensitivity determines glucose tolerance status in acromegalic patients. Clin Endocrinol (Oxf). 52. (5): 549-555.

Kofoed, EM. (2003). Growth hormone insensitivity associated with a STAT5b mutation. N Engl J Med. 349:1139-1147.

Kopchick, JJ; Parkinson, C; Stevens, EC. (2002). Growth hormone receptor antagonists: discovery, development, and use in patients with acromegaly. Endocr Rev. 23. (5): 623-646.

Kreutzer, J; Vance, ML; Lopes, MB. (2001). Surgical management of GH-secreting pituitary adenomas: an outcome study using modern remission criteria. J Clin Endocrinol Metab. 86. (9): 4072-4077.

Kwekkeboom, DJ; Krenning, EP; Bakker, WH; Oei, HY; Kooy, PPM; Lamberts SWJ. (1993). Somatostatin analogue scintigraphy in carcinoid tumours. Eur J Nucl Med. 20:283–92.

Ladas, SD; Thalassinos, NC; Ioannides, G; Raptis, SA. (1994). Does acromegaly really predispose to an increased prevalence of gastrointestinal tumours?. Clin Endocrinol (Oxf). 41:597-601.

Lamberts, SWJ. (1988). The role of somatostatin in the regulation of anterior pituitary hormone secretion and the use of its analogs in the treatment of human pituitary tumors. Endocr Rev. 9:417-436.

Lancranjan, I; Atkinson, AB and the Sandostatin LAR group. (1999). Results of a European multicenter study with Sandostatin LAR in acromegalic patients. Pituitary. 1:105-114.

Lanning, NJ; Carter Su, C. (2006). Recent advances in growth hormone signaling. Rev Endocr Metab Disord. 7:225-235.

Leavitt, J; Klein, I; Kendricks, F. (1983). Skin tags. a cutaneous marker for colonic polyps. Ann Intern Med. 98:928-930.

Le Roith, D; Bondy, C; Yakar, S; Liu, JL; Butler, A. (2001). The somatomedin hypothesis. Endocr Rev. 22(1), 53-74.

Leung, DW; Spencer, SA; Cachianes, G. (1987). Growth hormone receptor and serum binding protein: Purification, cloning, and expression. Nature. 330:537-543.

Levy A. (2000). Is monoclonality in pituitary adenomas synonymous with neoplasia? Clin Endocrinol (Oxf). 52:393–397.

Levy, A.(2001). Monoclonality of endocrine tumors: what does it mean? Trends Endocrinol Metab. 12:301–307.

Lewis, UJ; Dunn, JT; Bonewald, LF; Seavey, BK and VanderLaan, WP. (1978). A naturally occurring variant of human growth hormone. J Biol Chem. 253:2679-2687.

Lieberman, SA; Bjorkengren, AG; Hoffman, AR. (1992). Rheumatologic and skeletal changes in acromegaly. Endocrinol Metab Clin North Am. 21:615-631.

Lin, C; Lin, SC; Chang, CP. (1992). Pit-1-dependent expression of the receptor for growth hormone releasing factor mediates pituitary cell growth. Nature. 360:765-768.

Ludecke, DK; Abe; T. (2006). Transsphenoidal microsurgery for newly diagnosed acromegaly: a personal view after more than 1,000 operations. Neuroendocrinology. 83:230–239.

Maiza, JC; Vezzosi, D; Matta, M; Donadille, F; Loubes-Lacroix, F; Cournot, M; Bennet, A; Caron, P. (2007). Long-term (up to 18 years) effects on GH/IGF-1 hypersecretion and tumour size of primary somatostatin analogue (SSTa) therapy in patients with GH-secreting pituitary adenoma responsive to SSTa. Clin Endocrinol (Oxf). 67:282–28.

Marie, P. (1886). On two cases of acromegaly. Marked hypertrophy of the upper and lower limbs and the head. Rev Med. 6:297-333.

Marzullo, P; Ferone, D; Di Somma, C; Pivonello, R; Filippella, M; Lombardi, G; Colao, A. (1999). Efficacy of combined treatment with lanreotide and cabergoline in selected therapy-resistant acromegalic patients. Pituitary. 1:115–120.

McCarthy, TL; Centrella, M; Canalis, E. (1989). Regulatory effects of insulin-like growth factors I and II on bone collagen synthesis in rat calvarial cultures. Endocrinology. 124:301-309

Melmed, S; Braunstein, GD; Horvath, E. (1983). Pathophysiology of acromegaly. Endocr Rev. 4:271-290

Melmed, S. Acromegaly and cancer: not a problem?. (2001). J Clin Endocrinol Metab. 86:2929-2934.

Melmed, S. (2006). Medical progress: Acromegaly. N Engl J Med. 355(24):2558-73.

Melmed, S; Casanueva, FF; Cavagnini, F; Chanson, P; Frohman, L; Grossman, A; Ho, K; Kleinberg, D; Lamberts, S; Laws, E; Lombardi, G; Vance, ML; Werder, KV; Wass, J; Giustina, A. (2002). Guidelines for acromegaly management. J Clin Endocrinol Metab. 87(9):4054-8.

Melmed, S; Sternberg, R; Cook, D. (2005). A critical analysis of pituitary tumor shrinkage during primary medical therapy in acromegaly. J Clin Endocrinol Metab. 90:4405-4410.

Melmed, S; Colao, A; Barkan A; Molitch, M; Grossman, AB; Kleinberg; Clemmons, D; Chanson, P; Laws, E; Schlechte, J; Vance, ML; Ho, K and Giustina, A. (2009). Guidelines for Acromegaly Management: An Update J Clin Endocrinol Metab. 94(5):1509–1517.

Mendelson, WB. (1982). Studies of human growth hormone secretion in sleeping and waking. Int Rev Neurobiol. 23:367-389.

Mercado, M; Borges, F; Bouterfa, H; Chang, TC, ; Chervin A, ; Farrall AJ;, Patocs A;, Petersenn S; Podoba, J; Safari, M; Wardlaw, J. (2007). A prospective, multicentre study to investigate the efficacy, safety and tolerability of octreotide LAR (long-acting repeatable octreotide) in the primary therapy of patients with acromegaly. Clin Endocrinol (Oxf). 66:859–868.

Miell, JP; Taylor, AM; Zini, M; Maheshwari, HG; Ross RJM & Valcavi R. (1993). Effects of hypothyroidism and hyperthyroidism on insulin-like growth factors (IGFs) and growth hormone- and IGFbinding proteins. Journal of Clinical Endocrinology and Metabolism. 76:950–955.

Minniti, G; Moroni, C; Jaffrain-Rea ML. (1998). Prevalence of hypertension in acromegalic patients: clinical measurement versus 24-hour ambulatory blood pressure monitoring. Clin Endocrinol (Oxf). 48.(2): 149-152

Minniti, G; Jaffrain-Rea, ML; Osti, M; Esposito, V; Santoro, A; Solda, F; Gargiulo, P; Tamburrano, G; Enrici, RM. (2005). The long-term efficacy of conventional radiotherapy in patients with GH-secreting pituitary adenomas. Clin Endocrinol (Oxf). 62:210–216.

Mozid, AM; Tringali, G; Forsling, ML. (2003). Ghrelin is released from rat hypothalamic explants and stimulates corticotrophin releasing hormone and arginine vasopressin. Horm Metab Res. 35. 455-459.

Nabarro, JD. Acromegaly. (1987). Clin Endocrinol (Oxf). 26(4), 481-512.

Nasr, C; Mason, A; Mayberg, M; Staugaitis, SM; Asa, SL. (2006). Acromegaly and somatotroph hyperplasia with adenomatous transformation due to pituitary metastasis of a growth hormone releasing hormone-secreting pulmonary endocrine carcinoma. J Clin Endocrinol Metab. 91(12):4776–80.

Nomikos, P; Buchfelder, M; Fahlbusch, R. (2005). The outcome of surgery in 668 patients with acromegaly using current criteria of biochemical 'cure'. Eur J Endocrinol. 152:379–387.

Orme, SM; McNally, RJQ; Cartwright, RA; Belchetz PE. (1998). Mortality and cancer incidence in acromegaly: a retrospective cohort study. J Clin Endocrinol Metab. 83:2730–2734.

Painson, JC; Tannenbaum, GS. (1991). Sexual dimorphism of somatostatin and growth hormone releasing factor signaling in the control of pulsatile growth hormone secretion in the rat. Endocrinology. 128:2858-2866.

Parks, JS. (1989). Molecular biology of growth hormone. Acta Paed. Stand. [Suppl.] 349: 127-135.

Pascual, J; Freijanes, J; Berciano, J; Pesquera, C. (1991). Analgesic effect of octreotide in headache associated with acromegaly is not mediated by opioid mechanisms. Case report. Pain. 47:341-344.

Patel, YC. (1999). Somatostatin and its receptor family. Front Neuroendocrinol. 20. (3): 157-198.

Penalva, A; Pombo, M; Carballo, A. (1993). Influence of sex, age and adrenergic pathways on the growth hormone response to GHRP-6. Clin Endocrinol (Oxf). 38:87-91.

Peterfreund, RA; Vale, WW. (1984). Somatostatin analogs inhibit somatostatin secretion from cultured hypothalamus cells. Neuroendocrinology. 39:397-402.

Pietrobelli, DJ; Akopian, M; Olivieri, AO. (2001). Altered circadian blood pressure profile in patients with active acromegaly. Relationship with left ventricular mass and hormonal values. J Hum Hypertens.15.(9):601-605. 151. Pokrajac, A; Wark, G; Ellis, AR; Wear, J; Wieringa, GE; Trainer, PJ. (2007). Variation in GH and IGF-1 assays limits the applicability of international consensus criteria for local practice. Clin Endocrinol (Oxf). 67(1):65–70.

Pollock, BE; Jacob, JT; Brown, PD; Nippoldt, TB. (2007). Radiosurgery of growth hormone-producing pituitary adenomas: factors associated with biochemical remission. J Neurosurg. 106:833–838.

Raben, MS. (1958). Treatment of a pituitary dwarf with human growth hormone. J Clin Endocrinol Metab. 18:901-3.

Rajasoorya, C; Holdaway, IM; Wrightson, P; Scott, DJ; Ibbertson, HK. (1994). Determinants of clinical outcome and survival in acromegaly. Clin Endocrinol. 41:95–102.

Renehan, AG; Bhaskar, P; Painter, JE. (2000). The prevalence and characteristics of colorectal neoplasia in acromegaly. J Clin Endocrinol Metab. 85:3417-3424.

Renehan, AG; Zwahlen, M; Minder, C; O'Dwyer, ST; Shalet, SM & Egger, M. (2004). Insulin-like growth factor (IGF)-I, IGF binding protein-3, and cancer risk: systematic review and meta-regression analysis. Lancet. 363(9418), 1346-1353.

Rietveld, I; Janssen, JA; van Rossum, EF; Houwing-Duistermaat, JJ; Rivadeneira, F; Hofman, A; Pols, HA; van Duijn, CM; Lamberts, SW. (2004). A polymorphic CA repeat in the IGF-I gene is associated with gender-specific differences in body height, but has no effect on the secular trend in body height. Clin. Endocrinol. (Oxf) 61;195–203

Rimoin, DL. (1965). Pachydermoperiostosis (idiopathic clubbing and periostosis), genetic and physiologic considerations. N Engl J Med. 272:923–931.

Ritchie, CM; Atkinson, AB; Kennedy, AL. (1990). Ascertainment and natural history of treated acromegaly in Northern Ireland. Ulster Med J. 59: 55-62.

Roth, A; Cligg, SM; Yallow, CP. (1963). Secretion of human growth hormone: physiological and experimental modification. Metabolism. 12:557-559.

Ron, E; Gridley, G; Hrubee, Z. (1991). Acromegaly and gastrointestinal cancer. Cancer. 68:1673-1677.

Rosenow, F; Reuter, S; Deuss, U. (1996). Sleep apnoea in treated acromegaly: relative frequency and predisposing factors. Clin Endocrinol (Oxf). 45:563-569.

Sachar, EJ; Mushrush, G; Perlow, M. (1972). Growth hormone responses to l-dopa in depressed patients. Science. 178:1304-1305.

Sadoul, JL; Thyss, A; Freychet, P. (1992). Invasive mixed growth hormone/prolactin secreting pituitary tumour: complete shrinking by octreotide and bromocriptine, and lack of tumour growth relapse 20 months after octreotide withdrawal. Acta Endocrinol (Copenh). 126:179–183.

Selvarajah, D; Webster, J; Ross, R; Newell-Price, J. (2005). Effectiveness of adding dopamine agonist therapy to long-acting somatostatin analogues in the management of acromegaly. Eur J Endocrinol. 152:569–574.

Serri, O; Beauregard, C; Hardy, J. (2004)Long-term biochemical status and disease-related morbidity in 53 postoperative patients with acromegaly. Clin Endocrinol Metab. 89(2):658–1.

Shimon, I. (1997). Somatostatin receptor subtype specificity in human fetal pituitary cultures. Differential role of SSTR2 and SSTR5 for growth hormone, thyroid-stimulating hormone, and prolactin regulation. J. Clin. Invest. 99:789-798.

Shimon, I; Melmed, S. (1998). Management of pituitary tumors. Ann Intern Med. 129:472-483.

Shimon, I; Cohen, ZR; Ram, Z; Hadani, M. (2001). Transsphenoidal surgery for acromegaly: endocrinological follow-up of 98 patients. Neurosurgery. 48: 1239–1243.

Sugihara, H; Shibasaki, T; Tatsuguchi, A; Okajima, F; Wakita, S; Nakajima, Y. (2007). A non-acromegalic case of multiple endocrine neoplasia type 1 accompanied by a growth hormone-releasing hormone-producing pancreatic tumor. J Endocrinol Invest. 30(5):421–7.

Takahashi, Y; Kipnis DM; Daughaday, WH. (1968). Growth hormone secretion during sleep. J Clin Invest. 47:2079-2090.

Terzolo, M; Matrella, C; Boccuzzi, A. (1999). Twenty-four hour profile of blood pressure in patients with acromegaly. Correlation with demographic, clinical and hormonal features. J Endocrinol Invest. 22.(1): 48-54.

Thorner, MO; Perryman, RL; Cronin, MJ. (1982). Somatotroph hyperplasia: successful treatment of acromegaly by removal of a pancreatic islet tumor secreting a growth hormone releasing factor. J Clin Invest. 70:965–977.

Thorner, MO; Frohman, LA; Leong, DA. (1984). Extrahypothalamic growth hormone releasing factor (GRF) secretion is a rare cause of acromegaly: plasma GRF levels in 177 acromegalic patients. J Clin Endocrinol Metab. 59:846-849.

Trainer, PJ; Drake, WM; Katznelson, L; et al. 2000; Treatment of acromegaly with the growth hormone–receptor antagonist pegvisomant. N Engl J Med. 342:1171-1177.

Trtoman-Dickenson, B; Weetman, AP; Hughes, JMB. (1991). Upper airflow obstruction and pulmonary function in acromegaly: Relationship to disease activity. Q J Med. 79:527-533.

Turgut, S; Akın, F; Akcılar, R; Ayada, C; Turgut G. (2011). Angiotensin converting enzyme I/D, angiotensinogen M235T and AT1-R A/C1166 gene polymorphisms in patients with acromegaly. Mol Biol Rep. Jan;38(1):569-76

Ur, E; Mather, SJ; Bomanji, J. (1992). Pituitary imaging using a labelled somatostatin analogue in acromegaly. Clin Endocrinol (Oxf). 36:147-150.

Valcavi, R; Dieguez, C; Preece, M; Taylor, A; Portioli I & Scanlon MF. Effect of thyroxine replacement therapy on plasma insulin like growth factor 1 levels and growth hormone responsiveness to growth hormone releasing hormone in hypothyroid patients. (1987). Clinical Endocrinology. 27:85–90.

Valcavi, R; Zini, M; Portioli, I. (1992). Thyroid hormones and growth hormone secretion. Journal of Endocrinological Investigations. 15:313–330.

Valcavi, R; Dieguez, C; Zini, M; Muruais, C; Casanueva, F; Portioli I. (1993). Influence of hyperthyroidism on growth hormone secretion. Clin Endocrinol (Oxf). 38(5):515-22.

Vaessen, N; Heutink, P; Janssen, JA; Witteman, JC; Testers, L; Hofman, A; Lamberts, SW; Oostra, BA, ; Pols, HA; van Duijn, CM. (2001). A polymorphism in the gene for IGF-I: functional properties and risk for type 2 diabetes and myocardial infarction. Diabetes. 50; 637–642.

Van der Lely, AJ; De Herder, WW; Lamberts SW. (1997). The role of radiotherapy in acromegaly. J Clin Endocrinol Metab. 82:3185-3186.

Van der Lely, AJ; Hutson, RK; Trainer, PJ. (2001). Long-term treatment of acromegaly with pegvisomant, a growth hormone receptor antagonist. Lancet. 358. (9295):1754-1759.

Veldhuis, JD; Roemmich, JN; Richmond, EJ. (2006). Somatotropic and gonadotropic axes linkages in infancy, childhood, and the puberty-adult transition. Endocr Rev. 27:101-140.

Verde, GG; Santi, I; Chiodini, P. (1986). Serum type III procollagen propeptide levels in acromegalic patients. J Clin Endocrinol Metab. 63:1406-1410.

Vieira, Neto L; Taboada, GF; Corrêa, LL; Polo, J; Nascimento, AF; Chimelli, L. (2007). Acromegaly secondary to growth hormone releasing hormone secreted by an incidentally discovered pheochromocytoma. Endocr Pathol. 18(1):46–52.

Vigas, M; Malatinsky, J; Nemeth, S; Jurcovicova, J. (1977). α-Adrenergic control of growth hormone release during surgical stress in man. Metabolism. 26:399-402.

Wagenaar, AH; Harris, AG; van der Lely, AJ; Lamberts, SW. (1991). Dynamics of the acute effects of octreotide, bromocriptine and both drugs in combination on growth hormone secretion in acromegaly. Acta Endocrinol (Copenh). 125:637–642.

Weckbecker, G; Lewis, I; Albert, R; et al. (2003). Opportunities in somatostatin research: biological, chemical and therapeutic aspects. Nat Rev Drug Discov. 2:999-1017.

Wehrenberg, WB; Brazeau, P; Luben, R. (1982). Inhibition of the pulsatile secretion of growth hormone by monoclonal antibodies to the hypothalamic growth hormone releasing factor (GRF). Endocrinology. 111:2147-2148.

Weinstein, LS. (1991). Activating mutations of the stimulatory G protein in the McCune-Albright syndrome. N. Engl. J. Med. 325:1688-1695.

Wright, AD; Hill, DM; Lowery, C. (1970). Mortality in acromegaly. Quart J Med. 39:1–16.

Xu, BC; Wang, X; Darus, CJ; Kopchick, JJ. (1996) Growth hormone promotes the association of transcription factor STAT5 with the growth hormone receptor. J Biol Chem. 271:19768-19773.

Yamashita, S; Melmed, S. (1986). Insulin-like growth factor I action on rat anterior pituitary cells: Suppression of growth hormone secretion and messenger ribonucleic acid levels. Endocrinology.118:176-182.

Yamashita, S;Weiss, M; Melmed, S. (1986). Insulin-like growth factor I regulates growth hormone secretion and messenger ribonucleic acid levels in human pituitary tumor cells. J Clin Endocrinol Metab. 63:730-735.

4

Effects of Growth Hormone (GH) Overexpression in Signaling Cascades Involved in Promotion of Cell Proliferation and Survival

Lorena González, Johanna G. Miquet and Ana I. Sotelo
Instituto de Química y Fisicoquímica Biológica (UBA-CONICET), Facultad de Farmacia y Bioquímica, Universidad de Buenos Aires Argentina

1. Introduction

This chapter will describe the effects of long term exposure to growth hormone (GH) at the molecular level in the liver. Expression and activation of intermediates involved in GH-induced signaling were analyzed in transgenic mice overexpressing GH, as well as the influence of chronically elevated GH levels over Amend: epidermal growth factor receptor (EGFR) signaling. Several signaling mediators involved in cellular proliferation, survival and migration are altered in the liver of GH-transgenic mice. The molecular mechanisms underlying the pro-oncogenic pathology induced by prolonged exposure to elevated GH levels will be discussed.

1.1 Physiological actions of GH

Growth hormone (GH), also known as somatotropin, is the main regulator of postnatal body growth, but its actions are not limited to corporal stature. GH has important metabolic functions on carbohydrate, lipid and protein metabolism, as well as on tissue maintenance and repair, cardiac and immune function, mental agility and ageing. It exerts its actions both directly, and by means of endocrine and paracrine insulin-like growth factor (IGF) 1. At the cellular level, GH modulates proliferation, differentiation, motility and apoptosis.

GH secretion:

Growth hormone, part of the somatotropic axis, is mainly synthesized in somatotroph cells from the anterior pituitary. Growth hormone secretion is regulated centrally, through the hypothalamic-portal circulation, by hypothalamic peptides: its synthesis and release are promoted by growth-hormone releasing hormone (GHRH) and inhibited by somatostatin, and it is also stimulated by stomach-derived ghrelin. Stress, exercise, malnutrition, and anorexia also promote its secretion. By means of negative feedback, GH inhibits its own secretion: in the short central loop, GH acts on somatotroph cells to generate IGF1 locally, that in turn inhibits the cell; and it acts at the hypothalamic level to inhibit GHRH synthesis and release and to stimulate both synthesis and release of somatostatin. In the long peripheral loop, GH acts on the liver to generate most of circulating IGF1, which inhibits GH secretion by a dual mechanism: direct inhibition of the somatotrophs and stimulation of somatostatin release. GH is also produced locally in many tissues, acting in an autocrine and paracrine fashion. Central cholinergic stimulation increases the release of GH reducing the secretion of somatostatin. Glucocorticoids and metabolic substrates also affect GH secretion; treatment with glucocorticoids inhibits its release while fasting states with hypoglycemia, low circulating free fatty acids, and high circulating amino acid concentrations stimulate it.

GH secretion presents sexual dimorphism: the frequency of pulses is higher in females. The difference is most striking in rats, where secretion profile in males is characterized by high amplitude pulses every 3-4 h, with almost non-detectable values between pulses. Female rats, on the contrary, have more frequent lower amplitude pulses, and thus present baseline GH levels (Waxman & Frank, 2000). Humans, on the other hand, present higher values at night, during the first hours of sleep, and lower values in the early morning. GH secretory pattern conditions the sexually dimorphic gene expression in the liver, particularly of proteins involved in steroid and drug metabolism.

GH secretion presents age-dependency: circulating GH levels progressively rise during childhood, to achieve a maximum towards the end of adolescence in humans, and slowly diminish thereafter. By the sixth decade of life, they are only 20% of maximum (Turyn & Sotelo, 2004).

GH function:

Somatic growth: GH acts directly on bone and indirectly, through endocrine hepatic derived IGF1, as well as the locally produced factor. These growth promoting peptides act on the epiphyseal cartilage, inducing chondrocyte proliferation, which leads to longitudinal skeletal growth (Tritos & Biller, 2009). Longitudinal growth ceases when the epiphyses of the long bones fuse to the diaphyses. Oversecretion before this instance results in *gigantism*, whereas oversecretion afterwards results in *acromegaly*, characterized by abnormal growth of hands and feet, and roughening of the facial features: protrusion of brow and lower jaw, and nose enlargement. Lack of GH or GHR in humans results in severe short stature, reduced muscle mass, increased fat storage, decreased cortical bone mineral density and decreased fertility in females (Lichanska & Waters., 2008a). In animals, basically the same growth outcome can be observed, either in spontaneous mutants or in genetically engineered models. Notably, mice lacking GH or GHR live longer than their littermates (Bartke & Brown-Borg, 2004).

Besides its effects on skeletal growth, GH regulates body composition, increasing muscle mass and decreasing adipose content. The relationship between GH status and body composition is evidenced in patients and animal models lacking GH, which become obese. In humans, symptoms of GH deficiency resemble those of ageing, when GH levels decline: loss of muscular mass and tone, loss of bone mineral density, loss of strength, abdominal obesity (Perrini et al., 2010).

Metabolic actions: GH has important metabolic actions on lipid and carbohydrate metabolism. It presents both insulin-like and insulin-antagonistic actions, presumably the first are IGF1-mediated while the latter are directly exerted by the hormone, since the effects of IGF1 on lipolysis and gluconeogenesis are contrary to those of GH (Kaplan & Cohen, 2010). GH exerts lipolytic effects, principally at the visceral adipose tissue, resulting in an increase of circulating free fatty acids, by increasing adipose tissue hormone-sensitive lipase activity; at the same time, it inhibits glucose uptake in adipose tissue. On the other hand, in liver GH promotes triglyceride (TG) uptake and storage, and in skeletal muscle it induces TG uptake and utilization. GH also presents anabolic actions on protein metabolism, since it stimulates protein synthesis and inhibits its proteolysis (Vijayakumar et al., 2010).

The contrasting effects of GH and insulin on substrate metabolism depend on the nutritional status and food intake. Endogenous GH secretion is down-regulated by food intake, allowing insulin action on storage of nutrients. In a fasted state, GH secretion favors lipolysis. Between these two states, GH and insulin may act concomitantly to promote IGF1 production and therefore, protein synthesis. Usage of fatty acids as the energy source during fasting instead of glucose protects against excessive protein break-down. Thus, GH is both anabolic and anti-catabolic in protein metabolism (Jorgensen et al., 2010).

1.2 GH-signaling

1.2.1 Growth hormone receptor

Structure: GH exerts its functions by binding to its cognate receptor, the GHR. This receptor is a single-chain transmembrane glycoprotein which belongs to class I cytokine receptors. It is composed of three domains: the extracellular ligand-binding domain, arranged as two fibronectin type domains connected by a short flexible linker; the transmembrane domain; and the intracellular domain (ICD). The ICD has two motifs that bind tyrosine kinase JAK2, Box1 and Box2, and several tyrosine residues, which are substrates of JAK2 and become docking sites for phosphotyrosine binding molecules (Brooks et al., 2008). JAK2 is critical for GHR-signaling since GHR lacks intrinsic kinase activity. GHR is a member of the cytokine receptor superfamily, and is therefore structurally related to other members of this family, such as the receptors for prolactin, erythropoietin, thrombopoietin, leptin, interleukin 3, 5 and 6, granulocyte/macrophage colony-stimulating factor and interferon (Rosenfeld & Hwa, 2009; Lanning & Carter-Su, 2006).

GHR loss of function mutations: The GHR mediates GH growth-related functions, as mutations in the receptor lead to severe stature deficit, similar to the lack of the hormone. Laron syndrome is a genetic disorder characterized by growth retardation and very short stature at adulthood (>5 SD), patients also present impaired muscle and bone development, as well as obesity and steatosis (Brooks et al., 2008). It is associated with deletions or mutations principally at the extracellular ligand-binding domain of the receptor; as a GH insensitivity syndrome, it is concurrent with high GH but low IGF1 circulating levels.

GHR levels: Liver exhibits the highest GHR concentration, but it is also highly expressed in muscle, bone, kidney, mammary gland, adipose tissue, heart, intestine, lung, prostate, pancreas, cartilage, fibroblasts, and embryonic stem cells; in fact, GHR is expressed in almost every tissue of the body, indicating the relevance of GH action in every organ. Several factors regulate GHR concentration, including nutritional status and developmental stage. GHR levels are down-regulated by under-nutrition and fasting, while their levels gradually increase from birth to adulthood (Tiong & Herington, 1999). GH is a principal modulator of GHR, indeed it induces the synthesis of its own receptor (González et al., 2001; González et al., 2007).

GHR turnover: at least two different mechanisms participate in the down-regulation of the mature form of the GHR at the plasma membrane: ligand-independent endocytosis and proteolytic cleavage (Flores-Morales et al., 2006). The protein break-down consists of two steps: a metalloproteinase, the tumor necrosis factor-α converting enzyme (TACE), cleaves the extracellular portion of the receptor, close to the insertion point at the membrane. This generates the soluble form of the receptor, known as growth hormone binding protein (GHBP). After this process, the membrane-bound remnant is degraded by a γ-secretase complex, and targeted to proteasomal degradation (Flores-Morales et al., 2006; Zhang et al.,

2000; Wang et al., 2002; Cowan et al., 2005). This mechanism is believed responsible for GHBP release into circulation, but it is not expected to participate in termination of GH signaling since it is inhibited by ligand binding (Flores-Morales et al., 2006; Zhang et al., 2001). GHR endocytosis, which involves both clathrin-coated pits and caveolae, does not require ligand-binding although receptor occupation accelerates the process. Internalized receptors are mostly derived to lysosome and proteasome degradation, as they are not recycled to the membrane (Flores-Morales et al., 2006; Sachse et al., 2001; Lobie et al., 1999). GHR-internalization requires an intact ubiquitin conjugating system, although actual ubiquitination of the receptor does not seem to be required (Lanning & Carter-Su, 2006; van Kerkhof et al., 2007).

GHBP: Growth hormone circulates in plasma bound to specific proteins known as growth hormone-binding proteins (GHBP). The most important of these proteins, high affinity GHBP, coincides with the extracellular domain of the GHR, and is generated by two different mechanisms. While in humans and rabbits it surges after proteolytic processing of the mature receptor, in rodents it is the result of alternative splicing of the GHR pre-mRNA (Baumann, 2001). Lower affinity and high molecular weight GH-binding proteins are not related to the GHR (Kratzsch et al., 1996).

GHR nuclear localization: Apart from its expected localization at the cell surface and at the endoplasmic reticulum, GHR has also been found at the nucleus of several cells. This localization is not unique for the GHR, since other transmembrane receptors have also been described in the nuclear compartment. Nuclear GHR was found in cells exhibiting high proliferative status, associated with transformation and tumor progression (Brooks et al., 2008; Campbell-Conway et al., 2007). Autocrine GH is key to the action of nuclear GHR on cell proliferation (Brooks et al., 2008).

1.2.2 Signaling pathways induced by GH

Hormone binding: Compelling evidence suggests GHR exists as a preformed dimer on the cell surface. Growth hormone binds to the extracellular domain of the GHR dimer via two asymmetrically-placed binding sites on the hormone: high affinity site 1, and lower affinity site 2. Specificity of the dimerization partner is conferred by the extracellular domain of the receptor, while union of the two moieties is attained at the transmembrane level through leucine zipper-like interactions (Lichanska & Waters, 2008a). The current model posits ligand binding to homodimerized inactive receptor induces relative rotation of the intracellular domains, leading to proper alignment of tyrosine kinase JAK2 (Brown et al., 2005). The repositioning of the GHR induces JAK2, constitutively associated to the GHR, to become activated and thus phosphorylate not only other GHR-associated JAK2 molecules by trans-phosphorylation, but also modifies key tyrosine residues on the GHR, which become docking sites for SH2 (Src homology 2)-domain containing proteins (Rosenfeld & Hwa, 2009; Brooks et al., 2008). Autophosphorylation of JAK2 tyrosine-residues involves both activation of the catalytic site as well as modification of regulatory residues which may enhance or diminish kinase activity (Lanning & Carter-Su, 2007; Feng et al., 1997; Argetsinger et al., 2004; 2010).

Activated signaling pathways: Different signaling mediators are already preforming complexes with inactive receptor or are recruited to phosphotyrosines on activated GHR complex and bind to the complex by means of their phosphotyrosine binding modules, the PTB and the SH2-domains. GH activates at least three major signaling pathways, the signal transducers and activators of transcription (STATs), the mitogen activated protein kinase (MAPK) Erk1/2 and the phosphatidylinositol 3'-kinase (PI3K)/Akt pathways.

GH binding to its receptor triggers activation of STAT1, STAT3 and STAT5. These SH2-containing transcription factors are latent on the cytoplasm, become activated by tyrosine phosphorylation in one critical residue, and thus dissociate the receptor, dimerize and migrate to the nucleus as active dimers, where they bind specific DNA sequences to regulate the expression of multiple genes. STAT5 a and b are essential for many GH functions related to metabolism, body growth and sex-dependent liver gene regulation (Lanning & Carter-Su, 2006), indeed, STAT5b is regarded as the most relevant signaling mediator for GH actions, both direct and IGF1-mediated, as it regulates the transcription of the IGF1 gene (Woelfle et al., 2003a, 2003b; Woelfle & Rotwein, 2004). While it is not clear if STAT1 and STAT3 require GHR phosphorylation or bind to phosphotyrosine residues on the receptor, STAT5 can bind to several phosphotyrosine residues at the carboxi-terminal part of the intracellular domain of the receptor (Rowland et al., 2005; Lichanska & Waters, 2008a).

To date, there is no sufficient evidence relating the PI3K or the MAPK/Erk pathways with GH-induction of IGF1 transcription. Among the STATs, STAT5b has been regarded as the GH-mediator of IGF1 expression, but also of other important contributors to IGF1 function, as the acid labile subunit (ALS) and IGF1-binding protein 3 (IGF-BP3), both in rodents and in humans (Rosenfeld & Hwa, 2009; Woelfle & Rotwein, 2004). These two proteins complex IGF1 in circulation to modulate its bioavailability. Mutations in STAT5b have been associated with severe short stature in humans and reduced size in rodents, suggesting this mediator is crucial for GH-dependent skeletal growth (Udy et al., 1997; Kofoed et al., 2003; Rosenfeld et al., 2005).

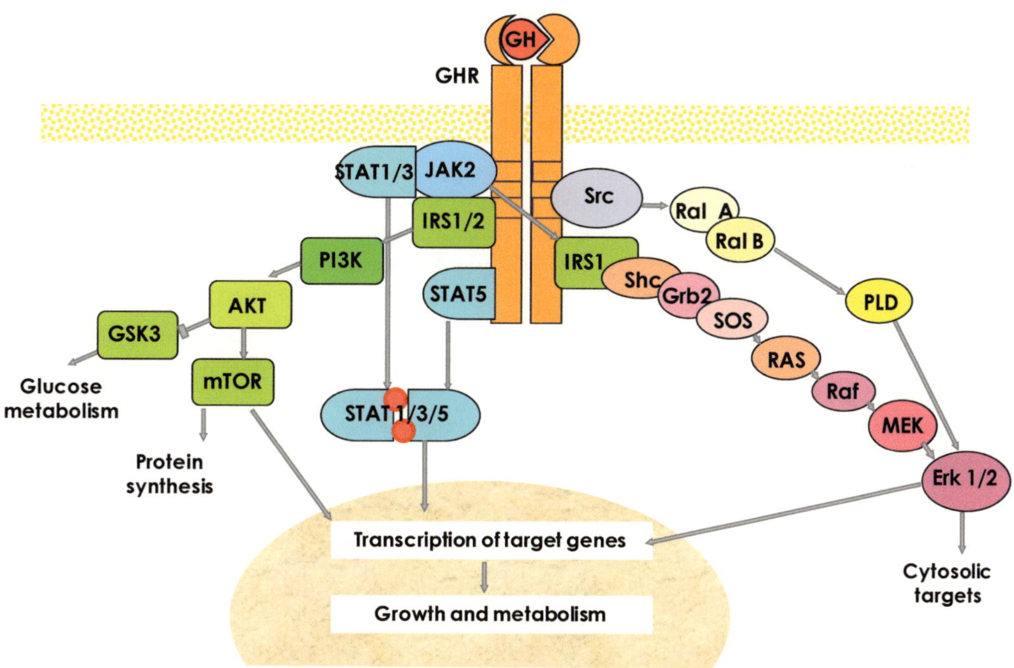

Fig. 1. Growth hormone signaling

GH activates the PI3K pathway, either by recruitment of insulin receptor substrates (IRS) 1, 2 and 3, or alternatively, by a CrkII-IRS1 interaction (Goh et al., 2000), or even by direct interaction of the PI3K to phosphotyrosine residues on the GHR (Lanning & Carter-Su, 2006; Moutoussamy et al., 1998). In either case, PI3K is recruited by binding of its p85 regulatory subunit to phosphotyrosine residues on its activated partners. This is a branching pathway, giving rise to multiple signals, which derive in protein and carbohydrate metabolism. Protein kinase B (PKB), a serine/threonine kinase most usually referred to as Akt, is one of PI3K principal downstream effectors. Akt activates mTOR (mammalian target of rapamycin), a protein-kinase that participates in the regulation of ribosomal protein translation, which leads to protein synthesis, among other substrates. Akt also participates in glucose metabolism, as it promotes glucose uptake and regulates glycogen synthesis. The IRSs/PI3K signaling cascade is the principal pathway activated by insulin and may therefore contribute to insulin-like actions of GH (Dominici et al., 2005).

The mitogen-activated protein kinase (MAPK) cascade participates in the control of cell proliferation, differentiation and migration. GH has been shown to activate the MAPK/Erk1/2 pathway by means of recruiting the adapter protein Shc (Src homology collagen) to the activated GHR-JAK2 complex, which becomes phosphorylated and thus binds Grb2, the guanine nucleotide exchange factor SOS, Ras, Raf, MEK (MAPK Erk kinase) and finally, the extracellular-regulated kinase (Erk) 1 and 2 (Lanning & Carter-Su, 2006). Recently, IRS-1 has been shown to act upstream of Shc/Grb activation of Erk1/2 (Wang et al., 2009). Alternatively, JAK2 was proposed to phosphorylate Grb2-binding site of the EGFR, allowing recruitment of Grb2 and activation of the pathway (Yamauchi et al. 1997; Lanning & Carter-Su, 2006). GH has also been shown to activate p38 and JNK/SAPK MAP kinases, other MAPK cascades (Zhu et al., 2001).

It is generally believed that activation of Erk1/2 rely on JAK2 activation, but it has also been reported to be activated by Src –another receptor-associated tyrosine kinase-, in a JAK2-independent fashion (Zhu et al., 2002; Rowlinson et al., 2008). GH-induced Src activation of Erk1/2 has been proposed to occur through an alternative mechanism, involving Ras-like small GTPases RalA and RalB and activation of phospholipase D (Zhu et al., 2002). The participation of JAK2 and Src in GH-mediated signal is dependent on cell type (Brooks & Waters, 2010), although the relative contribution of these cascades to GH signaling *in vivo* is controversial (Jin et al., 2008). Additionally, Erk1/2 have been shown to be activated by GH by another SKF (Src kinase family) member, Lyn, which signals through phospholipase C gamma and Ras (Rowlinson et al., 2008). Targeted mutation of Box1 –the JAK2 binding motif in GHR- in mice allows GH-induced activation of Src and Erk1/2 (Barclay et al., 2010) where JAK2 activation is abrogated, suggesting a minor contribution of this pathway to GH action. Moreover, it has recently been proposed that the conformational change the ligand impinges on the receptor conditions which signalling pathway becomes activated (Rowlinson et al., 2008).

1.2.3 Ending of the signal

GH is secreted episodically, thus the signaling elicited by each secretory burst must be readily counteracted to allow resensitization to a further pulse. Therefore, a critical balance between hormone signaling and its down-regulation is required. Described mechanisms of signaling attenuation involve blockage or removal of the phosphotyrosine residues in the activated GHR-complex by binding of inhibitory molecules or dephosphorylation, and ubiquitin-dependent GHR endocytosis (Lanning & Carter-Su, 2006).

Phosphatases: Since tyrosine phosphorylation is the primary event triggered upon ligand binding to receptor, it could be expected that removal of phosphorylation restores inactivated mediators. Several protein tyrosine phosphatases (PTPs) participate in GH-signaling termination, dephosphorylating not only GHR and JAK2 but also the STATs. Among these, the SH2 domain-containing protein tyrosine phosphatases SHP-1 and SHP-2 were the first described. While SHP-1 is preferentially expressed in hematopoietic cells, SHP2 is ubiquitously expressed (Murphy et al., 2010). SHP-1 is considered as a negative regulator of GH signaling, whereas SHP-2 has been regarded as a dual modulator, serving both positive and negative effects on GH signaling. It may act as a dephosphorylating enzyme, but it may also act as an adaptor protein binding to phosphotyrosine motifs by means of its SH2 domains. Mutation of SHP-2-binding residues on the GHR prolongs GH-induced phosphorylation of GHR, JAK2 and STAT5, thus suggesting negative regulation, while overexpression of catalytically inactive forms inhibited GH action (Lanning & Carter-Su, 2006; Stofega et al., 2000; Kim et al., 1998).
Other protein phosphatases have been shown to deactivate GHR-complex, namely, PTP-H1, PTP1, TC-PTP and PTP-1B (Pasquali et al., 2003); PTP-1B and PTP-H1 have also been shown to dephosphorylate STAT5 (Gu et al., 2003; Aoki & Matsuda, 2000). Catalytically inactive PTP-1B mutant mice present increased phosphorylation of JAK2 and STAT5-enhanced sensitivity to GH (Gu et al., 2003), while mice lacking the PTP-H1 catalytic domain show enhanced growth, with augmented hepatic mRNA IGF1 expression (Pilecka et al., 2007).
Suppressors of cytokine signaling (SOCS): SOCS proteins are regulators of the main signaling pathway induced by cytokines, the JAK/STAT pathway, therefore, they act to down-regulate the same signal that induced their expression, acting through a classical negative feedback loop (Flores-Morales et al., 2006). GH promotes transcription of four SOCS proteins, SOCS-1, -2, -3 and CIS (cytokine inducible suppressor), these proteins can be divided into two groups according to mechanism of action and to kinetics of appearance. SOCS-1 and SOCS-3 impede JAK2 activity once they are recruited to the GHR-JAK2 complex, whereas SOCS-2 and CIS bind to phosphotyrosine residues at the distal portion of the GHR, and thus interfere with STAT5 activation. SOCS-1 and -3 are rapidly but transiently induced after a GH stimulus, whereas CIS and SOCS-2 are induced after SOCS-1 and SOCS-3 mRNA levels diminish (Tollet-Egnell et al., 1999). Apart from the inhibitory mechanism, all SOCS proteins present a SOCS-box domain, by which they can associate an E3-ubiquitin-ligase complex that adds ubiquitin molecules to the SOCS-associated proteins, as JAK2 and GHR, to target them to proteasome degradation (Lanning & Carter-Su, 2006; Flores-Morales et al., 2006). SOCS-2 may also inhibit GH action indirectly, by limiting IGF1 signaling (Lanning & Carter-Su, 2006; Frutchman et al., 2005). Moreover, SOCS-2 was reported to target SOCS-3 for ubiquitination and protein degradation when it is associated to the signaling complex (Tannahill et al., 2005; Piessevaux et al., 2006), therefore contributing to cease the termination signal, and thus allow resensitization.

1.3 Therapeutical uses of GH

The use of growth hormone (GH) in clinical endocrine practice is expanding, and its role in the treatment of various clinical conditions is increasingly appreciated. GH has been used to treat children with GH deficiency (GHD) for more than 40 years. Human GH was originally obtained from cadaveric pituitaries and was available in limited quantities. From 1985, biosynthetic GH initially became available for prescription usage. Nowadays, human GH of recombinant DNA origin with an amino acid sequence identical to GH of pituitary origin is produced commercially by several pharmaceutical companies. These GH preparations contain minimal impurities, are apparently safe, and are readily available in unlimited supply. As a result, use of the hormone both in children and adults has expanded.

GH is used in children for the following pediatric conditions: growth hormone deficiency (GHD), Turner syndrome, chronic renal insufficiency, children born small for gestational age or intrauterine growth retardation, Prader-Willi syndrome and when the height deficit continues at puberty. GH is indicated in adult patients with growth hormone deficiency caused by pituitary disease from known causes, including pituitary tumor, pituitary surgical damage, hypothalamic disease, irradiation, trauma, and reconfirmed childhood GHD (Medical Guidelines for Clinical Practice for GH use in adults and children, American Association of Clinical Endocrinoloigists-2003 Update). GH usage has also been approved for the treatment of AIDS-related wasting.

In addition to the generally accepted therapeutic uses of human growth hormone, considerable interest exists in using GH treatment in various other conditions. The usefulness of GH treatment in adults who have completed their statural growth derives from the role of GH in the following processes: increasing bone density, increasing lean tissue, decreasing adipose tissue, strengthening cardiac contractility, recovering mood and motivation, increasing exercise capacity. Considering the anabolic actions of human growth hormone, it has become attractive as a potential agent for catabolic problems in a wide range of clinical conditions, including patients in an intensive care environment, burns, cystic fibrosis, inflammatory bowel disease, fertility alterations, osteoporosis, Down's syndrome, and also for people wishing to reverse the effects of ageing and to improve the athletic condition (Hadzović et al., 2004). These last two potential uses have received most attention as abuse of growth hormone. The definitions of the word abuse include "improper or excessive use." The classic form of "abuse" of human growth involves its use by athletes or bodybuilders to gain an unfair advantage over their competitors. The use of human growth hormone to increase the height of children who are already of normal height would also be considered abuse (Hintz, 2004). Another common form of use of human growth hormone outside the established indication is in its supposed action of diminishing or slowing the effects of ageing (Rudman et al., 1990). In addition to the lack of evidence for effectiveness of human growth hormone in these proposed uses, it causes side effects such as diabetes, carpal tunnel syndrome, fluid retention, joint and muscle pain and high blood pressure. Considering the increased incidence of leukemia and certain types of tumors reported in acromegalic patients, cancer onset is also a risk of GH use and abuse.

1.4 GH association with cancer development

Normal growth of a living organism depends on the rate of cell division and cell death. There is a strictly controlled balance between these processes. Organ and body size are determined by three fundamental processes: cell growth, cell division, and cell death, each regulated both by intracellular programs and by extracellular signaling molecules that control these programs. The cell decides its fate depending on the balance between survival and cell death which ensures that healthy functioning cells survive in appropriate environments while damaged or non-functioning cells are eliminated by programmed cell death (apoptosis). If this equilibrium is disturbed, one of two disorders might occur: the cells divide faster than they die which ultimately derives in tumor development or the cells divide slower than they die, which results in cell loss. One of the most important extracellular signaling molecules engaged in maintaining cell survival are the growth factors. When these proteins are overexpressed and when their receptors or signaling mediators are hyperactivated or overexpressed, cancer might arise.

The relevance of growth factors to the pathogenesis of human cancer has long been established. Several recent studies have suggested that, in addition to its effects on growth and metabolism, GH is involved in tumorigenesis and tumor progression. GH overexpression has been associated with cancer in animal models as well as in humans; indeed, acromegalic patients show an increased incidence of this pathology (Webb et al., 2002; Jenkins, 2004; Siegel & Tomer, 2005). Studies focusing on cancer incidence or cancer prevalence in acromegaly report 1.5 to 4-fold increased relative risk for acromegalic patients to develop tumors, mainly of the colon, breast, prostate, thyroid and hematological system (Siobhan & Shereen, 2008). However, as the main causes of death are cardiovascular and respiratory events, patients with uncontrolled acromegaly might succumb before developing recognizable cancer. On the contrary, a decreased incidence of cancer in the absence of growth hormone has been observed. In a worldwide survey of individuals with growth hormone deficiency or growth hormone receptor mutation, not even a single case of malignancy was reported, whereas first and second degree relatives reported a 10-24% incidence of malignancies (Brooks & Waters, 2010). Moreover, another study revealed that GHR deficiency in humans is associated with an important reduction of pro-ageing signaling, diabetes and cancer development (Guevara-Aguirre J, et al., 2011). Cancer risks of GH replacement therapy implies three possible situations: (1) tumor recurrence in children with previously treated cancer; (2) second neoplasms (SNs) in survivors of childhood cancer treated with GH; and (3) de-novo cancer in non-cancer patients treated with GH. The general evidence suggests no increased risk in case 1, but several and complex studies concluded that there is a very modest increase in cancer risk in treated GH-deficiency patients in situations 2 and 3 (Renehan & Brennan, 2008).

Concerning animal models, a large body of evidence has implicated GH with tumor progression. Absence or low GH levels are associated with reduced tendency to develop malignancies spontaneously (Anisimov, 2001; Ikeno et al., 2003) or in response to carcinogen administration (Styles et al., 1990; Pollak et al., 2001). For example, when nitrosomethylurea was administrated to GH-deficient dwarf rats, none of them developed tumors; however, when the tumorogenic drug was administrated to normal and GH-supplemented dwarf rats incidence and latency to tumor development was similar in both groups. Hormone replacement in these animals increased the tumor incidence towards normal levels, whereas discontinuation of GH treatment resulted in tumor regression (Shen et al., 2007). On the contrary, transgenic mice overexpressing GH are more susceptible to develop cancer and they have an increased incidence of hepatocellular carcinoma at advanced ages (Orian et al., 1990; Wanke et al., 1991; Snibson, 2002; Bartke, 2003).

2. Transgenic mice overexpressing growth hormone as a model to study the pre-neoplasic alterations induced by high GH levels

2.1 General characteristics of transgenic mice overexpressing GH

Transgenic technology allowed the genomic incorporation of heterologous GH genes (rat, human, ovine, bovine or human placental variant) under the control of different promoters, allowing the development of multiple lines of GH-transgenic mice. Mice that exhibit high levels of endogenous GH (pituitary mouse GH) were developed by transfection with the GH-releasing hormone (GHRH) gene (Bartke, 2003; Kopchick et al., 1999). Transgenic mice overexpressing GH have been extensively used to study the mechanisms of action of GH and as a model of acromegaly to investigate the effects of prolonged GH excess (Bollano et al., 2000; Colligan et al., 2002; Miquet et al., 2004; Dominici et al., 2005). Most of the GH-transgenic mice lines available were produced by standard microinjection techniques. Briefly, the DNA constructs (promoter fused to the coding sequences of GH gene) were injected in the male pronucleus of single cell embryos. Viable embryos were implanted into pseudopregnant females and the pregnancies were allowed to term. Offsprings positive for both integration and expression of the GH gene were used as founder animals for the development of individual transgenic lines. Mating of hemizygous transgenic males to normal females produced both normal and transgenic progeny, in approximately 1:1 ratio (McGrane et al., 1988, 1990; Bartke, 2003; Kopchick et al., 1999).

As the transgene is not controlled by its own promoter, GH is often expressed constitutively and in some cases ectopically, resulting in chronic exposure to high GH levels. The tissue and developmental stage expression of the GH transgene depends on the promoter used. For instance, genes under the control of the metallotionein I (MT) promoter are expressed in several tissues since fetal development, while the phosphoenolpyruvate carboxykinase (PEPCK) promoter leads to the expression of GH primarily in liver, kidney and adipose tissue just after birth. The expression of the transgene continues throughout the life of the animal and is not controlled by physiological mechanisms that modulate pituitary GH secretion (Mc Grane et al., 1988; McGrane et al., 1990; Kopchick et al., 1999; Bartke, 2003). The circulating GH levels vary depending on the transgenic line, but are usually extremely high and produce a consequent increase in IGF1 serum concentration (Kopchick et al., 1999).

Chronic overexpression of GH in transgenic mice leads to enhanced postnatal growth, achieving typically a 30-70% increase in adult body size compared to normal littermates, and in some lines transgenic mice almost double the size of their normal controls. Prolonged exposure to GH in these mice also leads to altered body composition, including reduced adiposity with increased lean body mass and organomegaly. Conditions of chronic elevation of GH, as seen in acromegaly, are often associated with hyperinsulinemia, insulin resistance and impaired glucose tolerance, which in some cases progress to diabetes; in fact, GH-transgenic mice have increased insulin levels with normoglycemia and insulin resistance. Prolonged exposure to high GH levels leads to several histo and physiopathological lesions in different organs in GH-transgenic mice, principally in the kidney, heart and liver (Quaife et al., 1989; Kopchick et al., 1999; Bartke et al., 2002; Bartke, 2003; Dominici et al., 2005).

The transgenic PEPCK-bGH line has been used to study the effects of prolonged exposure to high GH levels (McGrane et al., 1990; Valera et al., 1993; González et al., 2002; Dominici et al., 2005; Miquet et al., 2004). Transgenic mice present high GH and IGF1 serum levels, which result in an increment in both body and liver weight. While some organs are increased roughly in the proportion of the increase in body weight, the relative increase in liver weight is higher than the one observed for body weight, reflecting that transgenic mice exhibit hepatomegaly. Although transgenic mice displayed hyperinsulinemia, glucose levels were not altered, possibly reflecting a state of insulin resistance.

2.2 Hepatic alterations in GH-transgenic mice

As previously mentioned, chronic exposure to high GH levels in transgenic mice produces hepatomegaly. Studies performed in different lines of transgenic mice overexpressing GH revealed that the disproportional increase in liver size is due to hypertrophy and hyperplasia, with hepatocytes presenting morphological alterations such as large cellular and nuclear size, intranuclear inclusions and invaginations of nuclear membranes. Throughout lifespan, transgenic mice present high levels of hepatocellular replication, followed by the onset of hepatic inflammation, fibrosis and cirrhosis, which may derive in hepatocarcinoma at advanced ages. The preneoplasic liver pathology observed in the GH-overexpressing transgenic mice resembles that seen in human patients at high risk of developing liver cancer, which turns this animal model suitable for studies of hepatic cancer. The liver of GH-transgenic mice develops various degrees of necroinflammatory, cirrhotic, fibrotic and regenerative changes, all of which are factors known to predispose human individuals to hepatocarcinogenesis (Orian et al., 1989; 1990; Snibson et al., 1999; Snibson 2002; Bartke 2003). Moreover, high GH levels are observed in patients with liver conditions associated with increased risk of liver cancer (Hattori et al., 1992; Kratzsch et al., 1995). The liver lesions observed in GH overexpressing mice would not be attributed to the liver being one of the major sites of GH production in transgenic mice expressing heterologous GH genes because comparable abnormalities were observed in GH-releasing hormone trangenic mice, in which GH is homologous and secreted by the pituitary (Bartke, 2003). The increased susceptibility of transgenic mice overexpressing GH to develop liver cancer is believed to be a consequence of the direct action of GH in this organ rather than secondary to the elevated IGF1 levels. This is supported by the fact that IGF1 binding to hepatocytes is barely detectable (Barreca et al., 1992; Santos et al., 1994) and, moreover, IGF1 has been described to induce discrete metabolic effects and only a slight increase of DNA synthesis in liver (Hartmann et al., 1990; Kimura & Ogihara, 1998; Grunnet et al., 1999). Moreover, transgenic mice overexpressing IGF1 do not show the hepatic histopathological alterations observed in the liver of GH-overexpressing transgenic mice (Bartke, 2003).

3. Growth hormone signaling-pathways induced in liver of GH overexpressing transgenic mice

The JAK2/STAT5 signaling cascade is the principal signaling pathway activated by growth hormone. High continuous GH levels *in vivo* produce desensitization of this pathway in the liver. In both Mt-GHRH and PEPCK-bGH transgenic mice this desensitization was evidenced as a lack of activation after a massive stimulus with GH and no increase in the basal phosphorylation of STAT5, in spite of the very high GH concentration in their circulation (González et al., 2002; Miquet et al., 2004). This lack of response to GH was associated with elevated levels of the negative regulator CIS, a member of the family of suppressors of cytokine-signaling (SOCS) proteins, which is proposed to be a major factor responsible for the down-regulation of STAT5 signaling in the liver (Ram & Waxman, 2000; Landsman & Waxman, 2005).

The liver is one of the principal target organs of growth hormone, and GH overexpressing mice exhibit phenotypic characteristics that indicate GH is indeed acting in this tissue. For instance, absolute and relative liver weight is higher in GH-transgenic than in control mice, accompanied by pathological alterations in the liver (Orian et al., 1989; Quaife et al., 1989; Snibson, 2002; Bartke, 2003). Circulating levels of IGF1 and hepatic levels of IGF1 mRNA, which are primarily regulated by GH action in the liver, are increased in GH transgenic mice. Moreover, liver GHR expression is also increased, in accordance with the known ability of GH to upregulate its own receptor (Mathews et al. 1988; McGrane et al. 1990; González et al. 2001; Iida et al. 2004; González et al. 2007). As the JAK2/STAT5 signaling cascade is desensitized in the liver of GH-overexpressing mice, this pathway is probably not responsible for the proliferative effects of chronically elevated GH. Therefore, other signaling mediators induced by GH must be involved for the liver pathology observed in these animals. Studies performed in Mt-GHRH and PEPCK-bGH transgenic mice showed that these animals exhibit constitutive phosphorylation of STAT3 and upregulation of c-Src, FAK, EGFR, Akt, mTOR and Erk1/2 (Miquet et al., 2008). These molecules are all signaling mediators activated by GH that are involved in cell proliferation, differentiation, migration and survival, and their upregulation may represent alternative pathways to JAK2/STAT5 that are constitutively activated in the liver of transgenic mice overexpressing GH.

In several human cancers elevated protein levels and/or kinase activity of c-Src have been reported, and it was proposed that it could act by facilitating other signaling mediators action, including FAK and EGFR. A high proportion of breast cancers overexpress c-Src and members of the EGFR family, suggesting that they may interact to synergically promote cancer development and progression (Ishizawar & Parsons, 2004; Biscardi et al., 2000; Playford & Schaller, 2004). Importantly, EGFR upregulation was also found in hepatocellular carcinoma (Thomas & Zhu, 2005), and FAK overexpression was detected in several human tumor samples (Owens et al., 2005; Parsons, 2003; Ishizawar & Parsons, 2004; Playford & Schaller, 2004; Schlaepfer & Mitra, 2004). GH-transgenic mice show overexpression of c-Src, EGFR and FAK in liver, in accordance with the upregulation of these proteins that may be observed in human cancer (Miquet et al., 2008). Aberrant activation of STAT proteins is also related to cell transformation and oncogenesis. As mentioned before, GH-transgenic mice display increased basal activation of STAT3 in liver (Miquet et al., 2008). Constitutive activation of this protein has been found in many tumors with elevated activity of both c-Src and EGFR (Calò et al., 2003; Silva, 2004). Thus, higher STAT3 phosphorylation observed in transgenic mice, which also present elevated c-Src and EGFR levels, could be related to the increased kinase activity of c-Src they exhibit.

Akt is a crucial regulator of cellular proliferation, differentiation and metabolism, and has been implicated in the inhibition of apoptosis by several cytokines and growth factors. Akt is frequently activated or overexpressed in human cancers, probably cooperating with other oncogenic pathways to promote tumor progression by enhancing cell survival (Nicholson & Anderson, 2002). Signaling by the PI-3K/Akt/mTOR regulates mRNA translation, a crucial step for stimulation of protein synthesis (Proud, 2007). Altered mTOR signaling has been found in cancer, diabetes and obesity (Dann et al., 2007). Therefore, the upregulation of Akt and mTOR suggests that these kinases could contribute to the hepatic alterations transgenic mice exhibit. The MAP kinase proteins Erk1/2 are also involved in the control of the translational machinery and, thus, in the promotion of cell growth and proliferation (Proud, 2007). Erk1/2 were reported to be constitutively activated in many tumors and cancer derived cells (Chambard et al., 2007), so the increased levels of this kinase in transgenic mice liver could also contribute to the hepatic alterations observed.

Considering the well established association of the aforementioned signaling mediators with cancer, and taking into account their upregulation in the liver of GH-transgenic mice, it is reasonable to suggest that the described molecular alterations found in the liver of GH overexpressing transgenic mice may be implicated in the pathological alterations observed in these animals.

4. GH modulation of EGF signal

Among the growth factors and growth factor receptors that have been shown to be involved in the pathogenesis and progression of different carcinoma types is the epidermal growth factor (EGF) family of peptide growth factors and the EGF receptor (EGFR) (Ito et al., 2001; Normanno et al., 2001; 2006). EGF is a key regulatory factor in promoting cell proliferation and survival. Ligand binding to the receptor triggers several signaling pathways that activate different transcriptional programs in the nucleus which lead to the expression of proteins involved in cell cycle progression, apoptosis resistance, differentiation, adhesion, and cell migration.

4.1 The EGF family of receptors and EGF-induced signal transduction pathways

EGFR, also known as ErbB-1, belongs to a family of receptors, which comprises three additional proteins: ErbB-2, ErbB-3, and ErbB-4. These ErbB receptors are type I receptor tyrosine kinases that are activated by binding of growth factors of the EGF family. The ErbB receptors recognize different but structurally related growth factors and mediate processes in development, homeostasis and pathologies.

ErbB receptors consist of a heavily glycosylated and disulfide-bonded ectodomain that provides a ligand-binding site, a single transmembrane domain and a large cytoplasmatic region that encodes a tyrosine kinase and multiple phosphorylation sites. Upon ligand binding, the ErbB receptors form either homo or heterodimers (Jorissen et al., 2003). Except for certain constitutively active mutants, dimerization is induced by ligand binding and is essential for activation of their kinase domain. Dimerization and activation of the kinase domain results in trans-phosphorylation of the monomers. Subsequently, the activated receptor phosphorylates additional tyrosine residues on the C-terminal tail of the EGFR (Boeri Erba et al., 2005; Wu et al., 2006). Intracellular tyrosine kinases of the Src family such as c-Src and Abl are also capable of phosphorylating residues on the EGFR. Phosphorylated sites on the EGFR allow the association of proteins containing the Src homology 2 domain (SH2), like Grb2, Shc and Nck. These signaling mediators associate with additional proteins leading to their activation and the subsequent activation of other kinases or transcription factors. Post-receptor signaling by EGFR involves the activation of signaling pathways such as the MAPK Erk1/2 and p38, the PKC, the PI3K/Akt, and the STAT pathways (Jorissen et al., 2003; Henson & Gibson, 2006; Normanno et al., 2006). These signaling routes activate different transcriptional programs in the nucleus, leading to the expression of several genes involved in cell cycle progression, survival, differentiation, adhesion and migration.

As a consequence of ligand induced activation of the EGFR, it is endocytized and enters the endosomal pathway. In the absence of EGF stimulation, the receptor is recycled to the cell surface. On the contrary, after ligand binding, EGFR progresses from early to late endosomes and is subsequently degraded. EGFR was believed to trigger signal transduction pathways only when located at the cell membrane, however, recent studies suggest that signal is also propagated by internalized EGFR present in early or late endosomes (Burke et al., 2001). Moreover, it has been recently described that EGFR also acts at the nuclear level in response to stress and participates in cell proliferation and cell cycle and DNA repair processes (Dittmann et al., 2010).

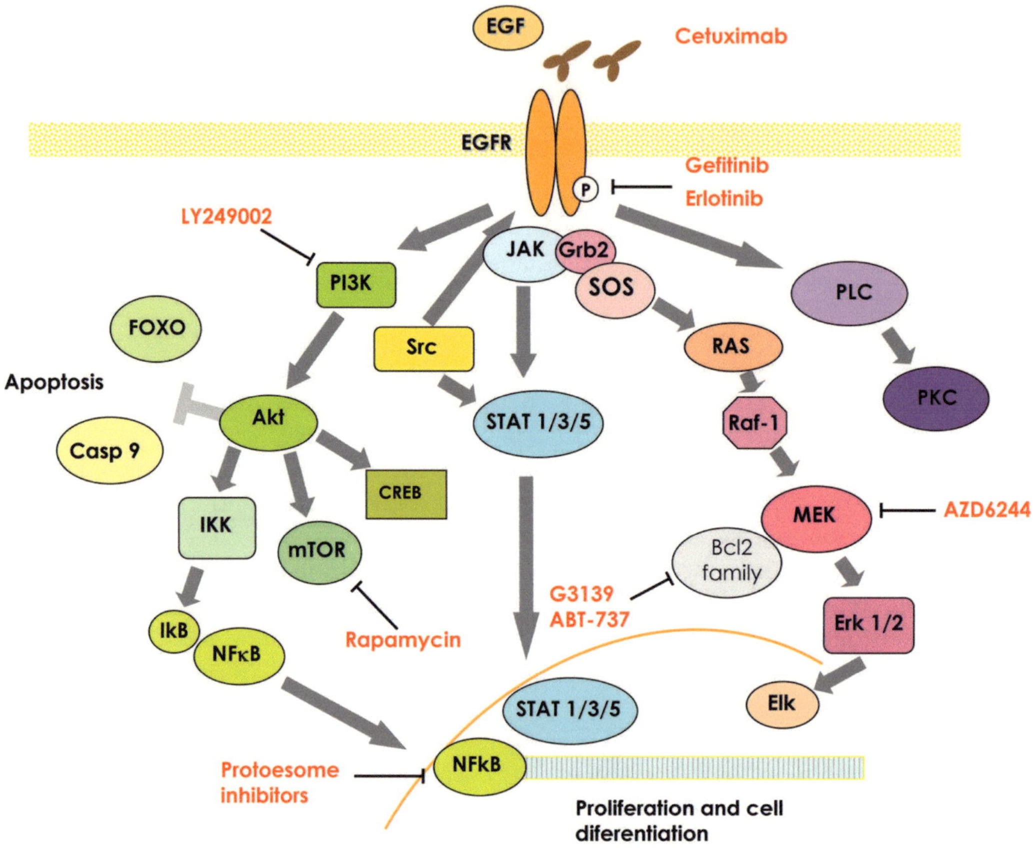

Fig. 2. Signal transduction pathways triggered by EGF.

4.2 EGFR and cancer

EGF receptor family members were first related to cancer in the early 1980s (Stoscheck et al., 1986). Since then, activation of EGFR has been implicated in the progression of different types of carcinomas (Ito et al., 2001; Normanno et al., 2001; 2006). The complexity of EGFR signal transduction and its importance for cell growth and survival explains the potential role of EGFR alterations in the development and maintenance of cancer. EGFR undergoes different alterations including gene amplification, structural rearrangements and somatic mutations in human carcinomas. In addition, some types of tumors produce an excess of EGF that leads to an increased activation of EGFR (Henson & Gibson, 2006). Besides the alterations in EGF receptor expression and ligand production, intracellular signaling cascades are often altered in cancer cells. All these alterations in EGF-mediated survival signaling can promote tumor processes like angiogenesis and metastasis and contribute to cancer progression and resistance to cancer therapies (Salomon et al., 1995). EGFR is overexpressed or hyperactivated in a variety of solid tumors, including colorectal cancer, non-small-cell lung cancer, squamous cell carcinoma of the head and neck, and also in ovarian, breast, liver, kidney, pancreatic and prostate cancer (Baselga, 2002; Lurje & Lenz, 2009). Moreover, aberrant EGFR expression or activity has been associated with disease progression, resistance to radiochemotherapy and poor survival.

Considering the relevance of EGFR and ErbB receptors for the development and progression of cancer, several anti-ErbB targeted therapies have been developed and are still under study. Specifically, ErbB1 or EGFR-targeted therapies can be classified into two major classes: the anti-EGFR monoclonal antibodies (MoAbs) and the EGFR–specific tyrosine kinase inhibitors (TKI). The anti-EGFR monoclonal antibodies, such as cetuximab, bind to the extracellular domain of the EGFR on the surface of tumor cells, thus preventing EGFR ligands from interacting and activating the receptor and ligand-induced internalization of the receptor. TKIs such as gefitinib and erlotinib block the binding of adenosine triphosphate (ATP) to the intracellular TK domain of the EGFR, which results in the inhibition of the tyrosine kinase activity of the receptor. Besides the drugs that target the EGFR itself, there is a second group of small molecular inhibitors that interfere with the activation of signaling mediators downstream the EGFR. Such molecules mainly target crucial proteins involved in the Ras/MEK/Erk and PI3K/Akt/mTOR pathways. Additionally, inhibitors of the transcriptional regulation of pro- and anti-apoptotic proteins are used. These molecules include proteosome inhibitors like BAY 11-7085, BAY 11-7082, soy isoflavone genistein, flavopiridol, which affect the NFκB signaling. Many of these substances are in various stages of clinical development and were proposed to be used in combination with standard chemotherapy (Lurje & Lenz, 2009). Antisense molecules that target the mRNA of the anti-apoptotic protein Bcl-2 like G3139 and Augmerosen interfere with pro-apoptotic pathways induced by EGF and could also be used as therapeutical agents. Moreover, peptides that mimic the BH3 only domain Bcl2 family members like ABT-737 interfere with anti-apoptotic pathways induced by EGF because they impede Bcl-2 association with pro-apoptotic Bcl-2 family members (Henson & Gibson, 2006).

4.3 EGFR and hepatocarcinoma (HCC)

Hepatocarcinoma (HCC) is a clear example of inflammation-related cancer because it mainly occurs in the context of persistent inflammation of the liver (Berasain et al., 2009). Indeed, the majority of HCCs slowly develop in a background of chronic hepatitis and cirrhosis, which are considered as preneoplastic conditions of the liver. A pro-inflammatory and proliferative microenvironment is a common feature of the preneoplastic liver regardless of the etiology. Upon tissue injury the liver triggers a defensive response to protect the organ and recover the lost parenchymal mass (Taub, 2004). This is a complex response that involves several cytokines and growth factors, among them the ErbB1 axis. Normal hepatocytes express high levels of EGFR, and EGFR ligands have a potent mitogenic effect on isolated or cultured hepatocytes. In the cases of acute and chronic liver injury and inflammation, the EGFR system plays an important role in liver regeneration and hepatocyte protection (Berasain et al., 2007). These pathological conditions are frequently associated with overexpression and overstimulation of the EGFR pathway (Berasain, 2009). Amplifications and mutations of the EGFR gene have been described in patients with HCC (Normanno et al., 2006) and sustained activation of EGFR was reported to induce the progression of HCC (Nalesnik et al., 1998; Ito et al., 2001). Moreover, pro-angiogenic roles of the EGFR have been described (Ueda et al., 2006). Currently, there are several studies in process concerning the use of anti-EGFR targeted therapies alone, or associated with other pharmacological agents, for the treatment of HCC (Berasain et al., 2007; Hu et al., 2011).

4.4 GH modulation of EGF signaling

EGF and GH signaling pathways share several signaling mediators. Both growth factors induce the JAK/STAT, MEK/Erk and PI3K/Akt pathways; however the degree in which each pathway is activated upon GH or EGF stimulus depends on the cell type and hormonal environment. In addition, GH regulates the expression of EGFR in the liver (Jansson et al., 1988, Johansson et al., 1989). Hypophysectomized and partially GH-deficient mutant mice showed reduced expression of the EGFR in liver (Johansson et al., 1989). When GH was administered to these animals, expression of the receptor was induced approaching EGFR levels found in normal controls (Johansson et al., 1989). Moreover, EGFR levels are increased in transgenic animals overexpressing GH, while its protein content is drastically diminished in mice lacking the GH receptor (GHR-KO mice) (Miquet et al., 2008; González et al., 2010).
GH has also been demonstrated to induce phosphorylation of the EGFR. EGFR phosphorylation at tyrosine residues 845, 992, 1068 and 1173 upon GH stimulation was described both in mice liver and in cell culture (Yamauchi et al., 1997; Kim et al. 1999, Huang et al., 2003). GH induced phosphorylation of the EGFR at tyrosine residue 1068 is mediated by JAK2 and allows Grb2 association and subsequent activation of Erk1/2 (Yamauchi et al., 1997). Another level of interaction between GH and EGF signaling involves GH-induced EGFR phosphorylation at threonine residues, which depends on Erk1/2 activity (Huang et al., 2004). Erk-dependent threonine phosphorylation of the EGFR reduces EGFR degradation, thus modulating EGFR trafficking and signaling (Frank, 2008).
Considering GH and EGF crosstalk and the relevance of EGFR in cancer, especially hepatocarcinoma, hepatic EGFR signaling was analyzed in two different *in vivo* models: GHR-KO mice, in which GH action is abolished, and the GH-transgenic mice. GHR-KO mice displayed diminished receptor activation due to EGFR down-regulation. Moreover, EGF-induced STAT5 and Erk1/2 phosphorylation was reduced in GHR-KO mice, while EGF did not activate STAT3 and Akt in these animals. On the other hand, overexpression of GH in transgenic mice induces EGFR up-regulation but this does not result in enhanced EGF signaling. Akt and Erk1/2 pathways showed diminished activation, while STAT3 and STAT5 activation was abrogated, indicating that GH differentially modulates EGF signaling pathways (González et al., 2010). The heterodesensitization produced by GH over EGF-induction of the STATs was related with diminished association between the EGFR and STAT3 or STAT5 in the liver from the GH-overexpressing transgenic mice. This suggested that recruitment of the STATs to activated EGFR might be inhibited. The increased association of STAT5 with SHP-2 phosphatase in transgenic mice could account for the observed desensitization of STAT5 signaling in this animal model, since this phosphatase is regarded as a negative regulator of STAT5 signaling (González et al., 2010).

5. Conclusion

Overexpression of GH has been associated with tumor promotion both in human and animal models. Chronic exposure to high GH levels induces hypertrophy and hyperplasia of hepatocytes, hepatic inflammation, fibrosis and even cirrhosis. These alterations comprise the preneoplastic liver pathology observed in the GH-overexpressing transgenic mice that might result in hepatocarcinoma at advance ages. Cancer cells show alterations in cytoskeletal organization, adhesion, motility, growth control and survival. Many of the signaling pathways implicated in these events are upregulated in the liver of mice that present high circulating levels of GH (Miquet et al., 2008) suggesting their role in the liver pathology observed in these animals. Overexpression and/or hyperactivation of these signaling mediators provide a molecular basis for the oncogenic potential of GH.

GH also modulates the expression and signaling of a growth factor receptor relevant for cancer development, the EGFR. The relevance of EGF-induced signaling cascades for tumor development should be further investigated to determine if the silencing of only certain signaling cascades, therefore altering the normal balance between mitogenic and apoptotic signals, might facilitate the onset of tumor.

6. References

Anisimov VN. 2001 Mutant and genetically modified mice as models for studying the relationship between aging and carcinogenesis. *Mech Ageing Dev.* 122: 1221-55.

Aoki N, Matsuda T. 2000 A cytosolic protein-tyrosine phosphatase PTP1B specifically dephosphorylates and deactivates prolactin-activated STAT5a and STAT5b. *J Biol Chem.* 275(50): 39718-26.

Argetsinger LS, Kouadio JL, Steen H, Stensballe A, Jensen ON, Carter-Su C. 2004 Autophosphorylation of JAK2 on tyrosines 221 and 570 regulates its activity. *Mol Cell Biol.* 24(11): 4955-67.

Argetsinger LS, Stuckey JA, Robertson SA, Koleva RI, Cline JM, Marto JA, Myers MG Jr, Carter-Su C. 2010 Tyrosines 868, 966, and 972 in the kinase domain of JAK2 are autophosphorylated and required for maximal JAK2 kinase activity. *Mol Endocrinol.* 24(5): 1062-76.

Barclay JL, Kerr LM, Arthur L, Rowland JE, Nelson CN, Ishikawa M, d'Aniello EM, White M, Noakes PG, Waters MJ. 2010 In vivo targeting of the growth hormone receptor (GHR) Box1 sequence demonstrates that the GHR does not signal exclusively through JAK2. *Mol Endocrinol.* 24(1): 204-17.

Barreca A, Voci A, Minuto F, de Marchis M, Cecchelli E, Fugassa E, Giordano G, Gallo G. 1992 Effect of epidermal growth factor on insulin-like growth factor-I (IGF- I) and IGF-binding protein synthesis by adult rat hepatocytes. *Mol Cell Endocrinol.* 84: 119-126.

Bartke A. 2003 Can growth hormone (GH) accelerate aging? Evidence from GH-transgenic mice. *Neuroendocrinology* 78: 210-216.

Bartke A, Brown-Borg H. 2004 Life extension in the dwarf mouse. *Curr Top Dev Biol.* 63: 189-225.

Bartke A, Chandrashekar V, Bailey B, Zaczek D, Turyn D. 2002 Consequences of growth hormone (GH) overexpression and GH resistance. *Neuropeptides.* 36(2-3): 201-208.

Baselga J. 2002 Why the epidermal growth factor receptor? The rationale for cancer therapy. *Oncologist.* 7 (suppl 4): 2-8.

Baumann G. 2001 Growth hormone bindingprotein 2001. *J Pediatr Endocrinol Metab.* 14(4): 355-75.

Berasain C, Castillo J, Prieto J, Avila MA. 2007 New molecular targets for hepatocellular carcinoma: the ErbB1 signaling system. *Liver International* 27(2): 174-85.

Berasain C, Perugorria MJ, Latasa MU, Castillo J, Goñi S, Santamaría M, Prieto J, Avila MA. 2009 The epidermal growth factor receptor: a link between inflammation and liver cancer. *Exp Biol Med (Maywood).* 234(7): 713-25.

Biscardi JS, Ishizawar RC, Silva CM, Parsons SJ. 2000 Tyrosine kinase signaling in breast cancer - Epidermal growth factor receptor and c-Src interactions in breast cancer. *Breast Cancer Res.* 2: 203-10.

Boeri Erba E, Bergatto E, Cabodi S, Silengo L, Tarone G, Defilippi P, Jensen ON. 2005 Systematic analysis of the epidermal growth factor receptor by mass spectrometry reveals stimulation-dependent multisite phosphorylation. *Mol Cell Proteomics.* 4: 1107-21.

Bollano E, Omerovic E, Bohlooly-y M, Kujacic V, Madhu B, Törnell J, Isaksson O, Soussi B, Schulze W, Fu ML, Matejka G, Waagstein F, Isgaard J. 2000 Impairment of cardiac function and bioenergetics in adult transgenic mice overexpressing the bovine growth hormone gene. *Endocrinology* 141(6): 2229-35.

Brooks AJ, Waters MJ. 2010 The growth hormone receptor: mechanism of activation and clinical implications. *Nature Rev Endocrinol.* 6: 515-25.

Brooks AJ, Wooh JW, Tunny KA, Waters MJ. 2008 Growth hormone receptor; mechanism of action. *Int J Biochem Cell Biol.* 40: 1984-89.

Brown RJ, Adams JJ, Pelekanos RA, Wan Y, McKinstry WJ, Palethorpe K, Seeber RM, Monks TA, Eidne KA, Parker MW, Waters MJ. 2005 Model for growth hormone receptor activation based on subunit rotation within a receptor dimer. *Nat Struct Mol Biol.* 12(9): 814-21.

Burke P, Schooler K, Wiley HS. 2001 Regulation of epidermal growth factor receptor signaling by endocytosis and intracellular trafficking. *Mol Biol Cell.* 12(6): 1897-1910.

Calò V, Migliavacca M, Bazan V, Macaluso M, Buscemi M, Gebbia N, Russo A. 2003 STAT proteins: From normal control of cellular events to tumorigenesis. *J Cell Physiol.* 197: 157-68.

Chambard JC, Lefloch R, Pouysségur J, Lenormand P. 2007 ERK implication in cell cycle regulation. *Biochim Biophys Acta.* 1773(8): 1299-310.

Colligan PB, Brown-Borg HM, Duan J, Ren BH, Ren J. 2002 Cardiac contractile function is enhanced in isolated ventricular myocytes from growth hormone transgenic mice. *J Endocrinol.* 73(2): 257-64

Conway-Campbell BL, Wooh JW, Brooks AJ, Gordon D, Brown RJ, Lichanska AM, Chin HS, Barton CL, Boyle GM, Parsons PG, Jans DA, Waters MJ. 2007 Nuclear targeting of the growth hormone receptor results in dysregulation of cell proliferation and tumorigenesis. *Proc Natl Acad Sci U S A.* 104(33): 13331-36.

Cowan JW, Wang X, Guan R, He K, Jiang J, Baumann G, Black RA, Wolfe MS, Frank SJ. 2005 Growth hormone receptor is a target for presenilin-dependent gamma-secretase cleavage. *J Biol Chem.* 280(19): 19331-42.

Dann SG, Selvaraj A, Thomas G. 2007 mTOR Complex1-S6K1 signaling: at the crossroads of obesity, diabetes and cancer. *Trends Mol Med.* 13(6): 252-59.

Dittmann K, Mayer C, Rodemann HP. 2010 Nuclear EGFR as novel therapeutic target: insights into nuclear translocation and function. *Strahlenther Onkol.* 186(1): 1-6.

Dominici FP, Argentino DP, Muñoz MC, Miquet JG, Sotelo AI, Turyn D. 2005 Influence of the crosstalk between growth hormone and insulin signalling on the modulation of insulin sensitivity. *Growth Horm IGF Res.* 15(5): 324-36.

Feng J, Witthuhn BA, Matsuda T, Kohlhuber F, Kerr IM, Ihle JN. 1997 Activation of Jak2 catalytic activity requires phosphorylation of Y1007 in the kinase activation loop. *Mol Cell Biol.* 17(5): 2497-501.

Flores-Morales A, Greenhalgh CJ, Norstedt G & Rico-Bautista E. 2006 Negative regulation of growth hormone receptor signaling. *Mol Endocrinol.* 20(2): 241-53.

Frank SJ. 2008 Mechanistic aspects of crosstalk between GH and PRL and ErbB receptor family signaling. *J Mammary Gland Biol Neoplasia.* 13(1): 119-29.

Fruchtman S, Simmons JG, Michaylira CZ, Miller ME, Greenhalgh CJ, Ney DM, Lund PK. 2005 Suppressor of cytokine signaling-2 modulates the fibrogenic actions of GH and IGF-I in intestinal mesenchymal cells. *Am J Physiol Gastrointest Liver Physiol.* 289(2): G342-50.

Goh EL, Zhu T, Yakar S, LeRoith D, Lobie PE. 2000 CrkII participation in the cellular effects of growth hormone and insulin-like growth factor-1. Phosphatidylinositol-3 kinase dependent and independent effects. *J Biol Chem.* 275(23): 17683-92.

González L, Curto LM, Miquet JG, Bartke A, Turyn D, Sotelo AI. 2007 Differential regulation of membrane associated-growth hormone binding protein (MA-GHBP) and growth hormone receptor (GHR) expression by growth hormone (GH) in mouse liver. *Growth Horm IGF Res.* 17(2): 104-12.

González L, Díaz ME, Miquet JG, Sotelo AI, Fernández D, Dominici FP, Bartke A and Turyn D. 2010 Growth hormone (GH) modulates hepatic epidermal growth factor (EGF) signaling in the mouse. *J Endocrinol.* 204: 299-309.

González L, Miquet JG, Sotelo AI, Bartke A & Turyn D. 2002 Cytokine-Inducible SH2 Protein Up-Regulation Is Associated with Desensitization of GH Signaling in GHRH-Transgenic Mice. *Endocrinology.* 143: 386-94.

González L, Sotelo AI, Bartke A, Turyn D. 2001 Growth hormone (GH) and estradiol regulation of membrane-associated GH binding protein and GH receptors in GH releasing hormone transgenic mice. *Growth Horm IGF Res.* 11(1): 34-40.

Grunnet N, Peng X, Tygstrup N. 1999 Growth factors and gene expression in cultured rat hepatocytes. *J Hepatol.* 31: 117-22.

Gu F, Dubé N, Kim JW, Cheng A, Ibarra-Sánchez MJ, Tremblay ML & Boisclair YR. 2003 Protein tyrosine phosphatase 1B attenuates growth hormone-mediated JAK2-STAT signaling. *Mol Cell Biol.* 23: 3753-62.

Hadzović A, Nakas-Ićindić E, Kucukalić-Selimović E, Salaka AU. 2004 Growth hormone (GH): usage and abuse. *Bosn J Basic Med Sci.* 4: 66-70.

Hartmann H, Schmitz F, Christ B, Jungermann K & Creutzfeldt W. 1990 Metabolic actions of insulin-like growth factor-I in cultured hepatocytes from adult rats. *Hepatology* 12: 1139-43.

Hattori N, Kurahachi H, Ikekubo K, Ishihara T, Moridera K, Hino M, Saiki Y, Imura H. 1992 Serum growth hormone-binding protein, insulin-like growth factor-I, and growth hormone in patients with liver cirrhosis. *Metabolism* 41(4): 377-81.

Henson ES, Gibson SB. 2006 Surviving cell death through epidermal growth factor (EGF) signal transduction pathways: implications for cancer therapy. *Cell Signal.* 18: 2089-97.

Hintz RL. 2004 Growth hormone: uses and abuses. *BMJ.* 328: 907-08.

Hu Y, Shen Y, Ji B, Wang L, Zhang Z, Zhang Y. 2011 Combinational RNAi gene therapy of hepatocellular carcinoma by targeting human EGFR and TERT. *Eur J Pharm Sci.* 42(4): 387-91.

Huang Y, Chang Y, Wang X, Jiang J, Frank SJ. 2004 Growth hormone alters epidermal growth factor receptor binding affinity via activation of extracellular signal-regulated kinases in 3T3-F442A cells. *Endocrinology.* 145: 3297-306.

Huang Y, Kim SO, Jiang J & Frank SJ. 2003 Growth hormone-induced phosphorylation of epidermal growth factor (EGF) receptor in 3T3-F442A cells. Modulation of EGF-induced trafficking and signaling. *J Biol Chem.* 278: 18902-13.

Iida K, del Rincon JP, Kim DS, Itoh E, Coschigano KT, Kopchick JJ, Thorner MO. 2004 Regulation of full-length and truncated growth hormone (GH) receptor by GH in tissues of lit/lit or bovine GH transgenic mice. *Am J Physiol Endocrinol Metab.* 287(3): E566-73.

Ikeno Y, Bronson RT, Hubbard GB, Lee S & Bartke A. 2003 Delayed occurrence of fatal neoplastic diseases in ames dwarf mice: correlation to extended longevity. *J Gerontol A Biol Sci Med Sci.* 58: 291-96.

Ishizawar R, Parsons SJ. 2004 c-Src and cooperating partners in human cancer. *Cancer Cell.* 6: 209-14.

Ito Y, Takeda T, Sakon M, Tsujimoto M, Higashiyama S, Noda K, Miyoshi E, Monden M, Matsuura N. 2001 Expression and clinical significance of erb-B receptor family in hepatocellular carcinoma. *Br J Cancer.* 84: 1377–83.

Jansson JO, Ekberg S, Hoath SB, Beamer WG & Frohman LA. 1988 Growth hormone enhances hepatic epidermal growth factor receptor concentration in mice. *J Clin Invest.* 82: 1871-76.

Jenkins PJ. 2004 Acromegaly and cancer. *Horm Res.* 62: 108-115.

Jin H, Lanning NJ, Carter-Su C. 2008 JAK2, but not Src family kinases, is required for STAT, ERK, and Akt signaling in response to growth hormone in preadipocytes and hepatoma cells. *Mol Endocrinol.* 22(8): 1825-41.

Johansson S, Husman B, Norstedt G, Andersson G. 1989 Growth hormone regulates the rodent hepatic epidermal growth factor receptor at a pretranslational level. *J Mol Endocrinol.* 3: 113-20.

Jørgensen JO, Rubeck KZ, Nielsen TS, Clasen BF, Vendelboe M, Hafstrøm TK, Madsen M, Lund S. 2010 Effects of GH in human muscle and fat. *Pediatr Nephrol.* 25(4): 705-709.

Jorissen RN, Walker F, Pouliot N, Garrett TP, Ward CW, Burgess AW. 2003 Epidermal growth factor receptor: mechanisms of activation and signalling. *Exp Cell Res.* 284: 31-53.

Kaplan SA, Cohen P. 2007 The somatomedin hypothesis 2007: 50 years later. *J Clin Endocrinol Metab.* 92(12): 4529-35.

Kim SO, Houtman JC, Jiang J, Ruppert JM, Bertics PJ, Frank SJ. 1999 Growth hormone-induced alteration in ErbB-2 phosphorylation status in 3T3-F442A fibroblasts. *J Biol Chem.* 274: 36015-24.

Kim SO, Jiang J, Yi W, Feng GS, Frank SJ. 1998 Involvement of the Src homology 2-containing tyrosine phosphatase SHP-2 in growth hormone signaling. *J Biol Chem.* 273(4): 2344-54.

Kimura M, Ogihara M. 1998 Effects of insulin-like growth factor I and II on DNA synthesis and proliferation in primary cultures of adult rat hepatocytes. *Eur J Pharmacol.* 354: 271-81.

Kofoed EM, Hwa V, Little B, Woods KA, Buckway CK, Tsubaki J, Pratt KL, Bezrodnik L, Jasper H, Tepper A, Heinrich JJ, Rosenfeld RG. 2003 Growth hormone insensitivity associated with a STAT5b mutation. *N Engl J Med.* 349(12): 1139-47.

Kopchick JJ, Bellush LL, Coschigano KT. 1999 Transgenic models of growth hormone action. *Annu Rev Nutr.* 19: 437-61.

Kratzsch J, Blum WF, Schenker E, Keller E. 1995 Regulation of growth hormone (GH), insulin-like growth factor (IGF)I, IGF binding proteins -1, -2, -3 and GH binding protein during progression of liver cirrhosis. *Exp Clin Endocrinol Diabetes.* 103(5): 285-91.

Kratzsch J, Selisko T, Birkenmeier G. 1996 Transformed alpha 2-macroglobulin as a low-affinity growth hormone-binding protein. *Acta Paediatr Suppl.* 417: 108-10.

Landsman T, Waxman DJ. 2005 Role of cytokine-induced SH2 domain-containing CIS in growth hormone receptor internalization. *J Biol Chem.* 280(45): 37471-80.

Lanning NJ, Carter-Su C. 2006 Recent advances in growth hormone signaling. *Rev Endocr Metab Disord.* 7: 225-235.

Lichanska AM, Waters MJ. 2008a New insights into growth hormone receptor function and clinical implications. *Horm Res.* 69(3): 138-45.

Lichanska AM, Waters MJ. 2008b How growth hormone controls growth, obesity and sexual dimorphism. *Trends Genet.* 24(1): 41-47.

Lobie PE, Sadir R, Graichen R, Mertani HC, Morel G. 1999 Caveolar internalization of growth hormone. *Exp Cell Res.* 246(1): 47-55.

Lurje G, Lenz H-J. 2009 EGFR signaling and drug discovery. *Oncology* 77: 400-410.

Mathews LS, Hammer RE, Brinster RL, Palmiter RD. 1988 Expression of insulin-like growth factor I in transgenic mice with elevated levels of growth hormone is correlated with growth. *Endocrinology* 123: 433-37.

McGrane MM, de Vente J, Yun J, Bloom J, Park E, Wynshaw-Boris A, Wagner T, Rottman FM, Hanson RW. 1988 Tissue-specific expression and dietary regulation of a chimeric phosphoenolpyruvate carboxykinase/bovine growth hormone gene in transgenic mice. *J Biol Chem.* 263(23): 11443-51.

McGrane MM, Yun JS, Moorman AF, Lamers WH, Hendrick GK, Arafah BM, Park EA, Wagner TE & Hanson RW. 1990 Metabolic effects of developmental, tissue-, and cell-specific expression of a chimeric phosphoenolpyruvate carboxykinase (GTP)/bovine growth hormone gene in transgenic mice. *J Biol Chem.* 265: 22371-79.

Medical Guidelines for Clinical Practice for GH use in adults and children, American Association of Clinical Endocrinoloigists-2003 Update.

Miquet JG, González L, Matos MN, Hansen C, Louis A, Bartke A, Turyn D, Sotelo AI. 2008 Transgenic mice overexpressing GH exhibit hepatic upregulation of GH-signaling mediators involved in cell proliferation. *J Endocrinol.* 198: 317-30.

Miquet JG, Sotelo AI, Bartke A, Turyn D. 2004 Suppression of growth hormone (GH) Janus tyrosine kinase 2/signal transducer and activator of transcription 5 signaling pathway in transgenic mice overexpressing bovine GH. *Endocrinology* 145: 2824-32.

Moutoussamy S, Renaudie F, Lago F, Kelly PA, Finidori J. 1998 Grb10 identified as a potential regulator of growth hormone (GH) signaling by cloning of GH receptor target proteins. *J Biol Chem*. 273(26): 15906-12.

Murphy JM, Tannahill GM, Hilton DJ, Greenhalgh CJ. 2010 The negative regulation of JAK/STAT signaling. Handbook of cell signaling, three volume set 2nd ed. Chapter 64 p467-480.

Nalesnik MA, Lee RG, Carr BI. 1998 Transforming growth factor alpha (TGFalpha) in hepatocellular carcinomas and adjacent hepatic parenchyma. *Hum Pathol*. 29(3): 228-34.

Nicholson KM, Anderson NG. 2002 The protein kinase B/Akt signaling pathway in human malignancy. *Cell Signal*. 14: 381-95.

Normanno N, Bianco C, De Luca A, Salomon DS. 2001 The role of EGF-related peptides in tumor growth. *Front Biosci.* 6: d685-d707.

Normanno N, De Luca A, Bianco C, Strizzi L, Mancino M, Maiello MR, Carotenuto A, De Feo G, Caponigro F, Salomon DS. 2006 Epidermal growth factor receptor (EGFR) signaling in cancer. *Gene*. 366: 2-16.

Orian JM, Lee CS, Weiss LM, Brandon MR. 1989 The expression of a metallothionein-ovine growth hormone fusion gene in transgenic mice does not impair fertility but results in pathological lesions in the liver. *Endocrinology* 124(1): 455-63.

Orian JM, Tamakoshi K, Mackay IR, Brandon MR. 1990 New murine model for hepatocellular carcinoma: transgenic mice expressing metallothionein-ovine growth hormone fusion gene. *J Natl Cancer Inst*. 82: 393-98.

Owens LV, Xu L, Craven RJ, Dent GA, Weiner TM, Kornberg L, Liu ET, Cance WG. 1995 Overexpression of the focal dhesion kinase (p125FAK) in invasive human tumors. *Cancer Res*. 55(13): 2752-55.

Parsons JT. 2003 Focal adhesion kinase: the first ten years. *J Cell Sci* 116: 1409-1416.

Pasquali C, Curchod M, Lchli S, Espanel X, Guerrier M, Arigoni F, Strous G, Hooft Van Huijsduijnen R. 2003 Identification of protein tyrosine phosphatases with specificity for the ligand-activated growth hormone receptor. *Mol Endocrinol*. 17(11): 2228–39.

Piessevaux J, Lavens D, Montoye T, Wauman J, Catteeuw D, Vandekerckhove J, Belsham D, Peelman F, Tavernier J. 2006 Functional cross-modulation between SOCS proteins can stimulate cytokine signaling. *J Biol Chem*. 281(44): 32953-66.

Perrini S, Laviola L, Carreira MC, Cignarelli A, Natalicchio A, Giorgino F. 2010 The GH/IGF1 axis and signaling pathways in the muscle and bone: mechanisms underlying age-related skeletal muscle wasting and osteoporosis. *J Endocrinol*. 205(3): 201-10.

Pilecka I, Patrignani C, Pescini R, Curchod ML, Perrin D, Xue Y, Yasenchak J, Clark A, Magnone MC, Zaratin P, Valenzuela D, Rommel C, Hooft van Huijsduijnen R. 2007 Protein-tyrosine phosphatase H1 controls growth hormone receptor signaling and systemic growth. *J Biol Chem*. 282(48): 35405-15.

Playford MP, Schaller MD. 2004 The interplay between Src and integrins in normal and tumor biology. *Oncogene* 23: 7928-46

Pollak M, Blouin MJ, Zhang JC, Kopchick JJ. 2001 Reduced mammary gland carcinogenesis in transgenic mice expressing a growth hormone antagonist. *Br J Cancer.* 85: 428-30.

Proud CG. 2007 Signalling to translation: how signal transduction pathways control the protein synthetic machinery. *Biochem. J.* 103: 217-34.

Quaife CJ, Mathews LS, Pinkert CA, Hammer RE, Brinster RL, Palmiter RD. 1989 Histopathology associated with elevated levels of growth hormone and insulin-like growth factor I in transgenic mice. *Endocrinology* 124: 40-48.

Ram PA, Waxman DJ. 2000 Role of the cytokine-inducible SH2 protein CIS in desensitization of STAT5b signaling by continuous growth hormone. *J Biol Chem.* 275: 39487-96.

Renehan AG, Brennan BM. 2008 Acromegaly, growth hormone and cancer risk. *Best Pract Res Clin Endocrinol Metab.* 4: 639-57.

Rosenfeld RG, Hwa V. 2009 The growth hormone cascade and its role in mammalian growth. *Horm Res.* 71 Suppl 2: 36-40.

Rosenfeld RG, Kofoed E, Buckway C, Little B, Woods KA, Tsubaki J, Pratt KA, Bezrodnik L, Jasper H, Tepper A, Heinrich JJ, Hwa V. 2005 Identification of the first patient with a confirmed mutation of the JAK-STAT system. *Pediatr Nephrol.* 20(3): 303-05.

Rowland JE, Lichanska AM, Kerr LM, White M, d'Aniello EM, Maher SL, Brown R, Teasdale RD, Noakes PG, Waters MJ. 2005 In vivo analysis of growth hormone receptor signaling domains and their associated transcripts. *Mol Cell Biol.* 25(1): 66-77. Erratum in: *Mol Cell Biol.* 2005 25(5): 2072.

Rowlinson SW, Yoshizato H, Barclay JL, Brooks AJ, Behncken SN, Kerr LM, Millard K, Palethorpe K, Nielsen K, Clyde-Smith J, Hancock JF, Waters MJ. 2008 An agonist-induced conformational change in the growth hormone receptor determines the choice of signalling pathway. *Nat Cell Biol.* 10(6): 740-47.

Rudman D, Feller AG, Nagraj HS Gergans GA, Lalitha PY, Goldberg AF, Schlenker RA, Cohn L, Rudman IW, Mattson DE. 1990 Effects of human GH in men over 60 years old. *N Engl J Med.* 323: 1-6.

Sachse M, van Kerkhof P, Strous GJ, Klumperman J. 2001 The ubiquitin-dependent endocytosis motif is required for efficient incorporation of growth hormone receptor in clathrin-coated pits, but not clathrin-coated lattices. *J Cell Sci.* 114(Pt 21): 3943-52.

Salomon DS, Brandt R, Ciardiello F, Normanno N. 1995 Epidermal growth factor-related peptides and their receptors inhuman malignancies. *Crit Rev Oncol Hematol.* 19: 183-32.

Santos A, Yusta B, Fernandez-Moreno MD, Blazquez E. 1994 Expression of insulin-like growth factor-I (IGF-I) receptor gene in rat brain and liver during development and in regenerating adult rat liver. *Mol Cell Endocrinol.* 101: 85-93.

Schlaepfer DD, Mitra SK. 2004 Multiple connections linf FAK to cell motility and invasion. *Curr Opin Genet Dev.* 14: 92-101.

Shen Q, Lantvit DD, Lin Q, Li Y, Christov K, Wang Z, Unterman TG, Mehta RG, Swanson SM. 2007 Advanced rat mammary cancers are growth hormone dependent. *Endocrinology* 148(10): 4536-44.

Siegel G & Tomer Y. 2005 Is there an association between acromegaly and thyroid carcinoma? A critical review of the literature. *Endocr Res.* 31: 51-58.

Silva CM. 2004 Role of STATs as downstream signal trasducers in Src family kinase-mediated tumorigenesis. *Oncogene* 23: 8017-23.

Siobhan L, Shereen E. 2008 Acromegaly: Re-thinking the cancer risk. *Rev Endocr Metab Disord.* 9: 41-58.

Snibson KJ. 2002 Hepatocellular kinetics and the expression of growth hormone (GH) in the livers and liver tumours of GH-transgenic mice. *Tissue Cell.* 34: 88-97.

Snibson KJ, Bhatal PS, Hardy CL, Brandon MR, Adams TE. 1999 High persistent hepatocellular proliferation and apoptosis precede hepatocarcinogenesis in growth hormone transgenic mice. *Liver* 19(3): 242-52.

Stofega MR, Herrington J, Billestrup N, Carter Su C. 2000 Mutation of the SHP-2 binding site in growth hormone (GH) receptor prolongs GH-promoted tyrosil phophorylation of GH receptor, JAK2 and STAT5B. *Mol Endocrinol.* 14: 1338-50.

Stoscheck CM, King LE Jr. 1986 Functional and structural characteristics of EGF and its receptor and their relationship to transforming proteins. *J Cell Biochem.* 31(2): 135-52.

Styles JA, Kelly MD, Pritchard NR, Foster JR. 1990 Effects produced by the non-genotoxic hepatocarcinogen methylclofenapate in dwarf mice: peroxisome induction uncoupled from DNA synthesis and nuclearity changes. *Carcinogenesis* 3: 387-91.

Tannahill GM, Elliott J, Barry AC, Hibbert L, Cacalano NA, Johnston JA. 2005 SOCS2 can enhance interleukin-2 (IL-2) and IL-3 signaling by accelerating SOCS3 degradation. *Mol Cell Biol.* 25: 9115-26.

Taub R. 2004 Liver regeneration: from myth to mechanism. *Nat Rev Mol Cell Biol.* 5(10): 836-47.

Tiong TS, Herington AC. 1992 Ontogeny of messenger RNA for the rat growth hormone receptor and serum binding protein. *Mol Cell Endocrinol.* 83(2-3): 133-41.

Tollet-Egnell P, Flores-Morales A, Stavréus-Evers A, Sahlin L, Norstedt G. 1999 Growth hormone regulation of SOCS-2, SOCS-3, and CIS messenger ribonucleic acid expression in the rat. *Endocrinology* 140(8): 3693-704.

Tritos NA, Biller BM. 2009 Growth hormone and bone. *Curr Opin Endocrinol Diabetes Obes.* 16(6): 415-22.

Turyn D, Sotelo AI. 2004 "Hormona de crecimiento", in "Hipófisis: fisiopatología", Stalldecker G. Ed. Midiciencia, Ch. 5, p. 91-114, ISBN 987-21376-1-7

Udy GB, Towers RP, Snell RG, Wilkins RJ, Park SH, Ram PA, Waxman DJ, Davey HW. 1997 Requirement of STAT5b for sexual dimorphism of body growth rates and liver gene expression. *Proc Natl Acad Sci U S A.* 94(14): 7239-44.

Ueda S, Basaki Y, Yoshie M, Ogawa K, Sakisaka S, Kuwano M, Ono M. 2006 PTEN/Akt signaling through epidermal growth factor receptor is prerequisite for angiogenesis by hepatocellular carcinoma cells that is susceptible to inhibition by gefitinib. *Cancer Res.* 66(10): 5346-53.

Valera A, Rodriguez-Gil JE, Yun JS, McGrane MM, Hanson RW, Bosch F. 1993 Glucose metabolism in transgenic mice containing a chimeric P-enolpyruvate carboxykinase/bovine growth hormone gene. *FASEB J.* 7(9): 791-800.

van Kerkhof P, Putters J, Strous GJ. 2007 The ubiquitin ligase SCF(betaTrCP) regulates the degradation of the growth hormone receptor. *J Biol Chem.* 282(28): 20475-83.

Vijayakumar A, Novosyadlyy R, Wu Y, Yakar S, LeRoith D. 2010 Biological effects of growth hormone on carbohydrate and lipid metabolism. *Growth Horm IGF Res.* 20(1): 1-7.

Wang X, He K, Gerhart M, Huang Y, Jiang J, Paxton RJ, Yang S, Lu C, Menon RK, Black RA, Baumann G, Frank SJ. 2002 Metalloprotease-mediated GH receptor proteolysis and GHBP shedding. Determination of extracellular domain stem region cleavage site. *J Biol Chem.* 277(52): 50510-19.

Wang X, Yang N, Deng L, Li X, Jiang J, Gan Y, Frank SJ. 2009 Interruption of growth hormone signaling via SHC and ERK in 3T3-F442A preadipocytes upon knockdown of insulin receptor substrate-1. *Mol Endocrinol.* 23(4): 486-96.

Wanke R, Hermanns W, Folger S, Wolf E, Brem G. 1991 Accelerated growth and visceral lesions in transgenic mice expressing foreign genes of the growth hormone family: an overview. *Pediatr Nephrol.* 5: 513-21.

Webb SM, Casanueva F, Wass JA. 2002 Oncological complications of excess GH in acromegaly. *Pituitary.* 5: 21-25.

Woelfle J, Rotwein P. 2004 In vivo regulation of growth hormone-stimulated gene transcription by STAT5b. *Am J Physiol Endocrinol Metab.* 286:E393–E401.

Woelfle J, Billiard J, Rotwein P. 2003a Acute control of insulin-like growth factor-I gene transcription by growth hormone through Stat5b. *J Biol Chem.* 278(25): 22696-702.

Woelfle J, Chia DJ, Rotwein P. 2003b Mechanisms of growth hormone (GH) action. Identification of conserved Stat5 binding sites that mediate GH-induced insulin-like growth factor-I gene activation. *J Biol Chem.* 278(51): 51261-66.

Woelfle J, Rotwein P. 2004 In vivo regulation of growth hormone-stimulated gene transcription by STAT5b. *Am J Physiol Endocrinol Metab.* 286(3): E393-401.

Wu SL, Kim J, Bandle RW, Liotta L, Petricoin E, Karger BL. 2006 Dynamic profiling of the post-translational modifications and interaction partners of epidermal growth factor receptor signaling after stimulation by epidermal growth factor using Extended Range Proteomic Analysis (ERPA). *Mol Cell Proteomics.* 9: 1610-27.

Yamauchi T, Ueki K, Tobe K, Tamemoto H, Sekine N, Wada M, Honjo M, Takahashi M, Takahashi T, Hirai H. 1997 Tyrosine phosphorylation of the EGF receptor by the kinase Jak2 is induced by growth hormone. *Nature* 390: 91-96.

Yamauchi T, Ueki K, Tobe K, Tamemoto H, Sekine N, Wada M, Honjo M, Takahashi M, Takahashi T, Hirai H, Tsushima T, Akanuma Y, Fujita T, Komuro I, Yazaki Y, Kadowaki T. 1998 Growth hormone-induced tyrosine phosphorylation of EGF receptor as an essential element leading to MAP kinase activation and gene expression. *Endocr J. Suppl* S27-31.

Zhang Y, Guan R, Jiang J, Kopchick JJ, Black RA, Baumann G, Frank SJ. 2001 Growth hormone (GH)-induced dimerization inhibits phorbol ester-stimulated GH receptor proteolysis. *J Biol Chem.* 276(27): 24565-73.

Zhang Y, Jiang J, Black RA, Baumann G, Frank SJ. 2000 Tumor necrosis factor-alpha converting enzyme (TACE) is a growth hormone binding protein (GHBP) sheddase: the metalloprotease TACE/ADAM-17 is critical for (PMA-induced) GH receptor proteolysis and GHBP generation. *Endocrinology* 141(12): 4342-48.

Zhu T, Goh EL, Graichen R, Ling L, Lobie PE. 2001 Signal transduction via the growth hormone receptor. *Cell Signal.* 13: 599–16.

Zhu T, Ling L, Lobie PE. 2002 Identification of a JAK2-independent pathway regulating growth hormone (GH)-stimulated p44/42 mitogen-activated protein kinase activity. GH activation of Ral and phospholipase D is Src-dependent. *J Biol Chem.* 277(47): 45592-603.

Part 3

The Thyroid Gland

5

Negative Regulation of the Thyrotropin β Gene by Thyroid Hormone

Shigekazu Sasaki, Akio Matsushita and Hirotoshi Nakamura
Second Division of Internal Medicine
Hamamatsu University School of Medicine
Japan

1. Introduction

Thyroid hormone (T3 and T4) is secreted from the thyroid gland, and is known to reduce the level of serum thyrotropin (thyroid-stimulating hormone, TSH) in the pituitary gland (Sarapura et al., 2002; Shupnik et al., 1989) (Fig. 1A). This is a typical example of negative feedback between the pituitary and endocrine organs, and is a key component of thyroid hormone homeostasis. TSH is one of the peptide hormones generated in the anterior pituitary, and is a heterodimer composed of an α chain (α-glycoprotein subunit, αGSU) and a β chain (TSHβ) (Shupnik et al., 1989). While αGSU is common to follicle stimulating hormone (FSH), luteinizing hormone (LH) and chorionic gonadotropin (CG), TSHβ is specific to TSH alone. Although the concentration of serum T4 is much higher than that of T3, T4 is converted to T3 by deiodinase (Dio) in the TSH-producing cells (thyrotrophs) of the pituitary (Christoffolete et al., 2006), and T3 exhibits biological activity as a thyroid hormone (Gereben et al., 2008). T3 inhibits expression of both *TSHβ* and *αGSU* at the transcriptional level (Shupnik et al., 1989). The magnitude of T3-induced repression of the *TSHβ* gene is greater than that of *αGSU*. Here, we provide an overview of the molecular mechanisms involved in T3-induced negative regulation of the *TSHβ* gene and its related genes.

2. Structure of T3 receptors (TRs)

T3 receptor (TR) belongs to the nuclear hormone receptor (NHR) superfamily, and is a ligand-dependent transcription factor (Cheng et al., 2010). TR is encoded by two separate alleles; *TRα* and *TRβ*. Through alternative splicing, the *TRα* gene generates TRα1 and TRα2, while the *TRβ* gene generates TRβ1 and TRβ2 (Fig. 2). While TRα1, TRβ1 and TRβ2 have T3-binding capacity, TRα2 does not bind T3. Hence, TRα1, TRβ1 and TRβ2 are thought to be the functional TRs. TRβ2 is expressed in limited organs including pituitary, hypothalamus and retina, while TRα1 and TRβ1 are ubiquitously expressed (Cheng et al., 2010). As in the case of other NHRs, TR consists of an N-terminal region (NTD), a central DNA binding domain (DBD), a hinge region and a C-terminal ligand binding domain (LBD) (Fig. 2).

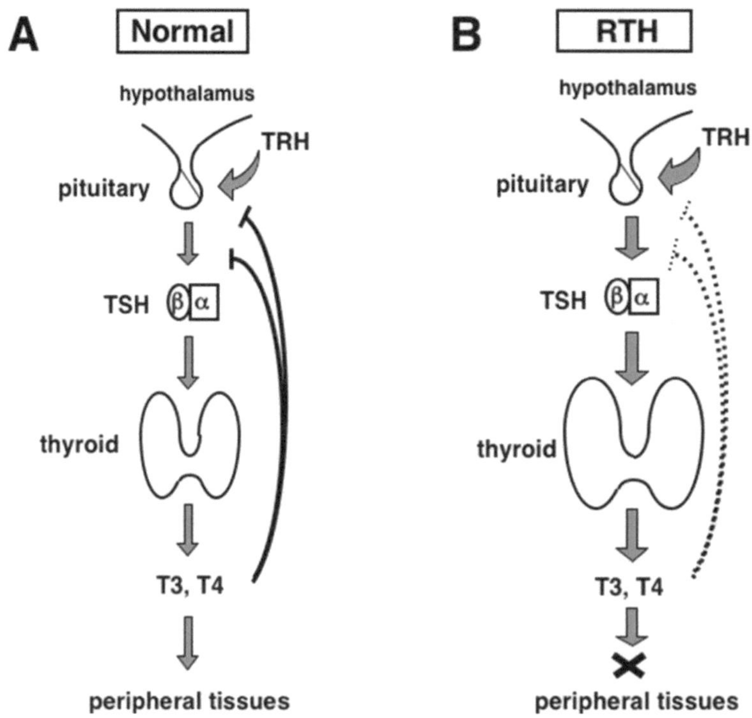

Fig. 1. Negative feedback loop in the hypothalamus-pituitary-thyroid axis and negative regulation of *TSHβ* and *αGSU*. A. The secretion of TSH (a heterodimer of TSHβ and αGSU subunits) in the anterior pituitary and TRH in the hypothalamus is inhibited by thyroid hormones (T3 and T4). β, TSHβ chain. α, αGSU chain. TRH, thyrotropin releasing hormone. Synthesis of TRH in hypothalamus is also negatively regulated by T3. B. In patients resistant to thyroid hormone (RTH), a negative feedback loop is impaired due to a defect in T3 receptor (TR) β. This finding provides the evidence for the involvement of TRβ in the negative regulation of the *TSHβ and αGSU* genes. Because of increased secretion of TSH, difuse goiters are often found in the patient with RTH.

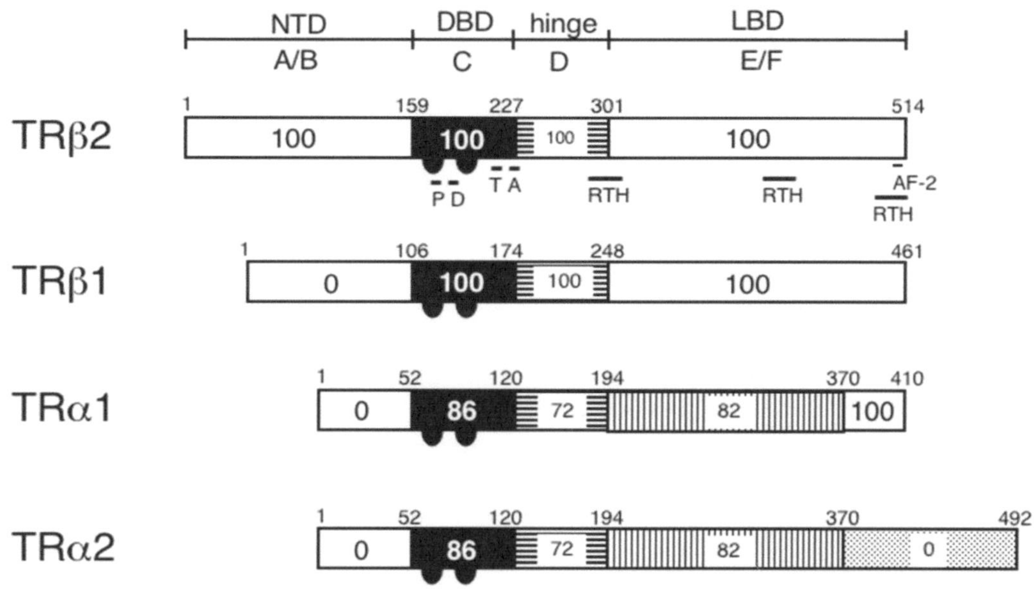

Fig. 2. Schematic representations of TR isoforms. TR consists of an N-terminal region (NTD, A/B domain), a central DNA-binding domain (DBD, C domain), a hinge region (D domain) and a C-terminal ligand binding domain (LBD, E/F domain). The numbers within the box represent the amino acid homology (%). While TRα1, TRβ1 and TRβ2 have T3-binding capacity, TRα2 does not bind T3. The P and D boxes are required for the recognition of half-site sequences (typically, AGGTCA) and the number of spacing nucleotides, respectively. The T and A boxes are involved in dimer formation and polarity of TR-RXR heterodimers on positive TRE (pTRE). P, Pbox. D, D box. T, Tbox. A, A box. RTH, three hot spots where mutations are frequently found in patients with RTH. AF-2, activation function 2.

3. Mechanism of positive regulation by T3

TR activates or inhibits the transcription of its target genes in a T3-dependent manner, and the molecular mechanism of T3-dependent activation (positive regulation) has been elucidated (Cheng et al., 2010) (Fig3A). Because findings in molecular mechanisms of positive regulation by T3 have greatly influenced the studies of negative regulation, it is necessary to outline the mechanism of T3-dependent positive regulation (Fig. 3A) before describing the negative regulation of the TSHβ gene (Fig. 3B). In the positive regulation, TR heterodimerizes with retinoid X receptor (RXR) at the T3-responsive element (TRE) of the gene, the transcription of which is positively regulated by T3-bound TR (T3/TR) (Cheng et al., 2010). In the absence of T3, TR-RXR heterodimers interact with co-repressors, including nuclear receptor co-repressor (NCoR) or silencing mediator for retinoid and thyroid hormone receptors (SMRT). These co-repressors recruit histone deacetylase (HDAC), which represses the transcription of the target genes. This repressive effect by unliganded TR is referred to as "silencing" and is thought to play an important role in the clinical symptoms in hypothyroidism (Astapova et al., 2008; Astapova et al., 2011). Upon T3 binding, the TR-RXR heterodimers release NCoR or SMRT and then recruit p160 family cofactors including steroid receptor coactivator-1 (SRC-1). The TR-RXR-p160 complex also recruits an additional coactivator, CBP/p300 (Chen et al., 1999; Glass and Rosenfeld, 2000; Huang et al., 2003). Both the p160 family and CBP/p300 have intrinsic histone acetyltransferase (HAT) activity and modify chromatin structure, resulting in the transactivation of the target genes (Fig. 3A).

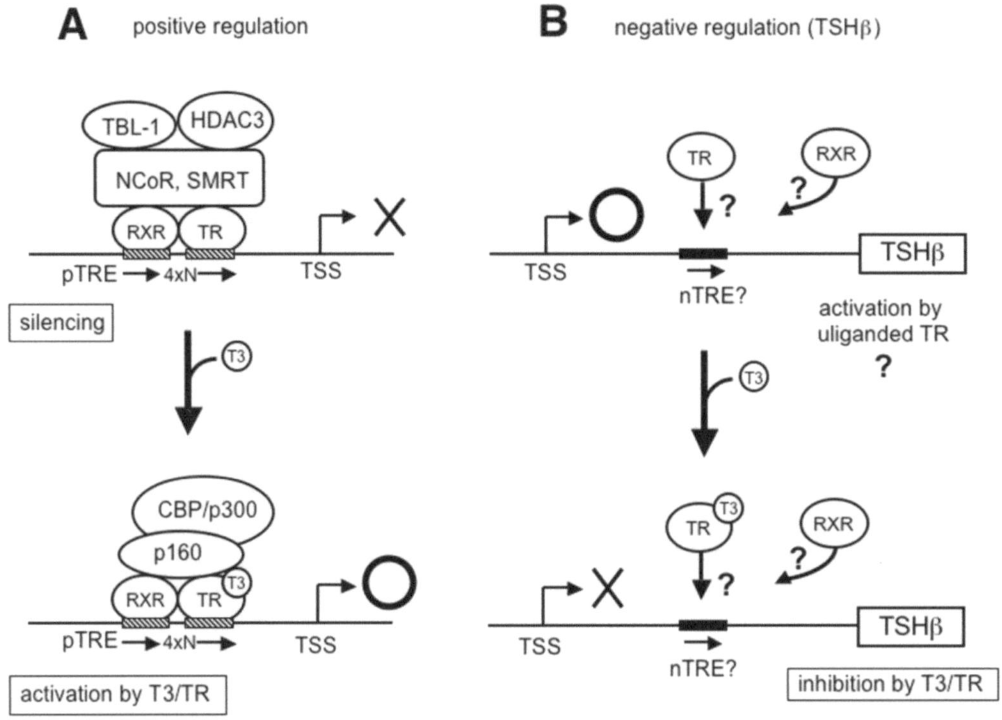

Fig. 3. Schematic representation of T3-dependent transactivation (positive regulation) (A) and transrepression (negative regulation) of the *TSHβ* gene (B). A. TR heterodimerizes with retinoid X receptor (RXR) on the T3-responsive element (TRE) of the gene, the transcription of which is positively regulated by T3-bound TR (T3/TR). Arrow, half-site sequence (typically, AGGTCA). 4xN, random four nucleotides for spacing. B. An nTRE (GGGTCA) has been postulated in the region immediately downstream to the transcription start site (TSS) of the *TSHβ* gene. In contrast to the mechanism for positive regulation, the molecular mechanism of negative regulation has been controversial (see text).

As shown in Fig. 3A, a typical TRE has a unique configuration designated as direct repeat 4 (DR4), in which the random four base pairs (spacer) are incorporated into tandem repeats of a hexameric half-site (Cheng et al., 2010; Umesono et al., 1991). Both the half-site sequence (typically AGGTCA) and the number of spacer nucleotides determine the specificity for DNA recognition by the TR-RXR heterodimer. Analogous to TR-RXR heterodimer binding at DR4, RXR heterodimerizes with vitamin D3 receptor (VDR) on direct repeats of half-sites spaced with 3 nucleotides (DR3) and it functions as a heterodimer partner for retinoic acid receptor (RAR) on direct repeats spaced with 5 nucleotides (DR5) (Cheng et al., 2010; Glass and Rosenfeld, 2000). In the studies of positive regulation by T3, monkey kidney-derived CV1 cells (Jensen et al., 1964) have been often used (Naar et al., 1991; Tillman et al., 1993; Umesono et al., 1991) because they possess endogenous RXR but not TR.

4. Involvement of TR in negative regulation of the *TSHβ* gene: Syndrome of thyroid hormone resistance (RTH)

Although the molecular mechanism in negative regulation of the *TSHβ* gene has been disputed (Lazar, 2003; Shupnik, 2000; Weitzel, 2008), it is apparent that TR plays a crucial role in it. Syndrome of resistance to thyroid hormone (RTH) is characterized by a reduced tissue response to T3 (Fig. 1B). The majority of patients with RTH have mutations in the LBD of the *TRβ* gene, of which amino acid sequence is shared by TRβ1 and TRβ2 proteins (Refetoff et al., 1993) (Fig. 2). These mutant TRβ1s and TRβ2s have defects in their T3-binding capacity but have intact DBDs capable of recognizing the TRE (Fig. 3A). Thus, they bind to the TRE and constitutively interact with NCoR or SMRT, even in the presence of T3, resulting in silencing. In the majority of patients with RTH, inheritance is usually autosomal dominant, and mutant *TRβ* is thought to interfere with T3-induced activation by wild-type TR bound to the TRE (dominant negative effect). Of note, patients with RTH also exhibit elevated secretion of TSH (syndrome of inappropriate secretion of TSH, SITSH) (Refetoff et al., 1993) (Fig. 1B). This finding provides evidence for the involvement of *TRβ* in the negative regulation of the *TSHβ and αGSU* genes. However, the mechanism downstream to TR has been unknown (Lazar, 2003; Shupnik, 2000; Weitzel, 2008). With regard to the mechanism of negative regulation of *TSHβ* and *αGSU*, the central question has been whether TR directly interacts and recognizes the DNA sequence of the *TSHβ* promoter, as identified for the TRE in positive regulation. Some theories indicate the direct binding of TR with DNA, while others favor models that are independent of a direct binding with DNA.

5. Direct binding of TR with DNA: Negative TRE (nTRE) hypothesis

Following the identification of the role of the TRE in the positive regulation of genes (hereafter, positive TRE, pTRE), some researchers have postulated a so-called negative TRE (nTRE) in the *TSHβ* (Fig. 3B) and *αGSU* genes (Chin et al., 1993; Shupnik, 2000; Wondisford et al., 1989). The observation that serum TSH levels increase in hypothyroidism led to the idea that unliganded TR may be the transcriptional activator for *TSHβ* (Fig. 3B, upper panel) and *αGSU*. If unliganded TR is the transcriptional activator on the nTRE of these genes, one may able to identify the nTRE as the sequence required for the transcriptional activation by unliganded TR. Based on this hypothesis, deletion analysis of the *TSHβ* promoter was performed using human kidney-derived 293 cells (Wondisford et al., 1989) and it was reported that the transcriptional activity of the this promoter was abolished after deletion of a short DNA sequence immediately downstream to the transcription start site (TSS) (Wondisford et al., 1989) (Fig. 4). This sequence (GGGTCA) has been postulated as the nTRE because it has homology with the consensus sequence of a half-site (AGGTCA). The nTRE hypothesis has been regarded as one of the principal models to explain the molecular mechanism of negative regulation of the *TSHβ* gene (Chin et al., 1993; Cohen and Wondisford, 2005), and has been regarded as a potential mechanism of T3-dependent negative regulation of other genes (Edwards et al., 1994; Kim et al., 2005; Lin et al., 2000; Santos et al., 2006; Wright et al., 1999). However, this raised several questions, as discussed below.

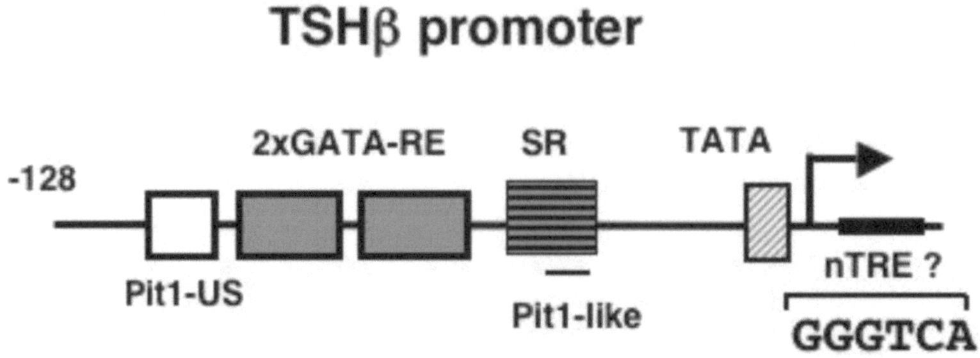

Fig. 4. Schematic representation of the *TSHβ* promoter. Pit1-US, functional Pit1-binding site. GATA-TRE, GATA-responsive element. SR, suppressor region. Pit1-like, the sequence similar to Pit1-binding site. TATA. TATA box. An nTRE (GGGTCA) has been postulated immediately downstream to the TSS.

5.1 Does TR heterodimerize with RXR on the nTRE?

While RXR is the obligate heterodimer partner for TR recognition of the pTRE (Fig. 3A), the involvement of RXR with the nTRE has not been determined (Fig. 3B). Although the nTRE sequence appears to be a single half-site, there remains the possibility that its flanking sequences may function as another half-site (Fig. 3B). However, if TR heterodimerizes with RXR on the nTRE, this configuration cannot be discriminated from that present on the pTRE (Fig. 3A), which may be functioning as a T3-dependent transcriptional activator but not an inhibitor. Previous results of reporter assays examining the effect of RXR overexpression on the *TSHβ* promoter have been controversial. Cohen et al. (Cohen et al., 1995) and Hallenbeck et al. (Hallenbeck et al., 1993) reported that RXR may antagonize inhibition of the *TSHβ* gene by T3/TR, while Safer et al. (Safer et al., 1997) reported that the requirement for RXR is different between TRβ1 and TRβ2. Nagaya et al. (Nagaya and Jameson, 1993) demonstrated that mutant TRβ1 (L428R) which is unable to dimerize with RXR failed to mediate T3-induced inhibition of the *αGSU* promoter, while Takeda et al. (Takeda et al., 1997) reported that overexpression of RXR had no effect on this promoter. According to Laflamme et al. (Laflamme et al., 2002) RXR enhances the negative regulation of the *TSHβ* gene by T3, and this effect is mediated by the RXR-LBD and but not the DBD, suggesting that RXR may act as a cofactor.

It was reported that the ligand for RXR (rexinoids) has inhibitory effect on *TSHβ* expression (Sherman et al., 1999). However, subsequent analysis revealed that the signaling pathway is mediated via a nt. -200/-149 region of the mouse *TSHβ* gene, which is different from the reported nTRE (GGGTCA at nt. +1/+6) (Sharma et al., 2006). While T3 inhibits the synthesis of thyrotropin releasing hormone (TRH) in hypothalamus (Fig 1A) and a nTRE is postulated in this gene (Hollenberg et al., 1995), rexinoids has no effect on its production (Sherman et al., 1999). It was reported that the transcription of the *TSHβ* gene is repressed in the CV1 cells treated with retinoic acid (RA) (Breen et al., 1995); however, its precise mechanism is unknown. Although all three RXRs, α, β and γ, are expressed in TSHoma cells, TtT97 (Sharma et al., 2006), double immunostaining studies of the hypothyroid rat pituitary using an antibodies against pituitary hormones and RXR suggest that RXRγ is predominantly expressed in thyrotrophs (Sugawara et al., 1995). Barros et al. (Barros et al., 1998) reported that no alteration in the serum level of TSH, T3 or T4 was observed in RXRα $^{(-/+)}$ mice or RXRγ $^{(-/-)}$ mice. The authors suggested that ablation of RXRs has little effect on the negative regulation of the *TSHβ* gene. Currently, there are few rationales to confirm the recognition of the nTRE by TR-RXR heterodimers.

5.2 Does TR bind to the nTRE as a monomer?

Gel shift assays indicate that TR monomers bind with the nTRE and that this interaction is abolished by RXR (Cohen et al., 1995). However, the hypothesis that TR binds with the nTRE as a monomer (Fig. 3B) also raises other questions which are difficult to answer. First, for the direct recognition of DNA sequence by DNA-binding transcription factors including NHRs, formation of a homo- or heterodimer is usually required. As expected, gel shift assays revealed that TR-monomer binding with single half-sites (i.e. nTRE) is much weaker than that of TR-RXR heterodimer binding to DR4 (Cohen et al., 1995). It should be noted that TSH synthesis in severe hypothyroidism is dramatically high (Fisher et al., 2000). Given that unliganded TR may maintain the basal activity of the *TSHβ* promoter in hypothyroidism, it is difficult to imagine that such a weak binding of TR monomer with the nTRE can achieve this high level of transcriptional activity. Second, there is ligand/NHR selectivity, i.e., the negative regulation of the *TSHβ* gene is clinically specific to T3 and partially estrogen (E2), but not other NHR ligands (Cohen and Wondisford, 2005). While, in positive regulation, the number of spacing nucleotides between half-sites is a critical factor in determining receptor specificity, it is unknown as to how TR selectively recognizes the nTRE DNA sequence in the *TSHβ* gene. Finally, it is not easy to explain why TR monomers on a single half-site can exhibit reverse functions, i.e. recruitment of co-activators in the absence of T3 and association with co-repressors in the presence of T3 (Fig. 3B). We proposed previously a model where TR is able to bind with reported nTRE only in the presence of T3 (Sasaki et al., 1999). Although the nTRE in the *TSHβ* gene was originally defined on the basis of the experiments with non-pituitary 293 cells (Wondisford et al., 1989), we and other investigators suggested the possibility that an unknown thyrotroph-specific factor may switch T3/TR on the nTRE from a transcriptional activator to an inhibitor (Sasaki et al., 1999; Shupnik, 2000; Wondisford et al., 1993). However, its existence has not been confirmed because of the limited number of cultured thyrotroph cell lines available (Ooi et al., 2004; Sarapura et al., 2002).

6. Models that do not postulate direct DNA binding of TR

The following hypotheses proposed models for T3-induced negative regulation without the involvement of direct DNA binding of TR.

6.1 NCoR or SMRT

There are many studies with regard to the involvement of NCoR or SMRT in the negative regulation by T3. It was reported that co-expression of NCoR and SMRT may enhance basal stimulation of the *TSHβ*, *αGSU* and *prepro-TRH* promoters in a TR-dependent manner (Tagami et al., 1997). With regard to the T3-induced negative regulation of the Rous sarcoma virus-derived 5′ truncated terminal repeat (RSV-LTR) (Berghagen et al., 2002) and the rat *CD44* gene (Kim et al., 2005), it was reported that NCoR and SMRT may function as transcriptional co-activators in the transcriptional regulation of these genes. According to

Tagami et al. (Tagami et al., 1999), unliganded TR in solution may squelch NCoR or SMRT from the transcription factor on the target promoter. Upon T3 binding, TR may release these co-repressors, resulting in their association with the DNA-binding transcription factor, which maintains the basal activity of the promoter of the target gene. However, this notion was tempered by following questions. First, the mechanism involved in the association of NCoR or SMRT with the target promoters is unknown. Second, it was undetermined whether the majority of NCoR and SMRT are sequestered by the relatively limited amount of intracellular TR (5000 to 10000 molecule/cell) (Oppenheimer et al., 1974). Third, NCoR and SMRT also interact with unliganded RAR and peroxisome proliferator-activated receptors (PPARs) (Nofsinger et al., 2008; Suzuki et al., 2010). It is unlikely that these NHRs also inhibit *TSHβ* or *αGSU* expression in the presence of cognate ligands. Finally, it was reported that the negative regulation by T3 is mediated by the mutant TRβ, AHT, of which interaction with co-repressors is impaired (Nakano et al., 2004). Using an experimental model similar to the mammalian two-hybrid assay, Wulf et al. (Wulf et al., 2008) also demonstrated that negative regulation by T3/TR is possible via the interaction of TR with a co-repressor. However, their experimental setting was completely artificial.
Amino acid sequence of TRβ2-NTD is unique and has low homology with that of TRβ1 or TRα1 (Fig. 2). The N-terminal domain of TRβ2 is known to neutralize the silencing activity of co-repressors in the context of TR-RXR heterodimers on the pTRE (Hollenberg et al., 1996; Yang et al., 1999), and the NTD of TRβ2 may have some role in the negative regulation of the *prepro-TRH* gene (Guissouma et al., 2002). However, the physiological relevance in the negative regulation of *TSHβ* gene is unknown. Of note, in vitro experiments showed that not only TRβ2 but also TRβ1 and TRα1 can inhibit the transcription of the *TSHβ* gene in a T3 dependent manner (Nakano et al., 2004). The findings in *TRβ/TRα*-double knockout mice (Gothe et al., 1999) indicates that TRα1 is partially involved in the negative regulation of *TSHβ* gene although its expression level is less than that of TRβ2 (see below).
The amino acid sequence required for the interaction of NCoR and SMRT with unliganded TR has been identified. Based on this information, mice harboring mutant SMRT (SMRTmRID) (Nofsinger et al., 2008) or mutant NCoR (NCoRΔID) (Astapova et al., 2011), which results in defective interaction with unliganded TR, were established. Importantly, the negative regulation of the *TSHβ* gene by T3 was not impaired in knock-in mice with SMRTmRID or NCoRΔID, although the latter exhibited a reduced amount of TR protein in the pituitary gland and reduced sensitivity for TSH by the thyroid gland. Likewise, TRH expression in the hypothalamus was not affected in NCoRΔID-knock-in mice (Astapova et al., 2011). This is supported by an *in vivo* study, which showed that the overexpression of these co-repressors is incompatible with physiological regulation of TRH (Becker et al., 2001). As in the cases of the *TSHβ* and *αGSU* genes, mRNA expression of the myosin heavy chain β subunit (*MHCβ*) gene in the heart is also repressed by T3/TR (Gupta, 2007). In NCoRΔID mice, T3-induced inhibition of *MHCβ* is maintained (Astapova et al., 2011). Moreover, Astapova et al, (Astapova et al., 2008) established a liver-specific NCoRΔID knock-in mouse. According to them, of 326 genes that are negatively regulated by T3 in the liver, only 3 genes were repressed in hypothyroid conditions, suggesting little effect of NCoR on the majority of the negatively regulated T3-target genes. While SMRTmRID- or NCoRΔID-knock-in mice survive, the global deletion of both the *NCoR* and *SMRT* genes are embryonic lethal (Jepsen et al., 2007). These findings suggest that NCoR and SMRT have important roles other than interaction with liganded NHRs. For example, they interact with

p53, Myc, MyoD Ptx1 and Foxo1 (Nofsinger et al., 2008). Thus, it is unlikely that T3-binding with TR affects the transcriptional regulation of all of the genes regulated by NCoR or SMRT *in vivo*.

6.2 CBP/p300 and p160 family

cAMP-response-element-binding protein-binding protein (CBP)/p300 is required for transactivation by multiple DNA-binding transcription factors including NFkB and AP-1, and functions as a coactivator for liganded NHRs (Kamei et al., 1996). As a model for the ligand-dependent inhibition by NHRs, it was proposed that liganded NHRs may attenuate the transactivation by DNA-binding transcription factors via interference of CBP/p300 function (Kamei et al., 1996). However, subsequent studies reported that inhibition by liganded NHR is not rescued by overexpression of these co-activators (De Bosscher et al., 1997; De Bosscher et al., 2001; Wu et al., 2004). It was also suggested that the CBP/p300-interacting surface on the NHR-LBD may be different from that required for T3-dependent inhibition (Saatcioglu et al., 1997; Valentine et al., 2000).

Although inappropriate overexpression of TSH is reported in SRC1-deficient mice (Takeuchi et al., 2002), it is difficult to determine what adaptive processes have occurred during pituitary development in SRC-1$^{(-/-)}$ mice since ablation of the SRC-1 gene also affects the expression of other p160 family members and TRs (Sadow et al., 2003; Xu et al., 1998). While p160 proteins are known to interact with multiple NHRs other than TR in a ligand-dependent manner, inhibition of the *TSHβ* gene or the *aGSU* gene is specific to T3, and partially estrogen (Cohen and Wondisford, 2005). In some patients with RTH, there are no mutations of the *TRβ* or *TRa* gene (non-TR RTH) (Refetoff and Dumitrescu, 2007; Refetoff et al., 1993). Although defects in cofactors that may mediate the negative regulation of the *TSHβ* gene have been postulated in these cases, linkage analyses with polymorphic markers showed that the involvement of SRC-1, NCoR, SMRT or RXRγ is unlikely (Reutrakul et al., 2000).

6.3 Protein-protein interaction of TR with DNA-binding transcription factors: Tethering model

In vitro binding assays, including gel shift assays, are limited in that the amount of TR and/or RXR used may not always reflect the *in vivo* situation. To overcome this problem, Shibusawa et al. (Shibusawa et al., 2003a; Shibusawa et al., 2003b) established mice in which TRβ is unable to bind DNA due to a mutation in its DBD. They reported that the negative regulation of the *TSHβ* gene is relieved in these mice. One may assume that this result provides evidence for the direct binding of TRβ with the nTRE because, in positive regulation, the pTRE is recognized by the TR-DBD. However, the function of the DBD of NHR is not limited to DNA recognition. It is known that the DBD also interacts with other DNA-binding transcription factors including NFkB (De Bosscher et al., 2003; Kalaitzidis and Gilmore, 2005; Kalkhoven et al., 1996; Ray and Prefontaine, 1994; Scheinman et al., 1995; Stein and Yang, 1995; Tao et al., 2001; Wissink et al., 1997), AP-1 (typically Jun/Fos heterodimers) (De Bosscher et al., 2001; Heck et al., 1994; Lopez et al., 1993; Schule et al., 1990; Webb et al., 1995), Nur77 (Martens et al., 2005) and GATA family transcription factors (Clabby et al., 2003; Matsushita et al., 2007), resulting in their inhibition by NHRs in a ligand-dependent fashion.

This kind of ligand-induced repression via protein–protein interactions is referred to as the "tethering mechanism" (De Bosscher et al., 2003; Herrlich, 2001; Nissen and Yamamoto, 2000; Pfahl, 1993). Thus, while mutation of the TRβ DBD abrogates the negative regulation of the *TSHβ* gene by T3, it does not always imply a direct interaction of the TR with DNA. Of note, there are ligand/receptor specificities in the repression by liganded NHRs via the tethering mechanism (Caldenhoven et al., 1995; Liden et al., 1997; Matsushita et al., 2007). Moreover, dimer formation is not always required for ligand-dependent inhibition via the tethering mechanism. A mutant glucocorticoid receptor (GR), A458T, is known to have a defect in dimer formation and therefore in glucocorticoid-responsive element-dependent transactivation. It was reported that functions that require cross-talk with other transcription factors, such as transrepression of the AP-1-driven genes, remain intact in this mutant GR (Herrlich, 2001; Reichardt et al., 1998). This raises again the question whether heterodimer formation of TR with RXR is necessary for the negative regulation of the *TSHβ* gene by T3.

7. Other possible mechanisms

Although T3 treatment is known to reduce the stability of TSHβ mRNA (Krane et al., 1991), the role of TR has not been clarified, and the involvement of similar mechanisms in the regulation of the αGSU mRNA have not been reported (Staton et al., 2000). A mechanism operating via anti-sense RNA was proposed to be involved in negative regulation of the MHCβ gene by T3 (Danzi and Klein, 2005; Haddad et al., 2003). In rat chromosome 15, the MHCβ gene is located upstream to the MHCα gene, which has a classic pTRE. It was reported that, in a T3-dependent manner, TR-RXR heterodimers at pTRE of the MHCα promoter may activate not only MHCα transcription but also synthesis of anti-sense RNA against the MHCβ gene, resulting in the antagonism of MHCβ expression. However, this kind of mechanism has not been reported in other negatively regulated genes including the TSHβ or the αGSU genes.

8. Artificial negative regulation by T3/TR

There have been at least two technical problems that have hindered the elucidation of the mechanism of negative regulation by T3/T.

8.1 pUC/pBR322-derived AP-1 site

As shown above, liganded NHRs, including T3/TR and liganded GR, inhibit the transcriptional activity of AP-1 via the tethering mechanism. Unexpectedly, a functional AP-1 site was identified in nt. 1/138 of pUC-derived plasmids and its activity is repressed by T3/TR (Lopez et al., 1993). More than 2000 plasmid constructs bearing the sequence identical to nt. 1/138 in the pUC18/19 vector were detected in the BLAST database. Interestingly, our computer search revealed that this site is also included in the pBR322 vector (Yanisch-Perron et al., 1985). In early molecular biology studies, both vectors were often utilized in “home-made plasmids”. Unfortunately, this AP-1 site was contaminated in some of the plasmids used for the analysis of *TSHβ* negative regulation by T3 (Hallenbeck et al., 1993; Wondisford et al., 1989).

8.2 Firefly luciferase gene

The firefly luciferase assay has been utilized in a variety of analyses of transcriptional regulation, including negative regulation of the *TSHβ* and the *αGSU* genes due to its advantage over the CAT assay (Misawa et al.). However, at least in CV1 cells (Tillman et al., 1993), JEG3 cells (Maia et al., 1996) and Hepa1-6 mouse hepatoma cells (Chan et al., 2008), firefly luciferase cDNA has been reported to function as a transcriptional regulatory sequence that mediates artificial negative regulation by T3/TR. The length of firefly luciferase cDNA (1653 bp) is much longer than that of the CAT gene (657 bp). A computer search predicts more than 250 potential sites for DNA-binding transcription factors in firefly luciferase cDNA (Liu and Brent, 2008). Misawa et al. (Misawa et al.) recently found that firefly luciferase cDNA behaves as a transcriptional enhancer that can be stimulated by the protein kinase C activator, phorbol 12-O-tetradecanoate-13-acetate (TPA), and that this activity is inhibited by T3/TR in CV1 and JEG3 cells. The cDNA sequences of modified firefly luciferase (luc+) (Annicotte et al., 2001; Paguio et al., 2005) and conventional Renilla luciferase (RL) (Ho and Strauss, 2004; Osborne and Tonissen, 2002; Zhuang et al., 2001) also harbor numerous short sequences that can be recognized by a variety of transcription factors. Modified luciferase genes, including hRluc (Zhuang et al., 2001) and Luc2 (Paguio et al., 2005), may be more reliable than firefly luciferase (Misawa et al.), presumably because the majority of predicted transcription factor binding sites were mutated.

8.3 Problems with artificial negative regulation in the identification of the nTREs by reporter assays

When a strong promoter is fused to firefly luciferase cDNA, the activity of this DNA sequence as a transcriptional regulatory element can be negligible. Nonetheless, one should remember that sequential deletion or mutation of the promoter sequence often reduces its transcriptional activity. Once the activity of the promoter becomes lower than that of the activity via the firefly luciferase gene, the overall activity of the reporter gene may represent that of the firefly luciferase cDNA, which can be artificially inhibited by T3/TR. For example, a deletion analysis to identify a nTRE in the *αGSU* gene was also carried out using the firefly luciferase reporter system in JEG3 cells (Madison et al., 1993). However, nTRE was not identified because T3-induced negative regulation was detected even a promoter that only has a TATA box and a TSS. There is the possibility that sequential deletion of DNA might reduce the transcription activity of the *αGSU* promoter, thereby permitting the firefly luciferase cDNA to function as a transcriptional regulatory element, resulting in artificial suppression by T3/TR. Using the luciferase reporter gene, it was previously proposed that the nTRE of the *TSHβ* gene may have a direct repeat configuration without spacing nucleotides (DR0) (Naar et al., 1991). The authors reported that a reduction in spacing nucleotide number may convert DR4 from a pTRE to a nTRE. Unexpectedly, this was not reproduced by the CAT-based reporter system (private communication from Dr. Kazuhiko Umesono). According to Tillman et al. (Tillman et al., 1993), deletion of spacing nucleotides might destroy the T3-dependent activation and allowed artificial repression by T3/TR via firefly luciferase cDNA.

Whereas firefly luciferase assay has broad linearity, careful interpretation and appropriate control are necessary in particular when the promoter activity before T3 addition is reduced in the course of deletion or mutation analysis (Misawa et al.). Although several nTREs in different genes have been suggested in the vicinity of TSSs, few of these reports excluded the possibility of T3-mediated artificial negative regulation by a reporter plasmid backbone.

9. TRβ2 is the main mediator for the negative regulation of the TSHβ gene by T3

There is one family with RTH in which the *TRβ* allele was globally deleted (Takeda et al., 1992). Elevated synthesis of TSH, i.e. SITSH, was found in a homozygote in this family, presumably due to the defect in TR signaling in the thyrotrophs. Likewise, mice deficient for the *TRβ* gene exhibit increased expression of *TSHβ* and *αGSU* in thyrotrophs (Forrest et al., 1996). These findings imply the involvement of TRβ in the negative regulation of these genes. Moreover, Abel et al. (Abel et al., 1999) reported that TRβ2-null mice develop a similar degree of central resistance to T3 similarly to TRβ-null mice, suggesting that, among TRβ1, TRβ2 and TRα1, TRβ2 is the main mediator for the inhibition of the *TSHβ* gene. This notion is compatible with our findings that the expression of TRβ2 is much higher than TRα1 or TRβ1 (Nakano et al., 2004) in the thyrotroph cell line, TαT1 (Yusta et al., 1998). The fact that no resistance to T3 is observed in mice deficient for the *TRα* gene (Fraichard et al., 1997; Wikstrom et al., 1998) indicates that TRα1 in thyrotrophs has a limited role in the negative feedback of the *TSHβ* gene by T3. It should be noted, however, that serum TSH levels in *TRβ/TRα*-double knockout mice (Gothe et al., 1999) is higher than *TRβ*-null mice (Forrest et al., 1996). Hence, the negative regulation of the *TSHβ* gene is partially mediated by TRα1 *in vivo.*

10. What is the mechanism that maintains the basal transcriptional activity of the *TSHβ* gene before T3 addition?

It is apparent that the negative regulation of the *TSHβ* gene by T3/TR can be observed only when its promoter is activated prior to T3 addition. However, previous studies have paid little attention to the mechanism of activation because some of the hypotheses mentioned above regard the basal transcriptional activity of the *TSHβ* gene to be maintained by unliganded TR. In addition, due to the limitation of the cell lines that recapitulate the thyrotroph phenotype (Ooi et al., 2004; Sarapura et al., 2002), the nTRE of the *TSHβ* gene has been studied using either kidney-derived 293 cells (Wondisford et al., 1989), COS cells (Carr et al., 1992) or somatotroph-derived GH3 cells (Sasaki et al., 1999). Of note, even in the presence of overexpressed TR, the magnitude of the basal transcriptional activity of the *TSHβ* gene prior to T3 addition is extremely low in these cell lines (Sasaki et al., 1999; Wondisford et al., 1989), and is almost negligible compared with that observed in the presence of the thyrotroph-specific transcription factors, Pit1 and GATA2 (Nakano et al., 2004) (see below).

11. Unliganded TR per se is not a transcriptional activator for the *TSHβ* gene

Because negative regulation has been regarded as the mirror image of the positive regulation, unliganded TR was thought to be a transcriptional activator (Wondisford et al., 1989). If this were the case, *TSHβ* and *αGSU* expression would be reduced in mice lacking the *TR* gene irrespective of serum T3 and T4 levels. However, as described above, their expression was not reduced but rather was increased in mice deficient for the *TRβ* gene (Abel et al., 1999; Forrest et al., 1996; Weiss et al., 1997) or both *TRα* and *TRβ* genes (Gothe et al., 1999). In the family with RTH, in which the *TRβ* allele is globally deleted (Takeda et al., 1992), elevation of serum TSH was also found in the homozygotes of this family. This again suggests that unliganded TRβ is not necessary for the activity of the *TSHβ* promoter in human and that the *TSHβ* gene is activated by factors other than unliganded TR.

12. GATA2 and Pit1 maintain basal *TSHβ* expression in thyrotrophs

It is known that a pituitary-specific transcription factor, Pit1 (Fig 5A), plays a critical role in *TSHβ* expression since its mutation causes combined pituitary hormone deficiency (CPHD), where the syntheses of TSHβ, prolactin and growth hormone are crippled or abolished (Cohen and Radovick, 2002).

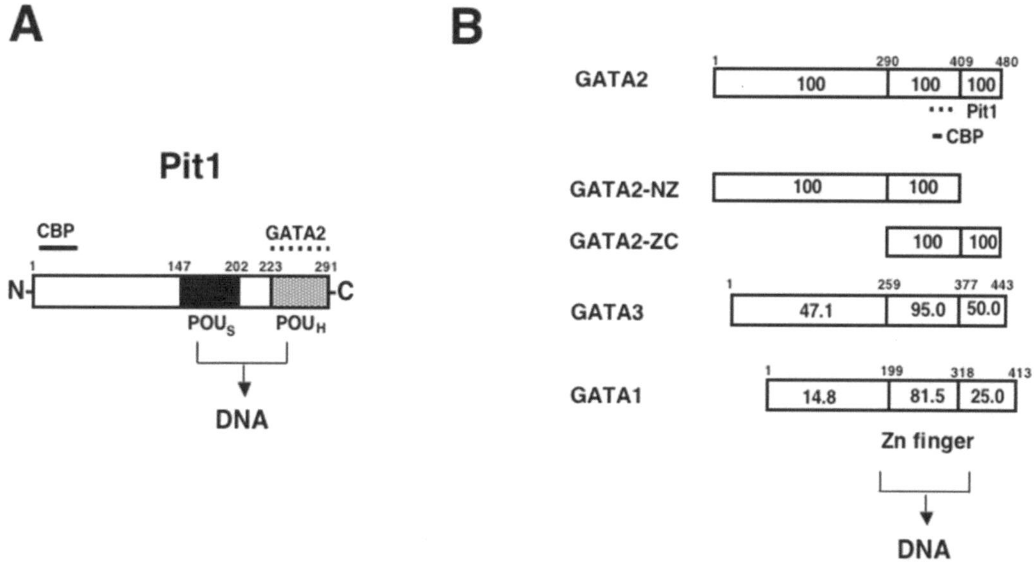

Fig. 5. Schematic representations of Pit1 (A) and GATA1, 2 and 3 (B). A. CBP, amino acid sequence interacting with CBP. POU_S, POU specific domain. POU_H. POU homeodomain. GATA, amino acid sequence interacting with GATA2. B. Structure of GATA1, 2, 3, GATA2-NZ and GATA2-ZC (see text). The numbers within the box represent the amino acid homology (%).

Promoter analysis of the *TSHβ* gene in TSHoma cells, TtT97, revealed that nt. -269 from the TSS is sufficient for thyrotroph-specific expression of this gene (Wood et al., 1990). As shown in Fig. 4, a functional Pit1-binding site is included in this region (Haugen et al., 1993) and was designated as Pit1-US (Kashiwabara et al., 2009). Interestingly, comparison of the pattern of DNA foot printing using nuclear extracts from TtT97 cells and that from GH3 cells revealed that this promoter region also has binding sites for the transcription factor, GATA2 (Fig 4 and 5B) (Gordon et al., 1997), which was originally identified to be involved in the gene regulation of a hematopoietic cell lineage (Shimizu and Yamamoto, 2005). Indeed, there are two GATA-responsive elements (GATA-REs) immediately downstream of the Pit1-US (Gordon et al., 1997). Subsequent analysis with various transgenic mice revealed that co-expression of Pit1 and GATA2 is crucial for the differentiation of thyrotrophs (Dasen et al., 1999).

13. GATA2, not Pit1, is the true activator that drives the promoter activity of *TSHβ*

Kashiwabara et al. (Kashiwabara et al., 2009) reported that the co-operation of Pit1 with GATA2 is strictly determined by the number of nucleotides between the Pit1-US and GATA-REs (Fig 4), and suggested the possibility that a configuration of the Pit1-US and GATA-REs may be critical for the recruitment of CBP/p300 (Fig 6).

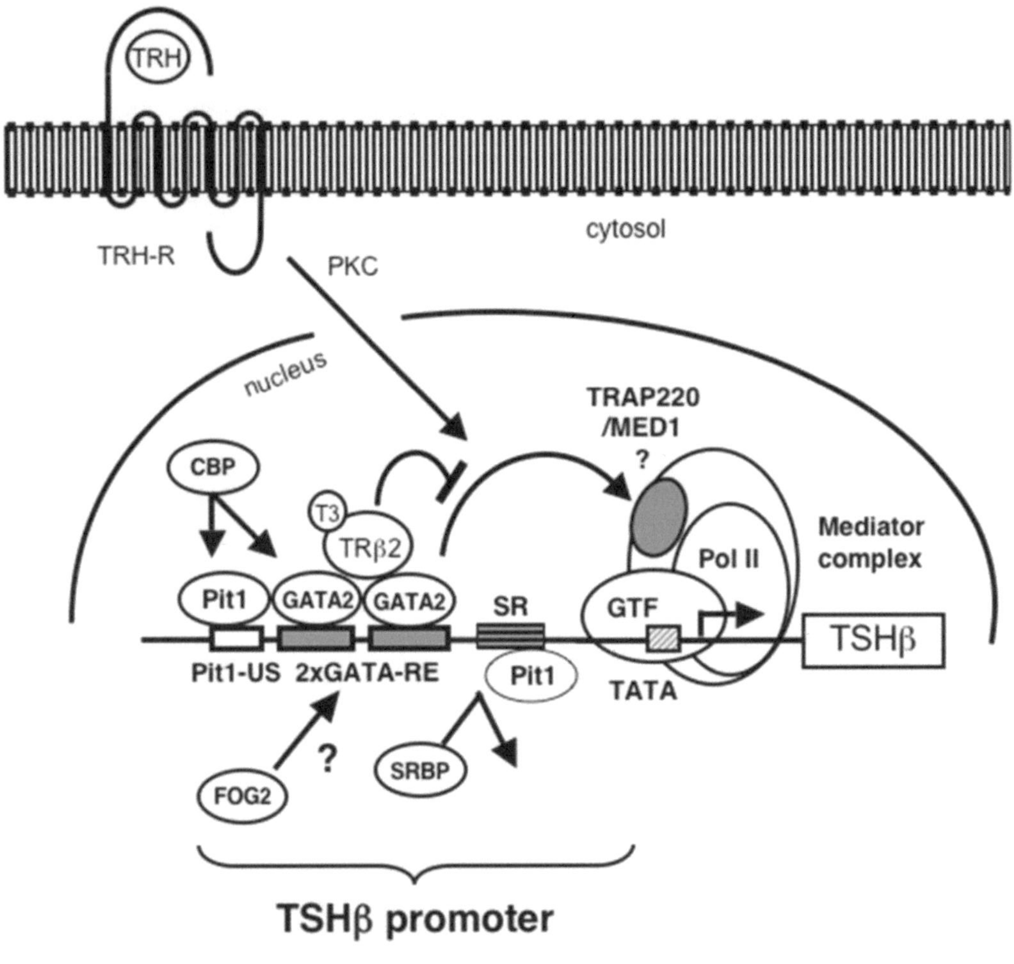

Fig. 6. Molecular mechanism of the transcriptional regulation of the TSHβ gene. A configuration of the Pit1-US and GATA-REs may be critical for the recruitment of CBP/p300. T3/TR represses the GATA2-dependent activation of the *TSHβ* promoter via a tethering mechanism. Pit1 binds with the Pit1-like element in SR and competes with SR binding protein (SRBP), resulting in protection of GATA2 functionality from inhibition by SR (de-repression). TRH-R, TRH receptor, FOG2, friend of GATA 2.

The authors also noticed that a 30bp region downstream from the GATA-REs is highly conserved among rat, mice and humans, and includes a sequence similar to the Pit1-binding site (Pit1-like element, Fig. 4). This sequence was designated the suppressor region (SR) because its deletion increased the transactivation by GATA2 and Pit1. Interestingly, deletion of the SR enabled GATA2 to transactivate the *TSHβ* gene without Pit1. Detailed analysis revealed that Pit1 binds with the Pit1-like element in the SR (Fig. 4) and competes with binding of SR binding protein (SRBP), resulting in protection of the GATA2 function from inhibition by SRBP (Fig 6). Thus, cooperation of Pit1 with GATA2 is not synergistic, but Pit1 protects GATA2 from inhibition by SR (de-repression). These findings not only provide an insight as to why *TSHβ* expression is restricted in thyrotrophs where Pit1 and GATA2 co-exist, but also imply that the true activator that drives the *TSHβ* promoter activity is GATA2 but not Pit1 (Kashiwabara et al., 2009).

14. Negative regulation of the *TSHβ* gene is not the mirror image of positive regulation

Gordon et al. (Gordon et al., 1997) reported that the *TSHβ* gene can be activated by Pit1 and GATA2 in CV1 cells. Because CV1 cells are kidney derived and has been utilized in the studies of positive regulation by T3/TR (Naar et al., 1991; Tillman et al., 1993; Umesono et al., 1991), Nakano et al. (Nakano et al., 2004) tested whether negative regulation of *TSHβ* by T3 may be simulated when TR is co-expressed with Pit1 and GATA2 in this cell line. They employed the CAT-based reporter gene, *TSHβ*-CAT (Sasaki et al., 1999), in which the pUC/pBR322-derived AP-1 element (Lopez et al., 1993) was deleted. Using this experimental system, Nakano et al. (Nakano et al., 2004) found the following results. First, T3-induced inhibition of the *TSHβ* gene was readily observed in CV1 cells transfected with Pit1, GATA2 and TRβ2. This implies that T3-induced negative regulation of the *TSHβ* gene does not require so-called thyrotroph specific factors except for Pit1, GATA2 and TR. Second, T3-induced inhibition was also detected with all three functional TRs, TRβ1, TRβ2 and TRα1, with TRβ2 exhibiting the most potent T3-dependent inhibition among them. This observation again supports the notion that TRβ2 is the principal TR that mediates negative regulation of the *TSHβ* gene (Abel et al., 1999). Third, without Pit1 or GATA2, unliganded TR did not transactivate the *TSHβ* promoter at all. This implies that unliganded TR alone is not the transcriptional activator. This notion is in line with the results of data from *TRβ*-knockout mice (Forrest et al., 1996) and *TRβ*/*TRα*-double knockout mice (Gothe et al., 1999). Therefore, in negative regulation of the *TSHβ* gene, T3/TR is a transcriptional repressor, but unliganded TR per se is not an activator. This is in contrast with positive regulation (Fig. 3A), where the T3-target genes are activated by T3/TR while it is repressed by unliganded TR (silencing). These findings run counter to the hypothesis that the negative regulation of this gene may be a mirror image of its positive regulation (Wondisford et al., 1989).

15. T3/TR represses GATA2-dependent activation of the *TSHβ* promoter via the tethering mechanism

The putative nTRE was defined by analysis of the *TSHβ* promoter in the absence of T3 (Wondisford et al., 1989). Because this was based on the hypothesis that unliganded TR may be a transcriptional activator, Matsushita et al. (Matsushita et al., 2007) re-evaluated the function of nTRE by deletion analysis of this promoter (Fig. 4) in the presence of Pit1, GATA2 and TR. Unexpectedly, we found that repression of the *TSHβ* promoter by T3/TRβ2 was maintained after the nTRE is completely deleted or mutated. Thus, the reported nTRE (Fig. 4) is dispensable for T3/TR-dependent inhibition. Moreover, repression by T3/TR was also observed even in a deletion construct that has only Pit1-US and two GATA-REs. These findings suggest that direct DNA binding of TR is unnecessary and that the mechanism for T3-dependent inhibition may be mediated by the crosstalk of T3/TR with Pit1 or GATA2 (Matsushita et al., 2007).

As mentioned above, the true activator that drives the TSHβ promoter is GATA2 but not Pit1 (Kashiwabara et al., 2009) and the deletion of SR enables GATA2 to transactivate the *TSHβ* promoter without Pit1. Using the reporter gene lacking for SR, Matsushita et al. (Matsushita et al., 2007) found that T3/TRβ2 inhibits the transactivation by GATA2 alone. Thus, GATA2 is thought to be the target of inhibition by T3/TR (Fig. 6). This notion is supported by the observation that T3/TRβ2 inhibits GATA2-induced activation of the *αGSU* promoter and the endothelin-1 (*ET-1*) promoter, both of which are known to bear a functional GATA-RE (Jorgensen et al., 2004; Steger et al., 1994; Dorfman et al., 1992). In addition, T3/TR inhibited the *CD34* gene-derived GATA-RE fused to a heterologous thymidine kinase promoter (Matsushita et al., 2007). Co-immunoprecipitation experiments and GST-pull down assays demonstrated that the DBD of TRβ2 interacts with the Zn finger domain of GATA2 *in vivo* in a T3-independent manner. Thus, the TR-DBD is involved in protein-protein interactions with GATA2 but not in direct binding of DNA (Matsushita et al., 2007). These results indicate that negative regulation of the *TSHβ* gene is mediated by tethering of T3/TR by GATA2 (Fig. 6).

16. Ligand/receptor specificity in negative regulation of the *TSHβ* gene

As discussed above, ligand/receptor specificity has been reported in ligand-dependent inhibition via the tethering mechanism (Caldenhoven et al., 1995; Liden et al., 1997). Matsushita et al. (Matsushita et al., 2007) found that GATA2-induced activity of the *TSHβ* promoter was specifically inhibited by T3/TR but not by RA/RAR or vitamins D3 (VD3)/VDR. This may reflect ligand selectivity *in vivo* in negative regulation of the *TSHβ* gene (Cohen and Wondisford, 2005). Of note, it is known that estrogen (E2) inhibits expression of the *TSHβ* gene (Cohen and Wondisford, 2005) at the transcriptional level, although its magnitude is smaller than that by T3. E2 is also known to reduce expression of the *αGSU* gene (Chaidarun et al., 1994; Shupnik et al., 1988), the promoter of which has a functional GATA-RE (Jorgensen et al., 2004; Steger et al., 1994). In agreement, the serum level of TSH in women has a tendency to elevate after the menopause (Nagayama et al., 2008). To explore the molecular mechanism underlying inhibition by E2, Nagayama et al. (Nagayama et al., 2008) tested the effect of E2-bound ERα (E2/ERα) using CV1 cells cotransfected with Pit1 and GATA2, and found that E2/ERα significantly inhibits activity of the *TSHβ* promoter. As predicted, the magnitude of inhibition by E2/ERα was approximately half of that by T3/TRβ2. They also found that E2/ERα directly interacts with GATA2, as shown for GATA1. Testosterone was reported to have the effect similar to estrogen, presumably due to the conversion of testosterone to estrogen (Ahlquist et al.,

1987). This may explain why elevation of serum TSH level is also found in aged men (Surks and Hollowell, 2007).

17. The role of GATA2 and TR in TRH signaling in thyrotrophs

TRH is processed from prepro-TRH and secreted from the hypothalamus (Fig. 1A). TRH signaling not only stimulates TSH secretion but also enhances expression of *TSHβ* and *αGSU* (Franklyn et al., 1986; Shupnik et al., 1986). To clarify the role of TRH-induced transactivation and T3/TR mediated inhibition in the hypothalamic-pituitary-thyroid (H-T-P) axis, various in *vivo* studies, including genetic ablation of these genes, have been performed (Forrest et al., 1996; Friedrichsen et al., 2004; Gothe et al., 1999; Mittag et al., 2009; Nikrodhanond et al., 2006; Shibusawa et al., 2000). Although the *in vivo* evidence observed in these experiments is definitely important, the experimental system using cultured cells has the advantage that the effect of individual hormone can be analyzed in detail without influence by a negative feedback loop.

17.1 TRH signaling-promoted *TSHβ* expression is mediated by GATA2

Although serum TSH levels are reduced in patient with CPHD who have mutations in the Pit1 gene (Cohen and Radovick, 2002), the involvement of Pit1 downstream of TRH signaling has been controversial (Ohba et al., 2011; Steinfelder et al., 1992a; Steinfelder et al., 1992b). Unfortunately, previous analyses have been performed without consideration of GATA2. Interestingly, the increase in *TSHβ* expression in hypothyroidism was impaired in mice with pituitary-specific ablation of the GATA2 gene (Charles et al., 2006). Because TRH synthesis in the hypothalamus is expected to increased in hypothyroidism (Fig. 1A) (Abel et al., 2001; Kakucska et al., 1992), this finding suggested the involvement of GATA2 in the TRH signaling pathway.

Using CV1, GH3 and TαT1 cells, Ohba et al. (Ohba et al., 2011) recently reported that TRH signaling potentiates GATA2/Pit1-induced transcriptional activity of the *TSHβ* gene. Additionally, experiments with a *TSHβ* promoter that lacks SR revealed that GATA2 but not Pit1 is the target of TRH signaling (Fig. 6). Similar results were obtained with GATA2-induced activation of the *αGSU* and *ET-1* promoters. It is known that the signal from TRH receptor activates protein kinase C (PKC) (Gershengorn and Osman, 1996; Sun et al., 2003). The PKC pathway is also known to enhance DNA binding of GATA2 with GATA-RE in the *αGSU* (Fowkes et al., 2002) and the *V-CAM1* promoters (Minami et al., 2003). Gel shift assays also suggested that DNA binding of GATA2 with the *TSHβ* promoter is facilitated by the TRH/PKC pathway (Ohba et al., 2011). Thus, GATA-REs seem to be the point of convergence for both activation and inhibition signals controlling TSHβ transcription. Although it has been postulated that TRH signaling in transactivation of the *TSHβ* gene may be mediated by unliganded TR on nTRE (Wondisford et al., 1993), Ohba et al. (Ohba et al., 2011) showed that unliganded TR without Pit1 or GATA2 failed to mediate the stimulating effect by TRH on this promoter and that reported nTRE (Fig. 4) is dispensable for activation of the TRH-induced transcription.

17.2 TRH-dependent activation vs. T3/TR-induced repression

The in vitro data demonstrated by Ohba et al. (Ohba et al., 2011) correlate well with the *in vivo* findings (Fig. 7).

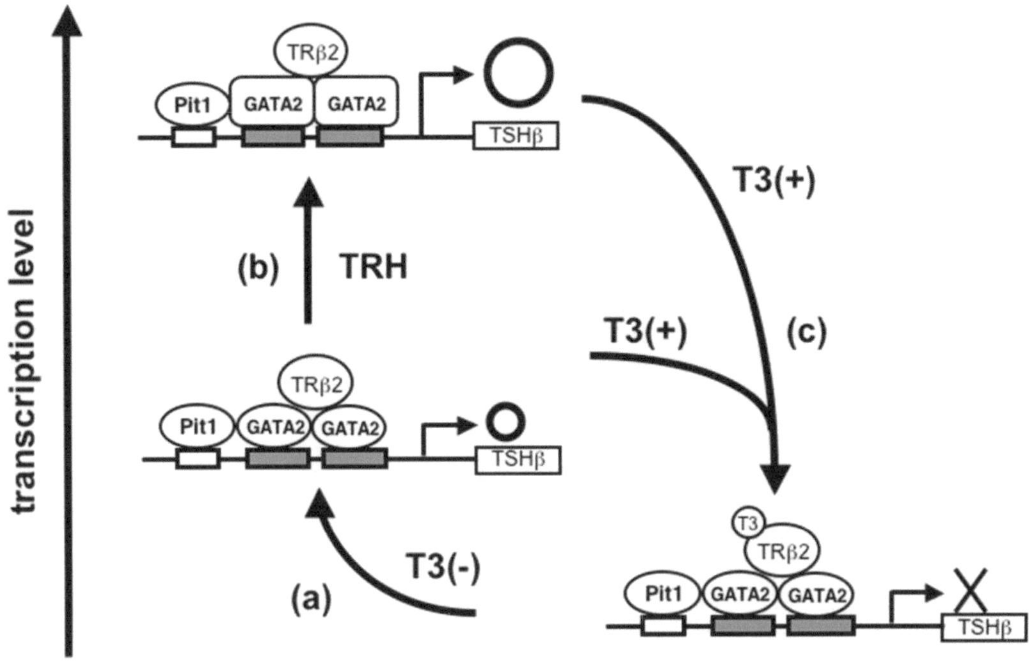

Fig. 7. Schematic representation of transcriptional regulation of the *TSHβ* gene by TRH signaling and T3/TR. With support by Pit1, GATA2 maintains the basal transcription of the *TSHβ* gene and mediates TRH/TRH-R1 signaling in hypothyroidism, while unliganded TR alone is not a transcriptional activator. Inhibition by T3/TR is dominant over activation by GATA2 even in the presence of TRH signaling. The release of T3/TR-induced repression (a) is more crucial for *TSHβ* expression than TRH signaling (b) since the inhibition by T3/TR is dominant over the stimulation by TRH (c). DNA binding of GATA2 with the *TSHβ* promoter is facilitated by the TRH pathway (b).

First, they showed that as long as T3 is at low concentrations or absent, expression of the *TSHβ* gene is maintained by Pit1 and GATA2 without stimulation by TRH signaling (Fig. 7(a)) (Gordon et al., 1997; Kashiwabara et al., 2009; Ohba et al., 2011). In agreement with this, the signaling and the number of TSHβ-positive cells in the pituitary of TRH-deficient mice were comparable with those of wild-type mice (Shibusawa et al., 2000). Second, given that unliganded TR is not a transcriptional activator, elevation of *TSHβ* expression in hypothyroidism should depend on TRH signaling but not on unliganded TR (Fig. 7(b)). Nikrodhanond et al. (Nikrodhanond et al., 2006) compared *TSHβ* expression in wild-type, TRH-, TRβ- and TRH/TRβ-double knockout mice and found that, in hypothyroidism, TSH expression predominantly depends on TRH signaling but not by unliganded TRβ. Since the authors regarded unliganded TRβ as the stimulator for the *TSHβ* gene, they mentioned that their findings were unexpected. However, their results are in agreement with the notion that unliganded TR is not the activator or mediator for the *TSHβ* gene in the absence or presence of TRH signaling. Finally, our data suggested that, in *TSHβ* transcription, the inhibitory effect by T3/TR is dominant over the TRH-induced stimulation (Fig. 7(c)) (Ohba et al., 2011). In accordance with this, an earlier study with human subjects indicated that continuous injection of TRH cannot release the inhibition of serum TSH in thyrotoxicosis (Chan et al.,

1979). Taking advantage of the fact that the Pax8-null mouse is an excellent animal model for congenital hypothyroidism (Friedrichsen et al., 2004), Mittag et al. (Mittag et al., 2009) demonstrated that thyrotroph differentiation in Pax8/TRH-R double-knockout mice is comparable with that in the hypothyroidism of mice homologous for a Pax8-null allele. Their results support the notion that release of T3/TR-induced inhibition (Fig. 7(a) is more critical for *TSHβ* expression than TRH signaling (Fig. 7(b)) because inhibition by T3/TR is dominant over stimulation by TRH (Fig. 7(c)).

18. Mechanism of T3/TR interference with GATA2 transactivating function

Negative regulation of the *TSHβ* gene is expected to provide an excellent experimental model to study transcriptional regulation since this promoter is activated by TRH signaling and repressed by T3/TR (Fig. 6). An important next step would be to investigate how T3/TR interferes with the transactivation function of GATA2. As pointed out above, the involvement of RXRs, TR-related coactivator (p160) or co-repressors (NCoR, SMRT) has been controversial. We favor another possibility; that TR may regulate the function of GATA2-related cofactors in a T3-dependent manner.

In pituitary-specific GATA2-null mice (Charles et al., 2006), the defect in *TSHβ* expression was partial and GATA3 expression was increased. Thus, GATA3 may be able to compensate for the reduction in GATA2 expression and there may be functional redundancy between GATA2 and GATA3. Amino acid homology between the Zn-finger domains of GATA1, GATA2 and GATA3 is well conserved (Fig. 5B) and plays a pivotal role in DNA recognition as well as cofactor interaction (Bates et al., 2008; Shimizu and Yamamoto, 2005). Consistent with this, our *in vitro* results show that GATA1, GATA2 and GATA3 have the capacity to mediate cooperation with Pit1 (Kashiwabara et al., 2009), TRH signaling-induced transactivation (Ohba et al., 2011) and inhibition by T3/TR (Matsushita et al., 2007). All these properties were also observed in the deletion mutant of GATA2 that lacks an N-terminal domain (GATA2-ZC) or a C-terminal domain (GATA2-NZ) (Fig. 5B). These findings suggest a critical role of the Zn-finger domain in GATA2 (GATA2-Zf) in *TSHβ* gene regulation. Besides CBP/p300, TR-associated protein (TRAP) 220/MED1 and Friend of GATA (FOG) 1 or 2 are known to interact with this domain. Of course, there is the possibility that other unknown factors may play a critical role in negative regulation by T3/TR and that there is interplay among various histone modifications to achieve local control of *TSHβ* gene transcription. Although the chromatin immunoprecipitation (ChIP) assay is expected to provide important information, the amount of endogenous GATA2 in TαT1 cells may not be sufficient for this approach (Ohba et al., 2011).

18.1 TRAP220/MED1 and Mediator complex

TRAP220/MED1 is a constituent of the Mediator complex that directly regulates the function of RNA polymerase II (Pol II) (Fig. 6) (Chadick and Asturias, 2005). The following findings indicate the involvement of TRAP220/MED1 in transactivation by the GATAs (Fig. 6). First, *in vitro* experiments show that TRAP220/MED1 interacts with GATA2-Zf (Gordon et al., 2006). Second, homozygous TRAP220/MED1-null mice are embryonic lethal due to an abnormality in cardiac function and its phenotype is reminiscent of that observed in mice deficient for the GATA family transcription factors (Crawford et al., 2002). Third, expression of the *TSHβ* gene is reduced in heterozygous TRAP220/MED-knockout mice (Ito et al., 2000), suggesting that TRAP220/MED1 is required for expression of the *TSHβ* gene, which is GATA2-dependent. Interestingly, TRAP220/MED1 possesses two LXXLL motives, which functions as an interface for interaction with the TR-LBD in a T3-dependent manner. Mutant TRAP220/MED1, which only has two LXXLL motives but lacks other transactivation domains, is reported to function as a dominant negative inhibitor against wild-type TRAP220/MED1 in T3-dependent positive regulation via TR-RXR heterodimers on the pTRE (Yuan and Gambee, 2000). Matsushita et al. (Matsushita et al., 2007) found that mutant MED1/TRAP220 also attenuates T3-induced inhibition of the *TSHβ* gene. It was reported that mutant TRAP220/MED1 specifically interferes with the activity of wild-type TRAP220/MED1 but not other LXXLL-type co-activators including the p160 family and CBP/p300 (Acevedo and Kraus, 2003). Thus, there is the possibility that TR may regulate the activity of a complex containing GATA2 and TRAP220/MED1 in a T3-dependent fashion. Given that inhibition by T3/TR targets the final step of GATA2-induced transactivation, i.e. TRAP220/MED1-Pol II complex, repression might occur downstream of or at the same point as TRH-induced activation. This may account for the findings that inhibition by T3/TR is dominant over TRH-induced activation of the *TSHβ* gene (Mittag et al., 2009; Ohba et al., 2011). *In vivo* experiments with mouse embryonic fibroblasts showed that the requirement of TRAP220/MED1 may be specific to TR, but not to RAR or VDR (Ito et al., 2000). Intriguingly, the binding of different activators triggers a specific conformational change in the Mediator complex, which may have a critical role in the regulation of Pol II (Chadick and Asturias, 2005).

18.2 FOG2 and chromatin-remodeling factors

The co-repressor, friend of GATA (FOG) 1 or 2 (Cantor and Orkin, 2005) may be involved in T3/TR-induced negative regulation via GATA2. FOG1 and FOG2 interact with the N-terminal Zn finger of the GATAs and recruit chromatin-remodeling factors (Fig. 6) (Hong et al., 2005; Roche et al., 2008; Rodriguez et al., 2005). In addition, FOG2 is expressed in non-hematopoietic tissues and interacts with TRβ (Rouf et al., 2008) and other NHRs (Clabby et al., 2003; Huggins et al., 2001). Matsushita et al. (Matsushita et al., 2007) generated a mutant GATA2 (C295A) which is predicted to have impaired interaction with the FOGs. Although the basal transcriptional activity of this mutant was also reduced (by approximately half) compared with wild-type GATA2, inhibition by T3/TR (fold repression) was significantly relieved in mutant GATA2.

19. Molecular mechanism of SITSH in RTH

As described above, patients with RTH exhibit SITSH (Refetoff et al., 1993). The mutant TRβ found in RTH patients is supposed to interact with GATA2 because it has an intact DBD, which is the interface for the Zn-finger domain of GATA2. Nakano et al. (Nakano et al., 2004) tested whether mutant TRβ2s identified in RTH patients exhibit a dominant negative effect on the negative regulation of the *TSHβ* gene using CV1 cells cotransfected with Pit1, GATA2 and wild-type TRβ2. As predicted, mutant TRβ2s blunted the T3-induced inhibition of the *TSHβ* gene by wild-type TRβ2. Although these findings are likely to be the result of dominant-negative interference of wild-type TRβ function by mutant TRβ, further studies are required with regard to its molecular mechanism. Following questions also remain. First, in patients with non-TR RTH (see above), no genetic abnormalities in the *TRβ* or *TRa* genes have been identified. Although linkage analysis of these patients showed no relation with NCoR, SMRT, SRC-1 or RXRγ (Reutrakul et al., 2000), an understanding of the transcriptional control mechanisms underlying non-TR RTH may provide an insight into the molecular basis of negative regulation of the *TSHβ* gene. Second, RTH is clinically classified as a generalized resistance to thyroid hormone (GRTH) and resistance of the pituitary to thyroid hormone (PRTH) (Refetoff et al., 1993). Patients with PRTH possess mutations similar or identical to those found in GRTH; however, PRTH patients display greater resistance to thyroid hormone in thyrotrophs compared to peripheral tissues, resulting in thyrotoxicosis. Currently, the mechanism of pituitary-dominant resistance in PRTH is unknown (Nakano et al., 2004).

20. Mechanism of logarithmic alterations in serum TSH by linear changes of T3/T4

TSH synthesis in the pituitary is dramatically altered by subtle changes in serum T3 and T4. Indeed, linear changes in the concentration of serum T4 and T3 correspond to logarithmic changes in serum TSH (Fekete and Lechan, 2007; Fisher et al., 2000; Kakucska et al., 1992). Such a sensitive alteration of *TSHβ* expression may be necessary for thyroid hormone homeostasis (Fig. 1A) because TSH signaling is thought to be one of the most critical determinants of T3 and T4 synthesis in the thyroid gland. In other words, serum TSH level has been regarded as most sensitive clinical marker for thyroid gland function. Indeed, SITSH is an important indicator for RTH.

With regard to the molecular mechanism of logarithmic changes in serum TSH, there are the following possibilities. First, T3/TR negatively regulates not only *TSHβ* and *aGSU* but also the prepro-TRH gene (Fig. 1A). Thus, the dual inhibitory mechanism at the hypothalamus and the pituitary may be important for the non-linear change of serum TSH level. Second, Pit1 expression may be negatively regulated by T3 (Sanchez-Pacheco et al., 1995). Because this was found in a somatotroph cell line, GH3 (Ooi et al., 2004), which lacks endogenous GATA2 (Gordon et al., 1997), an unknown pituitary factor may be involved in this inhibition. Third, expression of GATA2 in thyrotrophs may also be negatively regulated by T3. It was reported that there are two promoters in the *GATA2* gene, and that the distal one contains a GATA-RE (Kobayashi-Osaki et al., 2005). Therefore, there may be a positive feedback mechanism in the expression of *GATA2* and this mechanism is thought to be crucial in the differentiation of hematopoietic cell lineages. There is the possibility that, in thyrotrophs, T3/TR may interfere with the transactivation function of GATA2 not only on the *TSHβ* promoter but also on the GATA2 promoter. In addition, GATA2 protein may be quickly degraded by the ubiquitin system (its half life is approximately 30 min) (Minegishi et al., 2005). This may also contribute the drastic regulation of serum TSH level. Finally, there is the possibility that T3-induced inhibition of prepro-TRH expression in the hypothalamus may also be logarithmic (Fekete and Lechan, 2007; Kakucska et al., 1992). Although an nTRE was postulated in the prepro-TRH promoter (Hollenberg et al., 1995), the molecular mechanism of logarithmic inhibition of prepro-TRH expression by T3 is unknown.

The diagnoses of both subclinical hypo- and subclinical hyper-thyroidism also depend on the sensitive change in serum TSH level. Although serum free T3 and T4 levels are within normal range, subclinical hypo- or hyperthyroidism influence lipid metabolism (Walsh et al., 2005b) and cardiovascular function (Walsh et al., 2005a). In their pathogeneses, there may be the abnormality in the transcription of the gene which is negatively regulated by T3 as robustly as the TSHβ gene.

21. Other genes negatively regulated by T3/TR

Microarray analyses revealed that approximately 30 to 50% of T3-target genes are negatively regulated (Feng et al., 2000; Weitzel, 2008). Therefore, elucidation of negative regulation by T3 is thought to be the next frontier.

21.1 Reported nTREs in other T3-negatively regulated genes

In addition to the *TSHβ* gene, negative regulation by T3/TR has been reported in the genes for αGSU (Chatterjee et al., 1989; Pennathur et al., 1993), MHCβ (Edwards et al., 1994; Wright et al., 1999), prepro-TRH (Hollenberg et al., 1995; Satoh et al., 1996), RSV-LTR (Saatcioglu et al., 1993), rat Na, K-ATPase α3 subunit (Chin et al., 1998), Nm23-H1 (Lin et al., 2000), phospholamban (PBL) (Belakavadi et al., 2010), rat CD44 (Kim et al., 2005), superoxide dismutase-1 (Santos et al., 2006), deiodinase type 2 (Dio2) (Christoffolete et al., 2006) and β-amyloid precursor protein (Villa et al., 2004). In some of these genes, the existence of single half-sites homologous to the *TSHβ* nTRE have also been postulated (Chatterjee et al., 1989; Chin et al., 1998; Edwards et al., 1994; Hollenberg et al., 1995; Kim et al., 2005; Lin et al., 2000; Pennathur et al., 1993; Saatcioglu et al., 1993; Santos et al., 2006; Villa et al., 2004; Wright et al., 1999). However, there are few experimental studies that show the molecular mechanism by which these putative nTREs reverse the function of T3/TR from transcriptional activator to repressor. In *TRβ*- and/or *TRα1*-deficient mice, the expression of *αGSU* (Forrest et al., 1996; Gothe et al., 1999) in the pituitary, *prepro-TRH* in the hypothalamus (Abel et al., 2001; Dupre et al., 2004) and *MHCβ* in the heart (Mansen et al., 2001) are maintained, suggesting that, as in the case of the *TSHβ* gene, the basal activities of these genes are also maintained by a transcriptional activator other than unliganded TR. Thus, existence of nTREs in these genes should also be reconsidered.

21.2 Possible involvement of the tethering mechanism

If T3-dependent inhibition of these genes occurs via a tethering mechanism between a DNA-binding transcription factor and T3/TR, identification of such a transcription factor may provide an insight into the molecular mechanism of T3-induced inhibition. As discussed above, a functional GATA-RE in the *αGSU* promoter may be the target of suppression by T3/TR. GATA-REs are also predicted in the promoters of *Dio2* (Dentice et al., 2003), *MHCβ* (Hasegawa et al., 1997; Morimoto et al., 1999) and *PBL* (Belakavadi et al., 2010). *Dio* activity in the thyrotrophs regulates the intracellular concentration of T3, which is the determinant of negative regulation of the *TSHβ* gene (Escobar-Morreale et al., 1996). Although *Dio1* and *Dio2* are expressed in thyrotrophs, the inhibitory effect on TSH by T3 was relieved in mice deficient for *Dio2* but not *Dio1* (St Germain et al., 2005), indicating the crucial role of *Dio2* in the regulation of T3 concentration in the thyrotroph. Further studies may clarify the role of the predicted GATA-RE in the *Dio2* promoter (Dentice et al., 2003) and the complexity of the T3 sensing mechanism in regulation of the *TSHβ* gene (Christoffolete et al., 2006). Although it was previously reported that the GATA-RE in the *MHCβ* gene plays a role in its transcriptional activity (Hasegawa et al., 1997; Morimoto et al., 1999), other investigators suggested that it may not be functional (Vyas et al., 1999). Another study of the *MHCβ* promoter using rat neonatal cardiomyocytes suggests that the M-CAT site in this promoter is critical for its expression (Flink et al., 1992). M-CAT is the recognition site for the TEF family of transcription factors (Yoshida, 2008). TEF family transcription factors are the major target of α1 adrenaline signaling (Chen et al., 2004), which is known to mimic the cardiac phenotype seen in heart failure (Yoshida, 2008). Consistently, overexpression of TEF-1 in vivo exhibits a phenotype similar to that of chronic heart failure (Tsika et al., 2010). Our preliminary data suggests that T3/TR inhibits TEF-dependent transactivation of the *MHCβ* gene.

22. Negative regulation by liganded NHRs other than TR

A tethering mechanism has been reported in genes that are negatively regulated by liganded NHRs other than T3/TR. For example, the proopiomelanocortin (POMC) gene is activated by a transcription factor, Nur77, which is also the mediator of corticotropin-releasing hormone (CRH) signaling (Maira et al., 2003). Liganded GR interferes with this activity via a tethering mechanism (Martens et al., 2005). Moreover, a recent report suggested the involvement of chromatin remodeling factors in inhibition of the POMC gene by liganded GR (Bilodeau et al., 2006). Expression of parathyroid hormone (PTH) is inhibited by liganded VDR. PTH expression is maintained in the mice deficient for the VDR gene (Kim et al., 2007), suggesting that unliganded VDR is not the transcriptional activator for the PTH gene. A DNA-binding transcription factor, VDR interacting repressor (VDIR), binds with the promoter region of the *PTH* gene and activates its transcription (Kim et al., 2007). It was reported that VDR associates with VDIR (Kim et al., 2007; Murayama et al., 2004), resulting in VD3-dependent inhibition. A tethering mechanism between liganded VDR and VDIR also plays a role in negative regulation of human 1α(OH)ase (CYP27B1) expression by VD3 (Murayama et al., 2004). In this scenario, a chromatin remodeling factor complex (Kitagawa et al., 2003), and a DNA methylation-related proteins (Kim et al., 2009) may play crucial roles.

23. Conclusion

Negative feedback is the key component in homeostasis of hormones. A typical example is the inhibition of TSH synthesis by T3/TR. Although serum TSH levels are increased in hypothyroidism, observations in TR-knockout mice (Forrest et al., 1996; Gothe et al., 1999), human subjects with a deletion of the *TRβ* gene (Takeda et al., 1992) and *in vitro* experiments (Nakano et al., 2004) provide evidence that unliganded TR is not a transcriptional activator (Fig. 7). Moreover, deletion analysis of the *TSHβ* gene with co-expression of GATA2 and Pit1 revealed that a putative nTRE (Fig. 4) is dispensable for inhibition by T3/TR (Matsushita et al., 2007). Study of the *TSHβ* gene suggests the importance of a transcription factor that maintains the basal transcriptional activity of the promoter before ligand addition (Fig. 7). Identification of the factor required for the basal promoter activity may also be important and the first step in the analysis of other promoters that are repressed by T3/TR or other liganded NHRs. The factor may interact with NHRs. Once such a transcription factor is identified, it will be possible to study negative regulation using cells that express the factor and to carry out reporter analysis with co-transfection of its expression plasmid. For example, it will be possible to compare the mechanisms of positive and negative regulation using same cell line, for instance CV1 (Nakano et al., 2004). Information of the factor required for the basal promoter activity would be helpful to avoid artificial negative regulation mediated by plasmid backbones (for example a pUC/pBR322-derived AP-1 site or firefly luciferase cDNA). We are only just beginning to unravel some of complexities involved in negative regulation by liganded NHR including T3/TR.

24. References

Abel, E.D., Ahima, R.S., Boers, M.E., Elmquist, J.K. and Wondisford, F.E. (2001) Critical role for thyroid hormone receptor beta2 in the regulation of paraventricular thyrotropin-releasing hormone neurons. J Clin Invest, 107, 1017-1023.

Abel, E.D., Boers, M.E., Pazos-Moura, C., Moura, E., Kaulbach, H., Zakaria, M., Lowell, B., Radovick, S., Liberman, M.C. and Wondisford, F. (1999) Divergent roles for thyroid hormone receptor beta isoforms in the endocrine axis and auditory system. J Clin Invest, 104, 291-300.

Acevedo, M.L. and Kraus, W.L. (2003) Mediator and p300/CBP-steroid receptor coactivator complexes have distinct roles, but function synergistically, during estrogen receptor alpha-dependent transcription with chromatin templates. Mol Cell Biol, 23, 335-348.

Ahlquist, J.A., Franklyn, J.A., Wood, D.F., Balfour, N.J., Docherty, K., Sheppard, M.C. and Ramsden, D.B. (1987) Hormonal regulation of thyrotrophin synthesis and secretion. Horm Metab Res Suppl, 17, 86-89.

Annicotte, J.S., Schoonjans, K., Haby, C. and Auwerx, J. (2001) An E-box in pGL3 reporter vectors precludes their use for the study of sterol regulatory element-binding proteins. Biotechniques, 31, 993-994, 996.

Astapova, I., Lee, L.J., Morales, C., Tauber, S., Bilban, M. and Hollenberg, A.N. (2008) The nuclear corepressor, NCoR, regulates thyroid hormone action in vivo. Proc Natl Acad Sci U S A, 105, 19544-19549.

Astapova, I., Vella, K.R., Ramadoss, P., Holtz, K.A., Rodwin, B.A., Liao, X.H., Weiss, R.E., Rosenberg, M.A., Rosenzweig, A. and Hollenberg, A.N. (2011) The nuclear receptor corepressor (NCoR) controls thyroid hormone sensitivity and the set point of the hypothalamic-pituitary-thyroid axis. Mol Endocrinol, 25, 212-224.

Barros, A.C., Erway, L.C., Krezel, W., Curran, T., Kastner, P., Chambon, P. and Forrest, D. (1998) Absence of thyroid hormone receptor beta-retinoid X receptor interactions in auditory function and in the pituitary-thyroid axis. Neuroreport, 9, 2933-2937.

Bates, D.L., Chen, Y., Kim, G., Guo, L. and Chen, L. (2008) Crystal structures of multiple GATA zinc fingers bound to DNA reveal new insights into DNA recognition and self-association by GATA. J Mol Biol, 381, 1292-1306.

Becker, N., Seugnet, I., Guissouma, H., Dupre, S.M. and Demeneix, B.A. (2001) Nuclear corepressor and silencing mediator of retinoic and thyroid hormone receptors corepressor expression is incompatible with T(3)-dependent TRH regulation. Endocrinology, 142, 5321-5331.

Belakavadi, M., Saunders, J., Weisleder, N., Raghava, P.S. and Fondell, J.D. (2010) Repression of cardiac phospholamban gene expression is mediated by thyroid hormone receptor-{alpha}1 and involves targeted covalent histone modifications. Endocrinology, 151, 2946-2956.

Berghagen, H., Ragnhildstveit, E., Krogsrud, K., Thuestad, G., Apriletti, J. and Saatcioglu, F. (2002) Corepressor SMRT functions as a coactivator for thyroid hormone receptor T3Ralpha from a negative hormone response element. J Biol Chem, 277, 49517-49522.

Bilodeau, S., Vallette-Kasic, S., Gauthier, Y., Figarella-Branger, D., Brue, T., Berthelet, F., Lacroix, A., Batista, D., Stratakis, C., Hanson, J., Meij, B. and Drouin, J. (2006) Role of Brg1 and HDAC2 in GR trans-repression of the pituitary POMC gene and misexpression in Cushing disease. Genes Dev, 20, 2871-2886.

Breen, J.J., Matsuura, T., Ross, A.C. and Gurr, J.A. (1995) Regulation of thyroid-stimulating hormone beta-subunit and growth hormone messenger ribonucleic acid levels in the rat: effect of vitamin A status. Endocrinology, 136, 543-549.

Caldenhoven, E., Liden, J., Wissink, S., Van de Stolpe, A., Raaijmakers, J., Koenderman, L., Okret, S., Gustafsson, J.A. and Van der Saag, P.T. (1995) Negative cross-talk between RelA and the glucocorticoid receptor: a possible mechanism for the antiinflammatory action of glucocorticoids. Mol Endocrinol, 9, 401-412.

Cantor, A.B. and Orkin, S.H. (2005) Coregulation of GATA factors by the Friend of GATA (FOG) family of multitype zinc finger proteins. Semin Cell Dev Biol, 16, 117-128.

Carr, F.E., Kaseem, L.L. and Wong, N.C. (1992) Thyroid hormone inhibits thyrotropin gene expression via a position-independent negative L-triiodothyronine-responsive element. J Biol Chem, 267, 18689-18694.

Chadick, J.Z. and Asturias, F.J. (2005) Structure of eukaryotic Mediator complexes. Trends Biochem Sci, 30, 264-271.

Chaidarun, S.S., Eggo, M.C., Sheppard, M.C. and Stewart, P.M. (1994) Expression of epidermal growth factor (EGF), its receptor, and related oncoprotein (erbB-2) in human pituitary tumors and response to EGF in vitro. Endocrinology, 135, 2012-2021.

Chan, I.H., Borowsky, A.D. and Privalsky, M.L. (2008) A cautionary note as to the use of pBi-L and related luciferase/transgenic vectors in the study of thyroid endocrinology. Thyroid, 18, 665-666.

Chan, V., Wang, C. and Yeung, R.T. (1979) Thyrotropin: alpha- and beta-subunits of thyrotropin, and prolactin responses to four-hour constant infusions of thyrotropin-releasing hormone in normal subjects and patients with pituitary-thyroid disorders. J Clin Endocrinol Metab, 49, 127-131.

Charles, M.A., Saunders, T.L., Wood, W.M., Owens, K., Parlow, A.F., Camper, S.A., Ridgway, E.C. and Gordon, D.F. (2006) Pituitary-specific Gata2 knockout: effects on gonadotrope and thyrotrope function. Mol Endocrinol, 20, 1366-1377.

Chatterjee, V.K., Lee, J.K., Rentoumis, A. and Jameson, J.L. (1989) Negative regulation of the thyroid-stimulating hormone alpha gene by thyroid hormone: receptor interaction adjacent to the TATA box. Proc Natl Acad Sci U S A, 86, 9114-9118.

Chen, H., Lin, R.J., Xie, W., Wilpitz, D. and Evans, R.M. (1999) Regulation of hormone-induced histone hyperacetylation and gene activation via acetylation of an acetylase. Cell, 98, 675-686.

Chen, H.H., Mullett, S.J. and Stewart, A.F. (2004) Vgl-4, a novel member of the vestigial-like family of transcription cofactors, regulates alpha1-adrenergic activation of gene expression in cardiac myocytes. J Biol Chem, 279, 30800-30806.

Cheng, S.Y., Leonard, J.L. and Davis, P.J. (2010) Molecular aspects of thyroid hormone actions. Endocr Rev, 31, 139-170.

Chin, S., Apriletti, J. and Gick, G. (1998) Characterization of a negative thyroid hormone response element in the rat sodium, potassium-adenosine triphosphatase alpha3 gene promoter. Endocrinology, 139, 3423-3431.

Chin, W.W., Carr, F.E., Burnside, J. and Darling, D.S. (1993) Thyroid hormone regulation of thyrotropin gene expression. Recent Prog Horm Res, 48, 393-414.

Christoffolete, M.A., Ribeiro, R., Singru, P., Fekete, C., da Silva, W.S., Gordon, D.F., Huang, S.A., Crescenzi, A., Harney, J.W., Ridgway, E.C., Larsen, P.R., Lechan, R.M. and Bianco, A.C. (2006) Atypical expression of type 2 iodothyronine deiodinase in thyrotrophs explains the thyroxine-mediated pituitary thyrotropin feedback mechanism. Endocrinology, 147, 1735-1743.

Clabby, M.L., Robison, T.A., Quigley, H.F., Wilson, D.B. and Kelly, D.P. (2003) Retinoid X receptor alpha represses GATA-4-mediated transcription via a retinoid-dependent interaction with the cardiac-enriched repressor FOG-2. J Biol Chem, 278, 5760-5767.

Cohen, L.E. and Radovick, S. (2002) Molecular basis of combined pituitary hormone deficiencies. Endocr Rev, 23, 431-442.

Cohen, O., Flynn, T.R. and Wondisford, F.E. (1995) Ligand-dependent antagonism by retinoid X receptors of inhibitory thyroid hormone response elements. J Biol Chem, 270, 13899-13905.

Cohen, R.N. and Wondisford, F.E. (2005) Factors that control thyroid function: Thyrotropin. Werner and Ingbar's The Thyroid, Ninth Edition, pp159-197.

Crawford, S.E., Qi, C., Misra, P., Stellmach, V., Rao, M.S., Engel, J.D., Zhu, Y. and Reddy, J.K. (2002) Defects of the heart, eye, and megakaryocytes in peroxisome proliferator activator receptor-binding protein (PBP) null embryos implicate GATA family of transcription factors. J Biol Chem, 277, 3585-3592.

Danzi, S. and Klein, I. (2005) Posttranscriptional regulation of myosin heavy chain expression in the heart by triiodothyronine. Am J Physiol Heart Circ Physiol, 288, H455-460.

Dasen, J.S., O'Connell, S.M., Flynn, S.E., Treier, M., Gleiberman, A.S., Szeto, D.P., Hooshmand, F., Aggarwal, A.K. and Rosenfeld, M.G. (1999) Reciprocal interactions of Pit1 and GATA2 mediate signaling gradient-induced determination of pituitary cell types. Cell, 97, 587-598.

De Bosscher, K., Schmitz, M.L., Vanden Berghe, W., Plaisance, S., Fiers, W. and Haegeman, G. (1997) Glucocorticoid-mediated repression of nuclear factor-kappaB-dependent transcription involves direct interference with transactivation. Proc Natl Acad Sci U S A, 94, 13504-13509.

De Bosscher, K., Vanden Berghe, W. and Haegeman, G. (2001) Glucocorticoid repression of AP-1 is not mediated by competition for nuclear coactivators. Mol Endocrinol, 15, 219-227.

De Bosscher, K., Vanden Berghe, W. and Haegeman, G. (2003) The interplay between the glucocorticoid receptor and nuclear factor-kappaB or activator protein-1: molecular mechanisms for gene repression. Endocr Rev, 24, 488-522.

Dentice, M., Morisco, C., Vitale, M., Rossi, G., Fenzi, G. and Salvatore, D. (2003) The different cardiac expression of the type 2 iodothyronine deiodinase gene between human and rat is related to the differential response of the Dio2 genes to Nkx-2.5 and GATA-4 transcription factors. Mol Endocrinol, 17, 1508-1521.

Dorfman, D.M., Wilson, D.B., Bruns, G.A. and Orkin, S.H. (1992) Human transcription factor GATA-2. Evidence for regulation of preproendothelin-1 gene expression in endothelial cells. J Biol Chem, 267, 1279-1285.

Dupre, S.M., Guissouma, H., Flamant, F., Seugnet, I., Scanlan, T.S., Baxter, J.D., Samarut, J., Demeneix, B.A. and Becker, N. (2004) Both thyroid hormone receptor (TR)beta 1 and TR beta 2 isoforms contribute to the regulation of hypothalamic thyrotropin-releasing hormone. Endocrinology, 145, 2337-2345.

Edwards, J.G., Bahl, J.J., Flink, I.L., Cheng, S.Y. and Morkin, E. (1994) Thyroid hormone influences beta myosin heavy chain (beta MHC) expression. Biochem Biophys Res Commun, 199, 1482-1488.

Escobar-Morreale, H.F., del Rey, F.E., Obregon, M.J. and de Escobar, G.M. (1996) Only the combined treatment with thyroxine and triiodothyronine ensures euthyroidism in all tissues of the thyroidectomized rat. Endocrinology, 137, 2490-2502.

Fekete, C. and Lechan, R.M. (2007) Negative feedback regulation of hypophysiotropic thyrotropin-releasing hormone (TRH) synthesizing neurons: role of neuronal afferents and type 2 deiodinase. Front Neuroendocrinol, 28, 97-114.

Feng, X., Jiang, Y., Meltzer, P. and Yen, P.M. (2000) Thyroid hormone regulation of hepatic genes in vivo detected by complementary DNA microarray. Mol Endocrinol, 14, 947-955.

Fisher, D.A., Schoen, E.J., La Franchi, S., Mandel, S.H., Nelson, J.C., Carlton, E.I. and Goshi, J.H. (2000) The hypothalamic-pituitary-thyroid negative feedback control axis in children with treated congenital hypothyroidism. J Clin Endocrinol Metab, 85, 2722-2727.

Flink, I.L., Edwards, J.G., Bahl, J.J., Liew, C.C., Sole, M. and Morkin, E. (1992) Characterization of a strong positive cis-acting element of the human beta-myosin heavy chain gene in fetal rat heart cells. J Biol Chem, 267, 9917-9924.

Forrest, D., Hanebuth, E., Smeyne, R.J., Everds, N., Stewart, C.L., Wehner, J.M. and Curran, T. (1996) Recessive resistance to thyroid hormone in mice lacking thyroid hormone receptor beta: evidence for tissue-specific modulation of receptor function. Embo J, 15, 3006-3015.

Fowkes, R.C., King, P. and Burrin, J.M. (2002) Regulation of human glycoprotein hormone alpha-subunit gene transcription in LbetaT2 gonadotropes by protein kinase C and extracellular signal-regulated kinase 1/2. Biol Reprod, 67, 725-734.

Fraichard, A., Chassande, O., Plateroti, M., Roux, J.P., Trouillas, J., Dehay, C., Legrand, C., Gauthier, K., Kedinger, M., Malaval, L., Rousset, B. and Samarut, J. (1997) The T3R alpha gene encoding a thyroid hormone receptor is essential for post-natal development and thyroid hormone production. Embo J, 16, 4412-4420.

Franklyn, J.A., Wilson, M., Davis, J.R., Ramsden, D.B., Docherty, K. and Sheppard, M.C. (1986) Demonstration of thyrotrophin beta-subunit messenger RNA in rat pituitary cells in primary culture--evidence for regulation by thyrotrophin-releasing hormone and forskolin. J Endocrinol, 111, R1-2.

Friedrichsen, S., Christ, S., Heuer, H., Schafer, M.K., Parlow, A.F., Visser, T.J. and Bauer, K. (2004) Expression of pituitary hormones in the Pax8-/- mouse model of congenital hypothyroidism. Endocrinology, 145, 1276-1283.

Gereben, B., Zavacki, A.M., Ribich, S., Kim, B.W., Huang, S.A., Simonides, W.S., Zeold, A. and Bianco, A.C. (2008) Cellular and molecular basis of deiodinase-regulated thyroid hormone signaling. Endocr Rev, 29, 898-938.

Gershengorn, M.C. and Osman, R. (1996) Molecular and cellular biology of thyrotropin-releasing hormone receptors. Physiol Rev, 76, 175-191.

Glass, C.K. and Rosenfeld, M.G. (2000) The coregulator exchange in transcriptional functions of nuclear receptors. Genes Dev, 14, 121-141.

Gordon, D.F., Lewis, S.R., Haugen, B.R., James, R.A., McDermott, M.T., Wood, W.M. and Ridgway, E.C. (1997) Pit-1 and GATA-2 interact and functionally cooperate to activate the thyrotropin beta-subunit promoter. J Biol Chem, 272, 24339-24347.

Gordon, D.F., Tucker, E.A., Tundwal, K., Hall, H., Wood, W.M. and Ridgway, E.C. (2006) MED220/thyroid receptor-associated protein 220 functions as a transcriptional coactivator with Pit-1 and GATA-2 on the thyrotropin-beta promoter in thyrotropes. Mol Endocrinol, 20, 1073-1089.

Gothe, S., Wang, Z., Ng, L., Kindblom, J.M., Barros, A.C., Ohlsson, C., Vennstrom, B. and Forrest, D. (1999) Mice devoid of all known thyroid hormone receptors are viable but exhibit disorders of the pituitary-thyroid axis, growth, and bone maturation. Genes Dev, 13, 1329-1341.

Guissouma, H., Dupre, S.M., Becker, N., Jeannin, E., Seugnet, I., Desvergne, B. and Demeneix, B.A. (2002) Feedback on hypothalamic TRH transcription is dependent on thyroid hormone receptor N terminus. Mol Endocrinol, 16, 1652-1666.

Gupta, M.P. (2007) Factors controlling cardiac myosin-isoform shift during hypertrophy and heart failure. J Mol Cell Cardiol, 43, 388-403.

Haddad, F., Bodell, P.W., Qin, A.X., Giger, J.M. and Baldwin, K.M. (2003) Role of antisense RNA in coordinating cardiac myosin heavy chain gene switching. J Biol Chem, 278, 37132-37138.

Hallenbeck, P.L., Phyillaier, M. and Nikodem, V.M. (1993) Divergent effects of 9-cis-retinoic acid receptor on positive and negative thyroid hormone receptor-dependent gene expression. J Biol Chem, 268, 3825-3828.

Hasegawa, K., Lee, S.J., Jobe, S.M., Markham, B.E. and Kitsis, R.N. (1997) cis-Acting sequences that mediate induction of beta-myosin heavy chain gene expression during left ventricular hypertrophy due to aortic constriction. Circulation, 96, 3943-3953.

Haugen, B.R., Wood, W.M., Gordon, D.F. and Ridgway, E.C. (1993) A thyrotrope-specific variant of Pit-1 transactivates the thyrotropin beta promoter. J Biol Chem, 268, 20818-20824.

Heck, S., Kullmann, M., Gast, A., Ponta, H., Rahmsdorf, H.J., Herrlich, P. and Cato, A.C. (1994) A distinct modulating domain in glucocorticoid receptor monomers in the repression of activity of the transcription factor AP-1. Embo J, 13, 4087-4095.

Herrlich, P. (2001) Cross-talk between glucocorticoid receptor and AP-1. Oncogene, 20, 2465-2475.

Ho, C.K. and Strauss, J.F., 3rd. (2004) Activation of the control reporter plasmids pRL-TK and pRL-SV40 by multiple GATA transcription factors can lead to aberrant normalization of transfection efficiency. BMC Biotechnol, 4, 10.

Hollenberg, A.N., Monden, T., Flynn, T.R., Boers, M.E., Cohen, O. and Wondisford, F.E. (1995) The human thyrotropin-releasing hormone gene is regulated by thyroid hormone through two distinct classes of negative thyroid hormone response elements. Mol Endocrinol, 9, 540-550.

Hollenberg, A.N., Monden, T., Madura, J.P., Lee, K. and Wondisford, F.E. (1996) Function of nuclear co-repressor protein on thyroid hormone response elements is regulated by the receptor A/B domain. J Biol Chem, 271, 28516-28520.

Hong, W., Nakazawa, M., Chen, Y.Y., Kori, R., Vakoc, C.R., Rakowski, C. and Blobel, G.A. (2005) FOG-1 recruits the NuRD repressor complex to mediate transcriptional repression by GATA-1. Embo J, 24, 2367-2378.

Huang, Z.Q., Li, J., Sachs, L.M., Cole, P.A. and Wong, J. (2003) A role for cofactor-cofactor and cofactor-histone interactions in targeting p300, SWI/SNF and Mediator for transcription. Embo J, 22, 2146-2155.

Huggins, G.S., Bacani, C.J., Boltax, J., Aikawa, R. and Leiden, J.M. (2001) Friend of GATA 2 physically interacts with chicken ovalbumin upstream promoter-TF2 (COUP-TF2) and COUP-TF3 and represses COUP-TF2-dependent activation of the atrial natriuretic factor promoter. J Biol Chem, 276, 28029-28036.

Ito, M., Yuan, C.X., Okano, H.J., Darnell, R.B. and Roeder, R.G. (2000) Involvement of the TRAP220 component of the TRAP/SMCC coactivator complex in embryonic development and thyroid hormone action. Mol Cell, 5, 683-693.

Jensen, F.C., Girardi, A.J., Gilden, R.V. and Koprowski, H. (1964) Infection Of Human And Simian Tissue Cultures With Rous Sarcoma Virus. Proc Natl Acad Sci U S A, 52, 53-59.

Jepsen, K., Solum, D., Zhou, T., McEvilly, R.J., Kim, H.J., Glass, C.K., Hermanson, O. and Rosenfeld, M.G. (2007) SMRT-mediated repression of an H3K27 demethylase in progression from neural stem cell to neuron. Nature, 450, 415-419.

Jorgensen, J.S., Quirk, C.C. and Nilson, J.H. (2004) Multiple and overlapping combinatorial codes orchestrate hormonal responsiveness and dictate cell-specific expression of the genes encoding luteinizing hormone. Endocr Rev, 25, 521-542.

Kakucska, I., Rand, W. and Lechan, R.M. (1992) Thyrotropin-releasing hormone gene expression in the hypothalamic paraventricular nucleus is dependent upon feedback regulation by both triiodothyronine and thyroxine. Endocrinology, 130, 2845-2850.

Kalaitzidis, D. and Gilmore, T.D. (2005) Transcription factor cross-talk: the estrogen receptor and NF-kappaB. Trends Endocrinol Metab, 16, 46-52.

Kalkhoven, E., Wissink, S., van der Saag, P.T. and van der Burg, B. (1996) Negative interaction between the RelA(p65) subunit of NF-kappaB and the progesterone receptor. J Biol Chem, 271, 6217-6224.

Kamei, Y., Xu, L., Heinzel, T., Torchia, J., Kurokawa, R., Gloss, B., Lin, S.C., Heyman, R.A., Rose, D.W., Glass, C.K. and Rosenfeld, M.G. (1996) A CBP integrator complex mediates transcriptional activation and AP-1 inhibition by nuclear receptors. Cell, 85, 403-414.

Kashiwabara, Y., Sasaki, S., Matsushita, A., Nagayama, K., Ohba, K., Iwaki, H., Matsunaga, H., Suzuki, S., Misawa, H., Ishizuka, K., Oki, Y. and Nakamura, H. (2009) Functions of PIT1 in GATA2-dependent transactivation of the thyrotropin beta promoter. J Mol Endocrinol, 42, 225-237.

Kim, M.S., Fujiki, R., Murayama, A., Kitagawa, H., Yamaoka, K., Yamamoto, Y., Mihara, M., Takeyama, K. and Kato, S. (2007) 1Alpha,25(OH)2D3-induced transrepression by vitamin D receptor through E-box-type elements in the human parathyroid hormone gene promoter. Mol Endocrinol, 21, 334-342.

Kim, M.S., Kondo, T., Takada, I., Youn, M.Y., Yamamoto, Y., Takahashi, S., Matsumoto, T., Fujiyama, S., Shirode, Y., Yamaoka, I., Kitagawa, H., Takeyama, K., Shibuya, H., Ohtake, F. and Kato, S. (2009) DNA demethylation in hormone-induced transcriptional derepression. Nature, 461, 1007-1012.

Kim, S.W., Ho, S.C., Hong, S.J., Kim, K.M., So, E.C., Christoffolete, M. and Harney, J.W. (2005) A novel mechanism of thyroid hormone-dependent negative regulation by thyroid hormone receptor, nuclear receptor corepressor (NCoR), and GAGA-binding factor on the rat cD44 promoter. J Biol Chem, 280, 14545-14555.

Kinugawa, K., Yonekura, K., Ribeiro, R.C., Eto, Y., Aoyagi, T., Baxter, J.D., Camacho, S.A., Bristow, M.R., Long, C.S. and Simpson, P.C. (2001) Regulation of thyroid hormone receptor isoforms in physiological and pathological cardiac hypertrophy. Circ Res, 89, 591-598.

Kitagawa, H., Fujiki, R., Yoshimura, K., Mezaki, Y., Uematsu, Y., Matsui, D., Ogawa, S., Unno, K., Okubo, M., Tokita, A., Nakagawa, T., Ito, T., Ishimi, Y., Nagasawa, H., Matsumoto, T., Yanagisawa, J. and Kato, S. (2003) The chromatin-remodeling complex WINAC targets a nuclear receptor to promoters and is impaired in Williams syndrome. Cell, 113, 905-917.

Kobayashi-Osaki, M., Ohneda, O., Suzuki, N., Minegishi, N., Yokomizo, T., Takahashi, S., Lim, K.C., Engel, J.D. and Yamamoto, M. (2005) GATA motifs regulate early hematopoietic lineage-specific expression of the Gata2 gene. Mol Cell Biol, 25, 7005-7020.

Krane, I.M., Spindel, E.R. and Chin, W.W. (1991) Thyroid hormone decreases the stability and the poly(A) tract length of rat thyrotropin beta-subunit messenger RNA. Mol Endocrinol, 5, 469-475.

Laflamme, L., Hamann, G., Messier, N., Maltais, S. and Langlois, M.F. (2002) RXR acts as a coregulator in the regulation of genes of the hypothalamo-pituitary axis by thyroid hormone receptors. J Mol Endocrinol, 29, 61-72.

Lazar, M.A. (2003) Thyroid hormone action: a binding contract. J Clin Invest, 112, 497-499.

Liden, J., Delaunay, F., Rafter, I., Gustafsson, J. and Okret, S. (1997) A new function for the C-terminal zinc finger of the glucocorticoid receptor. Repression of RelA transactivation. J Biol Chem, 272, 21467-21472.

Lin, K.H., Shieh, H.Y. and Hsu, H.C. (2000) Negative regulation of the antimetastatic gene Nm23-H1 by thyroid hormone receptors. Endocrinology, 141, 2540-2547.

Liu, Y.Y. and Brent, G.A. (2008) Stealth sequences in reporter gene vectors confound studies of T3-regulated negative gene expression. Thyroid, 18, 593-595.

Lopez, G., Schaufele, F., Webb, P., Holloway, J.M., Baxter, J.D. and Kushner, P.J. (1993) Positive and negative modulation of Jun action by thyroid hormone receptor at a unique AP1 site. Mol Cell Biol, 13, 3042-3049.

Madison, L.D., Ahlquist, J.A., Rogers, S.D. and Jameson, J.L. (1993) Negative regulation of the glycoprotein hormone alpha gene promoter by thyroid hormone: mutagenesis of a proximal receptor binding site preserves transcriptional repression. Mol Cell Endocrinol, 94, 129-136.

Maia, A.L., Harney, J.W. and Larsen, P.R. (1996) Is there a negative TRE in the luciferase reporter cDNA? Thyroid, 6, 325-328.

Maira, M., Martens, C., Batsche, E., Gauthier, Y. and Drouin, J. (2003) Dimer-specific potentiation of NGFI-B (Nur77) transcriptional activity by the protein kinase A pathway and AF-1-dependent coactivator recruitment. Mol Cell Biol, 23, 763-776.

Mansen, A., Yu, F., Forrest, D., Larsson, L. and Vennstrom, B. (2001) TRs have common and isoform-specific functions in regulation of the cardiac myosin heavy chain genes. Mol Endocrinol, 15, 2106-2114.

Martens, C., Bilodeau, S., Maira, M., Gauthier, Y. and Drouin, J. (2005) Protein-protein interactions and transcriptional antagonism between the subfamily of NGFI-B/Nur77 orphan nuclear receptors and glucocorticoid receptor. Mol Endocrinol, 19, 885-897.

Matsushita, A., Sasaki, S., Kashiwabara, Y., Nagayama, K., Ohba, K., Iwaki, H., Misawa, H., Ishizuka, K. and Nakamura, H. (2007) Essential role of GATA2 in the negative regulation of thyrotropin beta gene by thyroid hormone and its receptors. Mol Endocrinol, 21, 865-884.

Minami, T., Abid, M.R., Zhang, J., King, G., Kodama, T. and Aird, W.C. (2003) Thrombin stimulation of vascular adhesion molecule-1 in endothelial cells is mediated by protein kinase C (PKC)-delta-NF-kappa B and PKC-zeta-GATA signaling pathways. J Biol Chem, 278, 6976-6984.

Minegishi, N., Suzuki, N., Kawatani, Y., Shimizu, R. and Yamamoto, M. (2005) Rapid turnover of GATA-2 via ubiquitin-proteasome protein degradation pathway. Genes Cells, 10, 693-704.

Misawa, H., Sasaki, S., Matsushita, A., Ohba, K., Iwaki, H., Matsunaga, H., Suzuki, S., Ishizuka, K., Oki, Y. and Nakamura, H. Liganded thyroid hormone receptor inhibits phorbol 12-O-tetradecanoate-13-acetate–induced enhancer activity via firefly luciferase cDNA. in submission.

Mittag, J., Friedrichsen, S., Strube, A., Heuer, H. and Bauer, K. (2009) Analysis of hypertrophic thyrotrophs in pituitaries of athyroid Pax8-/- mice. Endocrinology, 150, 4443-4449.

Morimoto, T., Hasegawa, K., Kaburagi, S., Kakita, T., Masutani, H., Kitsis, R.N., Matsumori, A. and Sasayama, S. (1999) GATA-5 is involved in leukemia inhibitory factor-responsive transcription of the beta-myosin heavy chain gene in cardiac myocytes. J Biol Chem, 274, 12811-12818.

Murayama, A., Kim, M.S., Yanagisawa, J., Takeyama, K. and Kato, S. (2004) Transrepression by a liganded nuclear receptor via a bHLH activator through co-regulator switching. Embo J, 23, 1598-1608.

Naar, A.M., Boutin, J.M., Lipkin, S.M., Yu, V.C., Holloway, J.M., Glass, C.K. and Rosenfeld, M.G. (1991) The orientation and spacing of core DNA-binding motifs dictate selective transcriptional responses to three nuclear receptors. Cell, 65, 1267-1279.

Nagaya, T. and Jameson, J.L. (1993) Thyroid hormone receptor dimerization is required for dominant negative inhibition by mutations that cause thyroid hormone resistance. J Biol Chem, 268, 15766-15771.

Nagayama, K., Sasaki, S., Matsushita, A., Ohba, K., Iwaki, H., Matsunaga, H., Suzuki, S., Misawa, H., Ishizuka, K., Oki, Y., Noh, J.Y. and Nakamura, H. (2008) Inhibition of GATA2-dependent transactivation of the TSHbeta gene by ligand-bound estrogen receptor alpha. J Endocrinol, 199, 113-125.

Nakano, K., Matsushita, A., Sasaki, S., Misawa, H., Nishiyama, K., Kashiwabara, Y. and Nakamura, H. (2004) Thyroid-hormone-dependent negative regulation of thyrotropin beta gene by thyroid hormone receptors: study with a new experimental system using CV1 cells. Biochem J, 378, 549-557.

Nikrodhanond, A.A., Ortiga-Carvalho, T.M., Shibusawa, N., Hashimoto, K., Liao, X.H., Refetoff, S., Yamada, M., Mori, M. and Wondisford, F.E. (2006) Dominant role of thyrotropin-releasing hormone in the hypothalamic-pituitary-thyroid axis. J Biol Chem, 281, 5000-5007.

Nissen, R.M. and Yamamoto, K.R. (2000) The glucocorticoid receptor inhibits NFkappaB by interfering with serine-2 phosphorylation of the RNA polymerase II carboxy-terminal domain. Genes Dev, 14, 2314-2329.

Nofsinger, R.R., Li, P., Hong, S.H., Jonker, J.W., Barish, G.D., Ying, H., Cheng, S.Y., Leblanc, M., Xu, W., Pei, L., Kang, Y.J., Nelson, M., Downes, M., Yu, R.T., Olefsky, J.M., Lee, C.H. and Evans, R.M. (2008) SMRT repression of nuclear receptors controls the adipogenic set point and metabolic homeostasis. Proc Natl Acad Sci U S A, 105, 20021-20026.

Ohba, K., Sasaki, S., Matsushita, A., Iwaki, H., Matsunaga, H., Suzuki, S., Ishizuka, K., Misawa, H., Oki, Y. and Nakamura, H. (2011) GATA2 mediates thyrotropin-releasing hormone-induced transcriptional activation of the thyrotropin beta gene. PLoS One, in press.

Ooi, G.T., Tawadros, N. and Escalona, R.M. (2004) Pituitary cell lines and their endocrine applications. Mol Cell Endocrinol, 228, 1-21.

Oppenheimer, J.H., Schwartz, H.L. and Surks, M.I. (1974) Tissue differences in the concentration of triiodothyronine nuclear binding sites in the rat: liver, kidney, pituitary, heart, brain, spleen, and testis. Endocrinology, 95, 897-903.

Osborne, S.A. and Tonissen, K.F. (2002) pRL-TK induction can cause misinterpretation of gene promoter activity. Biotechniques, 33, 1240-1242.

Paguio, A., Almond, B., Fan, F., Stecha, P., Garvin, D., Wood, M. and Wood, K. (2005) pGL4 Vectors: A New Generation of Luciferase Reporter Vectors. Promega Notes, 89, 7–10.

Pennathur, S., Madison, L.D., Kay, T.W. and Jameson, J.L. (1993) Localization of promoter sequences required for thyrotropin-releasing hormone and thyroid hormone responsiveness of the glycoprotein hormone alpha-gene in primary cultures of rat pituitary cells. Mol Endocrinol, 7, 797-805.

Pfahl, M. (1993) Nuclear receptor/AP-1 interaction. Endocr Rev, 14, 651-658.

Ray, A. and Prefontaine, K.E. (1994) Physical association and functional antagonism between the p65 subunit of transcription factor NF-kappa B and the glucocorticoid receptor. Proc Natl Acad Sci U S A, 91, 752-756.

Refetoff, S. and Dumitrescu, A.M. (2007) Syndromes of reduced sensitivity to thyroid hormone: genetic defects in hormone receptors, cell transporters and deiodination. Best Pract Res Clin Endocrinol Metab, 21, 277-305.

Refetoff, S., Weiss, R.E. and Usala, S.J. (1993) The syndromes of resistance to thyroid hormone. Endocr Rev, 14, 348-399.

Reichardt, H.M., Kaestner, K.H., Tuckermann, J., Kretz, O., Wessely, O., Bock, R., Gass, P., Schmid, W., Herrlich, P., Angel, P. and Schutz, G. (1998) DNA binding of the glucocorticoid receptor is not essential for survival. Cell, 93, 531-541.

Reutrakul, S., Sadow, P.M., Pannain, S., Pohlenz, J., Carvalho, G.A., Macchia, P.E., Weiss, R.E. and Refetoff, S. (2000) Search for abnormalities of nuclear corepressors, coactivators, and a coregulator in families with resistance to thyroid hormone without mutations in thyroid hormone receptor beta or alpha genes. J Clin Endocrinol Metab, 85, 3609-3617.

Roche, A.E., Bassett, B.J., Samant, S.A., Hong, W., Blobel, G.A. and Svensson, E.C. (2008) The zinc finger and C-terminal domains of MTA proteins are required for FOG-2-mediated transcriptional repression via the NuRD complex. J Mol Cell Cardiol, 44, 352-360.

Rodriguez, P., Bonte, E., Krijgsveld, J., Kolodziej, K.E., Guyot, B., Heck, A.J., Vyas, P., de Boer, E., Grosveld, F. and Strouboulis, J. (2005) GATA-1 forms distinct activating and repressive complexes in erythroid cells. Embo J, 24, 2354-2366.

Rouf, R., Greytak, S., Wooten, E.C., Wu, J., Boltax, J., Picard, M., Svensson, E.C., Dillmann, W.H., Patten, R.D. and Huggins, G.S. (2008) Increased FOG-2 in failing myocardium disrupts thyroid hormone-dependent SERCA2 gene transcription. Circ Res, 103, 493-501.

Saatcioglu, F., Deng, T. and Karin, M. (1993) A novel cis element mediating ligand-independent activation by c-ErbA: implications for hormonal regulation. Cell, 75, 1095-1105.

Saatcioglu, F., Lopez, G., West, B.L., Zandi, E., Feng, W., Lu, H., Esmaili, A., Apriletti, J.W., Kushner, P.J., Baxter, J.D. and Karin, M. (1997) Mutations in the conserved C-terminal sequence in thyroid hormone receptor dissociate hormone-dependent activation from interference with AP-1 activity. Mol Cell Biol, 17, 4687-4695.

Sadow, P.M., Koo, E., Chassande, O., Gauthier, K., Samarut, J., Xu, J., O'Malley, B.W., Seo, H., Murata, Y. and Weiss, R.E. (2003) Thyroid hormone receptor-specific interactions with steroid receptor coactivator-1 in the pituitary. Mol Endocrinol, 17, 882-894.

Safer, J.D., Langlois, M.F., Cohen, R., Monden, T., John-Hope, D., Madura, J., Hollenberg, A.N. and Wondisford, F.E. (1997) Isoform variable action among thyroid hormone receptor mutants provides insight into pituitary resistance to thyroid hormone. Mol Endocrinol, 11, 16-26.

Sanchez-Pacheco, A., Palomino, T. and Aranda, A. (1995) Negative regulation of expression of the pituitary-specific transcription factor GHF-1/Pit-1 by thyroid hormones through interference with promoter enhancer elements. Mol Cell Biol, 15, 6322-6330.

Santos, G.M., Afonso, V., Barra, G.B., Togashi, M., Webb, P., Neves, F.A., Lomri, N. and Lomri, A. (2006) Negative regulation of superoxide dismutase-1 promoter by thyroid hormone. Mol Pharmacol, 70, 793-800.

Sarapura, V.D., Samuels, M.H. and Ridgway, E.C. (2002) Thyroid-stimulating Hormone. The Pituitary, Second Edition, pp172-215.

Sasaki, S., Lesoon-Wood, L.A., Dey, A., Kuwata, T., Weintraub, B.D., Humphrey, G., Yang, W.M., Seto, E., Yen, P.M., Howard, B.H. and Ozato, K. (1999) Ligand-induced recruitment of a histone deacetylase in the negative-feedback regulation of the thyrotropin beta gene. Embo J, 18, 5389-5398.

Satoh, T., Yamada, M., Iwasaki, T. and Mori, M. (1996) Negative regulation of the gene for the preprothyrotropin-releasing hormone from the mouse by thyroid hormone requires additional factors in conjunction with thyroid hormone receptors. J Biol Chem, 271, 27919-27926.

Scheinman, R.I., Gualberto, A., Jewell, C.M., Cidlowski, J.A. and Baldwin, A.S., Jr. (1995) Characterization of mechanisms involved in transrepression of NF-kappa B by activated glucocorticoid receptors. Mol Cell Biol, 15, 943-953.

Schule, R., Rangarajan, P., Kliewer, S., Ransone, L.J., Bolado, J., Yang, N., Verma, I.M. and Evans, R.M. (1990) Functional antagonism between oncoprotein c-Jun and the glucocorticoid receptor. Cell, 62, 1217-1226.

Sharma, V., Hays, W.R., Wood, W.M., Pugazhenthi, U., St Germain, D.L., Bianco, A.C., Krezel, W., Chambon, P. and Haugen, B.R. (2006) Effects of rexinoids on thyrotrope function and the hypothalamic-pituitary-thyroid axis. Endocrinology, 147, 1438-1451.

Sherman, S.I., Gopal, J., Haugen, B.R., Chiu, A.C., Whaley, K., Nowlakha, P. and Duvic, M. (1999) Central hypothyroidism associated with retinoid X receptor-selective ligands. N Engl J Med, 340, 1075-1079.

Shibusawa, N., Hashimoto, K., Nikrodhanond, A.A., Liberman, M.C., Applebury, M.L., Liao, X.H., Robbins, J.T., Refetoff, S., Cohen, R.N. and Wondisford, F.E. (2003a) Thyroid hormone action in the absence of thyroid hormone receptor DNA-binding in vivo. J Clin Invest, 112, 588-597.

Shibusawa, N., Hollenberg, A.N. and Wondisford, F.E. (2003b) Thyroid hormone receptor DNA binding is required for both positive and negative gene regulation. J Biol Chem, 278, 732-738.

Shibusawa, N., Yamada, M., Hirato, J., Monden, T., Satoh, T. and Mori, M. (2000) Requirement of thyrotropin-releasing hormone for the postnatal functions of pituitary thyrotrophs: ontogeny study of congenital tertiary hypothyroidism in mice. Mol Endocrinol, 14, 137-146.

Shimizu, R. and Yamamoto, M. (2005) Gene expression regulation and domain function of hematopoietic GATA factors. Semin Cell Dev Biol, 16, 129-136.

Shupnik, M.A. (2000) Thyroid hormone suppression of pituitary hormone gene expression. Rev Endocr Metab Disord, 1, 35-42.

Shupnik, M.A., Gharib, S.D. and Chin, W.W. (1988) Estrogen suppresses rat gonadotropin gene transcription in vivo. Endocrinology, 122, 1842-1846.

Shupnik, M.A., Greenspan, S.L. and Ridgway, E.C. (1986) Transcriptional regulation of thyrotropin subunit genes by thyrotropin-releasing hormone and dopamine in pituitary cell culture. J Biol Chem, 261, 12675-12679.

Shupnik, M.A., Ridgway, E.C. and Chin, W.W. (1989) Molecular biology of thyrotropin. Endocr Rev, 10, 459-475.

St Germain, D.L., Hernandez, A., Schneider, M.J. and Galton, V.A. (2005) Insights into the role of deiodinases from studies of genetically modified animals. Thyroid, 15, 905-916.

Staton, J.M., Thomson, A.M. and Leedman, P.J. (2000) Hormonal regulation of mRNA stability and RNA-protein interactions in the pituitary. J Mol Endocrinol, 25, 17-34.

Steger, D.J., Hecht, J.H. and Mellon, P.L. (1994) GATA-binding proteins regulate the human gonadotropin alpha-subunit gene in the placenta and pituitary gland. Mol Cell Biol, 14, 5592-5602.

Stein, B. and Yang, M.X. (1995) Repression of the interleukin-6 promoter by estrogen receptor is mediated by NF-kappa B and C/EBP beta. Mol Cell Biol, 15, 4971-4979.

Steinfelder, H.J., Radovick, S., Mroczynski, M.A., Hauser, P., McClaskey, J.H., Weintraub, B.D. and Wondisford, F.E. (1992a) Role of a pituitary-specific transcription factor (pit-1/GHF-1) or a closely related protein in cAMP regulation of human thyrotropin-beta subunit gene expression. J Clin Invest, 89, 409-419.

Steinfelder, H.J., Radovick, S. and Wondisford, F.E. (1992b) Hormonal regulation of the thyrotropin beta-subunit gene by phosphorylation of the pituitary-specific transcription factor Pit-1. Proc Natl Acad Sci U S A, 89, 5942-5945.

Sugawara, A., Yen, P.M., Qi, Y., Lechan, R.M. and Chin, W.W. (1995) Isoform-specific retinoid-X receptor (RXR) antibodies detect differential expression of RXR proteins in the pituitary gland. Endocrinology, 136, 1766-1774.

Sun, Y., Lu, X. and Gershengorn, M.C. (2003) Thyrotropin-releasing hormone receptors -- similarities and differences. J Mol Endocrinol, 30, 87-97.

Surks, M.I. and Hollowell, J.G. (2007) Age-specific distribution of serum thyrotropin and antithyroid antibodies in the US population: implications for the prevalence of subclinical hypothyroidism. J Clin Endocrinol Metab, 92, 4575-4582.

Suzuki, S., Sasaki, S., Morita, H., Oki, Y., Turiya, D., Ito, T., Misawa, H., Ishizuka, K. and Nakamura, H. (2010) The role of the amino-terminal domain in the interaction of unliganded peroxisome proliferator-activated receptor gamma-2 with nuclear receptor co-repressor. J Mol Endocrinol, 45, 133-145.

Tagami, T., Madison, L.D., Nagaya, T. and Jameson, J.L. (1997) Nuclear receptor corepressors activate rather than suppress basal transcription of genes that are negatively regulated by thyroid hormone. Mol Cell Biol, 17, 2642-2648.

Tagami, T., Park, Y. and Jameson, J.L. (1999) Mechanisms that mediate negative regulation of the thyroid-stimulating hormone alpha gene by the thyroid hormone receptor. J Biol Chem, 274, 22345-22353.

Takeda, K., Sakurai, A., DeGroot, L.J. and Refetoff, S. (1992) Recessive inheritance of thyroid hormone resistance caused by complete deletion of the protein-coding region of the thyroid hormone receptor-beta gene. J Clin Endocrinol Metab, 74, 49-55.

Takeda, T., Nagasawa, T., Miyamoto, T., Hashizume, K. and DeGroot, L.J. (1997) The function of retinoid X receptors on negative thyroid hormone response elements. Mol Cell Endocrinol, 128, 85-96.

Takeuchi, Y., Murata, Y., Sadow, P., Hayashi, Y., Seo, H., Xu, J., O'Malley, B.W., Weiss, R.E. and Refetoff, S. (2002) Steroid receptor coactivator-1 deficiency causes variable alterations in the modulation of T(3)-regulated transcription of genes in vivo. Endocrinology, 143, 1346-1352.

Tao, Y., Williams-Skipp, C. and Scheinman, R.I. (2001) Mapping of glucocorticoid receptor DNA binding domain surfaces contributing to transrepression of NF-kappa B and induction of apoptosis. J Biol Chem, 276, 2329-2332.

Tillman, J.B., Crone, D.E., Kim, H.S., Sprung, C.N. and Spindler, S.R. (1993) Promoter independent down-regulation of the firefly luciferase gene by T3 and T3 receptor in CV1 cells. Mol Cell Endocrinol, 95, 101-109.

Trost, S.U., Swanson, E., Gloss, B., Wang-Iverson, D.B., Zhang, H., Volodarsky, T., Grover, G.J., Baxter, J.D., Chiellini, G., Scanlan, T.S. and Dillmann, W.H. (2000) The thyroid hormone receptor-beta-selective agonist GC-1 differentially affects plasma lipids and cardiac activity. Endocrinology, 141, 3057-3064.

Tsika, R.W., Ma, L., Kehat, I., Schramm, C., Simmer, G., Morgan, B., Fine, D.M., Hanft, L.M., McDonald, K.S., Molkentin, J.D., Krenz, M., Yang, S. and Ji, J. (2010) TEAD-1 overexpression in the mouse heart promotes an age-dependent heart dysfunction. J Biol Chem, 285, 13721-13735.

Umesono, K., Murakami, K.K., Thompson, C.C. and Evans, R.M. (1991) Direct repeats as selective response elements for the thyroid hormone, retinoic acid, and vitamin D3 receptors. Cell, 65, 1255-1266.

Valentine, J.E., Kalkhoven, E., White, R., Hoare, S. and Parker, M.G. (2000) Mutations in the estrogen receptor ligand binding domain discriminate between hormone-dependent transactivation and transrepression. J Biol Chem, 275, 25322-25329.

Villa, A., Santiago, J., Belandia, B. and Pascual, A. (2004) A response unit in the first exon of the beta-amyloid precursor protein gene containing thyroid hormone receptor and Sp1 binding sites mediates negative regulation by 3,5,3'-triiodothyronine. Mol Endocrinol, 18, 863-873.

Vyas, D.R., McCarthy, J.J. and Tsika, R.W. (1999) Nuclear protein binding at the beta-myosin heavy chain A/T-rich element is enriched following increased skeletal muscle activity. J Biol Chem, 274, 30832-30842.

Walsh, J.P., Bremner, A.P., Bulsara, M.K., O'Leary, P., Leedman, P.J., Feddema, P. and Michelangeli, V. (2005a) Subclinical thyroid dysfunction as a risk factor for cardiovascular disease. Arch Intern Med, 165, 2467-2472.

Walsh, J.P., Bremner, A.P., Bulsara, M.K., O'Leary, P., Leedman, P.J., Feddema, P. and Michelangeli, V. (2005b) Thyroid dysfunction and serum lipids: a community-based study. Clin Endocrinol (Oxf), 63, 670-675.

Webb, P., Lopez, G.N., Uht, R.M. and Kushner, P.J. (1995) Tamoxifen activation of the estrogen receptor/AP-1 pathway: potential origin for the cell-specific estrogen-like effects of antiestrogens. Mol Endocrinol, 9, 443-456.

Weiss, R.E., Forrest, D., Pohlenz, J., Cua, K., Curran, T. and Refetoff, S. (1997) Thyrotropin regulation by thyroid hormone in thyroid hormone receptor beta-deficient mice. Endocrinology, 138, 3624-3629.

Weitzel, J.M. (2008) To bind or not to bind - how to down-regulate target genes by liganded thyroid hormone receptor? Thyroid Res, 1, 4.

Wikstrom, L., Johansson, C., Salto, C., Barlow, C., Campos Barros, A., Baas, F., Forrest, D., Thoren, P. and Vennstrom, B. (1998) Abnormal heart rate and body temperature in mice lacking thyroid hormone receptor alpha 1. Embo J, 17, 455-461.

Wissink, S., van Heerde, E.C., Schmitz, M.L., Kalkhoven, E., van der Burg, B., Baeuerle, P.A. and van der Saag, P.T. (1997) Distinct domains of the RelA NF-kappaB subunit are required for negative cross-talk and direct interaction with the glucocorticoid receptor. J Biol Chem, 272, 22278-22284.

Wondisford, F.E., Farr, E.A., Radovick, S., Steinfelder, H.J., Moates, J.M., McClaskey, J.H. and Weintraub, B.D. (1989) Thyroid hormone inhibition of human thyrotropin beta-subunit gene expression is mediated by a cis-acting element located in the first exon. J Biol Chem, 264, 14601-14604.

Wondisford, F.E., Steinfelder, H.J., Nations, M. and Radovick, S. (1993) AP-1 antagonizes thyroid hormone receptor action on the thyrotropin beta-subunit gene. J Biol Chem, 268, 2749-2754.

Wood, W.M., Ocran, K.W., Kao, M.Y., Gordon, D.F., Alexander, L.M., Gutierrez-Hartmann, A. and Ridgway, E.C. (1990) Protein factors in thyrotropic tumor nuclear extracts bind to a region of the mouse thyrotropin beta-subunit promoter essential for expression in thyrotropes. Mol Endocrinol, 4, 1897-1904.

Wright, C.E., Haddad, F., Qin, A.X., Bodell, P.W. and Baldwin, K.M. (1999) In vivo regulation of beta-MHC gene in rodent heart: role of T3 and evidence for an upstream enhancer. Am J Physiol, 276, C883-891.

Wu, J., Li, Y., Dietz, J. and Lala, D.S. (2004) Repression of p65 transcriptional activation by the glucocorticoid receptor in the absence of receptor-coactivator interactions. Mol Endocrinol, 18, 53-62.

Wulf, A., Wetzel, M.G., Kebenko, M., Kroger, M., Harneit, A., Merz, J. and Weitzel, J.M. (2008) The role of thyroid hormone receptor DNA binding in negative thyroid hormone-mediated gene transcription. J Mol Endocrinol, 41, 25-34.

Xu, J., Qiu, Y., DeMayo, F.J., Tsai, S.Y., Tsai, M.J. and O'Malley, B.W. (1998) Partial hormone resistance in mice with disruption of the steroid receptor coactivator-1 (SRC-1) gene. Science, 279, 1922-1925.

Yang, Z., Hong, S.H. and Privalsky, M.L. (1999) Transcriptional anti-repression. Thyroid hormone receptor beta-2 recruits SMRT corepressor but interferes with subsequent assembly of a functional corepressor complex. J Biol Chem, 274, 37131-37138.

Yanisch-Perron, C., Vieira, J. and Messing, J. (1985) Improved M13 phage cloning vectors and host strains: nucleotide sequences of the M13mp18 and pUC19 vectors. Gene, 33, 103-119.

Yoshida, T. (2008) MCAT elements and the TEF-1 family of transcription factors in muscle development and disease. Arterioscler Thromb Vasc Biol, 28, 8-17.

Yuan, L.W. and Gambee, J.E. (2000) Phosphorylation of p300 at serine 89 by protein kinase C. J Biol Chem, 275, 40946-40951.

Yusta, B., Alarid, E.T., Gordon, D.F., Ridgway, E.C. and Mellon, P.L. (1998) The thyrotropin beta-subunit gene is repressed by thyroid hormone in a novel thyrotrope cell line, mouse T alphaT1 cells. Endocrinology, 139, 4476-4482.

Zhuang, Y., Butler, B., Hawkins, E., Paguio, A., Orr, L., Wood, M. and Wood, K. (2001) New Synthetic Renilla Gene and Assay System Increase Expression, Reliability and Sensitivity. Promega Notes, 79, 6-11.

6

Clinical Management of Thyroid Nodules in the Areas of Various Iodine Supply

Dorota Słowińska-Klencka[1], Bożena Popowicz[1],
Stanisław Sporny[2] and Mariusz Klencki[1]
[1]*Department of Morphometry of Endocrine Glands, Medical University of Lodz,*
[2]*Department of Dental Pathomorphology, Medical University of Lodz*
Poland

1. Introduction

The thyroid nodules constitute an important diagnostic problem mainly because various benign lesions must be distinguished from malignant neoplasms. This problem is of particular importance in endemic and postendemic areas where there are a lot of patients with multiple thyroid nodules. In such areas the majority of thyroid lesions is non-neoplastic and develop usually when diffuse goitre transforms into nodular one (Laurberg et al;. 2010, Słowińska-Klencka et al., 2002, 2008). Other non-neoplastic thyroid lesions may develop due to thyroiditis (acute thyroiditis, de Quervain disease, and autoimmune chronic thyroiditis). The frequency of revealing thyroid cancer - in comparison to malignancies in other organs - is relatively low. On the other hand, it is the most common cancer of endocrine glands, and the incidence of thyroid cancer is continuously increasing (Hughes et al., 2011; Sipos & Mazzaferri, 2010). This increase is partly related to the improvements to efficacy of preoperative diagnostics, but whatever is the nature of the observed higher incidence of the thyroid cancer it focuses the interests of physicians. It should be stressed that epidemiological assessments based on clinical data do not reflect the true incidence of the thyroid cancer, as it is found in as much as 30% of cadavers if the thyroid is serially examined during autopsy (Fukanaga & Yatani, 1975; Harach et al., 1985). In majority of such cases these cancers are subclinical papillary microcancers (with diameters below 10 mm) that are usually not diagnosed in alive patients. However, recently it has been shown that cytological examination of small thyroid lesions reveals invasive cancers (with the presence of cancer cells in lymph nodes and infiltration of the thyroid capsule) with a surprisingly high frequency (Chow et al. 2003; Kang et al., 2004; E.K. Kim et al., 2002; Lin et al., 2005; Nam-Goong et al., 2004; Papini et al., 2002, Słowińska-Klencka et al., 2008).

2. Influence of iodine supply on epidemiology of the thyroid lesions

Thyroid nodules can be revealed by palpation in 4–7% of adult patients in the areas of sufficient iodine supply, and in 10–15% in the areas of mild to moderate iodine deficiency (Hegedűs 2004; Knudsen et al., 2000; Tunbridge et al., 1977). The use of ultrasound (US) imaging raises ten times the rate of discovering thyroid lesions in comparison with palpatory examination (Ezzat et al., 1994; Tan et al., 1995). Many of these lesions do not exceed 10 mm in diameter. That increase poses diagnostic challenges particularly in endemic areas or areas with newly corrected iodine supply. We showed that, in such an area, focal lesions were found in the thyroid glands of nearly 80% of the examined patients, and the frequency of multinodular goitre, irrespective of the size of lesions, was considerably high - above 77%. Between infracentimetric nodules, found in more than 40% of all examined persons, the percentage of multiple lesions was even higher - above 80% (Słowińska-Klencka et al., 2008). This constitutes a major difference in comparison with countries with high iodine supply, where the thyroid lesions more frequently occur as single nodules (Feldt-Rasmussen, 2001; Frates et al. 2006; D.L. Kim 2008; E.K. Kim et al., 2002; Słowińska-Klencka et al., 2002).

The differences in iodine supply influence also the incidence of various pathological lesions in the thyroid (Laurberg et al. 2010). In endemic areas patients with nodular goitre and follicular neoplasms predominate. The introduction of iodine prophylaxis is related to a gradual decline in the occurrence of non-neoplastic nodular goitre as well as of follicular neoplasms; on the other hand, papillary cancer is diagnosed more frequently (Feldt-Rasmussen, 2001; Lind et al., 1998; Schmid 1989; Słowińska-Klencka et al., 2002; Solymosi et al., 2002). It should be remembered that the observed increase in the relative frequency of papillary carcinoma is partly attributed to the improving effectiveness of routine preoperative and postoperative morphological diagnostics that usually parallels introduction of iodine prophylaxis. It leads to more frequent revealing of papillary microcarcinoma and proper diagnosing of the follicular variant of papillary carcinoma without erroneous classification of such tumours into follicular carcinomas. The data from Sweden do not suggest any enhancing effect of iodisation on papillary carcinoma, since the increases in the incidence of such type of cancer were similar in both iodine-deficient and iodine-sufficient areas (Petteersson et al., 1996). Moreover, the correction of iodine deficiency rates virtually coincided in highly developed countries with the spread of thyroid ultrasound and biopsy, which have made diagnosis of clinically silent thyroid carcinoma more frequent. Thus, even though the incidence of thyroid carcinoma rose, the prognosis has significantly improved due to a shift towards differentiated forms of thyroid carcinomas that are diagnosed at earlier stages (Feldt-Rasmussen, 2001).

On the other hand, countries with high iodine supply are characterised by higher incidence of the thyroid autoimmune diseases, and especially of chronic thyroiditis. Our studies, carried to monitor side-effects of the introduction of iodine prophylaxis in Poland, showed that the occurrence of autoimmune stigmata in thyroid cytological smears were gradually increasing as iodine prophylaxis became more effective (Fig. 1) (Słowińska-Klencka et al., 2002; 2006). Similar observations were reported in a study from Greece by Doufas et al., (1999) and from Argentina by Harach & Williams (1995) (although during much longer intervals before and after introduction of iodine prophylaxis). It is believed that iodine intake might modulate the activity (and/or clinical expression) of thyroid autoimmune diseases in genetically susceptible individuals, but there is no evident proof that the amount of iodine intake - at least when in the range between iodine deficiency and full physiological doses - is involved in the de novo triggering of thyroid autoimmunity.

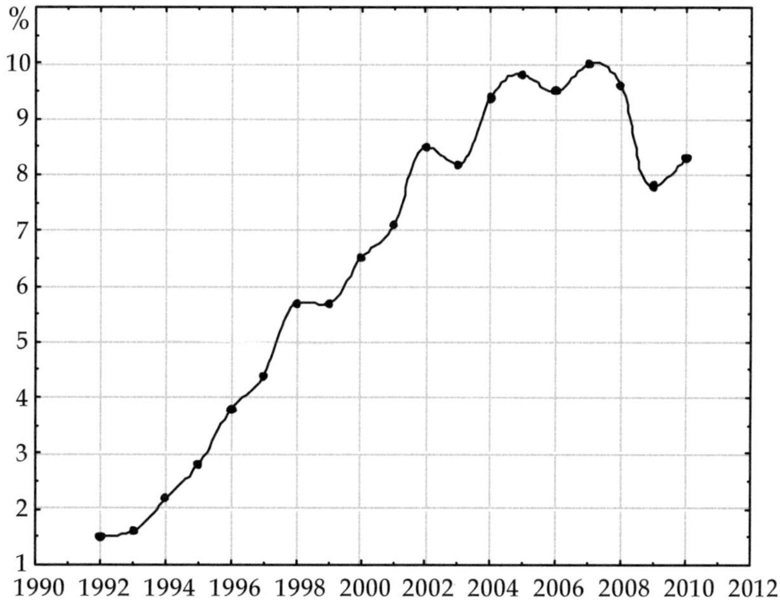

Fig. 1. The occurrence of chronic thyroiditis in cytological results in years 1992-2010 in one diagnostics centre in Poland. House-hold salt iodization was initiated in early 90's and in 1997 obligatory model of iodine prophylaxis (30 mg KI/kg of salt) was introduced.

3. Basic rules for diagnosing thyroid nodules

The need for an effective differential diagnostics of focal lesions in the thyroid comes from the necessity of an early diagnosis of thyroid cancer that even as a small lesion may show extrathyoidal invasiveness. The basic examination used for that purpose is fine-needle aspiration biopsy (FNAB). During the past years, many reports have been published indicating the usefulness of FNAB in the diagnosis of thyroid nodules. Fine-needle aspiration biopsy is a quick and, at the same time, the most sensitive examination in diagnosing thyroid nodules. The main advantages of FNAB are: the possibility of selecting patients for prompt surgical treatment, low invasiveness, and relatively low cost of examination (Faquin et al. 2011; Gharib et al., 2010; Lewis et al. 2009; Seningen et al., 2011). The management of thyroid nodule is usually based on cytological result which should always be interpreted together with other clinical data, mainly those related to the risk of cancer in the nodule. The clinical indications of the increased risk of cancer include: presence of hard painless nodule with diminished mobility (especially if the nodule causes hoarseness, dysphagia or dyspnoea), quick growth of the lesion as well as enlargement of the lymph nodes in the neck (Gharib et al., 2010; Wada et al., 2003). There are also other features of some importance in clinical suspicion of malignancy in a nodule: male sex, patient's age below 15-20 or above 60-70, history positive for neck irradiation or prolonged hyperstimulation of the thyroid with TSH (Belfiore et al., 1992; Hegedűs 2004; Kumar et al.; 1999; Samann et al., 1987; Schneider & Sarne, 2005). Familial history of thyroid cancer is of particular importance in relation to medullary cancer (MTC) as well as papillary cancer (PTC) (Kloos et al., 2009; Nose, 2011; Stoffer et al., 1986). The diagnosis of chronic thyroiditis is also of importance as it is considered to facilitate development of lymphoma of the

thyroid. Some investigators also believe that chronic thyroiditis is related to higher risk of papillary cancer (Azizi et al., 2011; Boi et al., 2005; Gul et al., 2010; Mukasa et al., 2011; Ruggiero et al., 2005; Shih et al., 2008; Singh et al., 1999; Słowińska-Klencka et al., 2006).
For proper interpretation of cytological smears it is also necessary to analyse the thyroid function and possible antithyroid treatment, as well as other laboratory results (like calcitonin serum concentration). Imaging examinations and oncological history (with possible chemo- and radiotherapy) should also be considered (Słowińska-Klencka et al., Gharib et al, 2010).

4. Role of ultrasound imaging in diagnostics of thyroid nodules

The thyroid ultrasonography (US) is the most common imaging examination of the gland. It allows to determine the precise size of the thyroid and to reveal non-palpable focal lesions. Despite of this, according to endocrine societies (American Thyroid Association - ATA, American Association of Clinical Endocrinologists - AACE and European Thyroid Association - ETA) guidelines, US is not recommended as a screening examination for patients without clinical data for the increased risk of cancer or clinical suspicion for any thyroid disease (Gharib et al, 2010).
Until recently, US was used in Europe more frequently than in the United States, and similarly US was more commonly used in Europe as a support to FNAB (Bennedbæk, 1999; Bennedbæk & Hegedüs 2000; Bonnema et al., 2000, 2002). At present it is proved that US assistance improves the diagnostic efficiency of FNAB in relation to both small and large, palpable lesions (Cesur et al., 2006). US allows to detect features suggestive of malignant growth and select the lesions to be recommended for FNAB. It also makes it possible to select the area of lesion optimal for FNAB (i.e. solid part free of areas of necrosis) and to choose the right gauge and length of the biopsy needle (Gharib et al., 2010). Because of its low invasiveness and possibility of multiple repeating in a patient, US is also useful for the assessment of goitre treatment effectiveness (both surgical and conservative) (Quadbeck et al., 2002). US examination is also used for diagnosing developmental disorders of the thyroid. In the cases of thyroid malignancy it allows to assess the completeness of thyroidectomy and the presence of possible local recurrence, as well as to control local lymph nodes (Frasoldati et al., 2003; Gharib et al., 2010; Hegedűs, 2001; Rago et al., 1998; Wong & Ahuja, 2005). It should be stressed that US does not allow by itself to differentiate between benign and malignant thyroid lesions (Gharib et al., 2010; Hegedűs, 2001).

4.1 Role of ultrasound imaging in selection of thyroid lesions for FNAB – A new approach

The precise indications for FNAB of thyroid lesions are still being investigated. The main criteria considered include sonographic features of nodules like the size, shape and echogenicity of lesions, the vascular pattern in Doppler imaging, the presence of microcalcifications and appearance of lesion's borders (Alexander et al., 2004; Frates et al., 2005; Gharib et al., 2010; Nam-Goong et al., 2004; Papini et al., 2002; 12–16; Tae et al., 2007). Current recommendations on the diagnostics of thyroid nodules take into consideration the similar frequency of revealing thyroid cancer in FNAB of small vs. large nodules (Berker et al., 2008; Nam-Goong et al., 2004; Papini et al., 2002), palpable vs. non-palpable nodules (Papini et al., 2002; Popowicz et al., 2009; Hagag et al., 1998) as well as solitary vs. multiple

nodules (Belfiore et al., 1992; Frates et al., 2006). In consequence, the recommendations focus on US features related to the increased risk of malignancy, and not on the size nor palpability of the nodule, which were important criteria in the previous recommendations.
Interestingly, attention is paid to US features allowing to identify invasive cancers including those growing in very small lesions. Some recent papers have brought convincing data on the high percentage of carcinomas (some of them with extrathyroidal invasion) in small lesions subjected to FNAB (Kang et al., 2004; E.K. Kim et al., 2002; S.J. Kim et al., 2003; Leenhardt et al., 1999; Lin et al., 2005; Nam-Goong et al., 2004; Papini et al., 2002). The majority of these reports come from the countries with natural high iodine supply (Japan, Korea) or those with long-established iodine prophylaxis. However, our data from the post-endemic region confirm these observations. In our material, the frequency of revealed small and large cancers was proportional to the frequency of the biopsied nodules of each size class, and approx. 1/3 of cytologically revealed thyroid microcancers metastasized to lymph nodes (Słowińska-Klencka et al., 2008).
Analysis of the reported studies justifies division of the known US features suggestive of malignancy into 2 groups of high and low specificity.
The highly specific US features in selection of thyroid lesions for FNAB include:
1. features of metastasis in the lymph nodes;
2. features of the thyroid capsule (or neighbouring organs) invasion;
3. microcalcifications (small, intranodular, punctate, hyperechoic spots with scanty or no posterior acoustic shadowing).

The features of lower specificity include:
1. irregular or microlobulated margins;
2. more tall (anteroposterior) than wide (transverse) shape;
3. marked hypoechogenicity;
4. chaotic arrangement or intranodular vascular images.

It should be stressed that the assessment of these features is yet not enough standardized, and because of their qualitative or semi-quantitative nature their reproducibility is not satisfactory (especially when sonographer lacks experience).
According to our observations and some other studies, there are differences in sensitivity and specificity of these features in respect of nodule size (Popowicz et al., 2008; Mazzaferri & Sipos, 2008). The influence of epidemiological situation (mainly iodine supply) on the specificity and sensitivity of these features is also underestimated.
The most sensitive feature of malignancy is hypoechogenicity, both for small and large lesions. Unfortunately, the specificity of this feature is low, especially in small nodules - majority of benign lesions (especially the small ones) is hypoechoic (Moon et al., 2008; Cappelli et al., 2006, 2007; Chan et al., 2003; Frates et al., 2005; 2006; E.K. Kim et al., 2002; Leenhardt et al., 1999; Lyshchik et al., 2005; Nam-Goong et al., 2004; Papini et al., 2002). Interestingly, in our material, all invasive microcarcinomas (with the signs of extrathyroidal growth or with spread to lymph nodes) were hypoechoic in the US examination (Popowicz et al., 2009). The role of hypoechogenicity, in revealing aggressive variants of microcarcinomas, was also indicated by Barbaro et al. (2005).
The most specific single feature is the presence of microcalcifications in the lesion (Cappelli et al., 2006, 2007; Chan et al., 2003; Frates et al., 2005, 2006; Iannuccilli et al., 2004; E.K. Kim et al., 2002; Moon et al., 2008; Nam-Goong et al., 2004; Papini et al., 2002; Rago et al., 2007). It increases tenfold the risk of cancer, but the sensitivity of this feature is low, particularly in

group of nodules not exceeding 10 mm (Popowicz et al., 2009). Similar results were obtained by Moon et al., (2008).

Less but still significantly predictive is the shape index (Alexander et al., 2004; Berker et al., 2008; Cappelli et al., 2006; E.K. Kim et al., 2002; Moon et al., 2008). Our analysis shows that the features describing the shape of lesion are useful mainly in the diagnostics of small nodules (Popowicz et al., 2009). Similar results with respect to the ratio of long to short axis of a lesion were reported by Berker et al. (Berker et al., 2008). The shape of larger lesions is a less sensitive feature probably because such lesions are more frequently partially cystic, and as such are more spherical even if benign.

With respect to the assessment of blood flow pattern, the published opinions are contradictory with some reporting that Doppler US is helpful (Papini et al., 2002; Moon et al., 2008; Cappelli et al., 2007; Chan et al., 2003; Lyshchik et al., 2005; Levine, 2006), and others reporting that Doppler US did not satisfactory improve diagnostic accuracy (Nam-Goong et al., 2004; Frates et al., 2003; Iannuccilli et al., 2004; Rago et al., 1998). Even though the logistic analysis of regression allows classification of intranodular vascular pattern as an independent feature suggesting malignancy, the OR is several times lower than for other features (Cappelli et al., 2007).

It is difficult to apprehend the role of lesion's borders assessment because there are significant differences in the definition of suspected appearance of borders. Some researchers, such as Nam-Gong et al., (2004), suggested that ill-defined nodules were important for predicting malignancies, while others (E.K. Kim et al., 2002, Cappelli et al., 2006, 2007 and Kang et al., 2004) suggested that irregular margins were important. Moreover, some authors reported that the presence of blurred margins was not significantly linked to malignancy of lesions (Leenhardt et al., 1999; Frates et al., 2006; Iannuccilli et al., 2004), or that well-defined margins were a common sonographic feature in papillary carcinomas (Chan et al., 2003).

Up to now, any single criterion of selecting lesions for FNAB was not found to be satisfactory. The analysis of usefulness of feature combinations brought diverse results, both in terms of specificity and sensitivity of such a set of features, and the possible reduction in the number of performed FNABs. This reduction is of particular importance in endemic areas where it determines economic effectiveness of cytological examination. Because of high predominance of benign thyroid lesions in such areas, the number of performed FNABs is very high in relation to the number of revealed cancers.

The current recommendations try to relate the indications for FNAB to predictive value of particular features and the size of lesion: the lower predictive value of a feature, the larger lesion that should be selected for FNAB (Gharib et al., 2010). However, in the setting of endemic goitre it is very difficult, if not impossible, to follow the recommendation to examine all solid hypoechoic lesions of diameter above 1 cm. Large number of such lesions makes their further selection a must. Thus it is important to underline the role of US examination in prioritization of lesions. In the cases of multiple thyroid nodules it is advisable to biopsy those lesions which are positive for a highly specific feature and those positive for several features of lower value.

The available recommendations suggest the number of lesions that should be biopsied in order to satisfactory exclude the risk of malignancy in the multiple nodular goitre (according to ATA/AACE/ETA – 2 lesions, and according to Polish recommendations, relating to postendemic area - 3-4 lesions) (Gharib et al., 2010; Sporny et al., 2010). However, such suggestions are the results of experts' consensus. There are few studies addressing this issue (Frates et al. 2006), and the mean number of lesions in goitre to be examined differs significantly between iodine rich and iodine deficient areas. Anyway it is justified to subject lesions to FNAB in the order resulting from the predictive value and number of positive US features.

In this context it should be mentioned that current recommendations indicate also negative features, i.e. those which allow to resign from biopsy. It is justified not to perform FNAB in the cases of purely cystic nodules, spongiform nodules, or autonomic nodules in patient with low TSH levels (Bonavita et al., 2009; Gharib et al., 2010).

The current recommendations underline the necessity of proper selection of the area within examined lesions that should be biopsied. In the case of cystic-solid lesions it is indicated to biopsy the solid part and to evaluate any fluid evacuated from the cystic part. Our experience shows that the use of cytological centrifuge for preparation of fluid significantly lowers the percentage of non-diagnostic outcomes (Słowińska-Klencka et al. 2004). In the case of solid lesions the biopsy of central part should be avoided as there is higher probability of necrosis in that area. In the case of large nodules it is recommended to perform at least 2 aspirations from various areas of the lesion.

4.2 Role of ultrasound imaging in diagnostics of thyroid lesions of size < 5 mm

The current recommendations distinguish the category of lesions of diameter below 5 mm. It is indicated to monitor such lesions with US examinations including the evaluation of features that can be helpful in revealing invasive microcancers or in making decision of FNAB. Such recommendation is based on several rationales: lower accuracy of US features evaluation in such small lesions, higher probability of missing lesion during aspiration (especially in dorsal location of lesion), and lower clinical aggressiveness of cancers smaller than 5 mm (Mazzaferri & Sipos, 2008). Obviously, there are exceptions related to particular indications for FNAB including: extrathyroidal growth of nodule (extracapsular invasion, lymph nodes involvement or metastases); positive history of neck irradiation in childhood or adolescence; papillary thyroid cancers, medullary thyroid cancers, or multiple endocrine neoplasia type 2 in first-degree relatives; previous thyroid surgery for cancer; increased calcitonin levels in the absence of interfering factors (Berker et al., 2008; Mazzaferri & Sipos, 2008; D.W. Kim et al., 2009; Kwak et al., 2008). Among features suggestive of the increased risk of invasive papillary cancer in lesion there are: shaping of the thyroid capsule by lesion or lesion abutting the capsule, and features of the lymph nodes involvement (Kwak et al., 2008; Ito & Miyauchi, 2009). It should be stressed that predictive value of the latter is very diverse, and the highest specificity is found for the presence of calcifications or cystic degeneration (relating to areas of necrosis) in the lymph nodes (Leboulleux et al., 2007; Sipos, 2009). Some investigators suggest that such data from US examination may be also useful in the selection of optimal treatment strategy, and according to Ito et al., (2003, 2009) careful US examinations of patients with small nodules may even allow refraining from surgical treatment in some cases of papillary microcancers. However, such management is not recommended by ATA, AACE nor ETA.

5. Efficacy of FNAB of thyroid nodules in the areas of various iodine supply

The above mentioned differences between areas of various iodine supply in the incidence of thyroid nodules, their solitary and multiple occurrence, as well as distribution of particular pathological lesions, significantly affect the efficacy of preoperative diagnoses of thyroid nodules.

Our group performed one of few studies on the effectiveness of FNAB of thyroid nodules in areas with newly corrected iodine supply. It was a retrospective analysis of US examination and FNAB on a large series of thyroid glands, performed in a single diagnostic centre. The analysis included the outcomes of FNABs performed in years 1985-2010, and obligatory iodine prophylaxis using household salt iodized with 30 mg KI/kg was established in Poland in 1997. Earlier, iodine prophylaxis was carried out with numerous discontinuations from 1930s until 1980, when it was dropped. In the years 1992–1993, a nationwide study performed in about 20 000 schoolchildren, showed that Poland was an area of mild or moderate iodine deficiency (Szybiński & Żarnecki, 1993). About this time salt iodization was partially reintroduced and iodine supply gradually increased. Reevaluation of iodine status of Polish population in early 2000s proved the efficacy of iodine prophylaxis by showing normalization of ioduria, rapid decrease in the incidence of goitre in schoolchildren and lowering the percentage of newborns with transient hyperthyrotropinemia (TSH> 5 mU/L) (Szybiński et al., 2008).

In total nearly 40,000 FNAB results were analysed, and in more than 6000 patients those results were verified by histopathological examination. It was found that in endemic areas the number of performed FNABs was very high in relation to the number of revealed cancers, despite of adhering to the recommendations for selection of lesions for FNAB. This is a consequence of high incidence of multiple mostly benign lesions. As a result, the frequency of outcomes in the category of benign lesions is higher than in iodine-rich areas. The suspicious or malignant lesions constitute < 10% of all cytological results (Słowińska-Klencka et al., 2002, 2008) while in areas of a long-term normal iodine supply this percentage reaches 20–30% (D.L. Kim et al., 2008; Nam-Goong et al., 2004). Moreover, in endemic or post-endemic areas the rate of malignant lesions in post-operative histopathological examination is relatively low. In our material, such rate was only 7% while in areas of high iodine supply it is several times higher. This difference results from a high number of patients in iodine-deficient areas who are referred to a surgeon not because of the suspicious FNAB outcome - only about 20% of the patients in our series - but because of large multinodular goitre, notwithstanding the benign outcome of FNAB (Słowińska-Klencka et al., 2008).

5.1 Efficacy of selection of thyroid nodules for FNAB in areas of various iodine supply

In endemic areas it is more difficult to select lesions that should be biopsied, and the probability of wrong selection affects especially small lesions. Small nodules are usually accompanied by other, often larger lesions, which are more frequently chosen for FNAB. As a result, the efficacy of preoperative diagnoses of small carcinomas in endemic areas is significantly lower than in the case of larger malignant tumours (Popowicz et al., 2009; Słowińska-Klencka et al., 2008). These differences are deepened by the fact that in the areas of iodine sufficiency the reported percentages of false negative (FN) results are falsely lowered, as FNAB outcomes are frequently verified not against histopathological examination but clinical follow-up. In such areas patients with cytologically diagnosed benign lesions, without goitre are not usually surgically treated, and as a result there may be some misdiagnosed cases of thyroid microcarcinomas in that group of patients (Theoharis et al., 2009). In endemic areas many patients are subjected to thyroidectomy because of large multinodular goitre and then some microcancers are revealed in lesions that were not selected for FNAB nor even identified in US examination.

In respect to described differences, in the regions of a high number of patients with multinodular goitre, it seems reasonable to use more powerful and rigorous criteria for selecting lesions for FNAB. Such criteria should allow to optimize the number of performed FNABs in relation to the number of revealed cancers and, in particular, should allow to diagnose invasive cancers. Our study showed that some indolent cancers, which probably never become aggressive, were revealed, but some invasive microcancers were missed (Popowicz et al., 2009; Słowińska-Klencka et al., 2008). It could be helpful to use the more specific set of features for diagnosing invasive thyroid carcinoma but an optimal definition of such a set is still being sought. E.K. Kim et al., (2002) reported that reduction number of performed FNABs by 47%, with 94% sensitivity and 66% specificity, could be achieved by selecting lesions fulfilling the shape criterion or those with microcalcifications, irregular or microlobulated margins or marked hypoechogenicity (relative to the strap muscles in the neck). Those data come from areas of high-iodine supply and low incidence of multinodular goitre. In our material from the area of recently corrected iodine supply, it was found that similar reduction in the number of performed FNABs is possible on the condition of exclusion of hypoechogenicity from the set of selection criteria. Examination of lesions more tall than wide only, or those with microcalcification or solitary ones, would allow limitation of the number of biopsies by 50% while keeping sensitivity above 80%. However, it would increase the risk of misdiagnosing small invasive thyroid cancers (in our material all invasive small cancers were hypoechoic) (Popowicz et al., 2009). It is possible that application of 'marked hypoechogenicity' feature would allow avoidance of that risk. In our material the achieving of above 90% sensitivity in the group of small lesions (<10 mm) was possible if all hypoechoic nodules or those with suspected shape were selected for FNAB. Such selection could lower the number of performed biopsies by 28%. The addition of all solitary nodules and all nodules with microcalcifications would not increase the number of examinations significantly, but would allow for biopsying 98% of malignant lesions (Popowicz et al., 2009). Similar results were reported by other authors who used the selection criteria as the shape of lesions jointly with other features from the US examination as the selection criteria. Cappelli et al., (2006) showed that 99% sensitivity can be achieved by aspiration of lesions more tall than wide and possessing at least two of the following features: hypoechogenicity, blurred margins and calcifications. The authors claimed that by applying such criteria, the number of performed FNABs could be lowered by 28%.

Most diagnostic algorithms suggest performing FNAB for solid, hypoechoic lesions with diameters over 10 mm, even in the absence of any other features suggesting the increased risk of cancer (Baloch et al., 2008; Gharib et al., 2010; Layfield et al., 2010). But in the case of large multinodular goitre, it is necessary to select large lesions for biopsy as well. Our studies showed that in the case of large nodules, the usefulness of sonographic features in selecting lesions for FNAB was less satisfactory than in the case of small ones. The sensitivity of selection of nearly 84% could be achieved by biopsying all hypoechoic or containing microcalcifications nodules or with the positive shape index, which would lower the number of FNAB by more than 55% (Popowicz et al., 2009).

It is also worth mentioning that in the majority of the reports, the influence of nodule size on the optimal set of features for selecting lesions for FNAB was not investigated. Only Cappelli et al., (2006) observed that the associations of US features with malignancy were similar in groups of large and small lesions. On the other hand, Lyshchik et al., (2005) and Berker et al., (2008) found that the usefulness of sonographic features in selecting lesions for FNAB in the group of larger nodules was lower than in the group of smaller ones, and that for thyroid nodules larger than 15 mm (Lyshchik) or than 10 mm (Berker) the only reliable criterion of cancer was hypoechogenicity. Moon et al., (2008) reported that a set of US features suggestive of malignancy (i.e. the presence of at least one of the findings including taller than wide shape, speculated margin, hypoechogenicity and the presence of calcifications) showed lower sensitivity and higher specificity for nodules >10 mm than for smaller nodules, which is in concordance with our data.

The discussed epidemiological differences may also attribute to the observed differences in the frequency of obtaining non-diagnostic material from small lesions. The data on the efficacy of FNAB in obtaining diagnostic cellular material from small thyroid lesions are equivocal. Some reports suggest that the smaller the size of aspirated lesion the higher the rate of inadequate specimens (Cesur et al., 2006; Lee et al., 2006; Sahin et al., 2006). Other reports from Japan and Korea suggest that if the staff performing FNAB of the thyroid is experienced enough, it is possible to aspirate reliably even very small lesions - with diameters of 2-3 mm (D.W. Kim, et al., 2009; Nam-Goong et al., 2004; Yang et al., 2002). In these Asian countries, specialists more often diagnose very small thyroid lesions which - because of the specific epidemiological situation - less frequently coexist with other larger lesions but are microcarcinomas more frequently than in the countries with low iodine supply.

5.2 Influence of iodine status of population on clinical interpretation of cytological results

The proper selection of lesions for biopsy is one of the important components influencing the effectiveness of this examination. Another is an epidemiological situation of examined populations which affects the incidences of follicular lesions (follicular adenomas and carcinomas as well as hyperplastic nodules in nodular goitre) and papillary cancers (Feldt-Rasmussen, 2001; Słowińska-Klencka et al., 2002).

FNAB does not allow for differentiation among certain forms of nodular goitre, follicular adenoma, follicular carcinoma and frequently also follicular variant of papillary carcinoma of the thyroid. This problem is the main limitation of FNAB diagnostics, especially in endemic regions. Consequently, in clinical practice, the cytological diagnoses of 'follicular neoplasm' and, especially, of 'Hürthle cell tumour' are frequently regarded as an indication for surgical treatment. However in the areas of long-term iodine deficiency, the consideration of 'follicular neoplasms' results as an indicator of malignancy yields a significant increase in false positive results. In our material, in which 'follicular neoplasm' corresponds more frequently to non-neoplastic hyperplastic nodules or follicular adenoma than to thyroid cancers, such interpretation puts false positive results in range 10-12% (Słowińska-Klencka et al., 2002, 2008). This is the reason for low positive predictive value of FNAB in such areas. In iodine-rich areas 'follicular neoplasm' diagnosis corresponds more frequently to follicular variant of papillary cancer.

Follicular cancer constituted 30% of all malignant tumours found in postoperative histopathological examination in patients who underwent FNAB at our centre before introduction of salt iodization, while 10 years later that percentage dropped to 6-7%. Parallel decrease in frequency of follicular adenoma was also observed. Papillary cancer constituted about 45% of all malignant tumours in the first period and 75% in the second one (Słowińska-Klencka et al., 2002, 2008). Such marked changes over relatively short time may be attributed not only to the increased iodine supply but also to erroneous classification of follicular variant of papillary cancer in the earlier period. As it was already mentioned, an introduction of iodine prophylaxis is often accompanied by the increased interest in the thyroid diseases what improves the standards of histopathological examination.

Analysis of the cytological results in our centre over the discussed period showed the gradual decrease in frequency of cytological results, applying to 'follicular neoplasm", while the frequency of diagnoses of oxyphilic variant of those neoplasms remained nearly constant (Fig. 2).

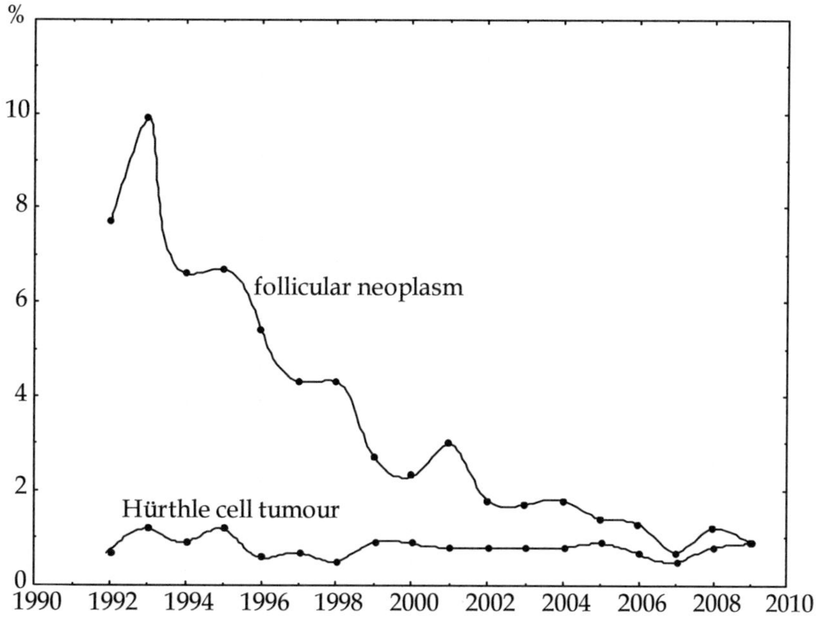

Fig. 2. The occurrence of cytological diagnoses of follicular neoplasm and Hürthle cell tumour

Interestingly, in the analysed period the risk of revealing cancer in postoperative histopathological examination in nodules diagnosed cytologically as 'follicular neoplasm' dropped from above 15% to below 8%. Those lesions more frequently were found to be hyperplastic nodules in histopathological examination. The decrease in occurrence of cancers in lesions with cytological diagnosis of 'follicular neoplasm' was more pronounced than the decrease in frequency of formulating this cytological diagnosis (Słowińska-Klencka et al., 2002, 2008). It should be kept in mind that such lowering of the risk of cancer is transient. In regions of recently established iodine prophylaxis the risk of thyroid cancer in a lesion described in FNAB as 'follicular neoplasm' is lower than in regions of constant sufficient iodine supply, where thyroid nodules are rarer but more frequently malignant (Baloch et al., 2002; Mihai et al., 2009).

Our data also show that if 'follicular neoplasm' in cytological outcome was assumed as a negative result with respect to cancer diagnosis it would cause a twofold increase in the number of undiagnosed cancers >10 mm and only 15% increase in the case of infracentimetric cancers. Thus, it seems that in the regions of recently normalized iodine supply, in patients with such cytological outcome the surgical treatment may be postponed only in the case of small lesions (Słowińska-Klencka et al., 2008).

Other reports also show that the size of lesion is important feature in the assessment of probability of thyroid cancer in patients with cytological diagnosis of follicular neoplasm. Lubitz et al., (2010), Mihai et al., 2009; Schlinkert et al., (1997) and Tutle et al., (1998) indicate that the size above 4 cm is significant; Baloch et al., (2002) - above 3 cm.

Concluding, it is reasonable to individualize indications for surgical treatment - particularly in countries with similar to Polish epidemiological situation, where the risk of cancer in lesion diagnosed as 'follicular neoplasm' is relatively low (<10%). It seems that in such cases small lesions can be treated conservatively providing the strict clinical follow-up is assured with US monitoring. It should be stressed that even in such areas the risk of cancer in the case of cytological diagnosis of 'Hürthle cell neoplasm' is high and reaches 20-30% (Słowińska-Klencka et al., 2002). The similar data on the difference in the risk of cancer between cytologically diagnosed follicular and oxyphilic neoplasms were reported by Sangalli et al., (2006) and Baloch et al., (2002). Thus, in our opinion, if FNAB outcome suggests 'Hürthle cell tumour' indications for surgical treatment are stronger. On the other hand, Pu et al., (2006), Sorrenti et al., (2009) and Theoharis et al., 2009 found no difference between such lesions regarding the rate of malignancy. However, Sorrenti et al., (2009) correctly mentions that more aggressive cancers tend to occur in patients with 'Hürthle cell neoplasm' than in persons with 'follicular neoplasm' diagnosed cytologically.

5.3 New classification of thyroid FNAB results - the impact on frequency of particular diagnoses from follicular lesions in postendemic area

The most recent recommendations for diagnostics of thyroid nodules permit centres with specific experience in thyroid cytology to divide diagnoses of follicular lesions into 'follicular lesion of undetermined significance' and 'follicular neoplasm' categories (Baloch et al., 2008; Gharib et al., 2010; Layfield et al., 2010). This distinction separates 2 cytologic groups at different risk for thyroid malignancy. At our centre similar distinction was introduced earlier - in some cases the cytopathologist tried to determine more precisely the benign character of the lesion by formulating the result as 'follicular neoplasm - probably adenoma' (Słowińska-Klencka et al., 2002). However, the current guidelines of National Institute of Cancer (NCI) assume wider definition of this particular diagnostic category. According to NCI 'follicular lesion of undetermined significance' is a heterogeneous category, which reflects the difficulty in the cytological diagnosis of the follicular lesions of the thyroid. It includes cases in which the cytomorphological findings are not representative of a benign lesion such as a hyperplastic / adenomatoid nodule, yet the degree of cellular or architectural atypia is not sufficient to render an interpretation of follicular neoplasm / suspicious for a follicular neoplasm or suspicious for malignancy. This diagnosis may also be used in thyroid FNAB specimens that are less than optimal due to limited cellularity, poor fixation and obscuring blood (Baloch et al., 2008; Layfield et al., 2010). The main reason for using this diagnostic category was to recommend a repeated FNAB in 3-12 months for these cases rather than surgical excision. The correlation of FNAB outcomes with the results of subsequent US examinations, or radionucleotide uptake studies may be helpful in improving the positive predictive value of that 'indeterminate' category.

We assessed the influence of the application of new classification of the thyroid cytological outcomes in postendemic area in respect to follicular lesions from which monomorphic thyroid follicular cells (tfc) (comprising oxyphilic cells) arranged in three-dimensional groups including microfollicles were aspirated. The analysis covered 2 periods: year 2009 and the period between May 2010 and February 2011. In the later period new classification of thyroid FNAB outcomes was used that was based on NCI classification with exclusion of cases with low cellularity from "follicular lesion of undetermined significance" subgroup. It was found that in both examined periods incidence of aspirates with monomorphic tfc was similar: 4.5% and 4.4% respectively. However the introduction of the subcategory of "follicular lesion of undetermined significance" significantly decreased the percentage of FNAB outcomes without diagnostic conclusion ($p<0.0001$, chi^2 test) (Table 1). Thus, it seems that the introduction of this new category of FNAB results makes it easier for endocrinologists to choose proper therapeutic options, especially in postendemic areas.

2009		V 2010 - II 2011	
Cytological results	**No/%**	**Cytological results**	**No/%**
Monomorphic tfc without conclusion	168/72.1%	Monomorphic tfc without conclusion - usually low cellularity smears	66/30.4%
Benign follicular nodule	10/4.3%	Benign follicular nodule	4/1.8%
Follicular neoplasm probably benign	6/2.6%	Follicular lesion of undetermined significance	106/48.9%
Follicular neoplasm	21/9.0%	Suspicious for a follicular neoplasm	21/9.7%
Follicular neoplasm Hürthle cell type probably benign	0/0.0%	Follicular lesion of undetermined significance Hürthle cell type	3/1.4%
Follicular neoplasm Hürthle cell type	28/12.0%	Suspicious for a follicular neoplasm Hürthle cell type	17/7.8%
Number of follicular lesions	233/100.0%	Number of follicular lesions	217/100.0%

Table 1. Comparison of cytological outcomes from thyroid nodules, where monomorphic tfc dominated in aspirates, formulated in 2 periods: year 2009 and between May 2010 and February 2011. In the later period new classification of thyroid FNAB outcomes was used.

Also Theoharis et al., (2009) found that the new approach of reporting thyroid FNA proposed by the NCI is advantageous in patients who may harbor a follicular or Hürthle cell neoplasm as it allows the reporting cytopathologists to express their level of concern of the possibility of an underlying malignancy to guide subsequent patient management.

5.4 Increased incidence of Hashimoto disease in endemic areas and the risk of FNAB false results

As it was already mentioned, the increase in iodine supply in endemic area is related to the increase in the incidence of chronic thyroiditis. It significantly affects the efficacy of morphological diagnostics of the thyroid. Noticeable anisocytosis of follicular cells observed in some cases of chronic thyroiditis can lead to an increased number of false positive (FP) results of FNAB. Additionally, marked hypoechogenecity and heterogeneity of the thyroid in US

scans poses difficulties in revealing any focal lesions. Another important issue is a coincidence of papillary cancer and chronic thyroiditis, which is indicated by numerous investigators, and makes cytological diagnostics of patients with Hashimoto disease even more challenging (Azizi et al., 2011; Cipolla et al., 2005; Gul et al., 2010; Liu et al., 2001; Mukasa et al., 2011; Ruggiero et al., 2005; Shih et al., 2008; Singh et al., 1999; Słowińska-Klencka et al., 2006).
In our material the frequency of papillary carcinoma diagnosed in postoperative histopathological examination was higher in the group of patients with cytologically confirmed chronic thyroiditis than in the group of patients with non-inflammatory benign lesion found in FANB (Słowińska-Klencka et al., 2006). There are also reports indicating the relation between the increased titres of antithyroid antibodies and the increased probability of obtaining FANB outcome which suggests or confirms thyroid malignancy (Boi et al., 2005). It was also shown that the risk of thyroid cancers is positively correlated to TSH levels even in its normal range (Boelaert et al., 2006, 2009), and chronic thyroiditis is main reason for the increase of TSH levels. Even without judging whether chronic thyroiditis facilitates the growth of papillary cancer, or rather lymphocytic infiltration is a kind of response to growing tumour, it can be concluded that patients with Hashimoto disease should be followed-up with a particular attention (Gul et al., 2010; Okayasu et al., 1995). It should be also kept in mind that chronic thyroiditis is regarded as a risk factor for malignant lymphoma of the thyroid (Holm et al., 1985; Matsuzuka et al., 1995).

5.5 Differences in statistical approach to the evaluation of FNAB efficacy

The differences described above in epidemiological situations of examined populations result in significant differences in the reported data on FP and false negative (FN) results, as well as sensitivity (from 65 to 98%) and specificity (from 72 to 100%) of the thyroid FNAB (Gharib et al., 2010). Another important source of these differences comes from the statistical approaches to the evaluation of FNAB data, which vary among authors, thus making the reported results hardly comparable (Słowińska-Klencka et al., 2002). Some authors exclude the so-called intermediate results (differently defined) from statistical analysis, while others exclude only the specific cases (e.g. exclusion from FP result, cases corresponding to follicular adenoma in histopathological examination or exclusion from FN results cases of papillary microcarcionomas incidentally found in postoperative histopathological examination) (Cap et al., 1999; La Rosa et al., 1991). This problem is further discussed in the papers by Lewis et al., (2009) and Theoharis et al., (2009).
There is a general agreement that in regions of endemic goitre (with an increased incidence of follicular neoplasms), a high number of FP results should be accepted and negative results should be optimised (Papanicolaou Society of Cytopathology, 1996). FN results may delay the institution of appropriate treatment. On the other hand, it should be kept in mind that the real rate of FN results of FNAB could be masked by the relatively high percentage of patients with cytologically diagnosed benign lesions who are not surgically treated, while differentiated carcinoma need not progress for years.

6. Rules of monitoring benign lesions – Its efficacy in relation to iodine supply

Cytological diagnosis of benign lesion is related to very low risk of malignancy (1–2% in the case of US-guided FNAB), on condition that such diagnosis is formulated only if smears satisfy strict quality criteria (Gharib et al., 2010). Assuming that these criteria were followed and the aspirated material was obtained from the examined lesion, there is no need to repeat FNAB unless changes in US image or other clinical data suggest the otherwise. It should be remembered that clinical decisions based on such cytological diagnosis should be limited to that particular lesion, and cannot be extended on other lesions. In the presence of any doubts it is justified to repeat FNAB after 6-12 months especially in lesions presenting some US features suggestive of malignancy (Kwak et al., 2010).

Opponents against performing control FNABs even in the cases of non-progressing nodule, indicate that such examination usually does not significantly change the cytological category of examined lesion, it lowers economic efficiency of thyroid diagnostics, and it unnecessarily stimulates the fear of cancer in patient (Aguilar et al., 1998; Lucas et al.; 1995; Merchant et al., 2000). On the other hand, there are proponents of control FNABs, who indicate that 1-3 control FNABs lower the risk of false negative results related to missing examined lesion (particularly small or dorsally located) (Flanagan et al., 2006; Gabalec et al., 2009; Hamburger 1987; Illouz et al. 2007; Orlandi et al. 2005). Some investigators suggest to perform follow-up FNA only in a selected group of patients with clinically suspicious symptoms (Chehade et al., 2001; Erdogan et al., 1998; Oertel et. al., 2007; van Roosmalen et al., 2010).

Analysis of our material showed that performing one control FNAB increases diagnostic efficacy of cytological examination in respect to diagnosing cancer. Next control FNABs do not change the cytological category of examined lesion if no US/clinical signs of progression are observed (Słowińska-Klencka et al., 2001). In the case of very long follow-up (10 years or more), it seems less rational to limit the number of performed FNABs to 1 or 2, but there are no recommendations addressing this question.

If quality criteria of smears are not satisfied FNAB should be classified as non-diagnostic. With such cytological outcome decision on surgical treatment must be based on the presence of clinical features suggesting the increased risk of cancer. If conservative treatment is undertaken, next biopsy should be performed within 3-12 months. Interpretation of non-diagnostic biopsy should include clinical context as some thyroid diseases are related to difficulties in obtaining material satisfying all quality criteria (e.g. chronic thyroiditis, colloid nodule). If two subsequent examinations give non-diagnostic material then an individual clinical assessment of the risk of cancer in the evaluated lesion should be performed. It seems that solid lesions should be more readily treated surgically while mixed, cystic-solid lesions may be observed (with possibility of surgical treatment in future). According to British Thyroid Association [BTA] (2007) guidelines, clinical attention should be increased if there are blood cells and histiocytes in smear and thyroid follicular cells are absent. BTA advises to regard such smears as more suspicious than those without follicular cells but with dominating colloid. According to our data, the frequency of histopathologically diagnosed neoplasms (both malignant and benign) in solid lesions is higher in the case of lesions from which non-diagnostic material was obtained twice in comparison with lesions that showed diagnostic material in the repeated (second) FNAB. No similar difference was noted in relation to malignant neoplasms only. However, the risk of diagnosing cancer in postoperative examination was higher than in lesions with diagnostic cytological outcome (classified as benign) - about 7% vs. 2%, respectively (Słowińska-Klencka et al., 2004). Others reported similar data (Orija et al., 2007). There is a general agreement that 'pure cystic' lesions should be treated conservatively because of low risk of malignancy.

Additional difficulty in areas of iodine deficiency is related to follow-up of multiple thyroid nodules which can be easily misidentified in control ultrasound examinations. As indications for FNAB are based on US features of revealed lesions, it is very important to clearly describe in US report as many identified lesions as possible, with precise description of their location, size and features used for selection to FNAB. The US report should not be limited to the description of a dominant lesion, and report of US-guided FNAB should allow to identify biopsied lesion in other diagnostic centre (Gharib et al., 2010). It is advisable to attach to FNAB result the US report with description of lesions that have been biopsied. Such joined report allows to compare US features of lesions during control examination. This is particularly important in endemic areas where it may be difficult to identify lesion among many others in multiple nodular goitre.

7. Conclusions

In the endemic areas the typical ultrasound criteria for selection of lesions for FNAB are inefficient. The number of performed FNABs is very high in relation to the number of revealed cancers, but in spite of this, some invasive cancers are missed. On the other hand, some indolent cancers, which probably never become aggressive, are revealed. In the regions of a high number of patients with multinodular goitre, it seems reasonable to use more powerful and rigorous criteria for selecting lesions for FNAB that would allow to improve diagnostic and economic effectiveness of biopsy. Such criteria must include features with higher predictive value instead of or along with features with high sensitivity but low specificity (like nodule hypoechogenecity).

In iodine-deficient areas in order to increase the chances of early detection of small invasive cancers, it seems particularly reasonable to follow up small lesions revealed in the thyroid with repeated US examinations. That allows detection of any significant changes in lesion image and lesion relationship with the thyroid capsule as well as evaluation of lymph nodes in the neck.

While clinically interpreting the results of cytological examination, the iodine status of examined population should be considered. Changes in the iodine status of a given population promptly influence the clinical significance of particular cytological results. In such circumstances, special attention is advised from both the cytologist and the thyroidologist.

Concluding, the clinical management of thyroid nodules in areas of high, sufficient or inadequate iodine supply is not fully comparable.

8. References

Aguilar, J.; Rodriguez, J.M.; Flores, B.; Sola, J.; Bas, A.; Soria, T.; Ramirez, P. & Parrilla, P. (1998). Value of repeated fine-needle aspiration cytology and cytologic experience on the management of thyroid nodules. *Otolaryngology Head and Neck Surgery* Vol.119, No.1, (July 1998), pp. 121–124, ISSN 1916-0216

Alexander, E.K.; Marqusee, E.; Orcutt, J.; Benson, C.B.; Frates, M.C.; Doubilet, P.M.; Cibas, E.S.; & Atri, A. (2004). Thyroid nodule shape and prediction of malignancy. *Thyroid,* Vol.14, No.11, (2004), pp. 953–958, ISSN 2042-0072

Azizi, G. & Malchoff, C.D. (2011). Autoimmune thyroid disease: a risk factor for thyroid cancer. *Endocrine Practice,* Vo.17, No.2, (March 2011), pp. 201-209, ISSN 1530-891X

Baloch, Z.W.; Fleisher, S.; LiVolsi, V.A. & Gupta P.K. (2002) Diagnosis of "follicular neoplasm": a gray zone in thyroid fine-needle aspiration cytology. *Diagnostic Cytopathology*, Vol.26, No.1, (January 2002), pp. 41–44, ISSN 8755-1039

Baloch, Z.W.; LiVolsi, V.A.; Asa, S.L.; Rosai, J.; Merino, M.J.; Randolph, G.; Vielh, P.; DeMay, R.M.; Sidawy, M.K. & Frable WJ. (2008). Diagnostic terminology and morphologic criteria for cytologic diagnosis of thyroid lesions: a synopsis of the National Cancer Institute Thyroid Fine-Needle Aspiration State of the Science Conference. *Diagnostic Cytopathology*, Vol.36, No.6, (June 2008), pp. 425-437, ISSN 8755-1039

Barbaro, D.; Simi, U.; Meucci, G.; Lapi, P.; Orsini, P. & Pasquini, C. (2005). Thyroid papillary cancers: microcarcinoma and carcinoma, incidental cancers and non-incidental cancers - are they different diseases? *Clinical Endocrinology*, Vol.63, No.5, (November 2005), pp. 577–5781, ISSN 0300-0664

Belfiore, A.; La Rosa, G.L.; La Porta, G.A.; Giuffrida, D.; Milazzo, G.; Lupo, L.; Regalbuto, C. & Vigneri, R. (1992). Cancer risk in patients with cold thyroid nodules: relevance of iodine intake, sex, age, and multinodularity. *The American Journal of Medicine*, Vol.93, No.4, (October 1992), pp. 363-369, ISSN 0002-9343

Bennedbæk, F.N.; Perrild, H. & Hegedűs, L. (1999). Diagnosis and treatment of the solitary thyroid nodule. Results of a European survey. *Clinical Endocrinology*, Vol.50, No.3, (1999), pp. 357-363, ISSN 0300-0664

Bennedbæk, F.N. & Hegedűs, L. (2000). Management of the solitary thyroid nodule: results of a North American survey. *Journal of Clinical Endocrinology and Metabolism*, Vol.85, No.7, (July 2000), pp. 2493-2498, ISSN 0021-972X

Berker, D.; Aydin, Y.; Ustun, I.; Gul, K.; Tutuncu, Y.; Isik, S.; Delibasi, T. & Guler, S. (2008). The value of fine-needle aspiration biopsy in subcentimeter thyroid nodules. *Thyroid*, Vol.18, No.6, (June 2008), pp. 603–608, ISSN 2042-0072

Boelaert, K. (2009). The association between serum TSH concentration and thyroid cancer. *Endocrine Related Cancer*, Vol.16, No.4, (December 2009), pp. 1065-1072, ISSN 1351-0088

Boi, F.; Lai, M.L.; Marziani, B.; Minerba, L.; Faa, G. & Mariotti, S. (2005). High prevalence of suspicious cytology in thyroid nodules associated with positive thyroid autoantibodies. *European Journal of Endocrinology*, Vol.153, No.5, (November 2005), pp. 637-642, ISSN 0804-4643

Bonavita, J.A.; Mayo, J.; Babb, J.; Bennett, G.; Oweity, T.; Macari, M. & Yee. J. (2009). Pattern recognition of benign nodules at ultrasound of the thyroid: which nodules can be left alone? *AJR. American Journal of Roentgenology*, Vol.193, No.1, (July 2009), pp. 207-213, ISSN 0361-803X

Bonnema, S.J.; Bennedbæk, F.N.; Wiersinga, W.M. & Hegedűs, L. (2000). Management of the nontoxic multinodular goitre: a European questionnaire study. *Clinical Endocrinology*, Vol.53, No.1, (July 2000), pp. 5-12, ISSN 0300-0664

Bonnema, S.J.; Bennedbæk, F.N.; Ladenson, P.W. & Hegedűs, L. (2002). Management of the nontoxic multinodular goiter: a North American survey. *Journal of Clinical Endocrinology and Metabolism*, Vol.87, No.1, (January 2002), pp. 112-127, ISSN 0021-972X

Cap, J.; Ryska, A.; Rehorkova, P.; Hovorkova, E.; Kerekes, Z. & Pohnetalova, D. (1999). Sensitivity and specificity of the fine needle aspiration biopsy of the thyroid:

clinical point of view. *Clinical Endocrinology,* Vol.51, No.4, (October 1999), pp. 509–515, ISSN 0300-0664

Cappelli, C.; Castellano, M.; Pirola, I.; Gandossi, E.; De Martino, E.; Cumetti, D.; Agosti, B. & Rosei, EA. (2006). Thyroid nodule shape suggests malignancy. *European Journal of Endocrinology,* Vol.155, No.1, (July 2006), pp. 27–31, ISSN 0804-4643

Cappelli, C.; Castellano, M.; Pirola, I.; Cumetti, D.; Agosti, B.; Gandossi, E. & Rosei, E.A. (2007). The predictive value of ultrasound findings in the management of thyroid nodules. *Quarterly Journal of Medicine,* Vol.100, No.1, (January 2007), pp. 29–35, ISSN 1460-2725

Cesur, M.; Corapcioglu, D.; Bulut, S.; Gursoy, A.; Yilmaz, A.E.; Erdogan, N. & Kamel, N. (2006). Comparison of palpation-guided fine-needle aspiration biopsy to ultrasound-guided fine-needle aspiration biopsy in the evaluation of thyroid nodules. *Thyroid,* Vol.16, No. 6, (June 2006), pp. 555–561, ISSN 2042-0072

Chan, B.K.; Desser, T.S.; McDougall, I.R.; Weigel, R.J. & Jeffrey, R.B. Jr. (2003). Common and uncommon sonographic features of papillary thyroid carcinoma. *Journal of Ultrasound in Medicine,* Vol.22, No.10, (October 2003), pp. 1083–1090, ISSN 0278-4297

Chehade, J.M.; Silverberg, A.B.; Kim, J.; Case, C. & Mooradian, A.D. (2001). Role of repeated fine-needle aspiration of thyroid nodules with benign cytologic features. *Endocrine Practice,* Vol.7, No.4, (July/August 2001), pp. 237–243, ISSN 1530-891X

Chow, S.M.; Law, S.C.; Chan, J.K.; Au, S.K.; Yau, S. & Lau, W.H. (2003). Papillary microcarcinoma of the thyroid - Prognostic significance of lymph node metastasis and multifocality. *Cancer,* Vol.98, No.1, (July 2003), pp. 31-40, ISSN 1097-0142

Cipolla, C.; Sandonato, L.; Graceffa, G.; Fricano, S.; Torcivia, A.; Vieni, S.; Latteri, S. & Latteri, M.A. (2005). Hashimoto thyroiditis coexistent with papillary thyroid carcinoma. *The American Surgeon,* Vol.71, No.10, (October 2005), pp. 874-878, ISSN 0003-1348

Doufas, A.G.; Mastorakos, G.; Chatziioannou, S.; Tseleni-Balafouta, S.; Piperingos, G.; Boukis, M.A.; Mantzos, E.; Caraiskos, C.S.; Mantzos, J.; Alevizaki, M. & Koutras, D.A. (1999). The predominant form of non-toxic goiter in Greece is now autoimmune thyroiditis. *European Journal of Endocrinology,* Vol.140, No.6, (June 1999), pp. 505–511, ISSN 0804-4643

Erdogan, M.F.; Kamel, N.; Aras, D.; Akdogan, A.; Baskal, N. & Erdogan, G. (1998). Value of re-aspiration in benign nodular thyroid disease. *Thyroid,* Vol.8, N.12, (December 1998), pp. 1087–1090, ISSN 2042-0072

Ezzat, S.; Sarti, D.A.; Cain, D.R. & Braunstein, G.D. (1994). Thyroid incidentalomas. Prevalence by palpation and ultrasonography. *Archives of Internal Medicine,* Vol.154, No.16 (August 1994), pp. 1838–1840, ISSN 0003-9926

Faquin, W.C. & Baloch, Z.W. (2010). Fine-needle aspiration of follicular patterned lesions of the thyroid: Diagnosis, management, and follow-up according to National Cancer Institute (NCI) recommendations. *Diagnostic Cytopathology* Vol.38, No.10, (October 2010), pp. 731-739, ISSN 8755-1039

Feldt-Rasmussen, U. (2001). Iodine and cancer. Thyroid, Vol.11, No.5, (May 2001), pp.483-485, ISSN 2042-0072

Flanagan, M.B.; Ohori, N.P.; Carty, S.E. & Hunt, J.L. (2006). Repeat thyroid nodule fine-needle aspiration in patients with initial benign cytologic results. *American Journal of Clinical Pathology*, Vol.125, No.5, (May 2006), pp. 698–702, ISSN 0002-9173

Frasoldati, A.; Pesenti, M.; Gallo, M.; Caroggio, A.; Salvo, D. & Valcavi, R. (2003). Diagnosis of neck recurrences in patients with differentiated thyroid carcinoma. *Cancer*, Vol.97, No.1, (January 2003), pp. 90-96, ISSN 1097-0142

Frates, M.C.; Benson, C.B.; Doubilet, P.M.; Cibas, E.S. & Marqusee, E. (2003). Can color Doppler sonography aid in the prediction of malignancy of thyroid nodules? *Journal of Ultrasound in Medicine*, Vol.22, No.2, (February 2003), pp. 127–131, ISSN 0278-4297

Frates, M.C.; Benson, C.B.; Charboneau, J.W.; Cibas, E.S.; Clark, O.H.; Coleman, B.G.; Cronan, J.J.; Doubilet, P.M.; Evans, D.B.; Goellner, J.R.; Hay, I.D.; Hertzberg, B.S.; Intenzo, C.M.; Jeffrey, R.B.; Langer, J.E.; Larsen, P.R.; Mandel, S.J.; Middleton, W.D.; Reading, C.C.; Sherman, S.I. & Tessler, F.N. (2005). Management of thyroid nodules detected at US: Society of Radiologists in Ultrasound consensus conference statement. *Radiology*, 2005 237, No.3, (December 2005), pp. 794–800, ISSN 0033-8419

Frates, M.C.; Benson, C.B.; Doubilet, P.M.; Kunreuther, E.; Contreras, M.; Cibas, E.S.; Orcutt, J.; Moore, F.D.Jr.; Larsen, P.R.; Marqusee, E. & Alexander, E.K. (2006). Prevalence and distribution of carcinoma in patients with solitary and multiple thyroid nodules on sonography. *Journal of Clinical Endocrinology and Metabolism*, 2006 91, No.9, (September 2006), pp. 3411–3417, ISSN 0021-972X

Fukunaga, F.H. & Yatani, R. (1975). Geographic pathology of occult thyroid carcinomas. *Cancer*, Vol. 36, No.3, (September 1975), pp. 1095-1099, ISSN 1097-0142

Gabalec, F.; Cáp, J.; Ryska, A.; Vasátko, T. & Ceeová, V. (2009). Benign fine-needle aspiration cytology of thyroid nodule: to repeat or not to repeat? *European Journal of Endocrinology*, Vol.161, No.6, (December 2009), pp. 933-937, ISSN 0804-4643

Gharib, H.; Papini, E.; Paschke, R.; Duick, D.S.; Valcavi, R.; Hegedüs, L. & Vitti, P. (2010) American Association of Clinical Endocrinologists, Associazione Medici Endocrinologi, and European Thyroid Association medical guidelines for clinical practice for the diagnosis and management of thyroid nodules. AACE/AME/ETA Task Force on Thyroid Nodules. *Endocrine Practice*, Vol.16, (Suppl 1), (May/June 2010), pp. 1-43, ISSN 1530-891X

Gul K, Dirikoc A, Kiyak G, Ersoy PE, Ugras NS, Ersoy R, Cakir B. (2010). The association between thyroid carcinoma and Hashimoto's thyroiditis: the ultrasonographic and histopathologic characteristics of malignant nodules. *Thyroid*, Vol.20, No.8, (August 2010), pp. 873-878, ISSN 2042-0072

Hagag, P.; Strauss, S. & Weiss, M. (1998). Role of ultrasound-guided fine-needle aspiration biopsy in evaluation of nonpalpable thyroid nodules *Thyroid*, Vol.8, No.11, (November 1998), pp. 989–995, ISSN 2042-0072

Hamburger, J.I. (1987). Consistency of sequential needle biopsy findings for thyroid nodules. *Archives of Internal Medicine*, Vol.147, No.1, (January 1987), pp. 97–99, ISSN 0003-9926

Harach, H.R.; Franssila, K.O. & Wasenius V.M. (1985). Occult papillary carcinoma of the thyroid. A "normal" finding in Finland. A systematic autopsy study. *Cancer*, Vol.56, No.3, (November 1985), pp. 531-538, ISSN 1097-0142

Harach, H.R. & Williams, E.D. (1995). Thyroid cancer and thyroiditis in the goitrous region of Salta, Argentina, before and after iodine prophylaxis. *Clinical Endocrinology,* Vol.43, No.6, (December 1995), pp. 701–706, ISSN 0300-0664

Hegedűs, L. (2004). The thyroid nodule. *New England Journal of Medicine,* 2004 351 pp. 1764–1771, ISSN 0028-4793

Hegedűs, L. (2001). Thyroid ultrasound. *Endocrinology and Metabolism Clinics of North America,* Vol.30, No.2, (June 2001), pp. 339-360, ISSN 0889-8529

Holm, L.E.; Blomgren, H. & Löwhagen, T. (1985). Cancer risks in patients with chronic lymphocytic thyroiditis. *New England Journal of Medicine,* Vol.312, No.10, (March 1985), pp. 601-604, ISSN 0028-4793

Hughes, D.T.; Haymart, M.R.; Miller, B.S.; Gauger, P.G. & Doherty, G.M. (2011). The most commonly occurring papillary thyroid cancer in the United States is now a microcarcinoma in a patient older than 45 years. *Thyroid,* Vol.21, No.3, (March 2011), pp. 231-236, ISSN 2042-0072

Iannuccilli, J.D.; Cronan, J.J. & Monchik, J.M. (2004). Risk for malignancy of thyroid nodules as assessed by sonographic criteria: the need for biopsy. *Journal of Ultrasound in Medicine*, Vol.23, No.11, (November 2004), pp. 1455–1464, ISSN 0278-4297

Illouz, F.; Rodien, P.; Saint-André, J.P.; Triau, S.; Laboureau-Soares, S.; Dubois, S.; Vielle, B.; Hamy, A. & Rohmer, V. (2007). Usefulness of repeated fine-needle cytology in the follow-up of non-operated thyroid nodules. *European Journal of Endocrinology,* Vol.156, No.3, (March 2007), pp. 303-308, ISSN 0804-4643

Ito, Y.; Uruno, T.; Nakano, K.; Takamura, Y.; Miya, A.; Kobayashi, K.; Yokozawa, T.; Matsuzuka, F.; Kuma, S.; Kuma, K. & Miyauchi, A. (2003). An observation trial without surgical treatment in patients with papillary microcarcinoma of the thyroid. *Thyroid*, Vol.13, No.4, (April 2003), pp. 381–387, ISSN 2042-0072

Ito, Y. & Miyauchi, A. (2009). Prognostic factors and therapeutic strategies for differentiated carcinomas of the thyroid. *Endocrine Journal,* Vol.56, No.6, (December 2009), pp. 177–192, ISSN 0918-8959

Kang, H.W.; No, J.H.; Chung, J.H.; Min, Y.K.; Lee, M.S.; Lee, M.K.; Yang, J.H. & Kim, K.W. (2004). Prevalence, clinical and ultrasonographic characteristics of thyroid incidentalomas. *Thyroid,* Vol.14, No.1, (January 2004), pp. 29-33, ISSN 2042-0072

Kim, D.L.; Song, K.H. & Kim, S.K. (2008). High prevalence of carcinoma in ultrasonography - guided fine needle aspiration cytology of thyroid nodules. *Endocrine Journal,* Vol.55, No.1, (March 2008), pp. 135–142, ISSN 0918-8959

Kim, D.W.; Lee, E.J.; Kim, S.H.; Kim, T.H.; Lee, S.H.; Kim, D.H. & Rho, M.H. (2009). Ultrasound-guided fine-needle aspiration biopsy of thyroid nodules: comparison in efficacy according to nodule size. *Thyroid,*Vol.19, No.1, (January 2009), pp. 27-31, ISSN 2042-0072

Kim, E.K.; Park, C.S.; Chung, W.Y.; Oh, K.K.; Kim, D.I.; Lee, J.T. & Yoo, H.S. (2002). New sonographic criteria for recommending fine-needle aspiration biopsy of nonpalpable solid nodules of the thyroid. *AJR. American Journal of Roentgenology,* Vol.178, No.3, (March 2002), pp. 687–691, ISSN 0361-803X

Kim, S.J.; Kim, E.K.; Park, C.S.; Chung, W.Y.; Oh, K.K. & Yoo, H.S. (2003). Ultrasound guided fine-needle aspiration biopsy in nonpalpable thyroid nodules: is it useful in infracentimetric nodules? *Yonsei Medical Journal,* 2003 44, No.4, (August 2003), pp. 635–640, ISSN 0513-5796

Kloos, R.T.; Eng, C.; Evans, D.B.; Francis, G.L.; Gagel, R.F.; Gharib, H.; Moley, J.F.; Pacini, F.; Ringel, M.D.; Schlumberger, M. & Wells, S.A.Jr. (2009). Medullary thyroid cancer: management guidelines of the American Thyroid Association. American Thyroid Association Guidelines Task Force, *Thyroid,* , Vol.19, No.6, (Jun 2009), pp. 565-612, ISSN 2042-0072

Knudsen, N.; Perrild, H.; Christiansen, E.; Rasmussen, S.; Dige-Petersen, H. & Jorgensen, T. (2000). Thyroid structure and size and two year follow-up of solitary cold thyroid nodules in an unselected population with borderline iodine deficiency. *European Journal of Endocrinology,* Vol.142, No.3, (March 2000), pp. 224–230, ISSN 0804-4643

Kumar, H.; Daykin, J.; Holder, R.; Watkinson, J.C.; Sheppard, M.C. & Franklyn, J.A. (1999). Gender, clinical findings, and serum thyrotropin measurements in the prediction of thyroid neoplasia in 1005 patients presenting with thyroid enlargement and investigated by fine-needle aspiration cytology. *Thyroid,* Vol.9, No.11, (November 1999), pp. 1105-1109, ISSN 2042-0072

Kwak, J.Y.; Kim, E.K.; Youk, J.H.; Kim, M.J.; Son, E.J.; Choi, S.H. & Oh, KK. (2008). Extrathyroid extension of well-differentiated papillary thyroid microcarcinoma on US. *Thyroid,* Vol.18, No.6, (June 2008), pp. 609–614, ISSN 2042-0072

Kwak, J.Y.; Koo, H.; Youk, J.; Kim, M.J.; Moon, H.J.; Son, E.J. & Kim, E.K. (2010). Value of US correlation of a thyroid nodule with initially benign cytologic results. *Radiology,* Vol.254, No.1, (January 2010), pp. 292-300, ISSN 0033-8419

La Rosa, G.L.; Belfiore, A.; Giuffrida, D.; Sicurella, C.; Ippolito, O.; Russo, G. & Verneri, R. (1991). Evaluation of the fine needle aspiration biopsy in the preoperative selection of cold thyroid nodules. *Cancer,* Vol.67, No.8, (April 1991), pp. 2137–2141, ISSN 1097-0142

Laurberg P, Cerqueira C, Ovesen L, Rasmussen LB, Perrild H, Andersen S, Pedersen IB, Carlé A. (2010). Iodine intake as a determinant of thyroid disorders in populations. *Best Practice and Research Clinical Endocrinology and Metabolism,* Vol.24, No.1, (February 2010), pp. 13-27, ISSN 1521-690X

Layfield, L.J.; Cibas, E.S. & Baloch, Z. (2010). Thyroid fine needle aspiration cytology: a review of the National Cancer Institute state of the science symposium. *Cytopathology,* Vol.21, No.2, (April 2010) pp. 75-85, ISSN 0956-5507

Leboulleux, S.; Girard, E.; Rose, M.; Travagli, J.P.; Sabbah, N.; Caillou, B.; Hartl, D.M.; Lassau, N.; Baudin, E. & Schlumberger M. (2007). Ultrasound criteria of malignancy for cervical lymph nodes in patients followed up for differentiated thyroid cancer. *Journal of Clinical Endocrinology and Metabolism,* Vol.92, No.9, (September 2007), pp. 3590-3594, ISSN 0021-972X

Lee, J.; Rhee, Y.; Lee, S.; Ahn, C.W.; Cha, B.S.; Kim, K.R.; Lee, H.C.; Kim, S.I.; Park, C.S. & Lim, S.K. (2006). Frequent aggressive behaviors of thyroid microcarcinomas in Korean patients. *Endocrine Journal,* Vol.53, No.5, (Ocrober 2006), pp. 627–632, ISSN 0918-8959

Leenhardt, L.; Hejblum, G.; Franc, B.; Fediaevsky, L.D.; Delbot, T.; Le Guillouzic, D.; Menegaux, F.; Guillausseau, C.; Hoang, C.; Turpin, G. & Aurengo, A. (1999). Indications and limits of ultrasound-guided cytology in the management of nonpalpable thyroid nodules. *Journal of Clinical Endocrinology and Metabolism,* 1999 Vol.84, No.1, (January 1999), pp. 24–28, ISSN 0021-972X

Levine, R.A. (2006). Value of Doppler ultrasonography in management of patients with follicular thyroid biopsy specimens. *Endocrine Practice,* 2006 12 pp. 270–274, ISSN 1530-891X

Lewis CM, Chang KP, Pitman M, Faquin WC, Randolph GW. (2009) Thyroid fine-needle aspiration biopsy: variability in reporting. *Thyroid,* Vol.19, No.7, (July 2009) pp. 717-723, ISSN 2042-0072

Lin,. J.D.; Chao, T.C.; Huang, B.Y.; Chen, S.T.; Chang, H.Y. & Hsueh, C. (2005). Thyroid cancer in the thyroid nodules evaluated by ultrasonography and fine-needle aspiration cytology. *Thyroid,* 2005 15 pp. 708–717, ISSN 2042-0072

Lind, P.; Langsteger, W.; Molnar, M.; Gallowitsch, H.J.; Mikosch, P. & Gomez, I. (1998). Epidemiology of thyroid diseases in iodine sufficiency. *Thyroid,* 1998 8 pp. 1179–1183, ISSN 2042-0072

Liu, L.H.; Bakhos, R. & Wojcik, E.M. (2001). Concomitant papillary thyroid carcinoma and Hashimoto's thyroiditis. *Seminars in diagnostic pathology,* Vol.18, No.2, (May 2001), pp. 99-103, ISSN 0740-2570

Lubitz, C.C.; Faquin, W.C.; Yang, J.; Mekel, M.; Gaz, R.D.; Parangi, S.; Randolph, G.W.; Hodin, R.A. & Stephen AE. (2010). Clinical and cytological features predictive of malignancy in thyroid follicular neoplasms. *Thyroid,* Vol.20, No.1, (January 2010), pp. 25-31, ISSN 2042-0072

Lucas, A.; Llatjo´s, M.; Salinas, I.; Reverter, J.; Pizarro, E. & Sanmarti, A. (1995). Fine-needle aspiration cytology of benign nodular thyroid disease. Value of re-aspiration. *European Journal of Endocrinology,* Vol.132, No.6, (June 1995), pp. 677–680, ISSN 0804-4643

Lyshchik, A.; Drozd, V.; Demidchik, Y. & Reiners, C. (2005). Diagnosis of thyroid cancer in children: value of gray-scale and power Doppler US. *Radiology,* Vol.235, No.2, (May 2005), pp. 604–613, ISSN 0033-8419

Matsuzuka, F.; Miyauchi, A.; Katayama, S. & Narabayashi I. (1995). Clinical aspects of primary thyroid lymphoma: diagnosis and treatment based on our experience of 119 cases. *Thyroid,* 1995; Vol.3, No.2, (Summer 1995), pp. 93-99, ISSN 2042-0072

Mazzaferri, E.L. & Sipos, J. (2008). Should all patients with subcentimeter thyroid nodules undergo fine-needle aspiration biopsy and preoperative neck ultrasonography to define the extent of tumor invasion? *Thyroid,* Vol.18, No.6, (June 2008), pp. 597–602, ISSN 2042-0072

Merchant, S.H.; Izquierdo, R. & Khurana, K.K. (2000). Is repeated fineneedle aspiration cytology useful in themanagement of patients with benign nodular thyroid disease? *Thyroid,* Vol.10, No.6, (June 2000), pp. 489–492, ISSN 2042-0072

Mihai, R.; Parker, A.J.; Roskell, D.& Sadler, G.P. (2009) One in four patients with follicular thyroid cytology (THY3) has a thyroid carcinoma. *Thyroid,* Vol.19, No.1, (January 2009), pp. 33-37, ISSN 2042-0072

Moon, W.J.; Jung, S.L.; Lee, J.H.; Na, D.G.; Baek, J.H.; Lee, Y.H.; Kim, J.; Kim, H.S.; Byun, J.S. & Lee, D.H. (2008). Benign and malignant thyroid nodules: US differentiation – multicenter retrospective study. *Radiology,* Vol.247, No.3, (June 2008), pp. 762–770, ISSN 0033-8419

Mukasa, K.; Noh, J.Y.; Kunii, Y.; Matsumoto, M.; Sato, S.; Yasuda, S.; Suzuki, M.; Ito, K. & Ito, K. (2011). Prevalence of malignant tumors and adenomatous lesions detected by ultrasonographic screening in patients with autoimmune thyroid diseases. Thyroid, Vol.21, No.1, (January 2011), pp. 37-41, ISSN 2042-0072

Nam-Goong, I.S.; Kim, H.Y.; Gong, G.; Lee, H.K.; Hong, S.J.; Kim, W.B. & Shong, Y.K. (2004). Ultrasonography-guided fine-needle aspiration of thyroid incidentaloma: correlation with pathological findings. *Clinical Endocrinology*, 2004; 60, No.1, (January 2004), pp. 21-28, ISSN 0300-0664

Nosé, V. (2011). Familial thyroid cancer: a review. *Modern Pathology*, Vol.24, Suppl 2 (April 2011), pp. 19-33 ISSN 0893-3952

Oertel, Y.C.; Miyahara-Felipe, L.; Mendoza, M.G. & Yu, K. (2007). Value of repeated fine needle aspirations of the thyroid: an analysis of over ten thousands FNA's. *Thyroid*, Vol.17, No.11, (November 2007), pp. 1061–1066, ISSN 2042-0072.

Okayasu, I.; Fujiwara, M.; Hara, Y.; Tanaka, Y. & Rose, N.R. (1995). Association of chronic lymphocytic thyroiditis andthyroid papillary carcinoma. A study of surgical cases among Japanese, and white and African Americans. *Cancer*, Vol.11, No.3, (December 1995), pp. 2312–2318, ISSN 1097-0142

Orija, I.B.; Piñeyro, M.; Biscotti, C.; Reddy, S.S. & Hamrahian, A.H. (2007). Value of repeating a nondiagnostic thyroid fine-needle aspiration biopsy. *Endocrine Practice*, Vol.13, No.7, (November/December 2007), pp 735–742, ISSN 1530-891X

Orlandi, A.; Puscar, A.; Capriata, E, & Fideleff, H. (2005). Repeated fine-needle aspiration of the thyroidin benign nodular thyroid disease: critical evaluation of long-term follow-up. *Thyroid*, Vol.15, No.3, (March 2005), pp. 274–278, ISSN 2042-0072

The Papanicolaou Society of Cytopathology Task Force on Standards of Practice. Guidelines of the Papanicolaou Society of Cytopathology for the examination of fine-needle aspiration specimens from thyroid nodules. *Modern Pathology*, Vol.9, No6 ,(June 1996), pp. 710–715, ISSN 0893-3952

Papini, E.; Guglielmi, R.; Bianchini, A.; Crescenzi A.; Taccogna, S.; Nardi, F.; Panunzi, C.; Rinaldi, R.; Toscano, V. & Pacella, C.M. (2002). Risk of malignancy in nonpalpable thyroid nodules: predictive value of ultrasound and color-Doppler features. *Journal of Clinical Endocrinology and Metabolism*, Vol.87, No.5, (May 2002), pp. 1941–1946, ISSN 0021-972X

Pettersson, B.; Coleman, M.P.; Ron, E. & Adami, H.O. (1996). Iodine supplementation in Sweden and regional trends in thyroid cancer incidence by histopathologic type. *International Journal of Cancer*, Vol.65, No.1, (January 1996), pp. 13–19, ISSN 0898-6924

Popowicz, B.; Klencki, M.; Lewiński, A. & Słowińska-Klencka, D. (2009). The usefulness of sonographic features in selection of thyroid nodules for biopsy in relation to the nodule's size. *European Journal of Endocrinology*, Vol.161, No.1, (January 2009), pp. 103–111, ISSN 0804-4643

Pu, R.;, Yang, J.; Wasserman, P.G.; Bhuiya, T.; Griffith, K.A. & Michael, C.W. (2006). Does Hurthle cell lesion-neoplasm predict malignancy more than follicular lesion-neoplasm on thyroid fine-needle aspiration? *Diagnostic Cytopathology* Vol.34, No, pp. 330–334, ISSN 8755-1039

Quadbeck, B.; Pruellage, J.; Roggenbuck, U.; Hirche, H.; Janssen, O.E.; Mann, K. & Hoermann, R. (2002). Long-term follow-up of thyroid nodule growth. *Experimental and Clinical Endocrinology and Diabetes*, Vol.110, No.7, (October 2002), pp. 348-354, ISSN 0947-7349

Rago, T.; Vitti, P.; Chiovato, L.; Mazzeo, S.; De Liperi, A.; Miccoli, P.; Viacava, P.; Bogazzi, F.; Martino, E. & Pinchera, A. (1998). Role of conventional ultrasonography and color flow-Doppler sonography in predicting malignancy in 'cold' thyroid nodules. *European Journal of Endocrinology,* Vol.138, No.1, (January 1998), pp. 41–46, ISSN 0804-4643

Rago, T.; Di Coscio, G.; Basolo, F.; Scutari, M.; Elisei, R.; Berti, P.; Miccoli, P.; Romani, R.; Faviana, P.; Pinchera, A. & Vitti, P. (2007). Combined clinical, thyroid ultrasound and cytological features help to predict thyroid malignancy in follicular and Hupsilonrthle cell thyroid lesions: results from a series of 505 consecutive patients. *Clinical Endocrinology,* Vol.66, No.1, (January 2007), pp. 13–20, ISSN 0300-0664

van Roosmalen, J.; van Hemel, B.; Suurmeijer, A.; Groen, H.; Ruitenbeek, T.; Links, T.P. & Plukker, J.T. (2010) Diagnostic value and cost considerations of routine fine-needle aspirations in the follow-up of thyroid nodules with benign readings. *Thyroid,*Vol.20, No.12, (December 2010), pp. 1359-1365, ISSN 2042-0072

Ruggiero, F.P.; Frauenhoffer, E. & Stack, Jr.B.C. (2005). Thyroid Lymphoma: A Single Institution's Experience. *Otolaryngology Head and Neck Surgery* Vol.133, No6, 888-896, ISSN 0194-5998

Sahin, M.; Sengul, A.; Berki, Z.; Tutuncu, N.B. & Guvener, N.D. (2006). Ultrasound-guided fine-needle aspiration biopsy and ultrasonographic features of infracentimetric nodules in patients with nodular goiter: correlation with pathological findings. *Endocrine Pathology,* Vol.17, No.1, (Spring 2006), pp. 67–74, ISSN 1046-3976

Sangalli, G.; Serio, G.; Zampatti, C.; Bellotti, M. & Lomuscio, G. (2006). Fine needle aspiration cytology of the thyroid: a comparison of 5469 cytological and final histological diagnoses. *Cytopathology,* Vol.17, No.5, (October 2006), pp. 245-250, ISSN 0956-5507

Schlinkert, R.T.; van Heerden, J.A.; Goellner, J.R.; Gharib, H.; Smith, S.L.; Rosales, R.F. & Weaver, A.L. (1997). Factors that predict malignant thyroid lesions when fine-needle aspiration is "suspicious for follicular neoplasm." *Mayo Clinic Proceedings* Vol.72, No.10 (October 1997), pp. 913–916, ISSN 0025-6196

Schmid, K.W. (1989). Clinicopathologic management of tumors of the thyroid gland in an endemic goiter area; combined use of preoperative fine needle aspiration biopsy and intraoperative frozen section. *Acta Cytologica,* 1989 33, No.1, (February 1989), pp. 27–30, ISSN 0001-5547

Schneider, A.B. & Sarne, D.H. (2005). Long-term risks for thyroid cancer and other neoplasms after exposure to radiation. *Nature Clinical Practice. Endocrinology & Metabolism,* Vol.1, No.2, (December 2005), pp. 82-91, ISSN 1745-8366

Seningen, J.L.; Nassar, A. & Henry, M.R. (2011). Correlation of thyroid nodule fine-needle aspiration cytology with corresponding histology at Mayo Clinic, 2001–2007: An institutional experience of 1,945 cases. *Diagnostic Cytopathology* Vol.39, No5, (May 2011), pp. in press, ISSN 8755-1039

Shih ML, Lee JA, Hsieh CB, Yu JC, Liu HD, Kebebew E, Clark OH, Duh QY. (2008). Thyroidectomy for Hashimoto's thyroiditis: complications and associated cancers. *Thyroid,* Vol.18, No.7, (July 2008), pp. 729-34, ISSN 2042-0072

Sidawy, M.K.; Del Vecchio, D.M. & Knoll, S.M. (1997). Fine-needle aspiration of thyroid nodules. Correlation between cytology and histology and evaluation discrepant cases. *Cancer Cytopathology*, Vol.81, No.4, (August 1997), pp. 253–259, ISSN 1934-662X

Singh, B.; Shaha, A.R.; Trivedi, H.; Carew, J.F.; Poluri, A. & Shah, J.P. (1999). Coexistent Hashimoto's thyroiditis with papillary thyroid carcinoma: impact on presentation, management, and outcome. *Surgery*, Vol.126, No.6, (December 1999), pp. 1070-1076, ISSN 0039-6060

Sipos, J.A. (2009). Advances in ultrasound for the diagnosis and management of thyroid cancer. *Thyroid*, Vol.19, No.12, (December 2009), pp. 1363-1372, ISSN 2042-0072

Sipos, J.A. & Mazzaferri, E.L. (2010) Thyroid cancer epidemiology and prognostic variables. *Clinical Oncology*, Vol.22, No.6, (August 2010), pp. 395-404, ISSN 0936-6555

Słowińska-Klencka, D.; Klencki M. & Lewiński A. (2001). Fine needle aspiration biopsy of the thyroid - routine control of benign nodules. *Proceedings of 5th European Congress of Endocrinology*, Turin, Italy, June, 2001

Słowinska-Klencka, D.; Klencki, M.; Sporny, S. & Lewinski, A. (2002). Fine needle aspiration biopsy of the thyroid in an area of endemic goitre: influence of restored sufficient iodine supplementation on the clinical significance of cytological results. *European Journal of Endocrinology*, Vol.146 No.1, (January 2002), pp. 19–26, ISSN 0804-4643

Słowińska-Klencka, D.; Klencki, M.; Sporny, S.; Popowicz, B.; Lewiński, A. (2003). Cytologic appearance of toxic nodular goiter after thyrostatic treatment. A karyometric study. *Analytical and Quantitative Cytology and Histology*, Vol. 25, No.1, (February 2003), pp. 39-46, ISSN 0884-6812

Słowińska-Klencka, D.; Sporny, S.; Klencki, M. & Lewiński, A. (2004). Nondiagnostic cytological outcome of thyroid biopsy and risk of thyroid malignancy. *Endocrine Pathology*, 2004; 15, No.1, (Spring 2004), pp. 65–75, ISSN 1046-3976

Słowińska-Klencka D, Sporny S, Klencki M, Popowicz B, Lewiński A. (2006). Chronic thyroiditis--current issue in the cytological diagnostics of the thyroid gland. *Endokrynologia Polsla - Polish Journal of Endocrinology*, Vol.57, No.4, (July/August 2006), pp. 299-306, ISSN 0423-104X

Słowińska-Klencka, D.; Popowicz, B.; Lewiński, A. & Klencki, M. (2008). The fine-needle aspiration biopsy efficacy of small thyroid nodules in the area of recently normalized iodine supply. *European Journal of Endocrinology*, Vol.159, No.6, (December 2008), pp. 747–754, ISSN 0804-4643

Solymosi, T.; Toth, G.L.; Gal, I.; Sajgo, C. & Szabolcs, I. (2002). Influence of iodine intake on the diagnostic power of fine-needle aspiration cytology of the thyroid gland. *Thyroid*, Vol.12, No.8, (August 2002), pp. 719–723, ISSN 2042-0072

Sorrenti, S.; Trimboli, P.; Catania, A.; Ulisse, S.; De Antoni, E. & D'Armiento, M (2009). Comparison of malignancy rate in thyroid nodules with cytology of indeterminate follicular or indeterminate Hürthle cell neoplasm. *Thyroid*, Vol.19, No.4, (April 2009), pp. 355-360, ISSN 2042-0072

Sporny, S.; Lange, D.; Sygut, J.; Kulig, A.; Olszewski, W.; Słowińska-Klencka, D.; Jarząb, B. (2010). Diagnosis and treatment of thyroid cancer — Polish guidelines. Part I. Diagnostics of nodular goitre and fine needle aspiration biopsy. *Endokrynologia Polska – Polish Journal of Endocrinology*, Vol.61, No.5, (September/October 2010), pp. 522-542, ISSN 0423-104X

Szybinski, Z. & Zarnecki, A. (1993). Prevalence of goiter, iodine deficiency and iodine prophylaxis in Poland. The results of the nation-wide study. *Endokrynologia Polska – Polish Journal of Endocrinology,* Vol.44, No.3, pp. 373–388, ISSN 0423-104X

Szybinski, Z.; Golkowski, F.; Buziak-Bereza, M.; Trofimiuk, M.; Przybylik- Mazurek, E.; Huszno, B.; Bandurska-Stankiewicz, E.; Bar-Andziak, E.; Dorant, B.; Kinalska, I.; Lewinski, A.; Klencki, M.; Rybakowa, M.; Sowinski, J.; Szewczyk, L.; Szponar, L. & Wasik, R. (2008). Effectiveness of the iodine prophylaxis model adopted in Poland. *Journal of Endocrinological Investigation*, Vol.31, No.4, (April 2008), pp. 309–313, ISSN 0391-4097

Tae, H.J.; Lim, D.J.; Baek, K.H.; Park, W.C.; Lee, Y.S.; Choi, J.E.; Lee, J.M.; Kang, M.I.; Cha, B.Y.; Son, H.Y.; Lee, K.W. & Kang, S.K. (2007). Diagnostic value of ultrasonography to distinguish between benign and malignant lesions in the management of thyroid nodules. *Thyroid*, Vol.17, No.5 (May 2007), pp. 461–466, ISSN 2042-0072

Tan, G.H.; Gharib, H. & Reading, C.C. (1995). Solitary thyroid nodule. Comparison between palpation and ultrasonography. *Archives of Internal Medicine*, Vol.155,No.22, (December 1995), pp. 2418–2423, ISSN 0003-9926

Theoharis, C.; Schofield, K.; Hammers, H.; Udelsman, R. & Chhieng, D.C. (2009). The Bethesda Thyroid Fine-Needle Aspiration Classification System: Year 1 at an Academic Institution. *Thyroid*, Vol.19, No.11, (November 2009), pp. 1215-1223, ISSN 2042-0072

Tunbridge, W.M.; Evered, D.C.; Hall, R.; Appleton, D.; Brewis, M.; Clark, F.; Evans, J.G.; Young, E.; Bird, T. & Smith, P.A. (1997). The spectrum of thyroid disease in a community: the Whickham survey. *Clinical Endocrinology*, 1977 7,No.6, (December 1977), pp. 481–493, ISSN 0300-0664

Tuttle, R.M.; Lemar, H.& Burch, H.B. (1998) Clinical features associated with an increased risk of thyroid malignancy in patients with follicular neoplasia by fine-needle aspiration. *Thyroid* Vol.8, No5. (May 1998), pp. 377–383, ISSN 2042-0072

Wada, N.; Duh, Q.Y.; Sugino, K.; Iwasaki, H.; Kameyama, K.; Mimura, T.; Ito, K.; Takami, H. & Takanashi, Y. (2003). Lymph node metastasis from 259 papillary thyroid microcarcinomas: frequency, pattern of occurrence and recurrence, and optimal strategy for neck dissection. *Annals of Surgery,* Vol.237, No.3, (March 2003), pp. 399-407, ISSN 0003-4932

Wong, K.T. & Ahuja, A.T. (2005). Ultrasound of thyroid cancer. *Cancer Imaging,* Vol.5, No,5, (December 200), pp. 157-166, ISSN 1740-5025

Yang, G.C.; LiVolsi, V.A. & Baloch, Z.W. (2002). Thyroid microcarcinoma: fine needle aspiration diagnosis and histologic follow-up. *International Journal of Surgical Pathology,* Vol.10, No.2, (April 2002), pp. 133–139, ISSN 1066-8969

7

Clinical Workup of Nodular and Mass Lesions of the Endocrine Organs

Xiaoqi Lin and Bing Zhu
Northwestern Memorial Hospital, Feinberg School of Medicine, Northwestern University
USA

1. Introduction

Fine needle aspiration (FNA) biopsy is a minimally invasive procedure that is widely used to evaluate nodular, mass, or cystic lesions of the endocrine organs, especially the thyroid glands. FNA biopsy can be performed without imaging guidance for palpable nodules or with guidance by ultrasound, computerized tomography (CT) scan, magnetic resonance imaging (MRI) scan, or endoscopic ultrasonography (EUS). FNA biopsy is used to make diagnoses of non-neoplastic lesions (infection, inflammation, and hyperplastic nodule), benign neoplasms, and malignancies. FNA biopsy is also used to distinguish primary neoplasms from metastatic malignancies. Immunohistochemical (IHC) stains and molecular assays can be performed on FNA biopsy materials, in order to make more accurate diagnoses and to determine the appropriateness of targeted treatment.

2. Clinical workup of thyroid nodules

2.1 Introduction

Thyroid nodules are a common clinical problem. Five to fifteen percentage of thyroid nodules are malignant depending on age, sex, radiation exposure history, family history, and other factors(Caruso and Mazzaferri 1991). In the United States, approximately 44,670 new cases of thyroid cancer were diagnosed and 1,690 deaths were caused by thyroid cancer in 2010(Jemal, Siegel et al. 2010). Autopsy examination showed that prevalence of micropapillary cancers was 13% in the United States(Harach, Franssila et al. 1985). The incidence of thyroid cancer is rising(Cooper, Doherty et al. 2009).

2.2 Clinical workup of thyroid nodules

Thyroid nodules can be detected by palpation (5% in women and 1% in men)(Vander, Gaston et al. 1968; Tunbridge, Evered et al. 1977), and are increasingly detected by ultrasound examination (19 - 67%)(Mazzaferri 1993; Tan and Gharib 1997) and other scanning techniques, such as fluorodeoxyglucose-positron emission tomography (^{18}FDG-PET)(Are, Hsu et al. 2007), sestamibi, CT scan, and MRI scans. Ultrasound should be performed in all patients with suspected thyroid nodules(Cooper, Doherty et al. 2009). A serum TSH level and ^{18}FDG-PET should be obtained(Cooper, Doherty et al. 2009). The risk of malignancy in ^{18}FDG-PET positive nodules is about 33%, and the cancers may be more aggressive(Are, Hsu et al. 2007). Therefore, these lesions require prompt evaluation. If the serum TSH is subnormal and diffuse or focal uptake on ^{18}FDG-PET scan is identified, a radionuclide thyroid scan using either technetium ^{99m}Tc pertechnetate or ^{123}I should be obtained to document whether the nodule is hyperfunctioning. No FNA evaluation is necessary(Cooper, Doherty et al. 2009). Higher serum TSH is associated with increased risk of malignancy in a thyroid nodule(Boelaert, Horacek et al. 2006) and prompts an FNA biopsy(Cooper, Doherty et al. 2009).

2.3 Fine needle aspiration biopsy of thyroid nodules

FNA has been demonstrated to be the most accurate and cost-effective method for evaluating thyroid nodules, which has resulted in a reduction of unnecessary thyroid surgery for patients with benign nodules and allowed appropriate triaging of patients with thyroid cancer to surgery. Before the routine use of thyroid FNA, only 14% of surgically resected thyroid nodules were malignant(Hamberger, Gharib et al. 1982). With current thyroid FNA practice, the percentage of malignancy in resected nodules exceeds 50%(Yassa, Cibas et al. 2007). Half of the malignant nodules were diagnosed by FNA cytology as malignant, and the other half had indeterminate cytology, a term used to describe atypia of undetermined significance (AUS), follicular neoplasm, and suspicious for malignancy(Yassa, Cibas et al. 2007). The sensitivity of FNA in diagnosis of malignancy is 66% in palpable thyroid nodules(Tee, Lowe et al. 2007). However, FNA diagnostic performance has varied across different studies. Core needle biopsy has a higher adequacy rate than FNA but seems less sensitive, especially for papillary carcinoma(Renshaw and Pinnar 2007). The combination of FNA with core needle biopsy seems to have the highest adequacy rate and sensitivity(Renshaw and Pinnar 2007). Every patient with a palpable thyroid nodule is a candidate for FNA biopsy and should undergo further evaluation to determine if an FNA is warranted. Before making the decision to proceed with an FNA, a serum thyrotropin level and thyroid ultrasound should be obtained.

Generally, only nodules >1 cm should be evaluated by clinical history, laboratory tests, ultrasound, and FNA, since they have a greater potential to be clinically significant cancers(Cooper, Doherty et al. 2009). Routine FNA is not recommended for nodules < 1 cm. Occasionally, there may be nodules <1 cm that require evaluation because of suspicious US findings, associated lymphadenopathy, a history of head and neck irradiation, or a history of thyroid cancer in one or more first-degree relatives(Cooper, Doherty et al. 2009). However, some nodules <1 cm that lack these warning signs eventually cause morbidity and mortality(Cooper, Doherty et al. 2009). These are rare, and given unfavorable cost-benefit considerations, attempts to diagnose and treat all small thyroid cancers in an effort to prevent these rare outcomes would likely cause more harm than good(Cooper, Doherty et al. 2009). Sonographic features suspicious for malignancy include presence of microcalcifications, hypoechogenicity, increased intranodular vascularity, irregular/lobulated infiltrative margins, an absent halo, nodal metastases, and a shape taller than the width measured in the transverse dimension(Cooper, Doherty et al. 2009). Microcalcifications are highly specific for PTC, but may be difficult to distinguish from colloid.

Thyroid FNA is performed with 27, 25 or 23 gauge needles with or without imaging guidance, however most are performed under ultrasound guidance. The solid area of thyroid nodules should be biopsied. Direct smears of FNA samples are preferred and cytospin or ThinPrep can be also used. The air-dried slides are stained with modified Giemsa stain for immediate interpretation for evaluation of adequacy. Alcohol fixed slides are stained with Papanicolaou stain, which is the ideal method to evaluate nuclear features for the diagnosis of papillary thyroid carcinoma.

Side effects of thyroid FNA include hemorrhage and infection. Acute thyroid hemorrhage may cause acute respiratory distress, which needs prompt intervention(Donatini, Masoni et al. 2010). Infarction in thyroid nodules can occur after FNA, which may interfere with histologic evaluation(Das, Janardan et al. 2009).

2.4 The Bethesda system for reporting thyroid cytopathology

In order for pathologists to better communicate thyroid FNA interpretations to referring physicians, the Bethesda System for Reporting Thyroid Cytopathology (TBSRTC) was developed in 2007(Cibas and Ali 2009). The 2007 National Cancer Institute (NCI) conference and 2009 35th European Congress of Cytology (ECC) reviewed and discussed 6 topics(Cibas and Ali 2009): (1) indications for thyroid FNA and pre-FNA requirements; (2) training and credentialing; (3) techniques for thyroid FNA; (4) diagnostic terminology and morphologic criteria; (5) utilization of ancillary studies in thyroid FNA; and (6) post-FNA testing and treat-pre-FNA requirements, training specifications, criteria for the selection of patients to undergo FNA, diagnostic categories and criteria, ancillary testing and post-FNA follow-up and treatment options. TBSTRC classified thyroid FNA findings into 6 categories (Table 1) (Cibas and Ali 2009).

Category	Subcategory
Nondiagnostic/unsatisfactory	Cystic fluid only, acellular/scant cellular specimen, and others (obscuring blood, clotting artifact, air drying artifact, poor fixation, poor preservation, etc.)
Benign	Consistent with a benign follicular nodule (adenomatoid/hyperplastic nodules, etc.), thyroiditis (lymphocytic, Hashimoto, granulomatous), and others
Atypia of undetermined significance (AUS) or follicular lesion of undetermined significance (FLUS)	Indeterminate for follicular neoplasm versus adenomatoid nodule, indeterminate for papillary thyroid carcinoma, suggestive of benign Hürthle cell nodule or lymphocytic thyroiditis, cyst-lining cells with atypia, follicular cells with nuclear enlargement and prominent nucleoli in patients with a history of radiation, carbimazole, or other pharmaceutical agents, reparative/reactive changes, atypical lymphoid infiltration, and others
Follicular neoplasm or suspicious for a follicular neoplasm	Specify if Hürthle cell (oncocytic) type
Suspicious for malignancy	Suspicious for papillary carcinoma, medullary carcinoma, metastatic carcinoma, lymphoma, and others
Malignant	Papillary thyroid carcinoma, poorly differentiated carcinoma, undifferentiated (anaplastic) carcinoma, medullary carcinoma, squamous cell carcinoma, carcinoma with mixed features (specify), metastatic carcinoma, non-Hodgkin lymphoma, and others

Table 1. The Bethesda system for reporting thyroid Cytopathology (TBSRTC)(Cibas and Ali 2009)

2.4.1 Category: Nondiagnostic/unsatisfactory

To be satisfactory for evaluation, a specimen should contain at least 6 groups of benign follicular cells and at least 10 cells in each group(Grant, Hay et al. 1989; Haider, Rakha et al. 2011), except for findings consistent with colloid nodule(Cibas and Ali 2009). Nondiagnostic/unsatisfactory cases should account less than 10% with a range from 2 – 20% of cases(Cibas and Ali 2009). Postoperative risk of malignancy in thyroid nodules with nondiagnostic cytology is 12% on average with a range from 0 - 32%(Cibas and Ali 2009; Wang, Friedman et al. 2010). The risk of malignancy for a cyst fluid only sample is 4%(Renshaw 2001). A repeated FNA aspiration with ultrasound guidance is recommended for nondiagnostic/unsatisfactory and clinically or sonographically worrisome cyst fluid only cases, and is diagnostic in 50 - 88% of cases(Renshaw 2001; Cooper, Doherty et al. 2009). Aspirates composed of pure colloid and lacking a cellular component should be considered benign rather than non-diagnostic(Layfield, Cibas et al. 2010).

2.4.2 Category: Benign

The FNA smears of hyperplastic/adenomatoid nodules typically show bland follicular cells as well as metaplastic Hürthle cells arranged in macrofollicles, normofollicles, and possibly microfollicles, and show moderate to abundant colloid (Figure 1). Abundant macrophages including hemosiderin-laden macrophages, proteinaceous material, hemolyzed red blood cells, reactive follicular cells, and stromal cells may be seen.

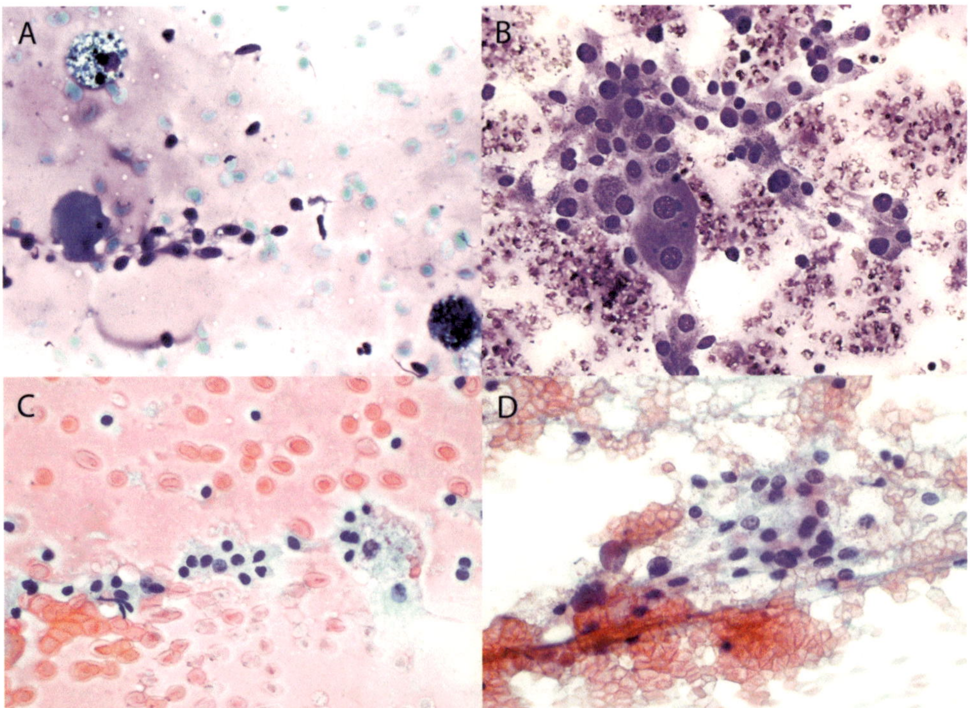

Fig. 1. Thyroid hyperplastic/adenomatoid nodule, FNA cytology, modified Giemsa (A and C) and Papanicolaou stain (B and D), 600x. Figures A and C show benign follicular cells in a background of abundant colloid with macrophages. Figures B and D show metaplastic Hürthle cells with moderate to abundant granular cytoplasm.

The FNA smears of chronic lymphocytic thyroiditis (Hashimoto's thyroiditis) typically show metaplastic Hürthle cells and follicular cells with possible reactive atypia (nuclear pseudoinclusions, nuclear grooves, prominent nucleoli), and abundant polymorphous lymphocytes and lymphohistiocytic aggregates (germinal centers) (Figure 2).

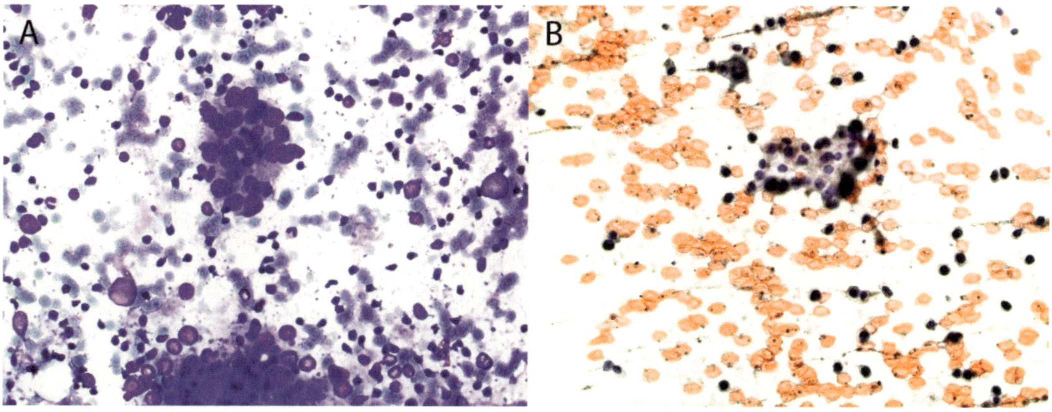

Fig. 2. Chronic lymphocytic thyroiditis, FNA cytology, modified Giemsa (A) and Papanicolaou stain (B), 400x. FNA smears show nests of metaplastic Hürthle cells infiltrated with lymphocytes, and background of polymorphous lymphocytes and lymphohistiocytic aggregates (follicular germinal center).

FNA results with benign cytology should account for 67 - 70% of cases(Cibas and Ali 2009). Postoperative risk of malignancy in thyroid nodules with benign cytology should be approximately 5% with a negative predictive value (NPV) of 95% according to the 2009 American Thyroid Association (ATA) guidelines(Cooper, Doherty et al. 2009) and 0 - 3% according to the 2007 TBSRTC(Layfield, Cibas et al. 2010) . Other studies showed an average of 6% with a range from 1 - 18% (Cibas and Ali 2009; Lewis, Chang et al. 2009; Wang, Friedman et al. 2010). Further immediate diagnostic studies or treatment are not routinely required(Cooper, Doherty et al. 2009). Some authors suggested that patients be followed up with repeated assessment by palpation or ultrasound at 6- to 18-month intervals and should be followed-up for at least 3 - 5 years(Layfield, Abrams et al. 2008; Cooper, Doherty et al. 2009). If the nodule shows significant growth (20% increase in nodule diameter with a minimum increase in two or more dimensions of at least 2 mm(Cooper, Doherty et al. 2009)) or shows "suspicious" sonographic changes, a repeated FNA is considered.

2.4.3 Category: Atypia of undetermined significance (AUS) or follicular lesion of undetermined significance (FLUS)

AUS/FLUS includes cases in which the cytomorphologic findings are not representative of a benign lesion such as a hyperplastic/adenomatoid nodule, yet the degree of cellular or architectural atypia is not sufficient to render an interpretation of follicular neoplasm/suspicious for a follicular neoplasm or suspicious for malignancy. This diagnosis may also be used in thyroid FNA specimens that are less than optimal due to limited cellularity, poor fixation and presence of obscuring blood. AUS cases account for 3 - 6% of thyroid FNAs(Yang, Schnadig et al. 2007; Yassa, Cibas et al. 2007). Postoperative risk of malignancy in nodules with atypical cytology is 16% on average with ranges from 5 -

48%(Cibas and Ali 2009; Wang, Friedman et al. 2010), and 5 - 15% according to 2007 TBSRTC(Layfield, Cibas et al. 2010). Patients with AUS cytology should be managed by undergoing an iodine[123] scan, especially if serum TSH level is low. If the scan is "hot", clinical follow-up with a repeated FNA in 3 - 6 months is recommended(Yassa, Cibas et al. 2007; Cibas and Ali 2009; Layfield, Cibas et al. 2010). Repeat FNA will result in definitive interpretation in most of cases, however a repeat diagnosis of AUS occurs in about 20% of cases(Yassa, Cibas et al. 2007). If the scan is "cold", the patient should be referred for surgery.

2.4.4 Category: Follicular neoplasm or suspicious for a follicular neoplasm

The category of follicular neoplasm or suspicious for a follicular neoplasm identifies a nodule that might be a follicular carcinoma (FC) and triages it for surgical lobectomy(Cibas and Ali 2009). The FNA smears are typically highly cellular, composed of abundant larger follicular cells arranged in microfollicles or trabeculae with crowding and nuclear overlapping, and have scant colloid (Figure 3)(Cibas and Ali 2009). FNA cytology cannot distinguish follicular carcinoma from benign follicular adenoma and sometimes adenomatoid nodule, because distinguishing a follicular carcinoma from follicular adenoma is based on identification of capsular invasion or vascular invasion of in the capsule. Distinguishing a follicular adenoma from adenomatoid nodule is based on the identification of entire capsulation. Diagnosis of follicular variant of papillary carcinoma is based on nuclear features, which, sometimes, is challenging.

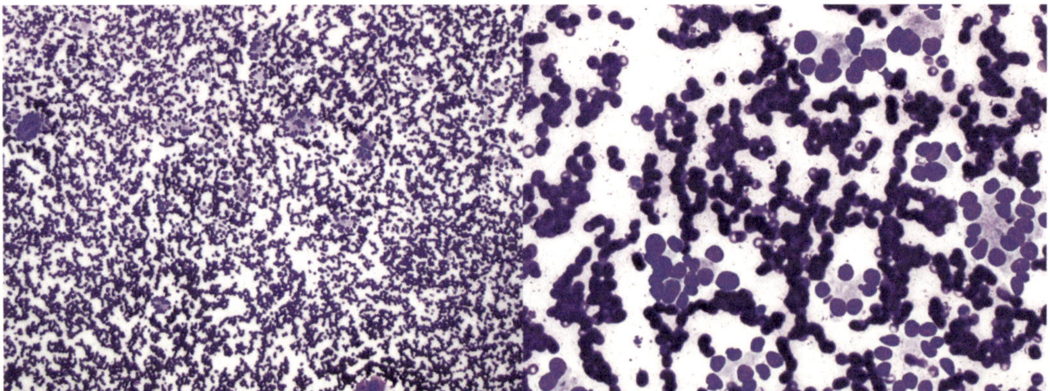

Fig. 3. Thyroid follicular lesion, FNA cytology, modified Giemsa stain, 100x (A) and 600x (B). FNA smears show abundant follicular cells arranged in microfollicles, and absence of colloid.

This category accounts for 9 - 30% of FNA specimens(Hegedus 2004; Mihai, Parker et al. 2009). Most cases in this category are benign follicular adenomas or adenomatoid nodules (up to 35%)(Yang, Schnadig et al. 2007). Postoperative risk of malignancy is 25% on average with a range from 14 - 49%(Cibas and Ali 2009; Wang, Friedman et al. 2010), and is 15 - 30% according to 2007 TBSRTC(Layfield, Cibas et al. 2010). Some cases are follicular carcinoma and others are follicular variant of papillary carcinoma(Yassa, Cibas et al. 2007). Hürthle cell variant should be specified due to different underlying genetics from follicular neoplasms. About 16% - 25% cases of Hürthle cell variant in this category are proven to be hyperplastic proliferations of Hürthle cells in nodular goiter or lymphocytic thyroiditis(Giorgadze, Rossi et al. 2004; Pu, Yang et al. 2006). About 15% to 45% of nodules are malignant, and the remainder of the neoplasms prove to be Hürthle cell adenomas(Giorgadze, Rossi et al. 2004; Pu, Yang et al. 2006). If the reading is "Hürthle cell neoplasm", either lobectomy/hemithyroidectomy or total thyroidectomy is recommended. When diagnosed by FNA as either Hürthle cell neoplasm or Hürthle cell lesion, males are much more likely to have malignant tumors than females(Wu, Clouse et al. 2008).

2.4.5 Category: Suspicious for malignancy

The "suspicious" category is used for those cases that show some nuclear features of papillary carcinoma or other malignancies, or have scant diagnostic cells due to sampling reason or small tumor (papillary microcarcinoma), but are not enough for diagnosis of malignancy. Postoperative risk of malignancy in thyroid nodules with suspicious for malignancy is 62% on average with a range from 42 - 87%, and is 65 - 75% according to 2007 TBSRTC(Layfield, Cibas et al. 2010). The rest are usually follicular adenoma(Yang, Schnadig et al. 2007; Yassa, Cibas et al. 2007; Cibas and Ali 2009; Wang, Friedman et al. 2010). Nodules called suspicious for papillary carcinoma are resected by lobectomy, near total thyroidectomy, or thyroidectomy(Cooper, Doherty et al. 2009; Layfield, Cibas et al. 2010).

2.4.6 Category: Malignant

The category of malignancy is used whenever the cytomorphologic features are conclusive for a malignancy. The diagnosis of papillary thyroid carcinoma by FNA biopsy depends on nuclear features of follicular cells (enlarged and elongated nuclei with nuclear pseudoinclusion, nuclear grooves, powdery chromatin), and architectures (papillary versus follicular) (Figure 4). Other FNA features include psammomatous calcification, and "gum"-like thick colloid.

The characteristic FNA features of undifferentiated (anaplastic) carcinoma are presence of pleomorphic, markedly atypical spindle cells (Figure 5).

The FNA features of thyroid medullary carcinoma are presence of pleomorphic polygonal tumor cells with characteristic neuroendocrine nuclear features "(salt and pepper") and granular cytoplasm, which are present in a single cell pattern, loosely cohesive clusters, follicular and papillary architecture (Figure 6). Serum calcitonin screening is useful in detection of C-cell hyperplasia and medullary thyroid cancer.

Large cell lymphoma is the predominant subtype, and consists of relatively monotonous populations of large, abnormal lymphoid cells(Morgen, Geddie et al. 2010). Marginal zone lymphoma is composed of small lymphocytes with plasmacytoid features(Morgen, Geddie et al. 2010). Amyloidosis may be seen.

The FNA features of metastatic malignancies vary depending on the primary organs and subtypes (Figure 7).

Approximately 3% to 7% of thyroid FNAs have conclusive features of malignancy, and most are papillary carcinomas(Yang, Schnadig et al. 2007; Cibas and Ali 2009). Postoperative risk of malignancy in thyroid nodules with malignant cytology averages 97% with a range from 93-100%(Cibas and Ali 2009; Layfield, Cibas et al. 2010; Wang, Friedman et al. 2010). Of the differentiated cancers, papillary cancer comprises about 85% of cases, follicular carcinoma comprises about 10%, and Hürthle cell carcinoma comprises 3%(Hundahl, Fleming et al. 1998). Lobectomy for follicular carcinoma and Hürthle cell carcinoma and near total and total thyroidectomy for papillary thyroid carcinoma is recommended. Postoperative radioiodine (RAI) remnant ablation is increasingly being used to eliminate the postsurgical thyroid remnant(Hay, Thompson et al. 2002). Thyroidectomy is not usually used for metastatic tumors, non-Hodgkin lymphomas, and undifferentiated carcinomas(Cibas and Ali 2009)

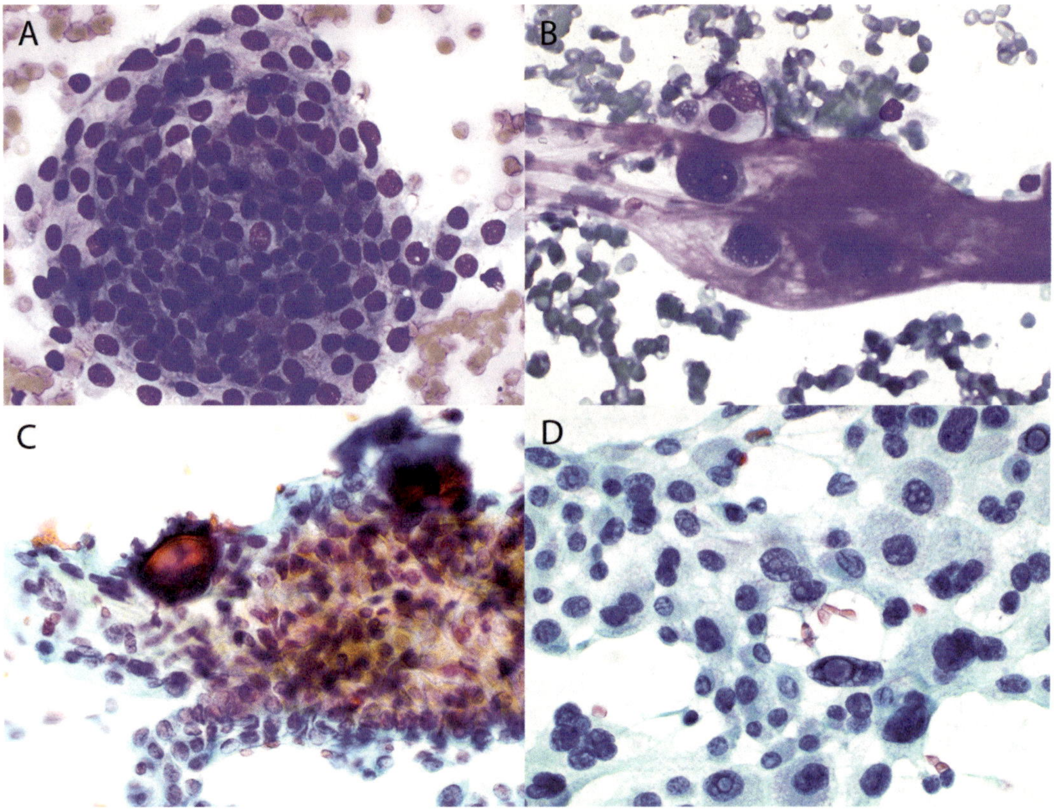

Fig. 4. Papillary thyroid carcinoma, FNA cytology, modified Giemsa (A and B) and Papanicolaou (C and D), 600x (A, B and D) and 400x (C). FNA smears show follicular cells arranged in true papillae with fibrovascular cores (C), swirling (A, papillary cap), singles (B) and cohesive clusters (D), with enlarged and elongated nuclei containing fine granular chromatin (powering), nuclear pseudoinclusion and nuclear grooves, and slightly dense cytoplasm (squamoid). Psammomatous calcification (C) and "chewing gum" dense colloid are seen (B).

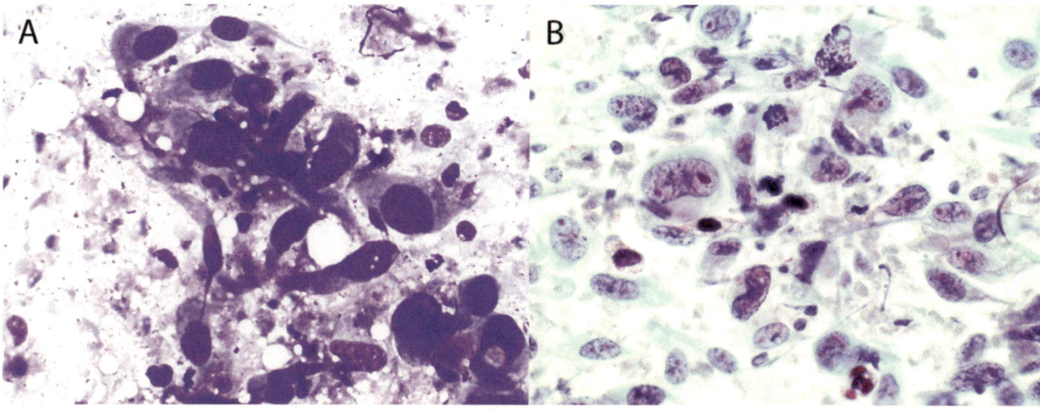

Fig. 5. Anaplastic thyroid carcinoma, FNA cytology, modifier Giemsa (A) and Papanicolaou stain (B), 600x. FNA smears show pleomorphic cells including bizarre spindle cells, atypical mitotic figure, and necrosis.

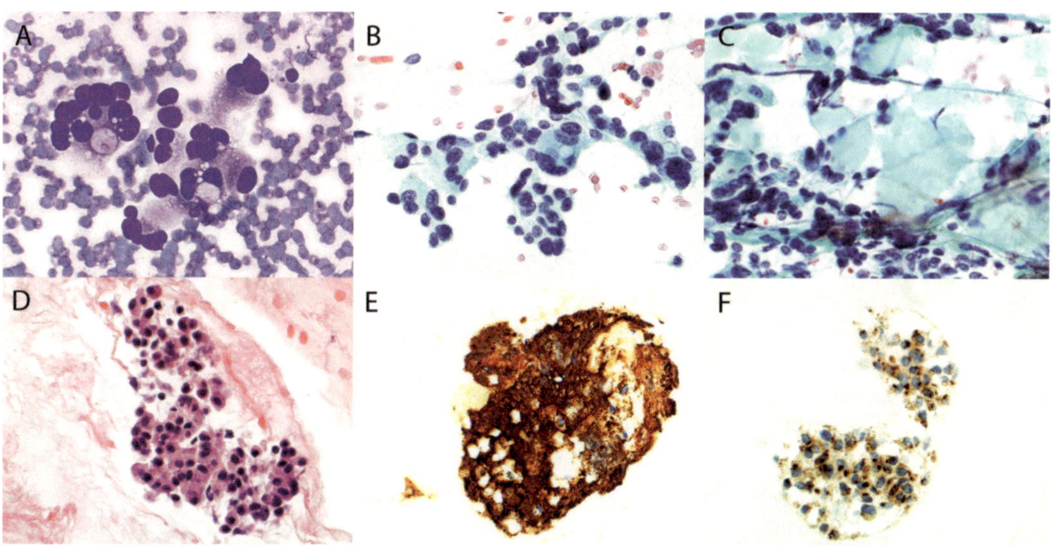

Fig. 6. Thyroid medullary carcinoma, FNA cytology. FNA smears (A: modified Giemsa stain, 600x; B and C: Papanicolaou stain, 600x) show pleomorphic epithelial cells that are present in loosely clusters and microacini/microfollicles, have round or oval nuclei containing granular and coarse ("salt and pepper") chromatin, some with prominent nucleoli, and scant to abundant cytoplasm, some with cytoplasmic granules. Amyloidosis is seen (C). Cellblock (D: H&E stain, 400x) shows tumor cells that form microacini/microfollicles and have scant to abundant eosinophilic cytoplasm. The tumor cells are positive for Calcitonin (E: 400x) and chromogranin (F: 400x) identified by immunohistochemical stains, confirming the diagnosis.

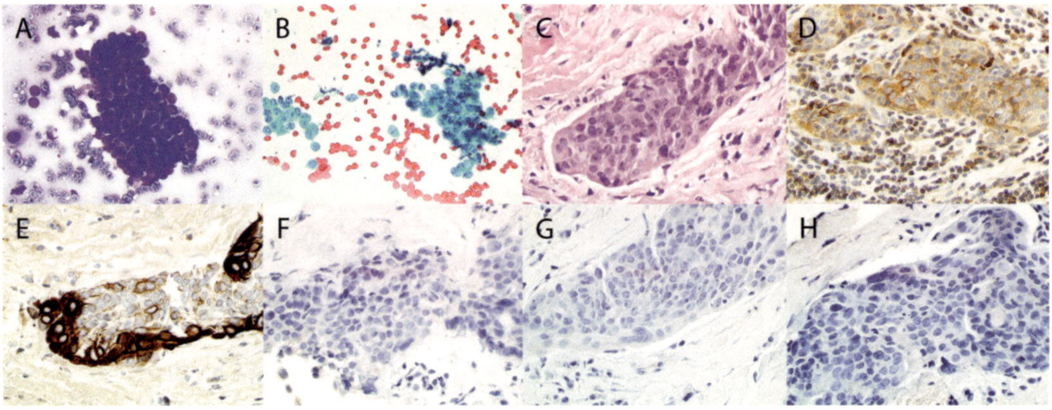

Fig. 7. Metastatic thymic carcinoma, FNA cytology. FNA smears (A: modified Giemsa stain, 600x and B: Papanicolaou stain, 600x) show cohesive three dimensional clusters of epithelial cells with round to oval nuclei containing prominent nucleoli, and scant cytoplasm. Cellblock (C: H&E stain, 600x) shows cohesive sheets of tumor cells with same cytomorphology as seen in FNA smears and surrounded by dense fibrous tissue. The tumor cells are positive for CD5 (D: 600x) and partially positive for CK7 (E: 600x), while are negative for thyroglobulin (F: 600x), calcitonin (G: 600x), and chromogranin (H: 600x), which confirms the diagnosis of thymic carcinoma, and exclude thymic neoplasm (follicular and medullary neoplasm), and parathyroid neoplasm.

2007 TBSRTC has been demonstrated to be excellent for reporting thyroid FNAs(Theoharis, Schofield et al. 2009). Each diagnostic category conveys specific risks of malignancy, which offers guidance for patient management. Routine second opinion review of indeterminate thyroid FNA biopsies can potentially obviate the need for diagnostic thyroidectomy in 25% of patients without increases in false negatives(Davidov, Trooskin et al. 2010). Routine second opinion review of FNA specimens increases sensitivity, specificity, positive predictive value, and negative predictive value(Tan, Kebebew et al. 2007).

2.5 Immunohistochemistry used in thyroid lesions

Immunohistochemical (IHC) stains are seldom used in thyroid FNA biopsy for follicular lesions. IHC can be performed on FNA cellblock or FNA smears.

Thyroid follicular neoplasms and medullary carcinomas are positive for TTF-1. Conventional papillary thyroid carcinoma is immunoreactive for p53 (76%), galectin-3 (100%), and EMA (50%), while are negative for p63(Koo, Shin et al. 2010). Diffuse sclerosing variant of papillary carcinoma is immunohistochemically positive for p63 (28.6%), p53 (42.9%) galectin-3 (16.3%), EMA (40.8%)(Koo, Shin et al. 2010), and BCL-2(Koo, Shin et al. 2010). Medullary thyroid carcinoma is positive for calcitonin.

Immunohistochemical stains for CD3, CD20, CD79a, PAX-5, CD5, CD10, CD23, cyclin D1 (BCL-1), BCL-1, BCL-6, alpha or lambda light chain, and other lymphoid markers are useful for diagnosis of lymphoma(Morgen, Geddie et al. 2010). Aliquot of FNA aspiration should be sent for flow cytometry analysis.

2.6 Molecular tests used in thyroid nodular lesions

Molecular tests can be performed on FNA specimens and can help in diagnosis and classification of thyroid nodules(Chudova, Wilde et al. 2010). Many molecular markers (e.g., galectin-3(Bartolazzi, Orlandi et al. 2008; Kato and Fahey 2009), cytokeratin, BRAF(Lin, Liu et al. 2006; Pizzolanti, Russo et al. 2007; Sapio, Posca et al. 2007; Kato and Fahey 2009; Nikiforov, Steward et al. 2009), RAS(Nikiforov, Steward et al. 2009), RET/PTC(Pizzolanti, Russo et al. 2007; Sapio, Posca et al. 2007; Kato and Fahey 2009; Nikiforov, Steward et al. 2009), TRK(Sapio, Posca et al. 2007), Pax8-PPARγ(Kato and Fahey 2009; Nikiforov, Steward et al. 2009), HBME-1(Kato and Fahey 2009), hTERT(Kato and Fahey 2009), miRNA(Kato and Fahey 2009), LOH at 10q23(Lin, Liu et al. 2006)) have been evaluated to improve diagnostic accuracy for indeterminate nodules(Sapio, Posca et al. 2007; Bartolazzi, Orlandi et al. 2008). Recent large prospective studies have confirmed the ability of genetic markers (BRAF, Ras, RET=PTC) and protein markers (galectin-3) to improve preoperative diagnostic accuracy for patients with indeterminate thyroid nodules diagnosed by FNA biopsy(Pizzolanti, Russo et al. 2007; Sapio, Posca et al. 2007; Bartolazzi, Orlandi et al. 2008; Franco, Martinez et al. 2009; Nikiforov, Steward et al. 2009). It is likely that some combination of molecular markers will be used in the future to optimize management of patients with indeterminate cytology on FNA specimens. BRAF mutations occur in approximately 44% (from 29 to 83% of papillary carcinoma, and can be used in diagnosis and as a target of treatment(Lassalle, Hofman et al. 2010). With more and more basic and clinical translational research, molecular tests as an adjunctive diagnostic tool will increase the diagnostic accuracy of FNA biopsy with cytologic diagnoses of AUS/FLUS, follicular neoplasm/suspicious for follicular neoplasm, and suspicious for malignancy. However, molecular markers (Galectin-3, CITED1, HBME-1, Ras, RET/PTC, and PAX8/PPARγ) have been identified in some histopathologically classified benign nodules(Arora, Scognamiglio et al. 2008). Follicular adenomas and Hürthle cell adenomas have similar gene expression profile as malignant tumors(Arora, Scognamiglio et al. 2008).

By detection of BRAF mutation and loss of heterozygosities (LOH), 66.7% papillary thyroid carcinomas (PTC), including 50% papillary microcarcinoma cases (<1 cm), were proved to be intrathyroid metastasis(Lin, Finkelstein et al. 2008). Patients with intrathyroid metastasis, including papillary microcarcinoma, had significantly increased lymph node metastasis(Lin, Finkelstein et al. 2008). LOHs of 17q21, 17p13, 10q23 and 22q13 may be important in predicting increased risk of lymph node metastasis(Lin, Finkelstein et al. 2008). LOH of 9p21 was found at the highest frequency in PTC (53.8%), followed by 1p36 (46.2%), 10q23 (34.6%), and 22q13 (34.6%)(Lin, Finkelstein et al. 2008). Papillary microcarcinoma had acquired similar genomic mutations as conventional PTC (>1 cm), but higher frequencies of mutations of B-RAF, 1p36, 18q, and 22q13 were found in the larger PTC, suggesting that they might play a role in the aggressiveness of PTC(Lin, Finkelstein et al. 2008). Different profiles of mutations were observed in conventional, follicular variant, and diffuse sclerosing variant of PTC, which might influence the different morphological appearances and clinical courses(Lin, Finkelstein et al. 2008). Therefore, molecular analysis can separate multifocal independent primary PTC from intrathyroid metastatic PTC, and may be more important than tumor size in predicting lymph node metastasis, aggressiveness, and prognosis of PTC(Lin, Finkelstein et al. 2008). Microarray analysis has be used in thyroid FNA specimens(Lubitz, Ugras et al. 2006).

3. Clinical workup of parathyroid lesions

3.1 Introduction

Primary hyperparathyroidism is a common problem encountered in clinical practice. Patients commonly present with elevated serum and urine calcium and parathyroid

hormone (PTH) concentration. In most cases, the diagnosis is relatively straightforward. However, when imaging studies fail to localize the parathyroid adenoma or hyperplasia, management can be challenging.
The gold standard to determine the cause of primary hyperparathyroidism is bilateral neck exploration. Minimally invasive parathyroidectomy is the preferred treatment of choice, but it requires the accurate localization of a parathyroid lesion by ultrasound imaging, Tc^{99}-sestamibi scan, and FNA combined with PTH test. Minimally invasive parathyroidectomy is not applicable in those patients who have coexisting thyroid cancers or nodules with suspicious cytology(Abraham, Duick et al. 2008) .

3.2 Clinical workup of parathyroid lesions

Ultrasound imaging and/or Tc^{99}-sestamibi scan are used to localize the abnormal parathyroid glands. For the detection of the incidentalomas, the positive predictive value (PPV) of thyroid ultrasound was 21.4%(Kwak, Kim et al. 2009). In the overall patients, the sensitivity and PPV of ultrasound, Tc^{99}-sestamibi scan, and ultrasound + Tc^{99}-sestamibi scan to localize parathyroid adenoma are 96% and 91%, 92% and 87%, and 95% and 94%, respectively(Erbil, Salmaslioglu et al. 2007). FNA biopsy is seldom used in evaluation of parathyroid lesions, especially those that can be visualized by ultrasound. Some authors suggested that FNA is valuable in patients who have a nondiagnostic Tc^{99}-sestamibi scan, with multiple enlarged parathyroid glands, prior failed surgery, differentiating parathyroid adenomas from posterior thyroid nodules, atypical location, and nonfunctioning parathyroid incidentalomas(Abraham, Duick et al. 2008; Vu and Erickson 2010). Cellular FNA specimens with features not typical for thyroid lesions should be triaged for PTH assay in the FNA rinse, which is useful to differentiate parathyroid lesions from thyroid lesions(Owens, Rekhtman et al. 2008; Ciuni, Ciuni et al. 2010; Lieu 2010). This technique is also used during operation(Lamont, McCarty et al. 2005).

3.3 Fine needle aspiration biopsy of parathyroid lesions

For the detection of the incidentalomas, the sensitivity of ultrasound guided FNA was 41.7%, specificity was 97.7%, accuracy was 85.7%, PPV was 83.3%, and negative predictive value (NPV) was 86%(Kwak, Kim et al. 2009). The sensitivity of FNA-parathyroid hormone test was 92.9%, specificity was 100%, accuracy was 94.4%, PPV was 100%, and NPV was 80%(Kwak, Kim et al. 2009). Overall, the sensitivity and positive predictive value of FNA-PTH assay to localize parathyroid adenoma is higher compared with ultrasound, Tc^{99}-sestamibi scan, and ultrasound + Tc^{99}-sestamibi scan(Erbil, Salmaslioglu et al. 2007).
FNA aspirates of parathyroid lesions are often cellular(Absher, Truong et al. 2002; Owens, Rekhtman et al. 2008). FNA cytomorphologic features include small and monotonous to moderately anisokaryotic cells that are present in cohesive cellular disorganized sheets, cords, cohesive three-dimensional groups, papillary fragments, and microfollicles (in 90% of parathyroid adenomas and absence in parathyroid hyperplasia), have round to oval hyperchromatic nuclei containing finely to coarsely granular chromatin and inconspicuous nucleoli, and have fragile, pale blue or finely granular cytoplasm with ill-defined borders(Absher, Truong et al. 2002; Liu, Gnepp et al. 2004; Owens, Rekhtman et al. 2008) (Figure 8). Isolated cells and naked nuclei are commonly present and sometimes predominate(Absher, Truong et al. 2002; Liu, Gnepp et al. 2004; Owens, Rekhtman et al. 2008), and rare case shows lymphoid-like smears(Absher, Truong et al. 2002). Prominent

nucleoli, mitotic figures, and karyolysis are seen in parathyroid carcinoma(Hara, Oyama et al. 1998). Nuclear pleomorphism is seen in 33% of parathyroid adenoma and absent in parathyroid hyperplasia(Liu, Gnepp et al. 2004). A granular smear background is usually present(Owens, Rekhtman et al. 2008). Oncocytic parathyroid adenoma is a rare benign neoplasm. It is challenging to distinguish from thyroid Hürthle cell lesion on FNA biopsy, and may be misinterpreted as suspicious for Hürthle cell neoplasm(Paker, Yilmazer et al. 2010) or Hürthle cell neoplasm. FNA reveals cellular smears containing monotonous oncocytic cells arranged in monolayered sheets, pseudopapillary structures and clusters within a rich vascular network(Paker, Yilmazer et al. 2010).

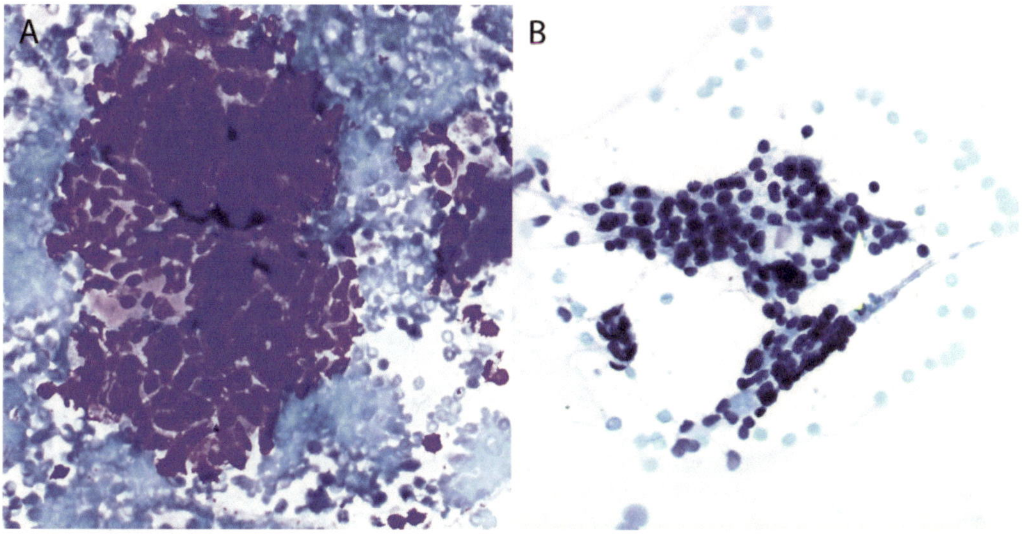

Fig. 8. Parathyroid adenoma, FNA cytology, modified Giemsa (A) and Papanicolaou stain (B), 600x. FNA smears show small and monotonous epithelial cells that are present in cohesive cellular disorganized sheets, three-dimensional groups and microfollicles, have round to oval hyperchromatic nuclei containing finely to coarsely granular chromatin and inconspicuous nucleoli, and have fragile, pale or finely granular cytoplasm with ill-defined borders.

Parathyroid cysts (PCS) are rare and rarely symptomatic except for swelling. PCS are divided into functional (hyperparathyroidism, hypercalcemia, and hypophosphatemia) and non-functional PCS that represent about 10% of PCS. The non-functional PCS are considered true PCS because their wall is lined by secretory epithelium, and the functioning PCS develop due to cystic degeneration of parathyroid gland adenomas. The ultrasound images demonstrate a cystic lesion. FNA aspirates clear liquid, which should be sent to chemistry laboratory to test PTH level(Absher, Truong et al. 2002; Ciuni, Ciuni et al. 2010; Lieu 2010). The first treatment is the aspiration FNA, which can be curative, but recurrences can be treated surgically(Ciuni, Ciuni et al. 2010).

FNA of parathyroid adenomas may cause severe fibrosis complicating surgery and final histologic diagnosis(Norman, Politz et al. 2007), which could be avoided by using fine bore needles (25 - 27 gauge) and fewer passes (1 to 2 passes)(Abraham, Duick et al. 2008). Needle track implantation of parathyroid carcinoma has been reported, although it is extremely rare(Agarwal, Dhingra et al. 2006).

3.4 Immunohistochemistry in parathyroid lesions

IHC stains for PTH, synaptophysin, chromagranin, NSE, and CD56 can be performed on FNA smears and cellblock for confirmation of parathyroid origin.

The FNA cytomorphology of parathyroid adenoma shares some features with thyroid lesions, which may lead to misinterpretation as thyroid follicular lesion/neoplasm, medullary carcinoma, papillary carcinoma, and thyroid cyst(Absher, Truong et al. 2002; Owens, Rekhtman et al. 2008; Lieu 2010). Therefore, a PTH assay of needle rinse and IHC studies should be ordered for any case with an FNA cytomorphology that is not typical for thyroid lesion, PCS develop due to absence of colloid, and is a highly cellular specimen.

4. Clinical workup of adrenal glands

4.1 Introduction

Adrenal gland is the fourth most frequent site of spread of tumors after lungs, liver, and bone(Willis 1973; Lloyd, Kawashima et al. 2004). Metastatic malignancies are far more common than primary malignancies of the adrenal gland(Lloyd, Kawashima et al. 2004). Adrenal metastases develop in 27% of patients dying with carcinomas(Abrams, Spiro et al. 1950; Lloyd, Kawashima et al. 2004). The most common primary sites are the breast, lung, kidney, stomach, pancreas, ovary, and colon. Adrenal glands are also often involved by disseminated infectious diseases.

The commonly encountered primary adrenal neoplasms include myelolipoma (2.5% of primary tumors)(Lam and Lo 2001), cortical adenoma (incidence, 1.5 – 7%)(Stewart 2002), cortical carcinoma (incidence, 1/1 million/year)(Lloyd, Tischler et al. 2004), and pheochromocytoma. Eighty five percent of adrenal cortical adenomas are nonfunctional(Stewart 2002), while 80% of adrenal cortical carcinomas are functional(Lloyd, Tischler et al. 2004). Adrenal cortical carcinoma is also associated with Li-Fraumeni syndrome, Beckwith-Wiedemann syndrome, and Carney complex. Pheochromocytoma is generally associated with clinical symptoms due to overproduction of catecholamines, intermittent, paroxysmal hypertension accompanied by sweating, palpitations, headache, diaphoresis, nervousness, nausea, vomiting, weakness, abdominal or chest pain.

4.2 Fine needle aspiration biopsy of adrenal lesions

FNA is often used to evaluate nodular or mass lesions of adrenal glands under the guidance of CT scan, ultrasound, EUS, and MRI scan. Application of FNA biopsy for incidentally discovered adrenal masses (incidentaloma) is controversial(Nurnberg 2005; Lumachi, Borsato et al. 2007; Quayle, Spitler et al. 2007). A thorough clinical history and radiographic studies (CT scan, MRI and norcholesterol scintigraphy) are very important in the work-up(Lumachi, Borsato et al. 2007). It may be difficult in some cases for FNA to distinguish benign (non-neoplastic or adenoma) from malignant adrenal cells with certainty(Tikkakoski, Taavitsainen et al. 1991), although a report stated that FNA cytology combined with clinical presentations (symptoms and endocrine function) and imaging studies (CT scan, MRI and norcholesterol scintigraphy) can increase diagnostic accuracy to 100%(Lumachi, Borsato et al. 2007). In addition, other reports stated that image-guided FNA cytology is a safe and sensitive procedure and should be performed in all patients with incidentally discovered adrenal masses with high sensitivity (83.3 - 100%), specificity (96.3 - 100%), positive predictive value (95.8 - 100%), negative predictive value (100%), and accuracy (97.6%)(Fassina, Borsato et al. 2000; Lumachi, Borsato et al. 2003).

The characteristic FNA cytologic features of myelolipoma are the presence of normal bone marrow hematopoietic cells (megakaryocytes, myeloid cells, and erythrocytic precursors) and mature adipose tissue in variable proportions(Settakorn, Sirivanichai et al. 1999) (Figure 9). The differential diagnosis includes well-differentiated liposarcoma and hematopoietic tumors.

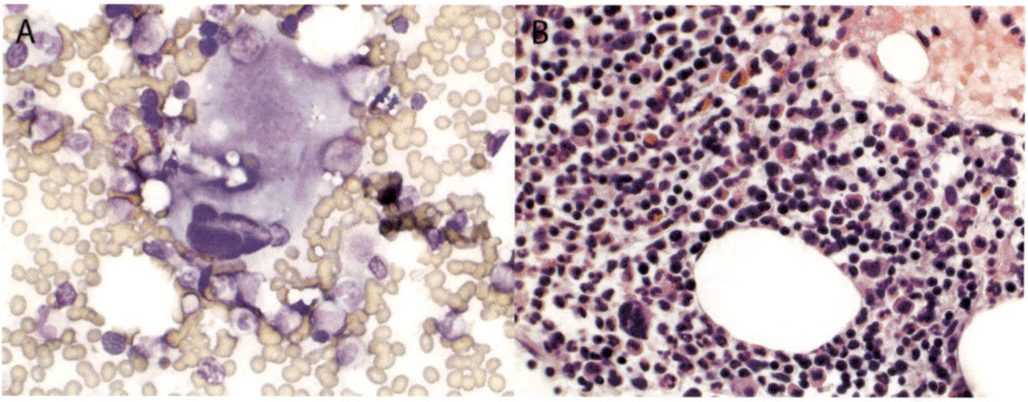

Fig. 9. Adrenal myelolipoma, FNA cytology. FNA smear (A: modified Giemsa stain, 600x) and cellblock (B: H&E stain, 600x) show trilineage of hematopoietic cells, similar to the cells seen in normal bone marrow (megakaryocytes, myeloid cells and red blood cell precursors), adipocytes, and fat droplets.

The characteristic FNA cytologic features of adrenal cortical neoplasm (adenoma and carcinoma) are the presence of loose aggregates, fascicles or microacini of polygonal cells with uniform or pleomorphic, round or oval nuclei containing granular chromatin and distinct nucleoli, and moderate to abundant, clear, delicate, vacuolated or granular cytoplasm with indistinct cell borders(Fassina, Borsato et al. 2000; Stelow, Debol et al. 2005; Ren, Guo et al. 2006) (Figure 10). Abundant naked nuclei and intranuclear pseudoinclusions may be present. A foamy background of lipid droplets is always seen. The cells of adrenal cortical adenoma are smaller and less pleomorphic than carcinoma. Mitoses and necrosis are more frequently seen in carcinoma. Differential diagnosis includes non-neoplastic adrenal cortex, nodular hyperplasia, pheochromocytoma, metastatic renal cell carcinoma, hepatocellular carcinoma, and small blue cell tumor (when aggregates of naked nuclei are present).

FNA biopsy should be performed carefully in cases that are clinically suspicious for pheochromocytoma due to possible fatal hypertensive crisis or hemorrhage. Therefore, biochemical testing for pheochromocytoma should be performed before biopsy of adrenal masses. The characteristic FNA findings of pheochromocytoma are presence of bland to pleomorphic epithelioid or spindle cells present singly or in discohesive nests (zellballen) and acinar-microglandular structures or rosettes(Jimenez-Heffernan, Vicandi et al. 2006) (Figure 11). The tumor cells have single or multiple eccentrically-located (plasmacytoid), round to oval nuclei with prominent nucleoli and granular chromatin(Jimenez-Heffernan, Vicandi et al. 2006). Large intranuclear inclusions, binucleation or multinucleation, and naked nuclei are commonly seen(Jimenez-Heffernan, Vicandi et al. 2006). The cytoplasm is abundant, and delicate, granular or "squamoid" with ill-defined cell borders(Jimenez-Heffernan, Vicandi et al. 2006). Hyaline globules and rarely melanin pigment may be seen in the cytoplasm. Differential diagnosis includes adrenal cortical neoplasm, metastatic adenocarcinoma, melanoma and neuroendocrine neoplasms.

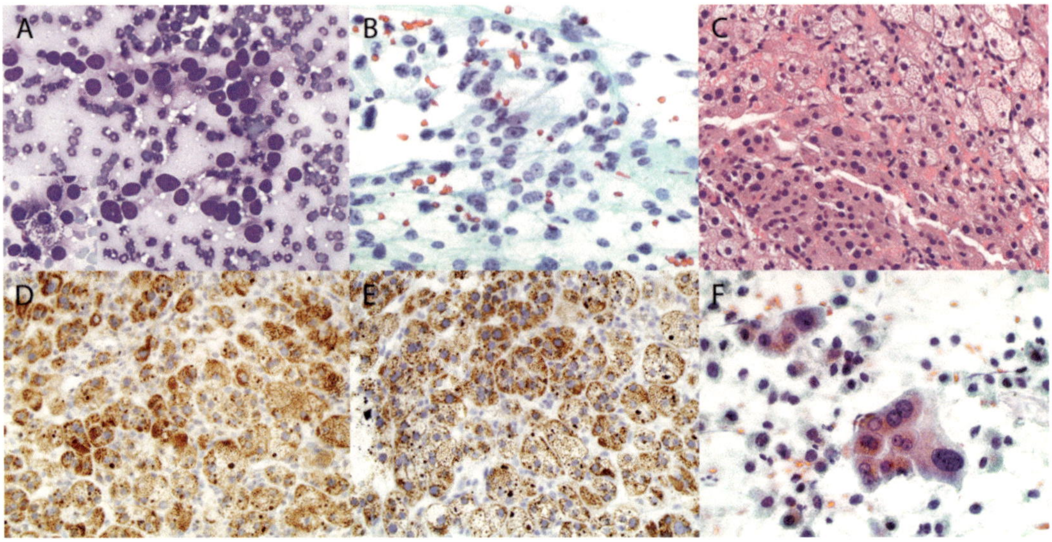

Fig. 10. Adrenal cortical neoplasms (adenoma, A to E, and carcinoma, F), FNA cytology. FNA smears (A: modified Giemsa stain, 600x; B: Papanicolaou stain, 600x) show loose aggregates or fascicles of polygonal cells with slightly pleomorphic, round or oval nuclei containing granular chromatin and distinct nucleoli, and moderate to abundant, clear, delicate, vacuolated or granular cytoplasm with indistinct cell borders. A foamy background of lipid droplets is seen. Cellblock (C: H&E stain, 600x) shows the sheets of polygonal cells with either granular or vacuolated cytoplasm. The tumor cells are positive for S-100 (D, 600x) and inhibin (E, 600x). The cells of adrenal cortical carcinoma are larger and more pleomorphic than adenoma (F: FNA smear, Papanicolaou stain, 600x).

FNA is an important tool to diagnose adrenal metastases. FNA findings vary depending on the primary site of the metastatic malignancies. Comparison with morphology of the known primary malignancy should be performed. Immunohistochemical stains are very useful in narrowing the differential diagnosis. Adrenal tumors are positive for melan A and inhibin and negative for epithelial membrane antigen (EMA).

When FNA smears show abundant inflammatory cells, benign adrenal glandular epithelial cells, necrosis or granulomas, an infectious lesion should be considered. An aliquot of FNA should be sent for culture, or molecular tests, and special stains (GMS, PAS, AFB, FITE, and GRAM) should be ordered on cytospin, smear, or cellblock.

Complications of adrenal FNA biopsy include hypertension, hematoma of liver, thorax and duodenum(Quijano and Drut 1989), and pneumothorax(Lumachi, Borsato et al. 2007).

4.3 Immunohistochemistry and special stains

The following special and IHC stains are useful in primary adrenal lesions. Special stains (chloroacetate esterase, myeloid peroxidase) or immunostains (factor VIII) are helpful to confirm the myeloid nature of the immature cells in myelolipoma. Adrenal cortical non-neoplastic and neoplastic cells are positive for inhibin, A103 and melan A, while negative for

CK7, CK20, and chromogranin. Pheochromocytoma cells are positive for chromogranin, synaptophysin and NSE, and are negative for EMA and cytokeratins. Sustentacular cells are positive for S-100.

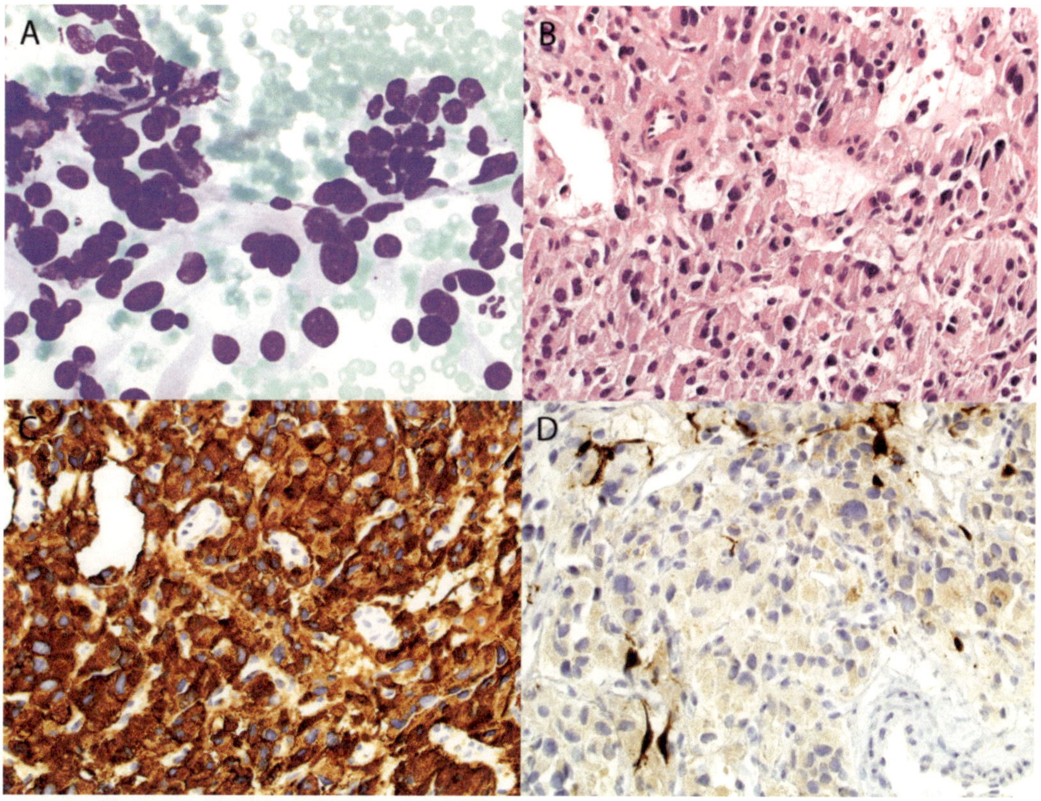

Fig. 11. Adrenal pheochromocytoma, FNA cytology. FNA smear shows pleomorphic epithelial cells present in loosely cohesive nests (zellballen), acinar/microglandular structures or rosettes. The tumor cells have single eccentrically-located (plasmacytoid), round to oval nuclei with prominent nucleoli and granular chromatin, naked nuclei, and abundant, delicate or granular cytoplasm with ill-defined cell borders. Cellblock (B: H&E stained, 600x) shows nests of epithelial cells with abundant eosinophilic granular cytoplasm that surrounded by spindle cells and capillaries. Tumor cells are positive for chromogranin (C: 600x), and surrounded spindle cells (sustentacular cells) are positive for S-100 (D: 600x).

5. Conclusion

In summary, a nodule or mass found in the endocrine organs should be evaluated thoroughly, no matter with or without clinical symptoms. Based on clinical presentation, past medical history, imaging studies, and laboratory tests, clinicians should evaluate if further investigation by FNA or needle core biopsy with accessory studies (special stains, IHC or molecular studies) is valuable for accurate diagnosis and making decision of suitable therapy (follow-up, surgical excision, chemotherapy including targeted chemotherapy, or radiation).

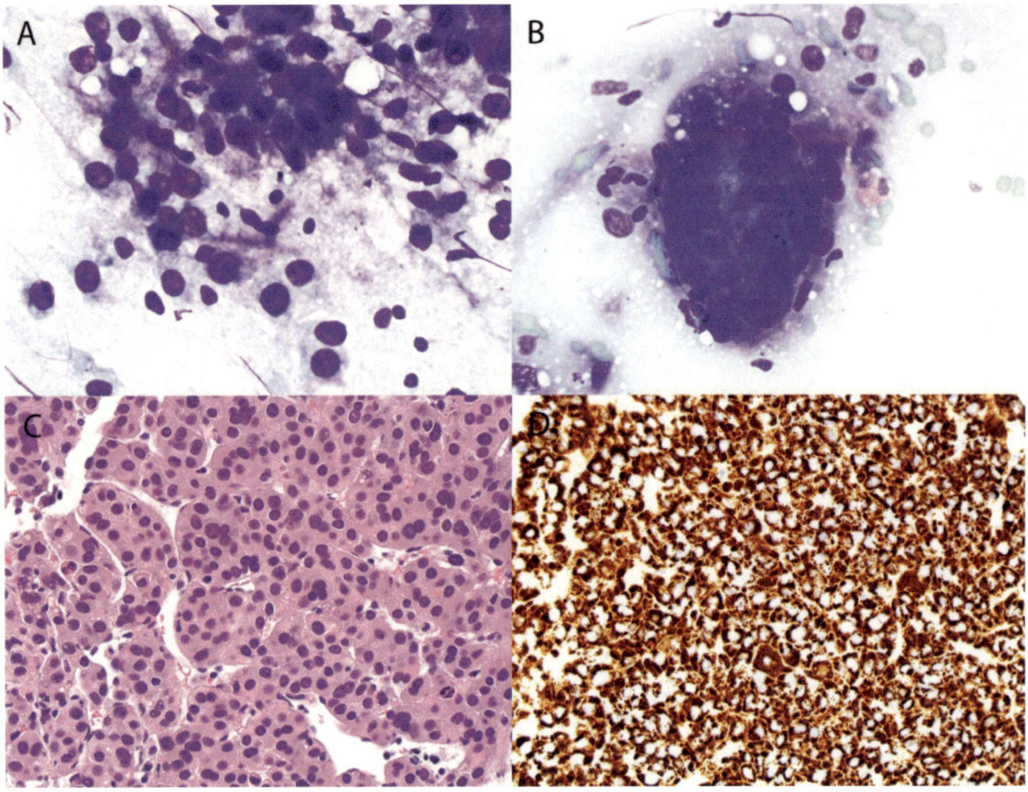

Fig. 12. Metastatic hepatocellular carcinoma to adrenal gland, FNA cytology. FNA smears (A and B, modified Giemsa stain, 600x) show loosely cohesive epithelial cells with round or oval hyperchromatic nuclei containing 1 to 3 prominent nucleoli and coarse chromatin, and fragile moderate granular cytoplasm (A), or cohesive 3 dimensional clusters of epithelial cells surrounded by endothelial cells of vessels (B). Cellblock (C: H&E stain, 600x) shows thickened or pseudoglandular epithelial cells with moderate granular cytoplasm and surrounded by endothelial cells, typical histologic features of hepatocellular carcinoma. The tumor cells are positive for HepPar-1, a marker for hepatocytes and hepatocellular neoplasms (D: 600x).

6. References

Abraham, D., D. S. Duick, et al. (2008). "Appropriate administration of fine-needle aspiration (FNA) biopsy on selective parathyroid adenomas is safe." Thyroid 18(5): 581-582; author reply 583-584.

Abrams, H. L., R. Spiro, et al. (1950). "Metastases in carcinoma; analysis of 1000 autopsied cases." Cancer 3(1): 74-85.

Absher, K. J., L. D. Truong, et al. (2002). "Parathyroid cytology: avoiding diagnostic pitfalls." Head Neck 24(2): 157-164.

Agarwal, G., S. Dhingra, et al. (2006). "Implantation of parathyroid carcinoma along fine needle aspiration track." Langenbecks Arch Surg 391(6): 623-626.

Are, C., J. F. Hsu, et al. (2007). "Histological aggressiveness of fluorodeoxyglucose positron-emission tomogram (FDG-PET)-detected incidental thyroid carcinomas." Annals of surgical oncology 14(11): 3210-3215.

Arora, N., T. Scognamiglio, et al. (2008). "Do benign thyroid nodules have malignant potential? An evidence-based review." World J Surg 32(7): 1237-1246.

Bartolazzi, A., F. Orlandi, et al. (2008). "Galectin-3-expression analysis in the surgical selection of follicular thyroid nodules with indeterminate fine-needle aspiration cytology: a prospective multicentre study." The lancet oncology 9(6): 543-549.

Boelaert, K., J. Horacek, et al. (2006). "Serum thyrotropin concentration as a novel predictor of malignancy in thyroid nodules investigated by fine-needle aspiration." The Journal of clinical endocrinology and metabolism 91(11): 4295-4301.

Caruso, D. R. and E. L. Mazzaferri (1991). "Fine needle aspiration biopsy in the management of thyroid nodules." Endocrinologist 1(1): 194-202.

Chudova, D., J. I. Wilde, et al. (2010). "Molecular classification of thyroid nodules using high-dimensionality genomic data." J Clin Endocrinol Metab 95(12): 5296-5304.

Cibas, E. S. and S. Z. Ali (2009). "The Bethesda System for Reporting Thyroid Cytopathology." Thyroid 19(11): 1159-1165.

Ciuni, R., S. Ciuni, et al. (2010). "[Parathyroid cyst. Case report]." Annali italiani di chirurgia 81(1): 49-52.

Cooper, D. S., G. M. Doherty, et al. (2009). "Revised American Thyroid Association management guidelines for patients with thyroid nodules and differentiated thyroid cancer." Thyroid 19(11): 1167-1214.

Das, D. K., C. Janardan, et al. (2009). "Infarction in a thyroid nodule after fine needle aspiration: report of 2 cases with a discussion of the cause of pitfalls in the histopathologic diagnosis of papillary thyroid carcinoma." Acta cytologica 53(5): 571-575.

Davidov, T., S. Z. Trooskin, et al. (2010). "Routine second-opinion cytopathology review of thyroid fine needle aspiration biopsies reduces diagnostic thyroidectomy." Surgery 148(6): 1294-1299; discussion 1299-1301.

Donatini, G., T. Masoni, et al. (2010). "Acute respiratory distress following fine needle aspiration of thyroid nodule: case report and review of the literature." Il Giornale di chirurgia 31(8-9): 387-389.

Erbil, Y., A. Salmaslioglu, et al. (2007). "Use of preoperative parathyroid fine-needle aspiration and parathormone assay in the primary hyperparathyroidism with concomitant thyroid nodules." Am J Surg 193(6): 665-671.

Fassina, A. S., S. Borsato, et al. (2000). "Fine needle aspiration cytology (FNAC) of adrenal masses." Cytopathology : official journal of the British Society for Clinical Cytology 11(5): 302-311.

Franco, C., V. Martinez, et al. (2009). "Molecular markers in thyroid fine-needle aspiration biopsy: a prospective study." Applied immunohistochemistry & molecular morphology : AIMM / official publication of the Society for Applied Immunohistochemistry 17(3): 211-215.

Giorgadze, T., E. D. Rossi, et al. (2004). "Does the fine-needle aspiration diagnosis of "Hurthle-cell neoplasm/follicular neoplasm with oncocytic features" denote increased risk of malignancy?" Diagn Cytopathol 31(5): 307-312.

Grant, C. S., I. D. Hay, et al. (1989). "Long-term follow-up of patients with benign thyroid fine-needle aspiration cytologic diagnoses." Surgery 106(6): 980-985; discussion 985-986.

Haider, A. S., E. A. Rakha, et al. (2011). "The impact of using defined criteria for adequacy of fine needle aspiration cytology of the thyroid in routine practice." Diagn Cytopathol 39(2): 81-86.

Hamberger, B., H. Gharib, et al. (1982). "Fine-needle aspiration biopsy of thyroid nodules. Impact on thyroid practice and cost of care." Am J Med 73(3): 381-384.

Hara, H., T. Oyama, et al. (1998). "Cytologic characteristics of parathyroid carcinoma: a case report." Diagn Cytopathol 18(3): 192-198.

Harach, H. R., K. O. Franssila, et al. (1985). "Occult papillary carcinoma of the thyroid. A "normal" finding in Finland. A systematic autopsy study." Cancer 56(3): 531-538.

Hay, I. D., G. B. Thompson, et al. (2002). "Papillary thyroid carcinoma managed at the Mayo Clinic during six decades (1940-1999): temporal trends in initial therapy and long-term outcome in 2444 consecutively treated patients." World journal of surgery 26(8): 879-885.

Hegedus, L. (2004). "Clinical practice. The thyroid nodule." The New England journal of medicine 351(17): 1764-1771.

Hundahl, S. A., I. D. Fleming, et al. (1998). "A National Cancer Data Base report on 53,856 cases of thyroid carcinoma treated in the U.S., 1985-1995 [see commetns]." Cancer 83(12): 2638-2648.

Jemal, A., R. Siegel, et al. (2010). "Cancer statistics, 2010." CA: a cancer journal for clinicians 60(5): 277-300.

Jimenez-Heffernan, J. A., B. Vicandi, et al. (2006). "Cytologic features of pheochromocytoma and retroperitoneal paraganglioma: a morphologic and immunohistochemical study of 13 cases." Acta Cytol 50(4): 372-378.

Kato, M. A. and T. J. Fahey, 3rd (2009). "Molecular markers in thyroid cancer diagnostics." The Surgical clinics of North America 89(5): 1139-1155.

Koo, J. S., E. Shin, et al. (2010). "Immunohistochemical characteristics of diffuse sclerosing variant of papillary carcinoma: comparison with conventional papillary carcinoma." APMIS : acta pathologica, microbiologica, et immunologica Scandinavica 118(10): 744-752.

Kwak, J. Y., E. K. Kim, et al. (2009). "Parathyroid incidentalomas detected on routine ultrasound-directed fine-needle aspiration biopsy in patients referred for thyroid nodules and the role of parathyroid hormone analysis in the samples." Thyroid 19(7): 743-748.

Lam, K. Y. and C. Y. Lo (2001). "Adrenal lipomatous tumours: a 30 year clinicopathological experience at a single institution." Journal of clinical pathology 54(9): 707-712.

Lamont, J. P., T. M. McCarty, et al. (2005). "Validation study of intraoperative fine-needle aspiration of parathyroid tissue with measurement of parathyroid hormone levels using the rapid intraoperative assay." Proceedings 18(3): 214-216.

Lassalle, S., V. Hofman, et al. (2010). "Clinical impact of the detection of BRAF mutations in thyroid pathology: potential usefulness as diagnostic, prognostic and theragnostic applications." Current medicinal chemistry 17(17): 1839-1850.

Layfield, L. J., J. Abrams, et al. (2008). "Post-thyroid FNA testing and treatment options: a synopsis of the National Cancer Institute Thyroid Fine Needle Aspiration State of the Science Conference." Diagn Cytopathol 36(6): 442-448.

Layfield, L. J., E. S. Cibas, et al. (2010). "Thyroid fine needle aspiration cytology: a review of the National Cancer Institute state of the science symposium." Cytopathology : official journal of the British Society for Clinical Cytology 21(2): 75-85.

Lewis, C. M., K. P. Chang, et al. (2009). "Thyroid fine-needle aspiration biopsy: variability in reporting." Thyroid 19(7): 717-723.

Lieu, D. (2010). "Cytopathologist-performed ultrasound-guided fine-needle aspiration of parathyroid lesions." Diagn Cytopathol 38(5): 327-332.

Lin, X., S. D. Finkelstein, et al. (2008). "Molecular analysis of multifocal papillary thyroid carcinoma." Journal of molecular endocrinology 41(4): 195-203.

Lin, X., Y. Liu, et al. (2006). "B-RAF and 10q23 loss of heterozygosity are valuable diagnostic molecular markers of follicular variant of papillary thyroid carcinoma in thyroid fine needle aspiration cytology initially classified as follicular lesion." Modern Pathology 19(supplement 1): 64A.

Liu, F., D. R. Gnepp, et al. (2004). "Fine needle aspiration of parathyroid lesions." Acta cytologica 48(2): 133-136.

Lloyd, R. V., A. Kawashima, et al. (2004). Secondary tumors. World Health Organization Classification of Tumors: Pathology & Genetics: Tumors of Endocrine Organs. R. A. DeLellis, R. V. Lloyd, P. U. Heitz and C. Eng. Lyon, IARC Press: 172-173.

Lloyd, R. V., A. S. Tischler, et al. (2004). Adrenal tumors: Introduction. World Health Organization Classification of tumors: Pathology & Genetics: Tumors of Endocrine Organs. R. A. DeLellis, R. V. Lloyd, P. U. Heitz and C. Eng. Lyon, IARC Press: 137-138.

Lubitz, C. C., S. K. Ugras, et al. (2006). "Microarray analysis of thyroid nodule fine-needle aspirates accurately classifies benign and malignant lesions." J Mol Diagn 8(4): 490-498; quiz 528.

Lumachi, F., S. Borsato, et al. (2003). "CT-scan, MRI and image-guided FNA cytology of incidental adrenal masses." European journal of surgical oncology : the journal of the European Society of Surgical Oncology and the British Association of Surgical Oncology 29(8): 689-692.

Lumachi, F., S. Borsato, et al. (2007). "High risk of malignancy in patients with incidentally discovered adrenal masses: accuracy of adrenal imaging and image-guided fine-needle aspiration cytology." Tumori 93(3): 269-274.

Mazzaferri, E. L. (1993). "Management of a solitary thyroid nodule." The New England journal of medicine 328(8): 553-559.

Mihai, R., A. J. Parker, et al. (2009). "One in four patients with follicular thyroid cytology (THY3) has a thyroid carcinoma." Thyroid : official journal of the American Thyroid Association 19(1): 33-37.

Morgen, E. K., W. Geddie, et al. (2010). "The role of fine-needle aspiration in the diagnosis of thyroid lymphoma: a retrospective study of nine cases and review of published series." Journal of clinical pathology 63(2): 129-133.

Nikiforov, Y. E., D. L. Steward, et al. (2009). "Molecular testing for mutations in improving the fine-needle aspiration diagnosis of thyroid nodules." The Journal of clinical endocrinology and metabolism 94(6): 2092-2098.

Norman, J., D. Politz, et al. (2007). "Diagnostic aspiration of parathyroid adenomas causes severe fibrosis complicating surgery and final histologic diagnosis." Thyroid 17(12): 1251-1255.

Nurnberg, D. (2005). "[Ultrasound of adrenal gland tumours and indications for fine needle biopsy (uFNB)]." Ultraschall in der Medizin 26(6): 458-469.

Owens, C. L., N. Rekhtman, et al. (2008). "Parathyroid hormone assay in fine-needle aspirate is useful in differentiating inadvertently sampled parathyroid tissue from thyroid lesions." Diagnostic cytopathology 36(4): 227-231.

Paker, I., D. Yilmazer, et al. (2010). "Intrathyroidal oncocytic parathyroid adenoma: a diagnostic pitfall on fine-needle aspiration." Diagn Cytopathol 38(11): 833-836.

Pizzolanti, G., L. Russo, et al. (2007). "Fine-needle aspiration molecular analysis for the diagnosis of papillary thyroid carcinoma through BRAF V600E mutation and RET/PTC rearrangement." Thyroid : official journal of the American Thyroid Association 17(11): 1109-1115.

Pu, R. T., J. Yang, et al. (2006). "Does Hurthle cell lesion/neoplasm predict malignancy more than follicular lesion/neoplasm on thyroid fine-needle aspiration?" Diagn Cytopathol 34(5): 330-334.

Quayle, F. J., J. A. Spitler, et al. (2007). "Needle biopsy of incidentally discovered adrenal masses is rarely informative and potentially hazardous." Surgery 142(4): 497-502; discussion 502-494.

Quijano, G. and R. Drut (1989). "Cytologic characteristics of Wilms' tumors in fine needle aspirates. A study of ten cases." Acta cytologica 33(2): 263-266.

Ren, R., M. Guo, et al. (2006). "Fine-needle aspiration of adrenal cortical carcinoma: cytologic spectrum and diagnostic challenges." Am J Clin Pathol 126(3): 389-398.

Renshaw, A. A. (2001). "Accuracy of thyroid fine-needle aspiration using receiver operator characteristic curves." Am J Clin Pathol 116(4): 477-482.

Renshaw, A. A. and N. Pinnar (2007). "Comparison of thyroid fine-needle aspiration and core needle biopsy." Am J Clin Pathol 128(3): 370-374.

Sapio, M. R., D. Posca, et al. (2007). "Detection of RET/PTC, TRK and BRAF mutations in preoperative diagnosis of thyroid nodules with indeterminate cytological findings." Clinical endocrinology 66(5): 678-683.

Settakorn, J., C. Sirivanichai, et al. (1999). "Fine-needle aspiration cytology of adrenal myelolipoma: case report and review of the literature." Diagnostic cytopathology 21(6): 409-412.

Stelow, E. B., S. M. Debol, et al. (2005). "Sampling of the adrenal glands by endoscopic ultrasound-guided fine-needle aspiration." Diagn Cytopathol 33(1): 26-30.

Stewart, P. M. (2002). The adrenal cortex. Williams Textbook of Endocrinology. P. R. Larsen, H. M. Kronenberg, s. Melmed and K. S. Polonsky. Philadelphia, Saunders: 491-551.

Tan, G. H. and H. Gharib (1997). "Thyroid incidentalomas: management approaches to nonpalpable nodules discovered incidentally on thyroid imaging." Annals of internal medicine 126(3): 226-231.

Tan, Y. Y., E. Kebebew, et al. (2007). "Does routine consultation of thyroid fine-needle aspiration cytology change surgical management?" J Am Coll Surg 205(1): 8-12.

Tee, Y. Y., A. J. Lowe, et al. (2007). "Fine-needle aspiration may miss a third of all malignancy in palpable thyroid nodules: a comprehensive literature review." Ann Surg 246(5): 714-720.

Theoharis, C. G., K. M. Schofield, et al. (2009). "The Bethesda thyroid fine-needle aspiration classification system: year 1 at an academic institution." Thyroid : official journal of the American Thyroid Association 19(11): 1215-1223.

Tikkakoski, T., M. Taavitsainen, et al. (1991). "Accuracy of adrenal biopsy guided by ultrasound and CT." Acta radiologica 32(5): 371-374.

Tunbridge, W. M., D. C. Evered, et al. (1977). "The spectrum of thyroid disease in a community: the Whickham survey." Clinical endocrinology 7(6): 481-493.

Vander, J. B., E. A. Gaston, et al. (1968). "The significance of nontoxic thyroid nodules. Final report of a 15-year study of the incidence of thyroid malignancy." Annals of internal medicine 69(3): 537-540.

Vu, D. H. and R. A. Erickson (2010). "Endoscopic ultrasound-guided fine-needle aspiration with aspirate assay to diagnose suspected mediastinal parathyroid adenomas." Endocrine practice : official journal of the American College of Endocrinology and the American Association of Clinical Endocrinologists 16(3): 437-440.

Wang, C. C., L. Friedman, et al. (2010). "A Large Multicenter Correlation Study of Thyroid Nodule Cytopathology and Histopathology." Thyroid : official journal of the American Thyroid Association.

Willis, R. V. (1973). The Spread of Tumors in the Human Body. London, Butterworth.

Wu, H. H., J. Clouse, et al. (2008). "Fine-needle aspiration cytology of Hurthle cell carcinoma of the thyroid." Diagn Cytopathol 36(3): 149-154.

Yang, J., V. Schnadig, et al. (2007). "Fine-needle aspiration of thyroid nodules: a study of 4703 patients with histologic and clinical correlations." Cancer 111(5): 306-315.

Yassa, L., E. S. Cibas, et al. (2007). "Long-term assessment of a multidisciplinary approach to thyroid nodule diagnostic evaluation." Cancer 111(6): 508-516.

8

Molecular Biology of Thyroid Cancer

Giuseppe Viglietto[1,2] and Carmela De Marco[1,2]
[1]*Department of Experimental and Clinical Medicine, University Magna Graecia, Catanzaro*
[2]*Institute for Genetic Research G. Salvatore, Ariano Irpino (AV)*
Italy

1. Introduction

Thyroid is a H-shaped gland localised in front of trachea at the base of the neck, whose main functions are the synthesis, the storage and the secretion of thyroid hormones under the control of the hypothalamic–pituitary axis. Thyroid is comprised of spherical follicles filled with colloid that are lined by cuboidal/flat epithelial cells denoted follicular cells (or thyrocytes). The other hormone-producing cells in the thyroid gland are scattered within follicles, and are denoted para-follicular cells (or C cells). Whereas follicular cells are responsible for iodine uptake and thyroid hormone synthesis, C cells are dedicated to the production of calcitonin (Dumont et al., 1992).

Cancers that arise in the thyroid gland represent the most common malignancy of the endocrine system and accounts for approximately 1% of all newly diagnosed cancer cases in Western countries, with estimates of annual incidence rates of 12 cases per 100,000 in North America and 5.6 new cases per 100,000 in Europe (Gilliland et al., 2009). Incidence rates of thyroid cancer widely vary worldwide, possibly because of inherent ethnic geographical or environmental differences that include iodine deficiency and radiation exposure. For instance the incidence of thyroid cancer is high in the Chinese and Filipino population of Hawaii (119 cases/million women and 45 cases/million men, respectively) and it is relatively low in Poland (14 cases/million women and 4 cases/million men, respectively) (Ain, 1995). The most common forms of thyroid carcinoma derive either from thyroid follicular epithelial cells or from C cells (Sherman, 2003). The former include well-differentiated carcinoma (WDTC) - divided into (PTC) and follicular thyroid carcinoma (FTC) -, poorly differentiated carcinoma (PDTC) and anaplastic thyroid carcinoma (ATC) (Rosai et al., 1992; DeLellis et al., 2004). PTC is the most frequent type of thyroid malignancy, and accounts for approximately 80-85% of all cases, FTC accounts for approximately 10-15% of all thyroid tumors whereas PDTC and ATC are rare aggressive malignancies (<2% of all thyroid cancer) that can develop either directly or from pre-existing well-differentiated PTC and FTC. Thyroid cancer derived from para-follicular C cells is denoted Medullary Thyroid Carcinoma (MTC). MTC is a relatively rare malignancy (<5%) and will not be discussed here. Most neoplasms derived from thyroid follicular epithelial cells are indolent tumours that can be effectively treated by surgical resection and/or radioactive-iodine administration. Usually, PTC and FTC are well-differentiated tumours with a fairly good prognosis that are generally curable with current treatments (Sherman,

2003). By contrast, PDTC and ATC represent partially or completely undifferentiated form of thyroid cancer that behave aggressively, and for which there is currently no effective treatment. Accordingly, patients with PDTC or ATC have a mean life expectancy of few months, representing the major therapeutic challenge for thyroid cancer therapy (Cornett et al., 2007). A study of nearly 16,000 patients in the United States estimated the survival rates for the various types of thyroid cancer to be 98% for PTC, 92% for FTC, and 13% for ATC. The main cause of thyroid cancer-related mortality is due to the surgical inoperability at diagnosis of many patients and to the frequent insensitivity exhibited by advanced thyroid cancer patients to radioiodine treatment. Therefore, there is the need for ameliorating the comprehension of thyroid tumorigenesis and for improving the treatment of patients with PDTC and ATC. This Chapter will focus on the mechanisms that underlie onset and progression of the more common neoplasms that originate from thyroid follicular cells and on novel targeted therapeutic strategies developed to treat thyroid cancer patients.

1.1 Epidemiology and risk factors of thyroid cancer

The main risk factors identified so far that contribute to the development of thyroid carcinoma are radiation exposure, reduced iodine intake, thyroiditis, hormonal factors and family history. Radiation exposure, especially if during infancy, represents the most important risk factor for PTC development, as demonstrated by several studies on the consequences of the explosions of atomic bombs of Hiroshima and Nagasaki (1945), nuclear testing in the Marshall Islands (1954) and Nevada (1951–1962), and of the more recent nuclear accident in Chernobyl (1986). Exposure to internal sources of ^{131}I as after the Chernobyl nuclear accident has led to a 3- to 75-fold increase in the incidence of PTC, with the highest effects most pronounced in children (Cardis et al., 2005). Similarly, exposure to external beam-radiation delivered between 1920 and 1950 for the treatment of benign conditions of the head and neck - such as thymic enlargement, tonsillitis, acne, and adenitis - and currently for Hodgkin's lymphoma, also has increased the risk of PTC of 3 to 9 fold per Gy. As suggested above, radiation exposure during childhood is more likely to produce thyroid neoplasia than similar exposure at a later age, because of the greater cellular mitotic activity shown by thyrocytes in the young. There is a linear relationship between radiation doses and the incidence of thyroid nodules and cancer. Most nodules tend to occur within 10 to 20 years of exposure, but the risk for development of malignant nodules may exist for over 40 years. The typical molecular lesion induced by radiation seems to be the chromosomal rearrangement as opposed to point mutation as a mode of aberrant gene activation associated to iodine deficiency (Ron et al., 1995).
A second risk factor for well-differentiated thyroid carcinoma is iodine deficiency (Sherman, 2003). Dietary iodine deficiency results in thyroid proliferation as a compensatory mechanism, which is the likely cause of goiter development. Interestingly, the incidence of FTC is higher in areas of iodine deficiency whereas PTC is the most frequent type of thyroid cancer in iodine-sufficient regions. However, the role of iodine in thyroid carcinogenesis is still unclear. Studies in experimental thyroid cancer systems have suggested that the role of iodine in thyroid carcinogenesis can be to modulate tumour morphology, causing the change from follicular to papillary morphology, more than decreasing overall tumor incidence (Yamashita et al., 1990). Another recognised risk factor that might predispose to the development of thyroid malignancies is the presence of some underlying inflammatory thyroid diseases (i.e. thyroiditis). Indeed, about a third of patients affected by thyroid

carcinoma present benign thyroid disease such as Hashimoto's disease, multinodular or adenomatoid goiter. Moreover, the finding that PTC frequently contains lymphocytic infiltration indicates that immunological factors might be involved in the initiation and/or progression of thyroid carcinoma. Recent studies have identified precursor lesions embedded inside chronic lymphocytic thyroiditis, though it remains to be determined whether this represents a reactive response or a prerequisite for tumorigenesis (Gasbarri et al., 2004). Thyroid cancer presents a marked sex- and age-specific incidence, being 2–4 times more frequent in females than in males (Gilliland et al, 2009; Sherman, 2003). This suggests that female hormones might regulate thyroid carcinogenesis. However, although it has been shown that oestrogen promotes the proliferation of thyrocytes there is no clear causal relationship between thyroid cancer and pregnancy or the use of exogenous sex hormones. Finally, the existence of a genetic component that may predispose to development of thyroid cancer has been also suggested. Family history with a parent or a sibling affected by follicular cell-derived thyroid carcinoma increases risk 3.2- and 6.2-fold, respectively (Hemminki et al., 2005). Putative susceptibility loci have been identified on chromosomes 1q21, 2q21, and 19p13.2.21. Other thyroid cancer susceptibility loci have been identified in familial tumour syndromes that predispose to PTC in association with papillary renal cell carcinoma (1q21), clear-cell renal-cell carcinoma ((3;8)(p14.2;q24.1)), and multinodular goiter (19p13.2) (Eng, 2000). Finally, familial thyroid cancers have been associated with inherited tumour syndromes that include familial Polyposis coli and the related Gardner and Turcot syndromes (associated with mutations in the adenomatosis polyposis coli gene (APC)), Cowden disease (associated with mutations in the phosphatase with tensin homology gene (PTEN)), Werner syndrome (associated with mutations in the WRN gene) and Carney complex (associated with mutations in the PRKAR1A gene, encoding the type 1A regulatory subunit of protein kinase) (Lindor & Greene, 2008).

1.2 Molecular pathogenesis of thyroid cancer

Tumors originating from thyroid follicular cells provide an excellent model to understand the development of human cancer. Thyroid nodules can be either benign tumors (hyperplastic goiter, adenoma) or malignant cancers. Knowledge of the molecular events that govern human thyroid tumorigenesis has grown considerably in the past twenty years leading to the identification of key genetic alterations and new oncogenic pathways implicated in cancer initiation and/or development (Nikiforova & Nikiforov 2008; Xing, 2008). In addition, it has become apparent that distinct molecular events are associated with specific stages of the multistep tumorigenic process, with a good genotype/phenotype correlation. In this section we will briefly review the pathological features of thyroid benign and malignant tumors, describing the molecular alterations identified so far.

1.2.1 Benign tumors

Goiter is an enlargement of the thyroid gland that is caused either by a primary thyroid disease or by aberrant stimulation of the gland due to an excess of blood hormone levels, autoantibodies or other factors. Thyroid adenomas represent benign epithelial tumours in which the cells are derived from the follicular epithelium and form recognizable follicular structures composed mostly of terminally differentiated thyrocytes (Figure 1). At the molecular levels, benign hyperfunctioning thyroid nodules as well as thyroid adenomas have been associated with activating mutations in the gene encoding the thyroid-stimulating hormone receptor (TSHR) or the GNAS1 gene encoding the GSα subunit of the TSHR-coupled guanine nucleotide-binding proteins (G-proteins). Both mutations constitutively activate the adenylyl cyclase-cyclic AMP (cAMP) cascade thereby regulating the growth of follicular cells (Krohn et al., 2005).

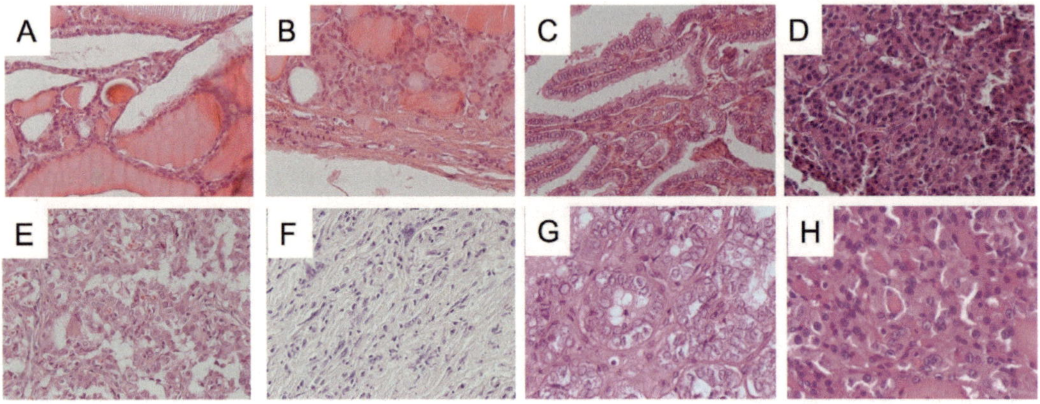

Fig. 1. Different histotypes of human thyroid cancer. A, Normal Thyroid. B, Adenoma. C, Classical Papillary Thyroid Carcinoma. D, Follicular Thyroid Carcinoma. E, Poorly Differentiated Thyroid Carcinoma. F, Anaplastic Thyroid Carcinoma; G. Typical PTC characterized by the presence of papillae, crowded nuclei with grooves and "ground glass" appearance. H, Hurthle-cell Thyroid Carcinoma. Courtesy of Dr. Renato Franco (INT Fondazione Pascale, Napoli, Italy).

1.2.2 Malignant cancers

Well-differentiated thyroid carcinomas are composed of differentiated follicular epithelial cells. Most well-differentiated thyroid cancers behave in an indolent manner and have an excellent prognosis. There are two main groups, PTC and FTC, each of which has several variants. PTC might occur in several histologic subtypes including classical form with papillary architecture, follicular variant, oncocytic variant (or Hurthle-cell variant), tall-cell variant or solid and cribriform types, each showing distinct patterns of growth and clinical behaviours (Rosai et al., 1992; DeLellis et al., 2004). The classical form of PTC is the most common and is a relative indolent disease with good prognosis. It is characterized by distinctive features such as the presence of papillae (consisting of a well-defined fibrovascular core surrounded by one or two layers of tumor cells), crowded nuclei with grooves and "ground glass" appearance, cytoplasmic pseudoinclusions caused by a redundant nuclear membrane, and Psammoma body (scarred and calcified remnants of infarcted papillae) (Figure 1C and G). Follicles and colloid are typically absent in PTC. The follicular variant accounts for approximately 10% of all PTC. It presents with cells organized into follicles rather than papillae, but at the cytological level, it displays the typical nuclear features of PTC. Overall survival and recurrence rates of follicular variant PTC are similar to those shown by the common type. By contrast, the tall-cell variant PTC is more aggressive, being characterized by cells with eosinophilic cytoplasm that are twice as tall as they are wide (Stojadinovic et al., 2001). In the tall-cell variant tumors tend to be large and invasive, and frequently patients present both local and distant metastases at the time of diagnosis.

The most studied pathway involved in PTC tumorigenesis is the RTK/RAS/BRAF/MAP kinase pathway, which is apparently essential for the development of PTC (Nikiforova & Nikiforov 2008; Xing, 2008). By contrast, this pathway seems to play a more limited role in FTC. At least three initiating events have been shown to occur in PTC: i) point mutations in the RAS genes; ii) point mutations in the BRAF gene; and iii) rearrangements of RET/PTC or neurotrophic tyrosine kinase receptor 1 (NTRK1) following radiation exposure (Nikiforova & Nikiforov 2008; Xing, 2008). The occurrence of mutually exclusive mutations of RET/PTC, TRK1, RAS or BRAF provides compelling genetic evidence for the critical role of the MAPK pathway in onset and/or progression of PTC. Unregulated activation of other tyrosine kinase receptors such as EGFR or MET may also represent a common step in the onset of PTC. See Table 1 for a summary of genetic alterations detected in thyroid cancer.

FTC is composed of well-differentiated follicular epithelial cells that lack the nuclear features of PTC that is characterized by haematogenous spread (Figure 1D). Typically, these tumors are encapsulated, and presents invasion along the capsule or across vascular endothelium (Rosai et al., 1992; DeLellis et al., 2004). Although cytologic features do not reliably allow discriminate between benign and malignant follicular lesions FTC may be distinguished from benign adenoma on the basis of the presence of invasive foci determined at the histological level. At difference with PTC, where the lack of a pre-malignant precursor has hindered the identification of the key steps in malignant transformation, it is generally hold that FTC may arise from benign thyroid adenoma as a result of transforming events. The two known initiating events in FTC are RAS mutations and the chromosomal translocation t(2;3)(q13;p25) that fuses the DNA binding domain of PAX8 to peroxisome proliferator-activated receptor (PPAR)γ (PAX8-PPARγ) (Nikiforova & Nikiforov 2008). Mutations in RAS, which are common in follicular adenomas, may lead to greater genomic instability, with increased allelic loss and more risk for transforming PAX8-PPARγ rearrangements that lead to development of FTC. Aberrant activation of the phosphatidylinositol-3 kinase (PI3K)/AKT pathway plays a fundamental role in FTC. Alterations within the PI3K/AKT pathway detected so far in thyroid tumors include mutations and genomic amplification/copy gain of the p110 catalytic subunit of PI3K (PIK3CA), PIK3CB, AKT1 and AKT2 and loss of PTEN through inactivating mutations, LOH or promoter methylation. Most of these genetic alterations are particularly common in FTC and in ATC but less common in PTC, in which the MAP kinase pathway, activated by the BRAF mutation or RET/PTC rearrangements, apparently plays a major role (Nikiforova & Nikiforov 2008; Xing, 2008). Many of these genetic alterations are mutually exclusive with increasing co-existence in ATC.

Variants of FTC include oncocytic (Hurthle-cell) and clear-cell types. Hurthle cell tumours are formed by cells containing numerous altered mitochondria, which confer the typical granular, eosinophilic appearance to their cytoplasm (Stojadinovic et al., 2001) (Figure 1H). Most Hurthle cell tumours have a follicular architecture and are diagnosed as adenoma or carcinoma on the basis of the same criteria applied to other follicular tumors - the identification of invasive behaviour. A Hurthle-cell variant of PTC also exists, though it is much less common than typical PTC. They present RET rearrangements and BRAF mutations and tends to be more aggressive than classical PTC (Cheung et al., 2000). Deletions and/or point mutations in mitochondrial DNA (mtDNA) are common in non-neoplastic and neoplastic thyroid cells that show morphological oncocytic changes (Yeh et al., 2000). However, although a role of mtDNA mutation in cell growth and tumorigenicity

TUMOUR TYPE	PREVALENCE	AGE (YEARS)	LYMPHNODE METASTASIS	DISTANT METASTASIS	SURVIVAL RATE (5 YEARS)	GENETIC ALTERATION
PTC	85-90%	20-50	< 50%	5-7%	> 90%	RET rearrangement (13-43%) BRAF mutation (29-69%) BRAF rearrangement (1%) NTRK1 rearrangement (5-13%) Ras mutation (0-21%) PIK3CA amplification (5-14%) PIK3CA mutation (0-3%) AKT1 amplification (n.d.) Akt1 mutation (n.d.)
FTC	< 10%	40-60	< 5%	20%	> 90%	Ras mutation (40-53%) PPARG rearrangement (25-63%) TP53 mutation (0-9%) PIK3CA amplification (24-28%) PIK3CA mutation (6-13%) AKT1 amplification (0-8.2%) AKT1 amplification (0-18.8%) Akt1 mutation (0%)
PDTC	0-7%	50-60	30-80%	30-80%	50%	RET rearrangement (0-13%) BRAF mutation (13-47%) Ras mutation (18-27%) CTNNB1 mutation (0-25%) TP53 mutation (17-38%) PIK3CA amplification (0-21%) PIK3CA mutation (5-21%) AKT1 mutation (0-16%)
ATC	2%	60-80	40%	20-50%	1-17%	BRAF mutation (10-35%) Ras mutation (20-60%) CTNNB1 mutation (66%) TP53 mutation (67-88%) PIK3CA amplification (0-42%) PIK3CA mutation (12-23%) AKT1 amplification (0-18.8%) Akt1 mutation (0%)

Table 1. Molecular alterations in thyroid carcinoma (from Kondo et al., 2006, modified).

has been reported in some studies, it is as yet unclear whether mtDNA mutation contributes to initiation and/or progression of thyroid cancer or only to the oncocytic phenotype. The finding of missense germ-line and somatic mutations in the GRIM19 (a nuclear gene located on chromosome 19p13.2) in oncocytic variant of FTC and PTC, but not in oncocytic adenoma or non-oncocytic carcinomas, suggests a dual function of this gene in mitochondrial metabolism and cell transformation (Maximo et al., 2005). PDTC shows loss of structural and functional differentiation, which implies they are intermediate between well-differentiated and undifferentiated thyroid carcinomas (Rosai et al., 1992; DeLellis et al., 2004; Cornett et al., 2007). Characteristically, these lesions show widely infiltrative growth, necrosis, vascular invasion and numerous mitotic figures (Figure 1E). Insular carcinomas are placed in this category. Typically, insular carcinoma is composed of small cells arranged in nests with numerous mitotic figures, necrosis, vascular invasion and infiltrative growth. ATC is composed, wholly or partially, of undifferentiated cells without the typical features of follicular-cell differentiation (Figure 1F). ATC develops from more differentiated tumors as a result of one or more dedifferentiating steps. Accordingly, half patients with ATC have either a prior or coexistent differentiated carcinoma (Rosai et al., 1992; DeLellis et al., 2004). ATC is a highly aggressive tumour, with a disease-specific mortality approaching 100% (Cornett et al., 2007). Patients with anaplastic carcinoma present with extensive local invasion, and distant metastases are found at disease presentation in 15 to 50% of patients. There is currently no effective treatment for ATC and death usually occurs within 1 year of diagnosis. ATC displays three main morphological patterns: squamoid, pleomorphic giant cell and spindle cell. At the molecular levels, it is apparent that tumors harboring mutant BRAF and RAS are prone to progress towards PDTC or ATC. According to this hypothesis, PDTC and ATC develop from more differentiated tumors as a result of one or more dedifferentiating steps. Particularly, loss of p53 and mutations of β-catenin, which are found with increasing incidence in PDTC and ATC compared to well-differentiated tumors, may serve as a direct molecular trigger of tumor dedifferentiation (Table 1) (Nikiforova & Nikiforov 2008).

In conclusion, the simplified view of thyroid tumorigenesis depicted here holds that genetic alterations in the PI3K/AKT pathway promote thyroid cell transformation to FTC and that rearrangements in genes that encode MAPK pathway effectors seem to be required for cell transformation to PTC. Indeed, mutually exclusive, activating events that involve the genes RET/PTC, NTRK1, BRAF or RAS are detectable in nearly 70% of all PTC. By contrast, accumulation of multiple genetic alterations that can activate both pathways promotes cancer progression to ATC. This provides a strong basis for the emerging development of novel genetic-based diagnostic, prognostic, and therapeutic strategies for thyroid cancer.

2. The normal thyroid gland

The identification of the molecular properties of cancer cells is a necessary condition for the comprehension of the biology of cancer cells and, consequently, for improving diagnostic techniques and performing more efficient therapies. Tumor cells originate from normal cells that have accumulated several mutations in their DNA, and that for this reason, have acquired the capability to grow independently of the normal physiological controls and have lost, in part or totally, the ability to differentiate properly. In the normal adult thyroid gland, thyroid follicular cells represent a relatively stable cell population with a very low rate of proliferation and cell death that can be resumed in response to appropriate stimuli (Dumont et al., 1992). In humans, the adult thyroid is made of approximately $2x10^9$ cells. The number of cell divisions required to generate an adult thyroid from the few precursor cells in the embryo is ~30 suggesting that each human thyrocyte divides about 5-6 times (i.e. once every 8 years) (Dumont et al., 1992). During the last decades, several cellular models that include rat thyroid cells lines as well as short-term primary cultures of dog and human thyrocytes, have been developed to investigate the mechanisms involved in the proliferation of normal thyroid cells (Medina and Santisteban, 2000; Kimura et al., 2001; Roger et al., 2010). Cell lines are simple systems that allow easy manipulation and for this reason they have represented the preferred system for *in vitro* studies of thyroid biology. Established rat thyroid cells present several properties compatible with those of "normal" differentiated thyrocytes: they are euploid, depend on TSH for growth and expression of differentiated functions, uptake iodide *in vitro*, express thyroid-specific differentiation markers (thyroglobulin, thyroperoxidase), do not grow in soft agar and are not tumorigenic in immunodeficient mice. However, several caveats must be underlined before definitive conclusions can be applied to human thyroid gland *in vivo* by extrapolating results from cultured murine or canine thyrocytes. First, the immortality itself of the cell lines indicates that they have lost some of the basic mechanisms of cell cycle control; moreover, the mechanisms that regulate cell cycle in rat, dog and human thyrocytes vary considerably (see below); finally, the effects of activated oncogenes (i.e. RAS) are sometimes very different when transfected into rat or human thyrocytes. The available data on cell cycle progression and signalling cascades involved in thyrocytes has led to the conclusion that the main regulators of thyroid growth and function are TSH and growth factors (i.e. insulin/IGF-

1). Thus it is possible to distinguish two major mitogenic pathways in thyrocytes, one that impinges on the TSHR/cAMP pathway and the other that acts through tyrosine kinase receptors of growth factors. However, the mechanisms whereby TSH/cAMP and growth factors regulate cell duplication and growth in rat, canine and human thyrocytes are mostly divergent, and will be described in detail below (Figure 2).

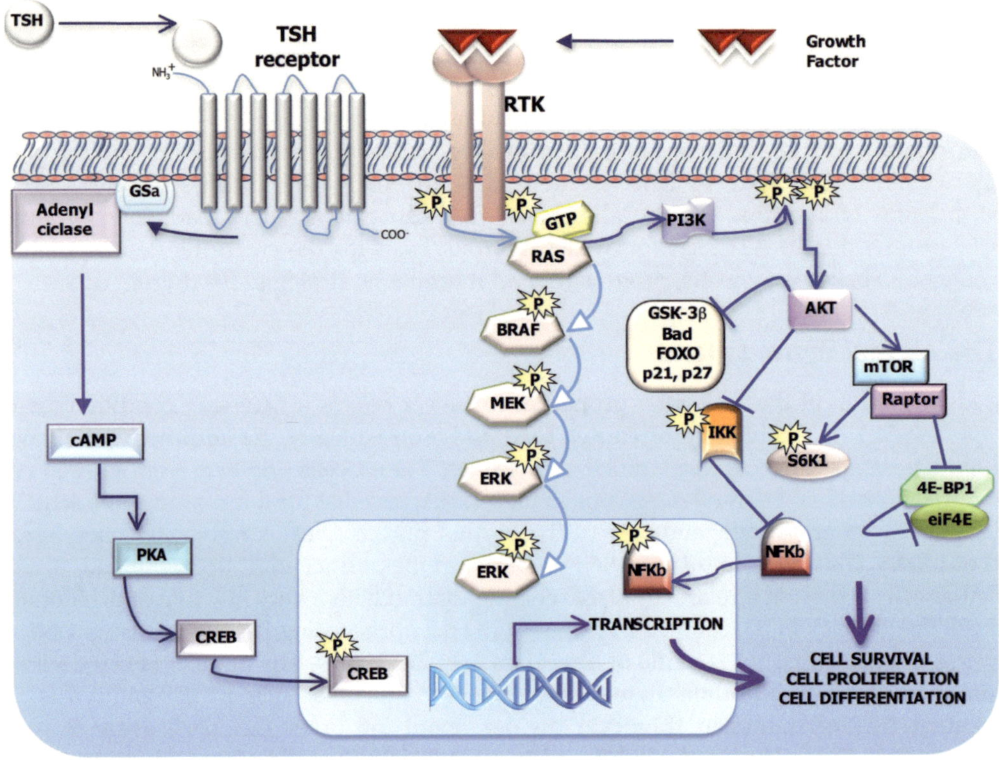

Fig. 2. Cell signalling pathways in normal thyrocytes. Thyrocytes express the TSHR and multiple growth factor receptors. TSH binds its cognate receptor and activates the G protein GSα, activating the adenylyl cyclase and increasing the level of cyclic AMP (cAMP). cAMP stimulates the cAMP-dependent protein kinase A (PKA), which in turn phosphorylates the nuclear transcription factor CREB. CREB activates the transcription of cAMP-responsive genes inducing proliferation and differentiation of thyroid follicular cells. Growth factors induce receptor-tyrosine kinase (RTK) dimerization, which results in phosphorylation of specific tyrosine residues within the cytoplasmic tail. Phosphorylated RTK activates RAS by inducing replacement of GDP with GTP. In turn, GTP-bound RAS activates the kinase BRAF and the downstream MAPK cascade. BRAF phosphorylates and activates the MAPK kinase (MEK), which phosphorylates extracellular signal-regulated kinase (ERK). Phosphorylated ERK migrates into the nucleus where it phosphorylates and activates multiple transcription factors (i.e. c-MYC, ELK1) that are involved in cell proliferation. Once activated, Akt phosphorylates a number of substrates in the cytoplasm and in the nucleus. Similarly, RTK activated PI3K signalling, which results in AKT activation. Active AKT phosphorylates and inactivates glycogen systhesis kinase-3 (GSK-3α and β), Bad, the forkhead family of transcription factors (FOXO), the CDK inhibitors p21CIP1 and p27KIP1, and conversely activate mTOR and IκB Kinases (IκKα and β).

2.1 Proliferative pathways in normal thyroid gland

So far, the most accurate model of thyroid cell cycle originated from studies performed in primary canine thyroid cells (Roger et al., 2010). Primary cultures of dog thyrocytes proliferate in monolayer culture in response to a combination of TSH, insulin, EGF and serum, though they arrest after few divisions. DNA synthesis in canine thyrocytes requires the simultaneous presence of TSH and insulin/IGF-1. Insulin or IGF-1 alone have minimal effects on DNA replication, though they support DNA synthesis and cell cycle progression induced by TSH, EGF, bFGF, or phorbol esters. By contrast, HGF is the only growth factor that acts as a full mitogen in dog thyrocytes, stimulating proliferation also in the absence of insulin/IGF-1. Established rat thyroid cell lines commonly used for the study of thyroid function and transformation are FRTL-5, PC Cl3 and WRT. FRTL-5 cells were obtained from 5-6 week old NIH Fisher 344 rats; PC Cl3 cells were obtained from 18-month old rats; WRT cells (Wistar Rat Thyroid) were established from 3-4 week old rats. Insulin/IGF-1 represents a powerful mitogen for all rat thyroid cells whereas TSH alone is not able to induce DNA synthesis in the absence of insulin it makes cells competent to respond to insulin/IGF-1, leading to the activation of MAPK and PI3K. A crucial question is how to apply the wealth of studies performed on rat and dog thyroid cells to the physiology of normal human thyrocytes. As indicated above, it appears that the canine model more accurately recapitulates the events that occur in human thyrocytes. In human primary cultures, TSH is able to induce DNA synthesis in serum-free primary cultures of adult and fetal human thyrocytes. The mitogenic effect of TSH is increased by the presence of IGF-1 or insulin, which alone weakly stimulate DNA synthesis. In thyrocytes derived from follicular adenomas, autocrine production of IGF-1 abrogates the dependence of proliferation from exogenous IGF-1. These different mitogenic stimuli exert their proliferative effects in thyrocytes by activating multiple cytoplasmic signalling cascades, which, in turn, impinge on the basic cell cycle machinery. As generally considered these mechanisms operate in the mid-to-late G1 phase of the cell cycle to promote progression through the restriction point. Typically, growth factors stimulate proliferation and inhibit differentiation. As in other cells, exposure of thyrocytes to EGF, FGF, IGF-1 or HGF activates RAS and MAPK, induces sustained expression of c-Jun and c-MYC, up-regulates cyclin D1 and down-regulates p27KIP1. On the contrary the effects exerted by TSH are in striking contrast with this general scheme. TSH induces proliferation of thyrocytes while maintaining the expression of the differentiative program. In doing so, TSH does not activate the RAS/MAPK cascade, repress c-MYC expression and increases the levels of cyclin D3 but not of cyclin D1. The differential use of cyclin D1 and cyclin D3 has been proposed to play a role in the different effects exerted by growth factors and TSH in thyrocytes (Roger et al., 2010).

2.1.1 The TSH/cAMP pathway

TSH is by far the most important physiological regulator of growth and function of thyrocytes. It is a glycoproteic hormone that recognizes a specific receptor on the thyrocyte surface, the TSH receptor (TSHR), a member of a broad class of G-protein-coupled receptors. The basic structure of these receptors comprises an extracellular segment at the N-terminus where the hormone binds, seven transmembrane helices, and three intracellular loops at the C-terminus (Vassart & Dumont, 1992). By binding to its cognate receptor TSH induces the coupling of different heterotrimeric guanine nucleotide-binding proteins (G-proteins) that include Gs, Gq/11, different subtypes of Gi and Go, G12 and G13, and cause the dissociation of the G protein into α and βγ subunits. TSH-mediated response involves activation of Gsα, which in turn, triggering the activation of adenylate cyclase, results in increased intracellular cAMP levels. cAMP is the main second messenger in thyroid cells, and activates protein kinase A (PKA), a ser/thr kinase that is required for differentiation and proliferation of thyroid cells. Activation of PKA occurs when cAMP binds to the regulatory subunits of PKA and displaces the catalytic subunits. Once activated, PKA promotes the phosphorylation and the activation of transcription factors such as CREB (**c**AMP **R**esponse **E**lement **B**inding protein), thus inducing the transcription of genes that are required for the control of growth and differentiation of thyroid follicular cells. Proliferation and differentiation are the most important effects exerted by cAMP in thyrocytes, and are mediated by PKA activation. *In vitro*, cAMP, or agents that mimic cAMP activity such as Forskolin or 8-bromo-cAMP, stimulate expression of thyroid-specific genes, iodine uptake, synthesis and secretion of thyroid hormones, and duplication of thyroid cells. TSH or cAMP can activate also PKA-independent pathways that include the cAMP-binding GTP-exchange factors (cAMP-GEFs or Epac) that function as exchange factors for the small GTPases RAP1, RAP2, and RAS, which, in turn, activates the RAF kinases, impinging into the ERK1/2 or p38MAPK pathways. On the other hand, Gβγ subunits have been demonstrated to regulate more than 20 effectors including phospholipases, adenylyl cyclases, ion channels, G protein-coupled receptor kinases, and PI3Ks.

2.1.2 The growth factor/tyrosine kinase receptor pathway

In addition to TSH, several growth factors (i.e. EGF, HGF, FGF, IGF-1, insulin) have been shown to regulate proliferation and differentiation of thyrocytes through the establishment of autocrine and/or paracrine loops (Dumont et al., 1992; Roger et al., 2010). These factors have been shown to mediate the local action of classic hormones such as TSH (Van der Laan et al., 1995). Indeed, at least 16 receptor-type tyrosine kinases are expressed in thyrocytes, with a possible role in regulating the growth and differentiated functions of thyroid cells. Binding of tyrosine kinase receptors by the cognate ligands activates the cytoplasmic kinase domain of the receptors and triggers downstream signal transduction pathways. Activated tyrosine kinase receptors promote the recruitment of the coupling complex Shc/Grb2/SOS that catalyzes the removal of GDP from one of the RAS proteins and the loading of GTP thus promoting RAS activation. RAS are small proteins with GTPase activity, which are the upstream regulators of several signalling pathways including RAF/MEK/ERK, PI3K/AKT and RalGDS/Ral (Shields et al., 2000). The active, GTP bound RAS recruits the RAF serine/threonine kinases to cell membrane, a gene family that consists of ARAF, BRAF and RAF-1 (CRAF). In turn, active RAF proteins phosphorylate and activate the Mitogen-activated protein kinase/Extracellular signal-regulated Kinases (MEKs), which phosphorylate and activate the serine/threonine **E**xtracellular-signal-**r**egulated **k**inases 1,2 (ERK). ERKs directly phosphorylate many transcription factors including Ets-1, c-Jun and c-Myc. ERKs can also phosphorylate and activate the 90 kDa ribosomal S6 kinase ($p90^{Rsk}$), which then leads to the activation of the transcription factor CREB (Shields et al., 2000). By altering the levels and activities of transcription factors, the MAPK pathway leads to altered transcription of genes that are important for the cell cycle. Many growth factors receptors such as PDGFR, EGFR, IGF-1R and insulin receptor activates also the PI3K/AKT pathway (Engelman et al., 2006). Accordingly, in thyroid cells IGF-1, EGF and HGF induces phosphorylation and activation of AKT and p70S6 (p70S6K) kinases downstream of phosphatidylinositol-3-kinase (PI3K). After ligand-induced activation of specific receptors, PI3K can be activated through one of two different mechanisms. First, activation of tyrosine kinase receptors generates phosphorylated tyrosine residues on the receptor that serve as docking sites for the p85 regulatory subunit of PI3K, which then recruits the p110 catalytic subunit to the complex, thus triggering downstream signalling. PDGFR and insulin receptor that have binding sites for p85 strongly activate PI3K upon binding to their ligands. Alternatively, GTP-bound RAS can activate PI3K by direct interaction with the catalytic subunit (Brasil et al., 2004). Activated PI3K converts phosphatidylinositol 4,5 biphosphate (PtdIns-3,4-P3) into phosphatidylinositol 3,4,5 phosphate (PtdIns-3,4,5-P3), which resulting in membrane localization of phosphoinositol-dependent kinase-1 (PDK1) via its pleckstrin homology (PH) domain. AKT is also recruited to the 3′ phosphorylated phosphatidylinositol-rich plasma membrane by its PH domain, where it is fully activated by phosphorylation at residues T308 and S473 by PDK1 and TORC2 complex, respectively. AKT is the primary mediator of PI3K-initiated signalling. Conversely, the PTEN and SHIP-1/2 phosphatases that remove the phosphate group from the 3′ position of the inositol ring of PtdIns-3,4,5-P3 are responsible for turning off PI3K signalling and antagonizing the activity of AKT (Carracedo & Pandolfi, 2008). AKT activation plays a fundamental role in the regulation of glucose metabolism, cell migration proliferation and survival by phosphorylation of a number of downstream substrates. Among these targets are: Bad, Bim, procaspase-9, IκKalpha, the forkhead family of transcription factors FOXO1, FOXO3a, GSK-3β, the ubiquitin ligases MDM2 and SKP2, the CDK inhibitors p21CIP1 and p27KIP1 and others. It is worth noting that AKT can either cause the activation of specific substrates (*e.g.*, MDM2, IκKalpha and CREB) or may mediate the inactivation of other proteins (*e.g.*, RAF, BRAF, p21CIP1, p27KIP1, BIM, BAD, procaspase-9, FOXO3a, and GSK-3β) (Manning & Cantley, 2007).

2.2 Biochemical aspects of signal transduction and cell cycle regulation in normal thyrocytes

Growth factors and TSH regulate cell cycle progression of thyrocytes with apparently different mechanisms (see Roger et al., 2010). In dog thyrocytes TSH does not activate RAS, PI3K, AKT or the different MAPKs but it activates mTOR. Conversely, insulin/IGF-1 strongly activates RAS, PI3K, AKT and the MAPKs. Interestingly, the observation that HGF, the ligand of the tyrosine kinase receptor MET, is the only growth factor that is able to stimulate both the MAPK- and the PI3K-dependent pathways, possibly explains why HGF is the only growth factor that acts as a full mitogen in dog thyrocytes, stimulating proliferation also in the absence of insulin. In dog thyroid cells, pRB phosphorylation is the critical event that regulates the passage through the restriction point. It has been convincingly shown that the complementary action of TSH and insulin converge on the activation of cyclin D3-CDK4 complexes, whose activity is required for pRB phophorylation and DNA synthesis in response to TSH and insulin. However, TSH-mediated proliferation of dog thyrocytes requires cyclin D3 and is independent of down-regulation of the cyclin-dependent kinase (CDK) inhibitor p27KIP1 whereas cyclin D3 is not required for growth factor-dependent proliferation. The current model holds that TSH (and cAMP) permits the passage through the restriction point by acting on the assembly, nuclear translocation and phosphorylation of an active cyclin D3-bound CDK4. This results in the redistribution of p27KIP1 from cyclin E/CDK2 to cyclin D3/CDK4 complexes, presumably allowing CDK2

activation and pRB phosphorylation (Roger et al., 2010). Conversely, IGF-1 or HGF induce cell cycle progression along G1 by increasing the levels of cyclin D1 and reducing those of p27KIP1.
Rat FRTL-5 cells proliferate rapidly (doubling time ~36-40 h) in the presence of serum and a six-hormone mixture (6H) containing TSH and high concentrations of insulin (that activate also IGF-1 receptors) (Medina & Santisteban, 2000). Insulin/IGF-1 are the only genuine mitogens for FRTL-5 whereas TSH makes cells competent to respond to insulin/IGF-1. bFGF, HGF as well as EGF are all able to induce robust DNA synthesis in synergy with TSH or insulin. In FRTL-5 cells proliferation induced by TSH or by cAMP requires RAS, AKT and PI3K signalling (Cass & Meinkoth, 2000; Ciullo et al., 2001). RAS activity is apparently necessary for TSH to induce the transition from quiescence to G1, though the ERK pathway seems not involved. Conversely, cAMP activates PKA and at the same time, influences the selection of RAS effectors (PI3K versus RAF). According to this model, PKA-phosphorylated p85 stabilizes the complex p110-p85 and thus facilitates the interaction between PI3K and RAS. In parallel, cAMP inhibits RAF/ERK signaling by decreasing RAF availability to RAS. Under these circumstances cAMP increases PI3K signaling (De Gregorio et al., 2007; Cosentino et al., 2007). Other studies have demonstrated that TSH/cAMP is able to activate ERKs and p38 MAPK, as well as to induce cyclin D1 and down-regulate the cyclin-dependent kinase inhibitor p27KIP1. Other rat thyroid cell lines - namely WRT and PC Cl3 cells - present discrepancies with FRTL-5. Similar to FRTL-5 cells, PC Cl3 cells are routinely maintained in a medium containing TSH and insulin. Insulin/IGF-1 stimulate proliferation and growth in size of PC Cl3 cells, and this effect is amplified by TSH (Kimura et al., 2001). Activation of the PI3K pathway by TSH in rat thyrocytes (WRT) and the involvement of cAMP in this pathway are controversial and depend on the specific cell type. In fact, TSH treatment leads to release of Gβγ dimers and subsequent activation of PI3K, one of the putative effectors of Gβγ dimers. Although debated, TSH has been shown to activate RAS and PI3K in WRT cells (Tsygankova et al., 2000). On the other hand, interference with RAS or PI3K activity impairs TSH-stimulated DNA synthesis. Through the activation of these pathways, TSH and serum deplete nuclear stores of p27KIP1, allowing activation of nuclear CDK2 and entry into S phase. TSH and serum regulate p27KIP1 in very different ways: TSH stimulated the nuclear accumulation of p27KIP1, whereas serum induced its nuclear export (Medina & Santisteban, 2000). DNA synthesis of PC Cl3 cells is also induced by FGF, phorbol esters (either in the presence or not of insulin) but not by EGF or HGF. WRT cells apparently proliferate in response to the activation of either the TSH/cAMP or insulin/IGF-1 cascades but are unresponsive to TPA, EGF and HGF (Roger et al., 2010). The PI3K pathway mediates most of the effects exerted by insulin/IGF-1 on cell cycle progression in rat thyrocytes. In fact, PI3K inhibitors impair insulin/IGF-1-dependent DNA synthesis and block the ability of insulin/IGF-1 to reduce p27KIP1 expression, to induce expression of cyclins D1 and E and to phosphorylate pRB (Roger, 2010). In serum-free primary cultures of adult and fetal human thyrocytes, TSH is able to induce DNA synthesis. However, the stimulation of DNA synthesis and/or proliferation by TSH decreases if thyrocytes originate from old people or cells exposed to high serum concentrations. In monolayer cultures, the effect of TSH is mimicked in large part, though not totally, by cAMP enhancers (forskolin, cholera toxin, (Bu)2 cAMP), with the mitogenic effect of TSH being increased by the presence of IGF-1 or insulin, which alone weakly stimulate DNA synthesis. In the absence of

exogenous insulin or IGF-1, the TSH-dependent DNA synthesis in human thyrocytes cultured with 1% serum is weak and depends on autocrine IGF production. The autocrine production of IGF-1 is further increased in thyrocytes derived from follicular adenomas, which abrogate dependence of proliferation from exogenous IGF (Roger, 2010).

3. Molecular biology of thyroid cancer

Cancer is a genetic disease in the sense that it affects genes. In the past decades many genes that have a causal role in thyroid cancer have been discovered and the pathways through which they act have been elucidated in their basic structures (Kondo et al., 2006; Nikiforova & Nikiforov 2008; Xing, 2008). The identification of the biochemical functions of these genes has allowed to highlight a small number of subverted pathways in follicular cell-derived tumors. Using both cell culture systems and experimental murine models of cancer it has become apparent that the malignant transformation of the thyroid follicular cell involves multiple genetic events that sequentially activate certain oncogenes (i.e. RAS, RET/PTC, NTRK1, BRAF, PIK3CA, AKT1) and inactivate specific tumour suppressors (i.e. p53, PTEN). These recurrent alterations are frequently mutually exclusive and occur in genes within relatively few critical pathways such as the TSH/cAMP, MAP kinase and the PI3K/AKT signalling cascades (Figure 3). The mitogenic and differentiating TSH/cAMP pathway is involved in hyperthyroidism whereas the mitogenic dedifferentiating growth factor-regulated MAPK pathway is involved in the development of thyroid cancer. On the other hand, recent evidences indicate that the constitutive activation of the PI3K/AKT pathway is implicated in the development of differentiated and poorly differentiated carcinomas.

3.1.1 The TSH/cAMP Pathway: Hyperfunctioning adenomas

As indicated, the TSH/cAMP pathway is the major regulator of follicular cell proliferation and function. Expectedly, the constitutive activation of this pathway plays a critical role in the pathogenesis of benign hyperfunctioning thyroid nodules and adenoma. Adenoma frequently displays gain-of-function mutations that confer constitutive activity to TSHR in 50–80% or GSα in 8% of cases, respectively. TSHR is encoded by a gene located on chromosome 14q31; GSα is encoded by GNAS1 gene located on chromosome 20q13. Similarly, mutations in TSHR or GNAS1 genes account for hyperfunctioning nodules in patients with multinodular goiters (Khron et al., 2005; Parma et al, 1993). Dominant activating mutations of the TSHR are also the cause of non-autoimmune hyperthyroidism, a common thyroid disorder. In adenoma, mutations are somatic and strongly activate the cAMP cascade in one cell, thus initiating a clonal expansion of the mutated cell that lead to autonomous tumor growth. Germline GNAS1 mutations are responsible for the McCune-Albright syndrome, a familial condition that include hyperthyroidism and growth hormone excess. In addition, inactivating mutations in the gene encoding PKA type 1-alpha regulatory subunit (PRKAR1A), have been identified in the Carney Complex syndrome, an autosomal dominant disease comprising myxomas of the heart and skin, hyperpigmentation of the skin and endocrine overactivity that has features overlapping those of the McCune-Albright syndrome (Lindor & Greene, 2008). The mutations of TSHR and GSα constitutively activate adenylyl cyclase leading to increased cAMP accumulation and TSH-independent proliferation. However, adoptive expression of TSHR induces neoplastic transformation of FRTL-5 cells as demonstrated by growth in semi-solid medium and tumorigenesis in nude mice whereas GSα does not. Accordingly, the constitutive activation of the cAMP cascade alone is apparently insufficient for the malignant transformation of thyroid follicular cells because: i) mutations of TSHR or GNAS1 are rarely detected in well-differentiated carcinomas; ii) hyper-functioning thyroid nodules rarely become malignant; and iii) patients with the McCune–Albright syndrome, which result from germline GNAS1 mutations, present low-incidence of thyroid cancer (Collins et al., 2003).

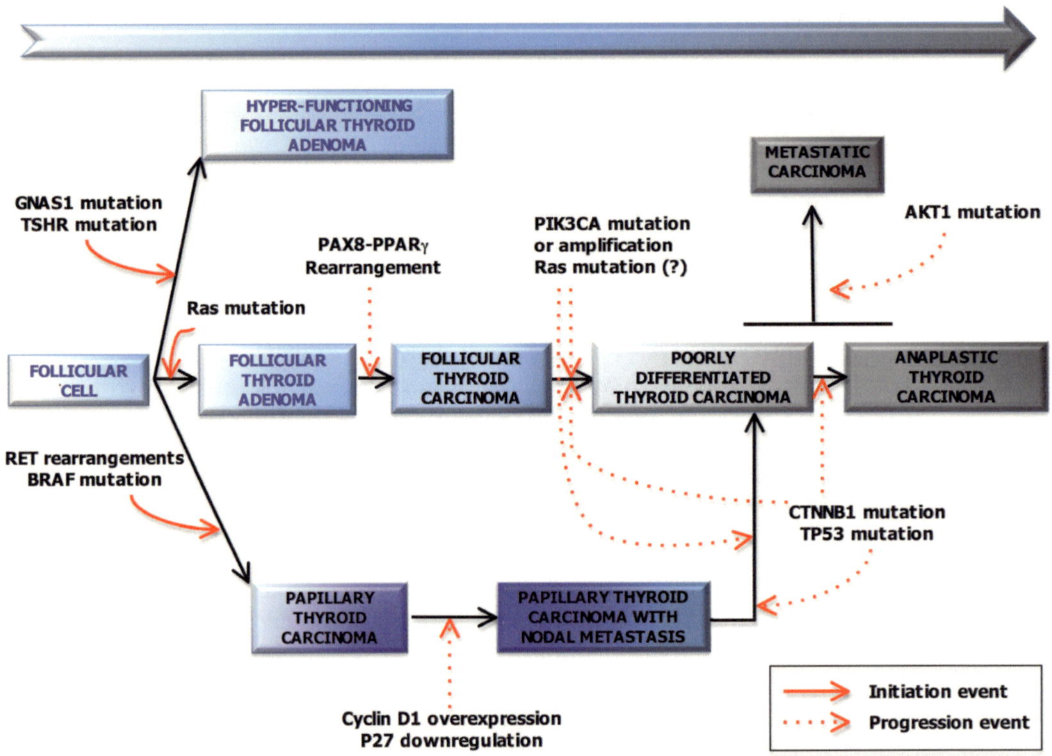

Fig. 3. The stepwise mechanism of thyroid carcinogenesis. Three distinct pathways have been proposed for the initiation of thyroid tumors including hyper-functioning follicular thyroid adenoma, FTC and PTC. Genetic defects that result in activation of RET or BRAF represent frequent early initiating events associated with radiation exposure that lead to PTC development. RAS mutations represent frequent early initiating events, associated with iodine deficiency, that lead to FTC development. By contrast, most PDTC and ATC are considered to derive from pre-existing well-differentiated thyroid carcinoma through the accumulation of additional genetic events that include nuclear accumulation of β-catenin (encoded by CTNNB1) and p53 inactivation.

Finally, more solid evidence on the role of the TSH/cAMP pathway in the transformation of thyroid follicular cells come from the study of transgenic mice (Kim and Zhu, 2009 and references therein). Murine strains modelling the constitutive activation of the cAMP-dependent mitogenic cascade in the thyroid gland provokes a phenotype very similar to the one seen in humans, with development of hyperplasia but not of overt tumors. In addition, mice made hypothyroid with antithyroid drugs do not develop thyroid cancer despite dramatic increase in serum TSH levels. Similarly, transgenic mice expressing the canine adenosine A2 receptor, which signals through G proteins and activates PKA as cAMP does, develop goiters and hyperthyroidism, but not thyroid cancer. Other mouse models that mimic TSHR overactivation via constitutive activation of GSα under control of the Tg promoter or with thyroid-specific expression of cholera toxin A1 subunit, develop goiters and hyperthyroidism, but not thyroid cancer. Finally, in a mouse model of PKA overactivation mice that are heterozygous for a null allele of the type 1a regulatory subunit of PKA (Prkar1a), develop PTC only sporadically and with long latency.

3.1.2 The RTK/RAS/BRAF/MAP kinase pathway: Papillary thyroid carcinomas

The most studied pathway involved in thyroid tumorigenesis is the RTK/RAS/BRAF/MAP kinase pathway, which seems to be essential for the development of PTC but apparently plays a more limited role in FTC. As in other tumors, these genetic events are mutually exclusive, providing compelling evidence for the requirement of this signalling system in PTC development (Figure 3).

Tyrosine kinase receptors

Tyrosine kinase receptors of growth factors regulate critical cellular functions required for tissue homeostasis such as cell proliferation, differentiation, survival, and apoptosis. Not surprisingly, signalling through these receptors is considered essential for initiation and progression of a broad spectrum of human tumours. Accordingly, certain subtypes of thyroid carcinomas are characterized by the aberrant activity of receptor-type tyrosine kinases (RET, NTRK1) that is consequent either to chromosomal rearrangements or to overexpression (EGFR, MET) (Kondo et al., 2006; Nikiforova & Nikiforov 2008; Xing et al., 2008). RET was the first activated receptor-tyrosine kinase to be identified in thyroid cancer. The RET proto-oncogene is located on chromosome 10q12 and encodes a tyrosine-kinase receptor protein with four cadherin-related motifs in the extracellular domain and a kinase in the cytoplasmic domain, whose expression and function is normally restricted to a subset of cells derived from the neural crest. RET is not normally expressed in follicular cells but is expressed in the developing central and peripheral nervous systems and is required for renal organogenesis and enteric neurogenesis (Fusco & Santoro, 2007). RET ligands include the glial cell line-derived neurotrophic factor (GDNF), and GDNF-like proteins such as Neurturin, Persephin, and Artemin. GDNF and GDNF-like proteins signal through a multi-component receptor system including the GPI-linked membrane receptor GDNF Family Receptors alpha (αGFRs), whose function is to bind the ligands and present them to the receptor, and RET, which operates as an intracellular signal transducing element (Airaksinen et al., 1999). RET activation is followed by dimerization, autophosphorylation at selected tyrosine residues and engagement of effectors through specific phosphorylated tyrosines. Activated RET triggers several downstream signal-transduction pathways including MAPK, PI3K and JNK (Fusco & Santoro, 2007). Different sites of tyrosine phosphorylation in the RET protein have been identified as docking sites for signalling molecules: Y905 that map in the kinase A loop mediates the recruitment of the SH2 domain-containing proteins Grb7 and Grb10; Y1015 mediates the association with phospholipase Cγ (PLCγ); and Y1062 that interacts with Shc and Frs2, which in turn, mediate RAS/RAF/MAPK activation. However, neither Y1015 nor Y1062 alone are apparently required for RET/PTC-induced effects on growth and apoptosis whereas, by contrast, there is an absolute requirement of Y1062 for RET/PTC-induced dedifferentiation (Knauf et al., 2003).

Chimeric oncogenes designated RET/PTC have been implicated in the development of PTC (Figure 4)(Fusco & Santoro, 2007). The RET/PTC oncogene is generated by chromosomal rearrangements resulting in the fusion of the RET tyrosine-kinase domain to the 5'-terminal region of heterologous genes. All rearrangements appear to be balanced inversions or translocations that involve the 3.0 kb intron 11 of RET. The RET/PTC rearrangement results from a fusion between the 3′-portion of RET that leaves intact the tyrosine kinase domain and the 5′-portion of various heterologous genes. All RET-fused genes provide putative dimerization domains to the chimeric RET/PTC genes. RET/PTC chimeric oncoproteins lack the signal peptide and the transmembrane domain, are expressed in the cytoplasm of follicular cells under the control of the newly acquired promoters, and show constitutive dimerization and ligand-independent activation of RET tyrosine kinase, which is essential for the transformation of thyroid cells. To date, at least 15 chimeric genes have been reported (Fusco & Santoro, 2007). The most common rearrangements are RET/PTC1, RET/PTC3 and RET/PTC2, respectively. RET/PTC1 and RET/PTC3 are generated by paracentric inversions at 10q between RET and H4 (OMIM #601985) or NCOA4 (ELE1) (OMIM 601984), respectively. RET/PTC2 is due to an interchromosomal translocation between chromosome 10 and chromosome 17 (Fusco & Santoro, 2007). Among human tumours, RET/PTC rearrangements were initially associated with PTC, radiation exposure and young age (Santoro et al., 1992; Ito et al., 1994). Reported frequencies of RET/PTC rearrangements in sporadic PTC vary widely among different countries. Depending on the detection method used and/or the geographical location of patients the frequency of RET/PTC rearrangements varies from 3% in Saudi Arabia to 59% in the United Kingdom; however a reasonable estimates of the frequency of RET/PTC rearrangements in adult patients is ~20%, with higher values in patients with a history of radiation exposure (50–80%). The high prevalence of RET/PTC rearrangements in children from the areas affected by nuclear disaster at Chernobyl indicates a role for radiation damage in the genesis of these paracentric inversions (Fusco & Santoro, 2007). Accordingly, exposure of cell lines to ionising radiation results in the expression of RET/PTC within hours, supporting a direct role for radiation in the recombination of RET (Ito et al., 1993).

There is compelling evidence that different RET/PTC rearrangements present variable oncogenic potential. Different types of RET/PTC are associated with distinct subtypes of PTC. RET/PTC1 tends to be more common in small indolent tumours with typical papillary growth and to have a more benign clinical course, whereas RET/PTC3 shows a strong correlation with subtypes believed to represent aggressive forms of papillary cancer such as the solid variant and, more recently, the tall cell variant (Nikiforov et al., 1997; Basolo et al., 2002). Accordingly, transgenic mice expressing RET/PTC1 under the control of the rat Tg promoter developed PTC (<50%) with a long latency period and with no distant metastasis. Similarly, transgenic mice expressing RET/PTC1 under the control of the bovine Tg promoter developed PTC. However, in both mouse strains metastases were absent indicating that RET-PTC1-depended cancers requires additional mutations (i.e. knockout of the tumor-suppressor p53) to result in metastasis (Kim and Zhu, 2009 and references therein). By contrast, RET/PTC3 mice develop PTC-like lesions that are similar to the human solid variant of PTC, and unlike RET-PTC1 mice, in about one-third of cases, develop axillary lymph node metastasis (Kim and Zhu, 2009 and references therein).

Although transgenic mouse models have shown that RET/PTC rearrangements can initiate thyroid carcinogenesis *in vitro,* the same studies have indicated that RET/PTC represents a weak tumour-initiating event, requiring additional genetic and/or epigenetic changes for clonal expansion of mutated cells. RET/PTC expression in thyroid cells induces dedifferentiation and apoptosis at the same time. However, at difference with RAS and BRAF, RET/PTC rearrangements do not induce genomic instability. Moreover, TSH-independence may develop in RET-positive tumours as a secondary adaptation during cancer progression since it has been shown that RET/PTC-transfected cells can acquire the capability to grow in a TSH-independent manner. Additional evidence demonstrating that RET/PTC rearrangements are tumour-initiating events is that they are present in microcarcinomas. Indeed a high frequency of RET/PTC rearrangements have been reported in 42-77% of the subclinical microcarcinomas detected at autopsy or in thyroidectomies for disorders other than cancer. In addition, RET alterations have been found in other early benign lesions such as follicular adenomas, benign thyroid nodules and Hashimoto's thyroiditis. The high frequency of RET rearrangements in microcarcinomas and in early benign lesions is consistent with the idea that they represent early events in the neoplastic processes. On the other hand, the low prevalence of RET rearrangements in poorly differentiated and undifferentiated thyroid carcinoma supports a minor role for RET/PTC in tumour progression (Fusco & Santoro, 2007).

The neurotrophic receptor-tyrosine kinase NTRK1 (also known as TRK and TRKA) was the second identified gene subjected to chromosomal rearrangement in thyroid cancer (Pierotti et al., 2001). The NTRK1 proto-oncogene is located on chromosome 1q22 and encodes the transmembrane tyrosine-kinase receptor for nerve growth factor (NGF). NTRK1 expression is typically restricted to neurons and regulates neuronal growth and survival. The activated receptor initiates several signal-transduction cascades including ERK, PI3K and the phospholipase-Cγ (PLCγ) pathways (Miller & Kaplan, 2001). Similar to RET, NTRK1 is activated in thyrocytes by chromosomal rearrangements that fuse the NTRK1 tyrosine kinase domain to the 5'-terminal region of heterologous genes. NTRK1 rearrangements have been detected in 5–13% of sporadic PTC but only in 3% of post-Chernobyl childhood PTC (Bongarzone et al., 1996). To date, three different rearrangements have been identified as chimeric oncogenes. The recombination events that cause the oncogenic activation of NTRK1 include an inversion fusing NTRK1 to non-muscular tropomyosine (TPM3) gene located at 1q31, a different intra-chromosomal rearrangement that juxtaposes NTRK1 to the 5′-end of a translocated promoter region (TPR) gene localized at 1q25 or to the 5′-sequence of a TRK-fused gene (TFG) localized on chromosome 3 (TRK-T1, TRK-T2 and TRK-T3 oncogenes, respectively). In all cases the resulting chimeric proteins exhibit ectopic expression and constitutive activation of the tyrosine kinase (Pierotti et al., 2001). The prevalence of each fusion type is nearly equal in sporadic PTC, whereas TPM3–NTRK1 is more frequent than other NTRK1 rearrangements in post-Chernobyl childhood PTC. The generation of TRK-T1 transgenic mouse model have demonstrated that, in contrast with *in vitro* results, TRK-T1 can initiate thyroid cancer. About half of the transgenic mice that expressed TRK-T1 developed thyroid cancer, either FTC or PTC, without distant metastasis (Kim and Zhu, 2009).

The receptor-tyrosine kinase MET (which is located on chromosome 7q31) encodes a two-subunit 190 kDa transmembrane protein that is the receptor for HGF. HGF is a powerful mitogen for thyrocytes and modulates thyroid cancer cell motility and invasiveness and promotes angiogenesis. MET is often overexpressed in PTC (77–93%), but is rare in other histological types of thyroid tumours (Di Renzo et al., 1995), though the pathogenetic significance of MET expression in papillary thyroid cancer remains to be identified. Some studies found MET overexpression associated with advanced tumor stages of thyroid carcinoma and histologic variants associated with poor prognosis while others showed decreased MET expression in poorly or undifferentiated tumors with an inverse correlation between MET expression and vascular invasion and distant metastases (Di Renzo et al., 1995). On the other hand, the finding that stromal cells of the thyroid secrete HGF suggests that MET may be involved in the stimulation of tumor growth through a paracrine mechanism. MET overexpression is apparently due to transcriptional or post-transcriptional mechanism. For example oncogenic RAS and RET/PTC have been shown to induce MET overexpression in thyroid follicular cells. Point mutations involving MET have also been detected in about 7% of well-differentiated thyroid carcinoma.

The epidermal growth factor receptor (EGFR) family includes EGFR (also known as ERBB1 or HER1), ERBB2 (also known as HER2), ERBB3 (also known as HER3) and ERBB4 (also known as HER4). All are involved in the transmission of signals that control cell growth and differentiation. Multiple ligands bind EGFR, ERBB3 or ERBB4, inducing rapid receptor dimerization, with a marked preference for ERBB2 as dimerization partner. EGFR and ERBB2 are often found in thyroid cancers (Kato et al., 2004). EGF stimulates the growth of human thyroid carcinoma cells and rat FRTL-5 cells *in vitro*. At difference with lung and breast carcinomas where EGFR mutations or ERBB2 amplification have been reported, respectively, neither activating mutations nor DNA amplification of EGFR were found in thyroid cancer. Conversely, thyroid tumors overexpress EGFRs and ligands, implicating EGFR signalling in thyroid tumorigenesis. Increased expression of EGFR correlates with poor prognosis in differentiated thyroid cancers whereas ERBB2 has no clear prognostic significance.

The Fibroblast growth factors (FGFs) and FGF receptors (FGFRs) are important regulators of angiogenesis and tumorigenesis (Grose & Dickson, 2005). At least 20 FGF ligands that signal through a complex family of receptor-tyrosine kinases, encoded by four distinct FGFR genes exist. So far, no mutations or rearrangements that involve members of the FGFR family have been identified in thyroid cancer. Conversely, FGFR1, FGFR3 and FGFR4 are overexpressed in thyroid carcinoma with FGFR4 expression restricted to the aggressive forms of thyroid carcinoma (St Bernard et al., 2005). In addition, the adoptive expression of FGFR3 in a human thyroid carcinoma cell line results in aberrant growth. As to the growth factors, expression of FGF2 (also known as basic FGF) is apparently increased in thyroid cancer and promotes mitogenic activity of rat thyroid follicular cells.

Vascular endothelial growth factor (VEGF) ligands — VEGFA, PlGF, VEGFB, VEGFC and VEGFD — are angiogenic growth factors that, by binding their cognate receptors on vascular cells, induce proliferation of endothelial and/or lymphatic cells. VEGFA, PlGF and VEGFB stimulates angiogenesis, whereas VEGFC and VEGFD promotes lymphangiogenesis (Bunone et al., 1999). Increased expression of VEGFA and PlGF has been frequently reported in thyroid goiters and carcinomas (Bunone et al., 1999). Conversely, the overexpression of VEGFC and VEGFD are implicated in development of the lymphatic system and correlates with the density of lymphatics and lymph-node metastasis of PTC (Hung et al., 2003).

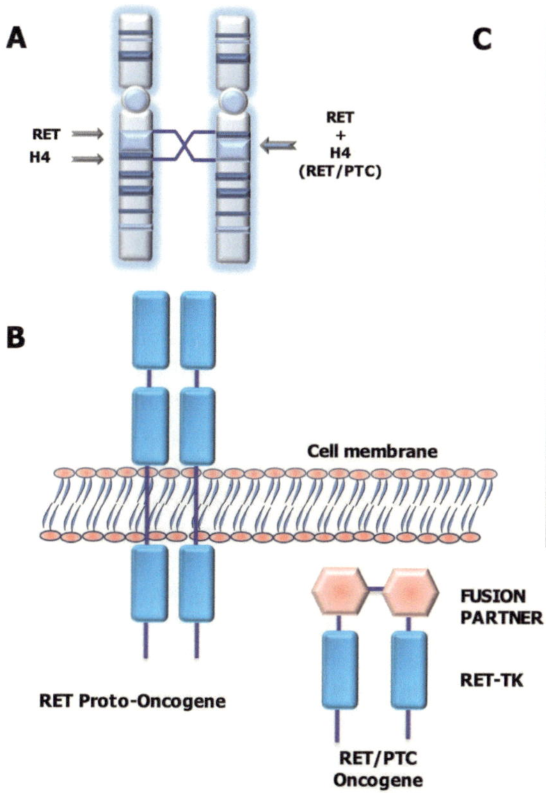

C

CHIMERIC ONCOPROTEIN	FUSION PARTNER	GENETIC LESION (*)
RET/PTC1	H4	inv10
RET/PTC2	PKA R1α	t(10;17)
RET/PTC3	RFG	inv10
RET/PTC4	RFG (ELE1/ARA70/Ncoa4)	inv10
RET/PTC5	RFG5 (golgin-84)	
RET/PTC6	HTIF1	t(7;10)
RET/PTC7	RFG7 (HTIFγ)	t(1;10)
RET/PTC8	KTN1	t(10;14)
RET/PTC9	RFG9	t(10;18)
RET/ELKS	ELKS	t(10;12)
RET/PCM1	PCM1	t(8;10)

* t: translocation
inv: inversion

Fig. 4. RET/PTC rearrangements in papillary thyroid carcinoma. A. Schematic representation of the molecular mechanism that generates PTC oncogene. B. A comparison between the RET proto-oncogene and the RET/PTC oncogene. C. A list of the different RET/PTC rearrangements identified.

The RAS G-protein

The RAS protooncogenes encode 21 kDa monomeric G-proteins, which transduce signals from a wide variety of growth factor receptors, particularly those of the tyrosine kinase family. Three RAS proto-oncogenes – HRAS (which is located on chromosome 11p11), KRAS (which is located on chromosome 12p12), and NRAS (which is located on chromosome 1p13) – are implicated in human cancer (Buday & Downward, 2008). The three RAS genes encode highly related proteins with GTPase activity that are located at the inner surface of the cell membrane and play a central role in the intracellular transduction of signals arising from cell membrane. In its inactive state, RAS is bound to guanosine diphosphate (GDP). Upon activation, it releases GDP, binds guanosine triphosphate (GTP), thus transiently activating downstream signalling and terminates signalling by hydrolizing GTP. RAS proteins convey signals from tyrosine kinase receptors and G-protein-coupled receptors (GPCRs) to different signalling pathways such as MAPK, PI3K and Ral-GDS, which activate the transcription of target genes resulting in the regulation of cell proliferation, migration and survival (Peyssonnaux & Eychene, 2001). Point mutations occurring in tumors affect the guanosine triphosphate (GTP)-binding domain (codons 12/13) or the GTPase domain (codon 61) and result in the replacement of specific amino acid residues that lock p21RAS in a constitutively active form of the protein. Such gain-of-function RAS mutations promote tumor development. Accordingly, it is estimated that around 30% of all human tumours contain a mutation in a RAS allele, which makes RAS genes the most mutated proto-oncogene in the human genome.

Oncogenic mutations involving all three RAS genes were among the first genetic alterations to be identified in tumours originating from the thyroid follicular epithelium and have been reported with variable frequency in thyroid neoplasms ranging from 7 to 62% (Vasko et al. 2003). Initially it has been proposed that RAS mutations might represent one of the early steps in the formation of thyroid cancer because they have been observed in benign tumours. However, more recent studies have demonstrated that RAS mutations are more represented in PDTC (55%) and ATC (52%) than in follicular adenomas and WDTC (5 to 10%), and that there exists a significant association between RAS mutations and poor survival (Garcia-Rostan et al., 2003). Although RAS mutations are not restricted to a specific thyroid tumour type they are more common in iodine-deficient and in lesions with follicular architecture, including FTC and follicular variant of PTC, and are rare in radiation-induced thyroid cancers of Chernobyl. RAS mutations are thought to be among the initiating molecular events in thyroid tumorigenesis. RAS mutants are able to activate both the PI3K/AKT and MAPK signalling cascades and, conversely, oncogenic transformation by mutant KRAS requires activation of both MAPK and PI3K/AKT pathways. Adoptive expression of HRAS-V12 into cultured rat thyroid cells promotes TSH-independent growth and dedifferentiation as a result of inhibition of the activity of TTF1 and PAX8, two transcription factors essential for the mainteinance of the thyroid differentiated state (De Vita et al., 2005). By contrast, adoptive expression of mutant RAS into human thyrocytes stimulate growth and differentiation (Gire et al., 2000). RAS activation in rat PC Cl3 cells displays also evidence of DNA damage, manifesting as chromosome misalignment, centrosome amplification and micronuclei formation and increased susceptibility to apoptosis (Saavedra et al., 2000). In the presence of TSH, HRAS-G12V also triggers the initiation of programmed cell death but, in the absence of TSH, acute expression of mutant RAS inhibits apoptosis and accelerates TSH-independent proliferation. The cells that loose TSH responsiveness and, at the same time, inactivate the RAS-dependent apoptotic cascade will undergo clonal expansion and tumor development (Shirokawa et al., 2000).

In vivo studies with transgenic mice have shown controversial results on the role of RAS in thyroid carcinogenesis (Kim and Zhu, 2009 and references therein). In some reports, mutant HRAS or KRAS alone are not apparently sufficient to induce cancer and it appears that additional genetic alterations are required for FTC development. Similarly, mice carrying mutant KRAS-G12V under the control of rat Tg promoter or KRAS-G12D under control of the endogenous KRAS promoter showed no sign of thyroid cancer, though another transgenic mouse strain expressing a mutated HRAS-G12V controlled by the bovine Tg promoter developed PTC. Conversely, targeting human NRAS with a mutation at codon 61 to thyroid follicular cells induced, in 30% of the transgenic mice, progressive changes from hyperplasia to adenoma and carcinoma that were of follicular or mixed histotype with large poorly differentiated areas closely resembling those observed in human patients.

The serine/threonine kinase BRAF

The proto-oncogene BRAF situated on 7q24 encodes a serine/threonine kinase that transduces regulatory signals through the RAS/RAF/MEK/ERK cascade. There are three isoforms of the RAF kinases in mammalian cells: ARAF, BRAF, and CRAF (also denoted

RAF1). BRAF is more efficient in phosphorylating MEKs than other RAF isoforms. RAF proteins play a critical role in the transduction of signals by growth factors, hormones and cytokines, being involved in the regulation of cell proliferation, differentiation and apoptosis (Peyssonnaux & Eychene, 2001). Expectedly, gain-of-function BRAF mutations provide an alternative route for the aberrant activation of ERK signalling that is implicated in the tumorigenesis of several human cancers – for example, melanoma and colon carcinoma (Davies et al., 2002). BRAF mutations represent the most common genetic change in PTC, having been detected in 29–83% PTC, especially in the aggressive tall-cell variant (55–100%), but not in FTC. In addition, BRAF mutations have also been observed in up to 13-15% of PDTC and 35% of ATC. By contrast, BRAF mutations are a relatively rare event in post-Chernobyl and sporadic childhood PTC. Interestingly, the frequency of BRAF mutations in ATC arising from pre-existing PTC is significantly higher than those arising from pre-existing FTC (Nikiforova et al., 2003). BRAF mutations are almost always exclusive to RAS genes mutations as well as to RET (RET/PTC) and NTRK1 rearrangements, altogether accounting for about 70% of PTC cases. BRAF mutations in PTC correlate with more advanced clinical stage, extrathyroidal extension and distant metastasis (Xing et al., 2005). Moreover, tumors with BRAF mutations are apparently unresponsive to ^{131}I treatment, pointing out that this genetic event is a new biological marker that predicts poor prognosis and resistance to treatment (Xing et al., 2005). This is consistent with the notion that BRAF mutations in human PTC are associated with decreased expression of iodine-metabolising genes (i.e. NIS, pendrin, Tg) and that, in addition, the conditional expression of BRAF-V600E in rat thyrocytes promotes down-regulation of TSHR, NIS, Tg, TTF-1 and PAX-8.

The great majority of BRAF mutations detected in PTC (>90%) are of a single type: a 1799T-A transition in exon 15 leading to the substitution of a valine by a glutamic acid at the position 600 (V600E), which one of the most prevalent somatic genetic events in human cancer (Figure 5). The V600E mutation of BRAF destabilise the inactive BRAF structure by generating repulsive electrostatic forces in the activation loop, thereby leading to a constitutive catalytic activation that stimulates ERK activity and transforms NIH3T3 cells. Interestingly, whereas the V600E mutation is common in classical and tall cell variant of PTC, the K601E mutation has been detected in the follicular variant. An alternative alteration of BRAF detected in radiation-associated thyroid cancers is a chromosomal rearrangement of BRAF (AKAP9–BRAF) (Ciampi et al., 2005). AKAP9-BRAF results from a paracentric inversion of the long arm of the chromosome 7 and leads to the fusion of the first 8 exons of the A-kinase anchor protein 9 (AKAP9) gene with the C-terminal coding region of the BRAF protooncogene. This fusion leads to a chimeric protein with constitutively activated BRAF kinase. The AKAP9-BRAF rearrangement has been reported in about 11% of post-Chernobyl, radiation-associated PTC whereas only 1% of sporadic PTC displays this mutation. Regardless of the mode of activation, these data highlight the crucial contribution of BRAF as an important effector in the role of MAPK activation and in thyroid tumorigenesis. BRAF mutations are thought to be a tumour-initiating event. BRAF concomitantly induces stimulation of DNA synthesis and apoptosis, resulting in no net growth in cell population. However, acute BRAF-V600E expression in PC Cl3 cells induces dedifferentiation and genomic instability, which, similarly to RAS, may facilitate the acquisition of secondary genetic or epigenetic events that may account for its aggressive properties (Mitsutake et al., 2005). In addition, the targeted expression of BRAF-V600E in thyroid cells of transgenic mice results in development of invasive PTC with poorly differentiated foci that closely recapitulate the phenotype of BRAF-positive PTC in humans. The BRAF-V600E mice had a 30% decrease in survival at 5 months (Kim and Zhu, 2009 and references therein).

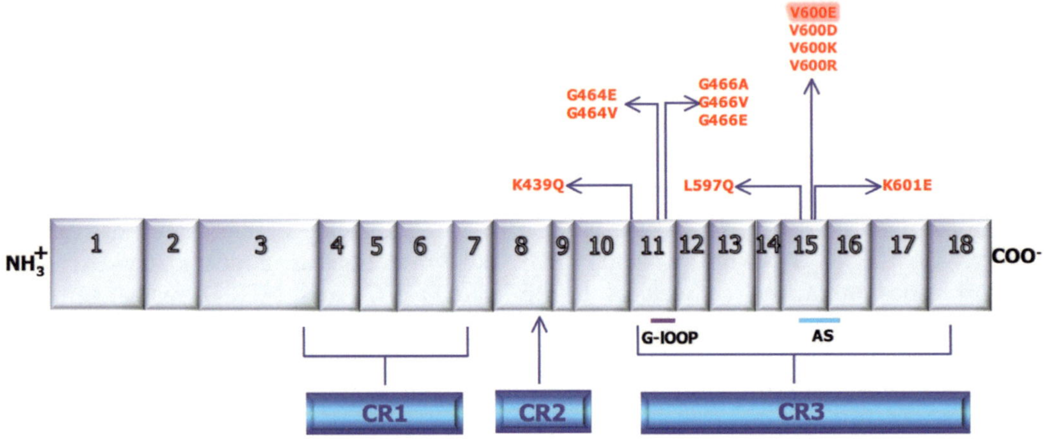

Fig. 5. BRAF mutations in thyroid cancer. The T1799A mutation accounts for about 90% of the more than 40 mutations identified in the BRAF gene so far. This mutation causes the V600E substitution in the BRAF protein that results in constitutive activation of the kinase and acquisition of oncogenic properties. Other BRAF mutations detected in human tumours are also reported. In thyroid cancer few other mutations that include the K601E have been reported.

3.1.3 The phosphatidylinositol 3-kinase (PI3K)/Akt pathway: Follicular thyroid carcinomas

Constitutive activation of the phosphatidylinositol-3-kinase (PI3K)/AKT signalling pathway plays a relevant in thyroid carcinogenesis (Bunney & Katan 2010). First, germline mutations of the tumor suppressor gene PTEN (phosphatase and tensin homologue deleted on chromosome 10) confer predisposition to Cowden disease, an autosomal dominant condition that causes hamartomatous neoplasms of the skin, gastrointestinal tract, thyroid, bones and predispose to CNS, breast and thyroid cancer (Hobert & Eng, 2009). Moreover, genetic alterations involving proteins within the PI3K/AKT pathway have been described in sporadic thyroid carcinomas, particularly in FTC and ATC (Ringel et al., 2001; García-Rostán et al., 2005; Ricarte-Filho et al., 2009). The reported alterations include genomic copy number gain or activating mutations of the gene encoding the catalytic subunit of PIK3CA, inactivating mutations, LOH or deletions of PTEN, and activating gain-of-function mutations in the AKT1 gene as discussed in detail below. The analysis of human thyroid cancer has also indicated that the PI3K/AKT pathway cooperates with MAPK signalling in the pathogenesis and progression of advanced or metastatic thyroid cancer.

PI3KCA mutations and amplifications

PI3Ks are a family of intracellular lipid kinases that generate the lipid second messenger PtdIns-3,4,5-P3 and PtdIns-3,4-P2. PI3K family members are grouped into three classes according to structure and substrate specificity (Engelman et al., 2006). Class I PI3Ks are heterodimeric molecules composed of a catalytic subunit known as p110 and a regulatory subunit denoted p85, which contains two SH2 (Src homology) domains that allow interaction with phosphotyrosines on activated tyrosine kinase receptors. This results in recruitment of the protein to the plasma membrane and activation of the enzymatic activity. There are three variants of the p110 catalytic subunit designated p110α, β, or δ, expressed by separate genes (PIK3CA, PIK3CB, and PIK3CD, respectively). By contrast, there are five variants of the p85 regulatory subunit, designated p85α, p55α, p50α, p85β, or p55γ; the first three regulatory subunits represent splice variants of the same gene (PIK3R1), and the other two are encoded by different genes (PIK3R2 and PIK3R3, respectively) (Vanhaesebroeck, & Waterfield, 1999). So far a central role in cancer has been demonstrated only for class IA PI3Ks, which transduce signals downstream of oncogenic tyrosine kinase receptors. PIK3CA, encoding the class IA PI3K catalytic subunit p110α, is the only PI3K gene identified with common gain-of-function mutations and gene amplification in human cancer (Vogt et al., 2007). Most mutations are located in hot spot regions that include the helical and the kinase domains of the gene encoding p110α that result in a mutant protein that becomes independent of the p85 regulatory subunit thus promoting proliferation, invasiveness, resistance to apoptosis, and malignant transformation (Bader et al., 2006). In thyroid cancer, gene amplification/copy number gain of the PIK3CA gene located at 3q26.3 is detected in 12-13% of follicular adenoma, 5-14% PTC, 24-28% FTC and up to 42% of ATC, though ethnic variation between Middle Eastern, Western or Asian populations has been reported (Wang et al., 2007; Liu et al., 2008). In addition to increased gene copy number, recent studies have reported the presence of activating mutations of PIK3CA in primary thyroid cancer and cancer-derived cell lines. PIK3CA mutations are rare in primary well-differentiated PTC (0-3%), more frequent in well-differentiated FTC (6-13%) and common in ATC (5-21%) (García-Rostán et al., 2005). Importantly, PIK3CA mutations are particularly common in the metastatic lesions of patients with radioactive-iodine refractory disease. This finding suggests an exclusive role for oncogenic mutant PIK3CA in promoting progression from more differentiated to less differentiated cancer. At present, it is not known whether PIK3CA mutations or amplification are sufficient to cause thyroid cancer *in vivo*. Mutant PIK3CA alleles are transforming in MCF-10 breast cells *in vitro* and in the chorioallantoic membrane of the chicken *in vivo*. However, transgenic mouse models indicated that activated PIK3CA mutant is able to induce fully malignant cancer in the lung but not in the ovary (Engelman et al., 2008). Therefore, further studies will be required to fully characterize the role of this oncogene in thyroid cancer development and progression.

PTEN mutations and loss of expression

PTEN is a tumour suppressor gene localized to chromosome 10q23 (Li et al., 1997). PTEN has been shown to have protein and lipid phosphatase activity. PTEN can dephosphorylate the D3 position of PtdIns-3,4-P2 and PtdIns-3,4,5-P3, the lipid products of the PI3K, thus antagonizing signalling through this pathway. Reportedly, cells lacking PTEN function exhibit a marked increase in the intracellular levels of PtdIns-3,4,5-P3 and AKT activation. PTEN represents a pivotal regulator of critical cellular functions such as proliferation and survival. A large body of evidence indicate that PTEN functions as a tumour suppressor in thyroid cancer. Loss of PTEN is a frequent finding in sporadic tumours, through mutations and LOH, reduced transcription caused by gene promoter hypermethylation, reduced translation via microRNA (miR21) overexpression or increased protein degradation (Bunney & Katan, 2010). Mutations of PTEN are uncommon in sporadic thyroid tumours (2% PTC;

7%FTC and 14% ATC, respectively). Moreover, allelic losses of the PTEN locus at 10q23.3, though frequent in adenoma and FTC (up to 25%), are not coupled with mutations in the second allele. Conversely, thyroid carcinoma frequently shows decreased expression of PTEN, at both mRNA and protein levels in <40% of well-differentiated thyroid carcinomas and in most ATC, in many cases through methylation of the PTEN gene promoter. Expectedly, PTEN inactivation in human tumors has been associated with increased AKT activity. Yet, in transgenic mice loss of PTEN and the subsequent activation of the PI3K/AKT pathway causes goiter and follicular adenoma but it appears not to be sufficient for malignant transformation of thyroid cells (Kim and Zhu, 2009 and references therein).

AKT1 mutations and amplification

The AKT kinases represent the primary downstream mediators of the effects of the PI3K pathway, and play a central role in both normal and pathological signalling (Brazil et al., 2004). In mammalian cells AKT comprises three highly homologous members (>80% protein sequence identity) termed AKT1/PKBα, AKT2/PKBβ and AKT3/PKBγ, encoded by three different genes located on chromosomes 14q32, 19q13 and 1q43, respectively. AKT kinases share the same structural organization, containing an N-terminal pleckstrin homology (PH) domain, a central catalytic domain and a C-terminal regulatory region. The PH domain of AKT can bind specifically to D3-phosphorylated phosphoinositides with high affinity and mediates kinase activation (Brazil et al., 2004). Despite their sequence similarity however, AKT isoforms are functionally distinct, as suggested by the different phenotypes of the corresponding knock-out mice. Also the expression of AKT1, AKT2 and AKT3 apparently contribute to the different roles of AKT isoforms. AKT1 and AKT2 are the principal isoforms expressed in the thyroid gland (Vasko et al, 2004).

Combining all the data from the existing literature, it appears that activation of the PI3K/AKT pathway in thyroid cancer, as detemined by S473 phosphorylation, is frequent and is associated with aggressive disease. Active AKT is observed more frequently in patients with undifferentiated cancer (40-50% of PTC and FTC; <93% of ATC, respectively) (Wang et al., 2007; Santarpia et al., 2008). Different mechanisms that cause the increased AKT signalling observed in thyroid cancer cells have been proposed. First, gain-of-function mutations of two different AKT isoforms have been reported to occur in human cancer (Carpten et al., 2007; Davies et al., 2008). A unique mutation at nucleotide 49 of the gene encoding AKT1 that results in the substitution of a lysine for glutamic acid at the amino acid 17 (AKT1-E17K) within the PH has been recently discovered. The E17K substitution allows membrane recruitment of AKT1 independent of PtdIns binding, increases its activity, and confers to AKT1 the capability to transform fibroblasts *in vitro* and induce leukaemia in mice. More recently, a mutation homologous to the E17K in AKT1 has been identified also in the PH domain of AKT3 in malignant melanoma (Davies et al., 2008). In thyroid cancer, the presence of a heterozygote E17K mutation in the AKT1 gene was observed at a relatively high frequency (9/55, 16%) in metastatic lesions of advanced cancer but not in the corresponding primary tumours, which suggested that AKT1 mutations were acquired during tumour progression (Ricarte-Filho et al., 2009). AKT1 mutations were most common in metastasis of tall cell variant PTC (17%), Hürthle cell carcinoma (33%), and poorly differentiated PTC (19%). Conversely, no mutation in the genes encoding AKT2 and AKT3 has been reported in thyroid cancer so far. In addition to mutations, an increase in the gene copy number of AKT1 in FTC (8%) and ATC (<19%) and of AKT2 in FTC (<22%), respectively, has also been reported (Liu et al., 2008). It is not yet known whether amplified

AKT1 differs from mutated AKT1 in its capability to activate downstream signalling. Recent studies have suggested that cellular compartimentalization of activated AKT may be important in determining its cellular effects. In particular, it was proposed that nuclear localization of activated AKT1 promotes invasion and migration in thyroid cancer cells. In invasive FTC phospho-AKT localizes primarily to the nucleus, whereas in PTC, it localizes to the cytoplasm, except for the cells at the invasive edge or in metastatic regions where it is localized also in cell nuclei (Vasko et al. 2004).

Although aberrant activation of the PI3K pathway has been identified in most thyroid cancers, relatively few transgenic mice that model dysregulation of the PI3K/AKT pathway in cancer have been generated (Kim and Zhu, 2009 and references therein). Recently, a mouse strain, in which Cre-mediated recombination was used to delete Pten in the thyrocytes has been reported. Conditional loss of Pten in the thyroid gland renders the thyrocytes highly susceptible to neoplastic transformation through mechanisms that include increased thyrocyte proliferation. Pten mutant mice developed diffuse goiter characterized by enlarged follicles, in the presence of normal TSH and T4 hormone levels. Loss of Pten resulted in a significant increase in the thyrocyte proliferative index and increased cell density in the thyroid gland, which was more prominent in female mice. By 10 months of age, more than 60% of the mutant females developed follicular adenomas. However, in these mice complete loss of Pten was not sufficient to cause invasive tumors. Subsequent studies by the same group revealed that the in vivo proliferative response to chronic PI3K activation relied on the activation of the mammalian target of rapamycin (mTOR)/S6K1 axis, and that mTOR inhibition restored normal proliferation rates in Pten mutant mice. mTOR functions as a key effector of PI3K-generated proliferative signals by increasing the levels of cyclins D1 and D3 proteins through post-transcriptional mechanisms, and mTOR inhibition effectively restored normal D-type cyclin protein levels and normal proliferation rates in thyrocytes. Recently, double-mutant mice were generated by crossing a mouse strain carrying a KRAS-G12D allele with mice carrying the thyroid-specific floxed Pten. The concurrent activation of KRAS-G12D and PI3K in thyroid follicular cells led to aggressive, invasive and metastatic FTC, indicating that PI3K activation allowed to fully realize the oncogenic potential of KRAS. Interestingly, combined pharmacological inhibition of PI3K and MAPK completely inhibited the growth of double mutant cancer cells, providing a compelling rationale for the simultaneous targeting of these pathways in thyroid cancer. These results indicate that, at difference with genes involved in the MAPK pathways (i.e. BRAF) the constitutive activation of PI3K signalling is probably insufficient by itself to initiate the growth of a malignat thyroid cancer, since loss of PTEN results in follicular adenoma; conversely, aberrant PI3K signalling may facilitate progression and dedifferentiation of tumour cells.

3.1.4 Genetic alterations in transcription factors: Follicular thyroid carcinomas

The PAX8/PPARγ rearrangement

The PAX8-PPARγ rearrangement is a chromosomal translocation t(2:3)(q13;p25) that contributes to the development of thyroid cancers (Kroll et al., 2000). PAX8 (paired-box gene 8) encodes a transcription factor required for the development of thyroid follicular cell lineage and the regulation of thyroid-specific gene expression, whereas PPARγ (Peroxisome Proliferator-Activated Receptor-γ), encoded by the PPARG gene located on chromosome

3p25, is a member of the steroid nuclear hormone receptor superfamily. PPARγ plays a role in adipogenesis and insulin sensitization, cell-cycle control, inflammation, atherosclerosis, apoptosis and carcinogenesis through its influence on gene expression (Desvergne et al., 1999). The PAX8-PPARγ rearrangement was first identified in thyroid neoplasms with a cytogenetically detectable translocation t(2;3)(q13;p25) that generates a chimeric gene encoding the DNA-binding domain of PAX8 and domains A–F of PPARγ. The function of this rearranged protein is not entirely elucidated, but it appears that the fusion product contributes to malignant transformation by acting as a dominant negative on the transcriptional activity of wild-type PPARγ (Gregory Powell et al., 2004). PAX8-PPARγ rearrangements are present in follicular adenoma (up to 30%), FTC (25-63%), in follicular variants of PTC, and in Hurthle cell cancers, with the initial indication that it correlates with a vasculo-invasive phenotype (Kroll et al., 2000; Nikiforova et al., 2003). Conversely, the presence of a PAX8-PPARγ rearrangement in follicular variant of PTC is controversial and, to date, it has not been detected in PDTC and ATC (Nikiforova et al., 2004). Together, RAS and PAX8-PPARγ mutations are identified in approximately 80% of FTC (Nikiforova et al., 2004). However, the finding that both RAS and PAX8-PPARγ mutations may be rarely detected in the same tumor, suggests that these cancers develop through at least two different molecular pathways and the finding that the PAX8-PPARγ oncoprotein, like RAS, is also detected in a sub-group of follicular adenoma supports the existence of a stepwise transition from adenoma to carcinoma.

3.1.5 Genetic alterations of cell-cycle regulators

Alteration of the basic mechanisms that regulate cell cycle is a hallmark of cancer (Hanahan & Weinberg 2000). Cell cycle is regulated by the sequential activation of several classes of proteins (cyclins, cyclin-dependent kinases (CDKs), CDK inhibitors, the family of retinoblastoma susceptibility proteins (pRB), E2F transcription factors). The factors that promote progression into cell cycle are the G1 cyclins (i.e. cyclin D1, cyclin E1), CDKs, and E2Fs whereas the factors that regulate negatively the G1-to-S transition are the pRB, the two families of CDK inhibitors (INK4, CIP/KIP, respectively) and the tumor suppressor TP53. Cyclin–CDK complexes promote cell-cycle progression through phosphorylation-dependent inactivation of pRB, which in turn releases E2F transcription factors and allows entrance into S phase. Particularly important for cancer development are the G1/S and the G2/M transitions as determined by the frequent observation of aberrant activity of the molecules involved in these processes. See Figure 6 for a summary of the genetic alterations of cell-cycle regulators observed in thyroid cancer.A reasonable anticipation is that the growth of well-differentiated thyroid carcinoma is relatively low compared with PDTC and ATC and that the altered expression and/or activity of cell-cycle regulators determine these differences in growth. Accordingly, the MIB-1 index is 1–3% in WDTC, 6–7% in PDTC and 14–52% in ATC (Katoh et al., 1995). A high-labeling index, as seen in ATC and poorly differentiated thyroid patients, correlated with persistent disease or death (Kjellman et al., 2003). Expectedly, as is the case with other common human carcinomas, a series of multiple alterations in cell cycle control-related gene products such as up-regulation of CDKs, down-regulation of CDK inhibitors or both, frequently contribute to the pathogenesis of thyroid cancer (Kondo et al. 2006). Cyclin D1 (which is encoded by CCND1 on chromosome 11q13) and cyclin E1 (which is encoded by CCNE1 on chromosome 19q12) are overexpressed in thyroid cancer. Overexpression of cyclin D1 is observed in approximately 30% of FTC and

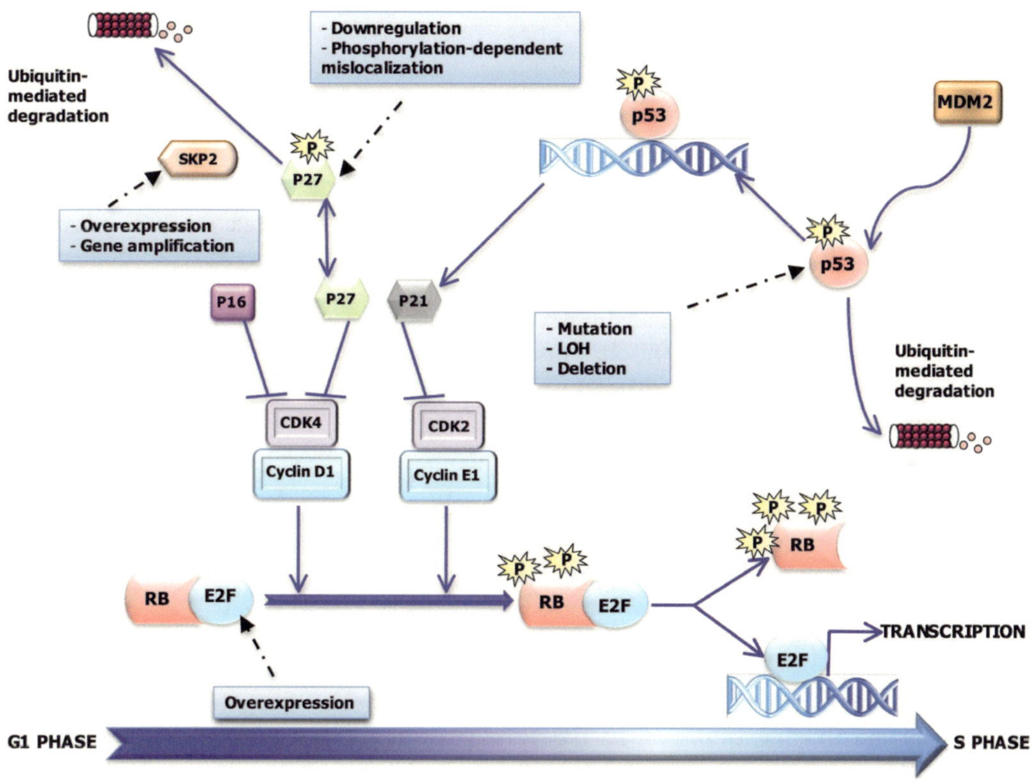

Fig. 6. Molecular alterations of cell-cycle regulators in thyroid cancer. The cyclin D1/CDK4 and cyclin E1/CDK2 cooperate to control the G1 to S phase transition through the phosphorylation of retinoblastoma protein (pRB). Hypophosphorylated pRB functions as a repressor of E2F transcription factors; conversely, inactivation of pRB through phosphorylation allows E2F activity. In particular, E2F activates the transcription of genes that are involved in the G1 to S phase transition, such as DNA polymerase and thymidine kinase. The CDK inhibitors p16INK4A, p21CIP1 and p27KIP1 impair the activity of cyclin/CDK complexes, thus preventing phosphorylation of pRB. Therefore, cyclins and CDKs function as oncogenes whereas CDK inhibitors function as tumour suppressors. The tumour suppressor TP53 induces cell-cycle arrest by up-regulating p21CIP1, another CDK inhibitor. The function of TP53, in turn, is controlled by negative regulators, including MDM2, which targets TP53 for ubiquitin-mediated degradation, constituting a feedback loop that maintains a low concentration of TP53 in the cells.

76% and PTC, respectively, having been correlated with metastatic dissemination of PTC (Lazzareschi et al., 1998). Similarly, cyclin E1 is overexpressed in a large number of thyroid carcinomas (Lazzareschi et al., 1998). At difference with other cancer types that show amplification or inversion of the locus containing CCND1, in thyroid cancers these genes are neither amplified nor rearranged (Lazzareschi et al., 1998). Therefore, overexpression of cyclins in thyroid tumours is a secondary effect that is induced by other genetic aberrations, such as RAS mutations or RET/PTC rearrangements. CDK inhibitors - both INK4 and CIP/KIP proteins - are commonly down-regulated in thyroid malignancies. Point mutations of CDKN2A on chromosome 9p21, which encodes p16INK4A, though common findings in glioma and melanoma, are rare in thyroid tumours. Alternatively, LOH in the chromosomal region spanning the CDKN2A locus is associated with FTC (27%) and ATC (50%), and methylation of 5' CpG islands of CDKN2A promoter is detected in 30% of thyroid neoplasms (Kondo et al., 2006 and references therein). As to the CIP/KIP proteins, normal and hyperplastic follicular cells show strong immunoreactivity for p27KIP1 (encoded by CDKN1B on chromosome 12p13), whereas its expression is significantly reduced in PTC, FTC and ATC (Erickson et al, 2000). P27 down-regulation in thyroid cancer depends on the over-expression of the ubiquitin-protein ligase Skp2, which is amplified in several thyroid tumors. Skp2 expression correlates with p27KIP1 down-regulation; forced expression of Skp2 circumvented serum-dependency and contact inhibition in Skp2-negative cells by promoting p27 degradation; and finally, the suppression of Skp2 expression drastically reduces proliferation of thyroid cancer cells. On the other hand, p27KIP1 that normally resides in the nucleus, is frequently inactivated by mislocalizion to the cytoplasm, a mechanism linked to AKT-dependent phosphorylation. P21CIP1, another CIP/KIP inhibitor encoded by CDKN1A gene on chromosome 6p21, is expressed in 40% of well-differentiated PTC 7% of PDTC, and not in ATC. On average, 10-13% of thyroid malignancies harbour CDKN1A deletions on chromosome 6p21 (Shi et al., 1996). The expression pattern of pRB in benign and malignant thyroid lesions is controversial. Although one group has reported the presence of inactivating mutation in the gene encoding pRB1 (located on chromosome 13q14) in 55% of thyroid carcinomas this has not been confirmed by other investigators. The main targets of pRB are represented by the E2F transcription factors, which consists of six members: E2F1–E2F6. E2F-regulated genes are repressed by pRB proteins; such a repression is alleviated by CDK-dependent phosphorylation of pRB. E2F1, but not other members of this family, is up-regulated in 35–89% of WDTC, 34% of PDTC and 67% of ATC (Volante et al., 2002). As part of the cell cycle surveillance system, the G2 spindle checkpoint protects the cell from genomic instability. Entry into mitosis is blocked by the G2 checkpoint that ensures that chromosomes are not segregated to daughter cells when DNA is damaged. Thyroid cell transformation is accompanied by the overexpression of a cell proliferation/genetic instability-related gene cluster that includes Polo-like kinase 1 (PLK1), a protein kinases involved in in several G2- and M-phase–related events such as centrosome maturation, proper spindle formation, cyclin B/Cdk1 activation, anaphase-promoting complex/cyclosome (APC/C) activation, chromosome segregation, and cytokinesis (Salvatore et al., 2006). ATC, but not normal thyroid, cells are dependent on PLK1 for survival. RNAi-mediated PLK1 knock-down caused mitotic arrest associated with 4N DNA content and massive mitotic cell death (Nappi et al., 2009). Other alterations implicated in the G2/M transition include overexpression of the Aurora A-C kinases in ATC cell lines and tumors (Sorrentino et al. 2005) and the mitotic spindle assembly checkpoint genes hBUB1, hBUBR1 and hMAD2 (Wada et al. 2008).

ANIMAL MODELS OF THYROID CANCER					
	MOUSE LINE	STRAIN	PATHOLOGY	METASTASIS	THYROID FUNCTION
PTC	RET/PTC1	CS57BL/6J	22% WITH PTC	NO	NA
	RET/PTC1	FVB/N	100% WITH MULTIFOCAL PTC	NO	NORMAL/HYPOTHYROIDISM
	RET/PTC3	C3H/He	31% WITH PTC BY 3 MONTHS	LYMPH NODES	NA
	$BRAF^{V600E}$ (Tg-BRAF2)	FVB/N	93% WITH PTC BY 3 MONTHS	LYMPH NODES	TSH INCREASED
	$BRAF^{V600E}$ (Tg-BRAF3)	FVB/N	25% WITH PTC AT 3 MONTHS	NO	TSH INCREASED
	TRK-T1	B6C3F1	23% WITH PTC-LIKE CANCER	NO	NA
	$H\text{-}Ras^{G12V}$	MIXED	3 OUT OF 4 MICE DEVELOPED PTC	UNCLEAR	NORMAL T4 LEVEL
	$Prkar1a^{D2/+}$	MIXED	95% WITH PTC-LIKE CANCER	NO	NA
FTC	$K\text{-}Ras^{G12V}$	C57BL/6J, DBA/2	2% WITH FTC	NO	NORMAL
	Pten -/-	FVB/N x 129Sv	FTC IN FEMALES	NO	NORMAL TSH AND T4 LEVELS
	$N\text{-}Ras^{Glu61Lys}$	FOUNDERS x C57BL/6J	11% ADENOMA, 29,5% FTC/MIXED	LIVER, LUNG, BONE	ELEVATED TSH
	$K\text{-}Ras^{G12D}$ Pten -/-	129SV	100% FTC WITH LOCAL INVASION	LUNG	LOW TSH/HIGH T4
	$TRb^{PV/PV}$	C57BL/6J x 129Sv	100% FTC	LUNG	ELEVATED TSH, T3 AND T4
	1b-adrenergic receptor	FOUNDERS x C57BL/6J	3 OUT OF 6 LINES WITH GOITER AND FTC	LUNG	ELEVATED T4
	$Rap1b^{G12V}$	FVB (Taconic)	FTC AFTER TREATMENT WITH A GOITROGEN	NO	NORMAL

Table 2. Animal models of thyroid carcinomas (from Kim and Zhu, 2009, modified).

3.1.6 Genetic alterations in anaplastic thyroid carcinomas

The tumour-suppressor gene TP53

Most of the mutations discussed so far are mainly found in differentiated thyroid cancers and are believed not to be sufficient by themselves to trigger the progression to PDTC and ATC. By contrast, mutations of TP53, a tumor suppressor gene located on chromosome 17, are common features of PDTC or ATC, and could be responsible for the loss of differentiation observed during tumor progression. In thyroid cancers, TP53 mutations occur in 17–38% of PDTC and 67–88% of ATC, respectively, and only in isolated cases of differentiated PTC and FTC (Nikiforov, 2008 and references therein). TP53 is a key gatekeeper that plays a role in cell cycle regulation, apoptosis, genomic stability, and inhibition of angiogenesis. In its anti-cancer role, TP53 can induce growth arrest by holding the cell cycle at the G1/S or G2/M points following DNA damage recognition, which prevents replication of cells with damaged DNA and allows the DNA repair proteins to have time to fix the damage and resume the cell cycle. Alternatively, TP53 can initiate the programmed cell death if DNA damage proves to be irreparable Activation of wild-type TP53 can lead to G1 cell-cycle arrest through transcriptional induction of the CDK inhibitor p21CIP1, or apoptotic cell death by activating transcription of pro-apoptotic molecules such as BAX and FAS. Loss-of- function mutations of TP53 impair its transcriptional activity and induce genomic instability, owing to weakened DNA repair systems, and subsequent cancer progression.

β-catenin mutations

β-catenin, encoded by the CTNNB1 gene on chromosome 3p22–21.3, plays a role in cell adhesion and transcription. In normal cells, most β-catenin protein is bound to E-cadherin (encoded by the CDH1 gene on chromosome 16q22) in the cytoplasmic portion of adherens junctions, thus fulfilling an essential role in cell adhesion. This binding sequesters β-catenin from the nucleus and restrains its growth-promoting role. β-catenin is a critical regulator of cell proliferation induced by Wnt signalling, promoting transcription of cyclin D1 and MYC (Cadigan & Peifer, 2009). The cellular abundance of β-catenin is finely modulated through proteasomal degradation. This process occurs through the action of a multicomponent complex that includes APC - encoded by the APC gene inactivated in familial adenomatous polyposis –the scaffold protein Axin and the Glycogen Synthase Kinase-3 (GSK), which phosphorylates β-catenin and targets it for polyubiquitination and degradation. Activation of the Wnt pathway inhibits GSK-3-dependent phosphorylation of β-catenin as well as its subsequent proteosomal degradation, allowing β-catenin to translocate to the nucleus and function as a transcriptional effector of Wnt. In cancer cells the growth-promoting activity of β-catenin is enhanced either by reducing its binding to E-cadherin (e.g. due to decreased CDH1 expression), or when APC-Axin-GSK3β-mediated degradation of β-catenin is defective due to inactivating mutations of APC and/or CTNNB1 or to overactive Wnt signalling. Such mutations disrupt phosphorylation sites of β-catenin and lead to protein stabilization. Mutations and abnormal nuclear localization of β-catenin have been observed, along with overexpression of its target genes c-Myc and cyclin D1, in thyroid malignancies (Ishigaki et al., 2002). Although increased levels of cytoplasmic β-catenin are observed in most thyroid cancer cells, mutations of β-catenin that lead to nuclear localization of the protein are limited to PDTC and ATC suggesting a role in tumor progression (Garcia-Rostan et al., 2001). On the other hand, E-cadherin is highly expressed in normal thyroid and benign adenoma but its expression is consistently decreased in cancer, especially in recurrent or metastatic carcinomas. Mutations of CDH1 are infrequent in undifferentiated cancer; conversely loss of E-cadherin is due to aberrant methylation of the CDH1 promoter (Kato et al., 2002). Another observation that supports a role of the APC–β-catenin pathway in the development of thyroid cancer is that familial adenomatous polyposis (FAP) and its variant, Gardner syndrome, which confers a markedly increased risk of development of PTC are caused by germline mutations in the APC gene. However, it appears that the aberrant nuclear localization of β-catenin observed in thyroid carcinoma is more likely induced by CTNNB1 mutations rather than APC mutations.

3.1.7 Genetic alterations of microRNA in thyroid cancer

MicroRNAs (miRs) are a class of 19–23 nucleotide-long non-coding RNAs that negatively regulate gene expression through either the inhibition of mRNA translation or the induction of its degradation (Ambros 2004). MiRs are transcribed by RNA polymerase II in the nucleus, are transported into the cytoplasm by the Exportin system where they are incorporated into the RISC, thus acquiring the ability to bind to the 3' untranslated region (UTR) of the target mRNAs causing mRNA degradation or the block of translation (Ambros 2004, Bartel 2004). At present it is estimated that there are 300–1000 microRNAs, each of which may bind to several hundred mRNA targets. MiRs are involved in a wide range of basic processes such as cell proliferation, development and apoptosis (Bartel 2004). MiRs are abnormally expressed in many types of human cancer and can act as oncogenes or tumor suppressor genes or, in some cases, can perform both functions (Calin & Croce 2006,). Recent studies have shown that miRs may also contribute to onset and/progression of thyroid malignancies. Most studies have focused on the analysis of miR expression profile of PTC by 'miRCHIP' microarray. Several miRs including miR-221, -222, -146, -21, -155, -181a, and -181b have been shown to be up-regulated in PTC compared with the normal thyroid (Pallante et al., 2005). In particular miR-221, -222, and -181b have been proposed to represent a signature for PTC. MiR-221 and -222 represent the most consistently up-regulated miRs in PTC. They are very similar in sequence, clustered on chromosome X, and are likely transcribed as polycistronic transcripts (Ciafrè et al. 2005). Adoptive expression of miR-221/222 significantly modifies proliferation of thyrocytes, increasing G1- to S-phase transition through the reduction of p27KIP1 protein levels (Visone et al. 2007a). However, the mechanism by which these miRs are upregulated in PTC is still under investigation, since no gene amplification or changes in the methylation status has yet been found. Although most of the studies conducted so far have focused on miR expression in PTC, Nikiforova et al. (2008) reported on a signature specifically associated with follicular adenoma and FTC. The most highly up-regulated miRs in conventional FTC were miR-187, -224, -155, -222, and -221, and those in oncocytic variants were miR-187, -221, -339, -183, -222, and -197. In a different study, four miRs that are differentially expressed between FTC and adenoma (miR-192, -197, -328, and -346) have been identified (Weber et al. 2006). Inhibition of miR-197 and - 346 in human thyroid cancer cells (FTC133) caused growth arrest (Weber et al. 2006). MiR-21 targets E2F and inhibits PTEN. Recent data indicate that specific miRs are associated with different histological types of thyroid. MiR-187 is expressed at high levels in PTC harboring RET/PTC rearrangements whereas miR-221 and -222 are found at the highest level in BRAF- and RAS-positive PTC and those with no known mutations. Conversely, RAS-positive PTC expresses high amount of miR-146. In ATC samples and cell lines the miR-17–92 cluster containing seven miRs as well as miR-106a and -106b are overexpressed (Takakura et al. 2008). Antisense inhibition of miRs 17-3p, -17-5p, and -19a causes cell cycle arrest, and suggests an oncogenic role for these miRs. MiR-19a and -19b in the cluster have PTEN as a target, and miR-106a and -106b have E2F1 as a target, thus suggesting that there are multiple potential therapeutic targets in the miR-17–92 cluster (Takakura et al. 2008). On the other hand, four miRs (-30d, -125b, -26a, and 30a-5p) have been shown to be under-expressed in ATC but not in PTC (Visone et al. 2007b). MiR-26a and -125b target HMGA1 and HMGA2, two proteins causally involved in thyroid cell transformation. In addition, miR-138 that targets hTERT is reduced in ATC (Visone et al., 2007b). In conclusion, the studies of miRs expression and function indicate that each of the three principal types of thyroid cancer has several distinct miRs already and hold promise to improve the evaluation and management of these tumors.

4. Targeted therapy of thyroid cancer

The current treatment of patients with differentiated thyroid cancer includes surgery, radioactive iodine administration and thyroid hormone suppression therapy and is, in most cases, effective. Accordingly, survival rates for patients with local differentiated thyroid carcinoma are excellent. By contrast, treatment of patients with advanced thyroid cancer continues to represent a significant challenge for clinical oncologists. These patients are not responsive to standard treatment and require additional therapies. However, the efficacy of cytotoxic chemotherapy is poor and that of external beam radiation has not been established yet. It is likely that this scenario has just started to change because of the introduction of targeted therapies - especially tyrosine kinase inhibitors - for the treatment of advanced thyroid cancer (Santoro & Carlomagno, 2006). Tyrosine kinase inhibitors cause tumor shrinkage and/or disease stabilization. The rationale for the development of specific inhibitors of the oncogenes that initiate cancer is based on the hypothesis denoted the "oncogene addiction" (Weinstein &, Joe, 2008). According to this hypothesis, the initiating genetic alteration that hits a normal cell and starts the transformation process becomes essential for the survival of cancer cells. Thus, inhibition of the oncogene that initiates a certain cancer is expected to lead to either tumor stabilization or regression. For this reason, a lot of interest arose in the therapeutic potential of kinase inhibitors for thyroid cancer patients. The prevalence of activating BRAF mutations, RET/PTC rearrangements and RAS mutations that is reflected into consequent downstream activation of ERKs, suggests that activation of the MAP kinase pathway may be an obligatory step in the transformation of thyrocytes. Therefore, such dependency may represent a potential Achilles heel of cancer cells. Since thyroid cancer cells are apparently "addicted" to aberrant MAP kinase signalling, several small molecules that target this pathway are currently being developed (Sherman, 2009). Several lines of evidence suggest that RET/PTC can be a good target. The quinazoline low molecular weight tyrosine kinase inhibitor ZD6474 (Vandetanib), a potent inhibitor of the VEGF receptor-2 (flk-1/KDR), has also been shown to inhibit the enzymatic and transforming activity of RET/PTC oncoproteins and to block the growth of RET/PTC3-induced tumours in nude mice (Carlomagno et al., 2002). Multiple phase II clinical trials testing the efficacy of ZD6474 in patients with metastatic medullary thyroid cancer, as well as metastatic papillary cancer are currently underway. In the case of patients with metastatic familial medullary thyroid carcinoma one of these clinical trials demonstrated partial response in 17% of patients and stable disease in another 33% (Sherman, 2008a).

BRAF represents another valuable therapeutic candidate for treatment of thyroid cancer due to the high frequency of BRAF mutation in thyroid tumors and its association with tumor dedifferentiation and resistance to the conventional radioiodine therapy. The biaryl urea Sorafenib (BAY 43-9006) is a potent inhibitor of BRAF, VEGFR and RET (Wilhelm et al., 2004). Sorafenib has shown cytostatic effects in thyroid tumor cells lines, both with and without the presence of BRAF mutations (Salvatore et al., 2006). In xenografts, daily administration of sorafenib inhibits phospho-MEK activity, attenuates tumour growth, and reduces Ki67/MIB-1 staining. Sorafenib received approval from the US Food and Drug Administration for the treatment of metastastic renal cancer, a malignancy where BRAF mutations have not been observed. In this case, it is believed that the clinical efficacy of sorafenib may derive more from its anti-VEGF activity than from BRAF block. Data from multiple clinical studies for the treatment of advanced thyroid cancer with sorafenib have been reported (Gupta-Abramson et al., 2008; Hoftijzer et al., 2009; Kloos et al., 2009). Three phase II studies have been conducted to determine the efficacy of sorafenib in advanced thyroid carcinomas of follicular origin. Despite its promising preclinical properties, the preliminary efficacy data for sorafenib in patients with thyroid cancer appear modest. This drug was shown to have a partial response in some patients with progressive PTC. Currently, phase II clinical trials are underway using BAY 43-9006 in the treatment of ATC and metastatic MTC. Preliminary results of the trial in patients with progressive PTC have shown minimal or partial response in some patients. However, several second-generation small molecule inhibitors of BRAF and MEK that exhibit *in vitro* activity exceeding that of

sorafenib are currently being investigated. Presumably, these and other emerging RAF inhibitors may provide a more robust effect against MAP kinase activity in clinical trials.
Another strategy to block growth of thyroid tumor is through the inhibition of angiogenesis (Ferrara & Kerbel, 2005). This results in reduced delivery of oxygen and nutrients to tumor cells and a reduced removal of waste and CO2, which ultimately compromises cell viability. VEGF is a stimulator of angiogenesis that substantially contributes to tumor progression. AMG 706 is an ATP-competitive inhibitor of VEGFR1, VEGFR2 and VEGFR3 that inhibits VEGF-induced cell proliferation and vascular permeability, thus inducing tumour regression *in vivo* (Polverino et al. 2006). AMG 706 has shown encouraging anti-tumour activity in a subset of patients with iodine-refractory metastatic thyroid cancer in a phase I study.
Axitinib is an oral tyrosine kinase inhibitor that effectively blocks VEGFR1, VEGFR2 and VEGFR3 at subnanomolar concentrations. As AMG 706, it also appears to inhibit c-KIT and PDGFRβ. A multicenter phase II study examined the efficacy of axitinib in advanced or metastatic thyroid carcinoma (Cohen et al., 2008a). Among the 45 evaluable patients, 30% experienced a partial response and 38% presented stable disease lasting more than 16 weeks, yielding an objective response rate of 30% and a disease control rate of 68%.
Motesanib diphosphate is an oral inhibitor that blocks VEGFRs at nanomolar concentrations (VEGFR1 IC50 of 2 nM; VEGFR2 IC50 of 3 nM; VEGFR3 IC50 of 6 nM) (Sherman et al., 2008b). Moreover, it appears to inhibit c-KIT (IC50 of 8 nM), PDGFRβ (IC50 of 84 nM) and RET (IC50 of 59 nM) either wild type or mutated. A multicenter phase II study examined the efficacy of motesanib in locally advanced or metastatic, radioiodine-resistant differentiated thyroid cancer (Sherman et al., 2008b; Schlumberger et al., 2009). The study yielded an objective response rate of 14% and a disease control rate of 81%. The median estimate of progression-free survival was 40 weeks.
Finally, sunitinib is an oral inhibitor that inhibits VEGFR1 (IC50 of 2 nM), VEGFR2 (IC50 of 9 nM), VEGFR3 (IC50 of 17 nM), RET (IC50 of 41 nM), RET/PTCs (for RET/PTC3 IC50 of 224 nM) and PDRGRβ (IC50of 2nM) (Kim et al., 2006). In an initial phase II study 43 patients with metastatic, iodine-refractory thyroid carcinoma of all histological sub-types were enrolled (Cohen et al., 2008b). Partial response was observed in 13% of patients, stable disease in 68%, and progressive disease in 10%, yielding an objective response rate of 13% and a disease control rate of 81%. As the results of additional ongoing clinical trials are expected to be available in the near future, it is expected to reach a more precise assessment of the role of such molecular inhibitors, administered alone or in combination, in the therapy of thyroid cancer.

5. Conclusions

In conclusion, our increasing understanding of the biology of thyroid follicular cancer is leading to the development of novel and promising therapies. Tumour-initiating events have been identified in a high proportion of the most frequent types of thyroid cancer - PTC, FTC, and ATC. All the genetic alterations identified so far converge in few signalling cascades - the RTK/RAS, the BRAF/MAPK and the PI3K/AKT pathways, respectively. This provides a strong basis for the development of novel gene-based diagnostic, prognostic, and therapeutic strategies. In fact, the treatment of advanced thyroid cancer is changing dramatically following the development of kinase inhibitors. It remains to be determined whether combinations of targeted therapies with chemotherapy or radiotherapy will improve response rates. The results of the on-going clinical trials, as well as the new agents in development, will likely contribute to improve the lives of patients with advanced thyroid cancer.

6. References

Ain, K.B. (1995). Papillary thyroid carcinoma. Etiology, assessment, and therapy. *Endocrinology and Metabolism Clinics of North America*, Vol.24, No.4, (December 1995), pp. 711-760, ISSN 0889-8529.

Airaksinen, M.S., Titievsky, A. & Saarma, M. (1999). GDNF family neurotrophic factor signaling: four masters, one servant? *Molecular and cellular neurosciences*,Vol.13, No.5, (May 1999), pp. 313-325, ISSN 1044-7431.

Ambros, V. (2004). The functions of animal microRNAs. *Nature*, Vol.431, No.7006, (September 2004), pp. 350–355, ISSN 0028-0836.

Bader, A.G., Kang, S. & Vogt, P.K. (2006). Cancer-specific mutations in PIK3CA are oncogenic *in vivo*. *Proceedings of the National Academy of Sciences of the United States of America*, Vol.103, No.5, (January 2006), pp. 1475-9, ISSN 0027-8424.

Bartel, D.P. (2004). MicroRNAs: genomics, biogenesis, mechanism, and function. *Cell*, Vol.116, No.2, (January 2004), pp. 281–297, ISSN 0092-8674.

Basolo, F., Giannini, R., Monaco, C., Melillo, R.M., Carlomagno, F., Pancrazi, M., Salvatore, G., Chiappetta, G., Pacini, F., Elisei, R., Miccoli, P., Pinchera, A., Fusco, A. & Santoro, M. (2002). Potent mitogenicity of the RET/PTC3 oncogene correlates with its prevalence in tall-cell variant of papillary thyroid carcinoma. *The American journal of pathology*, Vol.160, No.1, (January 2002), pp. 247-254, ISSN 0002-9440.

Bongarzone, I., Fugazzola, L., Vigneri, P., Mariani, L., Mondellini, P., Pacini, F., Basolo, F., Pinchera, A., Pilotti, S. & Pierotti, M.A. (1996). Age-related activation of the tyrosine kinase receptor protooncogenes RET and NTRK1 in papillary thyroid carcinoma. *The Journal of clinical endocrinology and metabolism*,Vol.81, No.5, (May 1996), pp. 2006-2009, ISSN 0021-972X.

Brazil, D.P., Yang, Z.Z. & Hemmings, B.A. (2004). Advances in protein kinase B signalling: AKTion on multiple fronts. *Trends in biochemical sciences*, Vol.29, No.5, (May 2004), pp. 233-242, ISSN 0968-0004.

Buday, L. & Downward, J. (2008). Many faces of Ras activation. *Biochimica et biophysica acta*, Vol.1786, No.2, (December 2008), pp. 178-187, ISSN 0006-3002.

Bunney, T.D. & Katan, M. (2010). Phosphoinositide signalling in cancer: beyond PI3K and PTEN. *Nature reviews. Cancer*, Vol.10, No.5, (May 2010), pp. 342-352, ISSN 1474-175X.

Bunone, G., Vigneri, P., Mariani, L., Butó, S., Collini, P., Pilotti, S., Pierotti, M.A. & Bongarzone, I.(1999). Expression of angiogenesis stimulators and inhibitors in human thyroid tumors and correlation with clinical pathological features. *The American journal of pathology*, Vol.155, No.6, (December 1999), pp. 1967-1976, ISSN 0002-9440.

Cadigan, K.M. & Peifer, M. (2009). Wnt signaling from development to disease: insights from model systems. *Cold Spring Harbor perspectives in biology*, Vol.1, No.2, (August 2009), pp. a002881, ISSN 1943-0264 .

Calin, G.A. & Croce, C.M. (2006). MicroRNA signatures in human cancers. *Nature Reviews. Cancer*, Vol.6, No.11, (November 2006), pp. 857–866, ISSN 1474-175X.

Cardis, E., Kesminierne, A., Ivanov, V., Malakhova, I., Shibata, Y., Khrouch, V., Drozdovitch, V., Maceika, E., Zvonova, I., Vlassov, O., Bouville, A., Goulko, G., Hoshi, M., Abrosimov, A., Anoshko, J., Astakhova, L., Chekin, S., Demidchik, E., Galanti, R., Ito, M., Korobova, E., Lushnikov, E., Maksioutov, M., Masyakin, V., Nerovnia, A., Parshin, V., Parshkov, E., Piliptsevich, N., Pinchera, A., Polyakov, S., Shabeka, N., Suonio, E., Tenet, V., Tsyb, A., Yamashita, S. & Williams D. (2005). Risk of thyroid cancer after exposur e to 131-I in childhood. *Journal of the National Cancer Institut*, Vol.97, No.10 (May 2005), pp. 724-732, ISSN 1052-6773.

Carlomagno, F., Vitagliano, D., Guida, T., Ciardiello, F., Tortora, G., Vecchio, G., Ryan, A.J., Fontanini, G., Fusco, A. & Santoro, M. (2002). ZD6474, an orally available inhibitor of KDR tyrosine kinase activity, efficiently blocks oncogenic RET kinases. *Cancer Research*, Vol.62, No.24, (December 2002), pp. 7284-7290, ISSN 0008-5472.

Carpten, J.D., Faber, A.L., Horn, C., Donoho, G.P., Briggs, S.L., Robbins, C.M., Hostetter, G., Boguslawski, S., Moses, T.Y., Savage, S., Uhlik, K., Lin, A., Du, J., Qian, Y.W., Zeckner, D.J., Tucker-Kellogg, G., Touchman, J., Patel, K., Mousses, S., Bittner, M., Schevitz, R., Lai, M.H., Blanchard, K.L. & Thomas, J.E. (2007). A transforming mutation in the pleckstrin homology domain of AKT1 in cancer. *Nature*, Vol.448, No.7152, (July 2007), pp. 439-444, ISSN 0028-0836.

Carracedo, A. & Pandolfi, P.P. (2008). The PTEN–PI3K pathway: of feedbacks and cross-talks. *Oncogene*, Vol.27, No.41, (September 2008), pp. 5527-5541, ISSN 0950-9232.

Cass, L.A. & Meinkoth, J.L. (2000). Ras signaling through PI3K confers hormone-independent proliferation that is compatible with differentiation. *Oncogene*, Vol.19, No.7, (February 2000), pp. 924-932, ISSN 0950-9232.

Cheung, C.C., Ezzat, S., Ramyar, L., Freeman, J.L. & Asa, S.L. (2000). Molecular basis of Hurthle cell papillare thyroid carcinoma. *The Journal of clinical endocrinology and metabolism*, Vol.85, No.2, (February 2000), pp. 878–882, ISSN 0021-972X.

Ciafrè, S.A., Galardi, S., Mangiola, A., Ferracin, M., Liu, C.G., Sabatino, G., Negrini, M., Maira, G., Croce, C.M. & Farace, M.G. (2005). Extensive modulation of a set of microRNAs in primary glioblastoma. *Biochemical and Biophysical Research Communications*, Vol.334, No.4, (September 2005), pp. 1351–1358, ISSN 0006-291X.

Ciampi, R., Knauf, J.A., Kerler, R., Gandhi, M., Zhu, Z., Nikiforova, M.N., Rabes, H.M., Fagin, J.A. & Nikiforov, Y.E. (2005). Oncogenic AKAP9–BRAF fusion is a novel mechanism of MAPK pathway activation in thyroid cancer.The *Journal of Clinical Investigation*, Vol.115, No.1, (January 2005), pp. 94–101, ISSN 0021-9738.

Ciullo, G., Diez-Roux, M., Di Domenico, A., Migliaccio & Avvedimento, E.V. (2001). Avvedimento: cAMP signaling selectively influences Ras effectors pathways. *Oncogene*, Vol.20, No.10, (March 2001), pp. 1186-1192, ISSN 0950-9232.

Cohen, E.E., Needles, B.M., Cullen, K.J., Wong, S.J., Wade, J.L., Ivy, S.P., Villaflor, V.M., Seiwert, T.Y., Nichols, K. & Vokes, E.E. (2008b). Phase 2 study of sunitinib in refractory thyroid cancer. *Journal of Clinical Oncology*, Vol.26, No.15S, (May 2008), pp. 6025, ISSN 0732-183X.

Cohen, E.E., Rosen, L.S., Vokes, E.E., Kies, M.S., Forastiere, A.A., Worden, F.P., Kane, M.A., Sherman, E., Kim, S., Bycott, P., Tortorici, M., Shalinsky, D.R., Liau, K.F. & Cohen, R.B. (2008a). Axitinib is an active treatment for all histologic subtypes of advanced thyroid cancer: results from a phase II study. *Journal of Clinical Oncology,* Vol.26, No.29, (October 2008), pp. 4708-4713, ISSN 0732-183X.

Collins, M.T., Sarlis, N.J., Merino, M.J., Monroe, J., Crawford, S.E., Krakoff, J.A., Guthrie, L.C., Bonat, S., Robey, P.G. & Shenker, A. (2003). Thyroid carcinoma in the McCune–Albright syndrome: contributory role of activating Gs⟨ mutations. *The Journal of clinical endocrinology and metabolism,* Vol.88, No.9, (September 2003), pp. 4413–4417, ISSN 0021-972X.

Cornett, W.R., Sharma, A.K., Day, T.A., Richardson, M.S., Hoda, R.S., van Heerden, J.A. & Fernandes, J.K. (2007). Anaplastic thyroid carcinoma: an overview. *Current Oncology Reports*, Vol.9, No.2, (January 2007), pp. 152-158, ISSN 1523-3790.

Cosentino, C., Di Domenico, M., Porcellini, A., Cuozzo, C., De Gregorio, G., Santillo, M.R., Agnese, S., Di Stasio, R., Feliciello, A., Migliaccio, A. &. Avvedimento, E.V. (2006). p85 regulatory subunit of PI3K mediates cAMP-PKA and estrogens biological effects on growth and survival. *Oncogene*, Vol.26, No.14, (March 2007), pp. 2095-2103, ISSN 0950-9232.

Davies, H., Bignell, G.R., Cox, C., Stephens, P., Edkins, S., Clegg, S., Teague, J., Woffendin, H., Garnett, M.J., Bottomley, W., Davis, N., Dicks, E., Ewing, R., Floyd, Y., Gray, K., Hall, S., Hawes, R., Hughes, J., Kosmidou, V., Menzies, A., Mould, C., Parker, A., Stevens, C., Watt, S., Hooper, S., Wilson, R., Jayatilake, H., Gusterson, B.A., Cooper, C., Shipley, J., Hargrave, D., Pritchard-Jones, K., Maitland, N., Chenevix-Trench, G., Riggins, G.J., Bigner, D.D., Palmieri, G., Cossu, A., Flanagan, A., Nicholson, A., Ho, J.W., Leung, S.Y., Yuen, S.T., Weber, B.L., Seigler, H.F., Darrow, T.L., Paterson, H., Marais, R., Marshall, C.J., Wooster, R., Stratton, M.R. & Futreal, P.A. (2002). Mutations of the BRAF gene in human cancer. *Nature*, Vol.417, No.6892, (June 2002), pp. 949–954, ISSN 0028-0836.

Davies, M.A., Stemke-Hale, K., Tellez, C., Calderone, C.L., Deng, W., Prieto, V.G., Lazar, A.J., Gershenwald, J.E. & Mills, G.B. (2008). A novel AKT3 mutation in melanoma tumours and cell lines. *British Journal of Cancer*, Vol.99, No.8, (October 2008), pp. 1265-1268, ISSN 0007-0920.

De Gregorio, G., Coppa, A., Cosentino, C., Ucci, S., Messina, S., Nicolussi, A., D'Inzeo, S., Di Pardo, A., Avvedimento, E.V. & Porcellini, A. (2006). The p85 regulatory subunit of PI3K mediates TSH-cAMP-PKA growth and survival signals. *Oncogene*, Vol.26, No.14, (March 2007), pp. 2039-2047, ISSN 0950-9232.

De Vita, G., Bauer, L., da Costa, V.M., De Felice, M., Baratta, M.G., De Menna, M. & Di Lauro, R. (2004). Dose-dependent inhibition of thyroid differentiation by RAS oncogenes. *Molecular Endocrinology*, Vol.19, No.1, (January 2005), pp. 76-89, ISSN 0888-8809.

DeLellis, R.A., Lloyd, R.V., Heitz, P.U. & Eng, C. (2004). *Pathology and Genetics of Tumours of Endocrine Organs,* IARC Press, ISBN 9789283224167, Lyon.

Desvergne, B. & Wahli, W. (1999). Peroxisome proliferator activated receptors: nuclear control of metabolism. *Endocrine Reviews*, Vol.20, No.5, (October 1999), pp. 649–688, ISSN 0163-769X.

Di Renzo, M.F., Olivero, M., Serini, G., Orlandi, F., Pilotti, S., Belfiore, A., Costantino, A., Vigneri, R., Angeli. A., Pierotti, M.A., et al. (1995). Overexpression of the c-MET/HGF receptor in human thyroid carcinomas derived from the follicular epithelium. *Journal of endocrinological investigation*, Vol.18, No.2, (February 1995), pp.134-139, ISSN 0391-4097.

Dumont, JE., Lamy, F., Roger, P. & Maenhaut, C. (1992). Physiological and pathological regulation of thyroid cell proliferation and differentiation by thyrotropin and other factors. *Physiological Reviews*, Vol.72, No.3, (July 1992), pp. 667-697, ISSN 0031-9333.

Eng, C. (2000). Familial papillary thyroid cancer—many syndromes, too many genes? *The Journal of clinical endocrinology and metabolism*, Vol.85, No.5, (May 2000), pp. 1755–1757, ISSN 0021-972X.

Engelman, J.A., Luo, J. & Cantley, L.C. (2006). The evolution of phosphatidylinositol 3-kinases as regulators of growth and metabolism. *Nature reviews. Genetics*, Vol.7, No.8, (August 2006), pp. 606-619, ISSN 1471-0056.

Engelman, J.A., Chen, L., Tan, X., Crosby, K., Guimaraes, A.R., Upadhyay, R., Maira, M., McNamara, K., Perera, S.A., Song, Y., Chirieac, L.R., Kaur, R., Lightbown, A., Simendinger, J., Li, T., Padera, R.F., García-Echeverría, C., Weissleder, R., Mahmood, U., Cantley, L.C. & Wong, K.K. (2008). Effective use of PI3K and MEK inhibitors to treat mutant Kras G12D and PIK3CA H1047R murine lung cancers. *Nature Medicine*, Vol.14, No.12, (December 2008), pp. 1351-1356, ISSN 1078-8956.

Erickson, L.A., Yousef, O.M., Jin, L., Lohse, C.M., Pankratz, V.S. & Lloyd, R.V. (2000). p27kip1 expression distinguishes papillary hyperplasia in Graves' disease from papillare thyroid carcinoma. *Mod Pathol*, Vol.13, No.9, (September 2000), pp. 1014–1019, ISSN 0893-3952.

Ferrara, N. & Kerbel, R.S. (2005). Angiogenesis as a therapeutic target. *Nature*, Vol.438, No.7070, (December 2005), pp. 967-974, ISSN 0028-0836.

Fusco, A. & Santoro, M. (2007). 20 years of RET/PTC in thyroid cancer: clinico-pathological correlations. *Arquivos brasileiros de endocrinologia e metabologia*, Vol.51, No.5, (July 2007), pp. 731-735, ISSN 0004-2730.

Garcia-Rostan, G., Camp, R.L., Herrero, A., Carcangiu, M.L., Rimm, D.L. & Tallini, G.(2001). ®-catenin dysregulation in thyroid neoplasms: down-regulation, aberrant nuclear expression, and CTNNB1 exon 3 mutations are markers for aggressive tumor phenotypes and poor prognosis. *The American journal of pathology*, Vol.158, No.3, (March 2001), pp. 987–996, ISSN 0002-9440.

García-Rostán, G., Costa, A.M., Pereira-Castro, I., Salvatore, G., Hernandez, R., Hermsem, M.J., Herrero, A., Fusco, A., Cameselle-Teijeiro, J. & Santoro, M. (2005). Mutation of the PIK3CA gene in anaplastic thyroid cancer. *Cancer Research*, Vol.65, No.22, (November 2005), pp. 10199-10207, ISSN 0008-5472.

Gasbarri, A., Sciacchitano, S., Marasco, A,. Papotti, M., Di Napoli, A., Marzullo, A., Yushkov, P., Ruco, L. & Bartolazzi, A. (2004). Detection and molecular characterisation of thyroid cancer precursor lesions in a specific subset of Hashimoto's thyroiditis. *British Journal of Cancer*, Vol.91, No.6, (September 2004), pp. 1096–1104, ISSN 0007-0920.

Gilliland, F.D., Hunt, W.C., Morris, D.M. & Key, C.R. (December 2009). Thyroid cancer-UK incidence statistics, In: *UK Cancer Research*, 10.12.2009, Available from: http://info.cancerresearchuk.org/cancerstats/types/thyroid/incidence/uk-thyroid-cancer-incidence-statistics.

Gire, V. & Wynford-Thomas, D. (2000). RAS oncogene activation induces proliferation in normal human thyroid epithelial cells without loss of differentiation. *Oncogene*, Vol.9, No.6, (February 2000), pp. 737-44, ISSN 0950-9232.

Gregory Powell, J., Wang, X., Allard, B.L., Sahin, M., Wang, X.L., Hay, I.D., Hiddinga, H.J., Deshpande, S.S., Kroll, T.G., Grebe, S.K., Eberhardt, N.L. & McIver, B. (2004). The PAX8–PPARγ fusion oncoprotein transforms immortalized human thyrocytes through a mechanism probably involving wild-type PPARγ inhibition. *Oncogene*, Vol.23, No.20, (April 2004), pp. 3634–3641, ISSN 0950-9232.

Grose, R. & Dickson, C. (2005). Fibroblast growth factor signaling in tumorigenesis. *Cytokine & growth factor reviews*, Vol.16, No.2, (April 2005), pp. 179-186, ISSN 1359-6101.

Gupta-Abramson, V., Troxel, A.B., Nellore, A., Puttaswamy, K., Redlinger, M., Ransone, K., Mandel, S.J., Flaherty, K.T., Loevner, L.A., O'Dwyer, P.J. & Brose, M.S. (2008). Phase II trial of sorafenib in advanced thyroid cancer. *Journal of Clinical Oncology*, Vol.26, No.29, (October 2008), pp. 4714-4719, ISSN 0732-183X.

Hanahan, D. & Weinberg, R.A. (2000). The hallmarks of cancer. *Cell*, Vol.100, No.1, (January 2000), pp. 57-70, ISSN 0092-8674.

Hemminki, K., Eng, C. & Chen, B. (2005). Familial risks for nonmedullary thyroid cancer. *The Journal of clinical endocrinology and metabolism*. Vol.90, No.10, (October 2005), pp. 5747–5753, ISSN 0021-972X.

Hobert, J.A. & Eng, C. (2009). PTEN hamartoma tumor syndrome: an overview. *Genet Med*, Vol.11, No.10, (October 2009), pp. 687-694, ISSN 1098-3600.

Hoftijzer, H., Heemstra, K.A., Morreau, H., Stokkel, M.P., Corssmit, E.P., Gelderblom, H., Weijers, K., Pereira, A.M., Huijberts, M., Kapiteijn, E., Romijn, J.A. & Smit, J.W. (2009). Beneficial effects of sorafenib on tumor progression, but not on radioiodine uptake, in patients with differentiated thyroid carcinoma. *European journal of endocrinology*, Vol.161, No.6, (December 2009), pp. 923-931, ISSN 0804-464.

Hung, C.J., Ginzinger, D.G., Zarnegar, R., Kanauchi, H., Wong, M.G., Kebebew, E., Clark, O.H. & Duh, Q.Y. (2003). Expression of vascular endothelial growth factor-C in benign and malignant thyroid tumors. *The Journal of clinical endocrinology and metabolism*, Vol.88, No.8, (August 2003), pp. 3694-3699, ISSN 0021-972X.

Ishigaki, K., Namba, H., Nakashima, M., Nakayama, T., Mitsutake, N., Hayashi, T., Maeda, S., Ichinose, M., Kanematsu, T. & Yamashita, S. (2002). Aberrant localization of β-catenin correlates with overexpression of its target gene in human papillary thyroid cancer. *The Journal of clinical endocrinology and metabolism*, Vol.87, No.7, (July 2002), pp. 3433–3440, ISSN 0021-972X.

Ito, T., Seyama, T., Iwamoto, K.S., Hayashi, T., Mizuno, T., Tsuyama, N., Dohi, K., Nakamura, N. & Akiyama, M. (1993). In vitro irradiation is able to cause RET oncogene rearrangement. *Cancer Research*, Vol.53, No.13, (July 1993), pp. 2940-2943, ISSN 0008-5472.

Ito, T., Seyama, T., Iwamoto, K.S., Mizuno, T., Tronko, N.D., Komissarenko, I.V., Cherstovoy, E.D., Satow, Y., Takeichi, N., Dohi, K. & Akiyama, M. (1994). Activated RET oncogene in thyroid cancers of children from areas contaminated by Chernobyl accident. *Lancet*, Vol.344, No.8917, (July 1994), pp. 259, ISSN 0140-6736.

Kato, N., Tsuchiya, T., Tamura, G. & Motoyama, T. (2002). E-cadherin expression in follicular carcinoma of the thyroid. *Pathology International*, Vol.52, No.1, (January 2002), pp. 13–18, ISSN 1320-5463.

Kato, S., Kobayashi, T., Yamada, K., Nishii, K., Sawada, H., Ishiguro, H., Itoh, M., Funahashi, H. & Nagasaka, A. (2004). Expression of erbB receptors mRNA in thyroid tissues. Biochimica et biophysica acta, Vol.1673, No.3, (August 2004), pp. 194-200, ISSN 0006-3002.

Katoh, R., Bray, C.E., Suzuki, K., Komiyama, A., Hemmi, A., Kawaoi, A., Oyama, T., Sugai, T. & Sasou, S. (1995). Growth activity in hyperplastic and neoplastic human thyroid determined by an immunohistochemical staining procedure using monoclonal antibody MIB-1. *Human Pathology*, Vol.26, No.2, (February 1995), pp.139–146, ISSN 0046-8177.

Kim, C.S. & Zhu, Z. (2009). Lessons from mouse models of thyroid cancer. *Thyroid,* Vol.9, No.12, (December 2009), pp.1317-1331, ISSN 1050-7256.

Kim, D.W., Jo, Y.S., Jung, H.S., Chung, H.K., Song, J.H., Park, K.C., Hwang, J.H., Rha, S.Y., Kweon, G.R., Lee, S.J., Jo, K.W. & Shong, M. (2006). An orally administered multitarget tyrosine kinase inhibitor, SU11248, is a novel potent inhibitor of thyroid oncogenic RET/papillary thyroid cancer kinases. *Journal of Clinical Oncology,* Vol.91, No.10, (October 2006), pp. 4070-4076, ISSN 0732-183X.

Kimura, T., van Keymeulen, A., Golstein, J., Fusco, A., Dumont, J.E. & Roger, P.P. (2001). Regulation of thyroid cell proliferation by TSH and other factors: a critical evaluation of in vitro models. *Endocrine Reviews*, Vol.22, No.5, (October 2001), pp. 631-56, ISSN 0163-769X.

Kjellman, P., Wallin, G., Höög, A., Auer, G., Larsson, C. & Zedenius, J. (2003). MIB-1 index in thyroid tumors: a predictor of the clinical course in papillary thyroid carcinoma. *Thyroid*, Vol.13, No.4, (April 2003), pp. 371–380, ISSN 1050-7256.

Kloos, R.T., Ringel, M.D., Knopp, M.V., Hall, N.C., King, M., Stevens, R., Liang, J., Wakely, P.E.Jr, Vasko, V.V., Saji, M., Rittenberry, J., Wei, L., Arbogast, D., Collamore, M., Wright, J.J., Grever, M. & Shah, M.H. (2009). Phase II trial of sorafenib in metastatic thyroid cancer. *Journal of Clinical Oncology*, Vol.27, No.10, (April 2009), pp. 1675-1684, ISSN 0732-183X.

Knauf, J.A., Kuroda, H., Basu, S. & Fagin, J.A. (2003). RET/PTC-induced dedifferentiation of thyroid cells is mediated through Y1062 signaling through SHC-RAS-MAP kinase. *Oncogene*, Vol.22, No.28, (July 2003), pp. 4406-4412, ISSN 0950-9232.

Kondo, T., Ezzat, S. & Asa, S.L. (2006). Pathogenetic mechanisms in thyroid follicular-cell neoplasia. *Nature Reviews. Cancer,* Vol.6, No.4, (April 2006), pp. 292–306, ISSN 1474-175X.

Krohn, K., Führer, D., Bayer, Y., Eszlinger, M., Brauer, V., Neumann, S. & Paschke, R.(2004). Molecular pathogenesis of euthyroid and toxic multinodular goiter. *Endocrine Reviews,* Vol.26, No.4, (June 2005), pp. 504–524, ISSN 0163-769X.

Kroll, T.G., Sarraf, P., Pecciarini, L., Chen, C.J., Mueller, E., Spiegelman, B.M. & Fletcher, J.A. (2000). PAX8–PPARγ1 fusion oncogene in human thyroid carcinoma. *Science,* Vol.289, No.5483, (August 2000), pp. 1357–1360, ISSN 0036-8075.

Lazzereschi, D., Sambuco, L., Carnovale Scalzo, C., Ranieri, A., Mincione, G., Nardi, F. & Colletta, G. (1998). Cyclin D1 and Cyclin E expression in malignant thyroid cells and in human thyroid carcinomas. *International Journal of Cancer,* Vol.76, No.6, (June 1998), pp. 806–811, ISSN 0020-7136.

Li, J., Yen, C., Liaw, D., Podsypanina, K., Bose, S., Wang, S.I., Puc, J., Miliaresis, C., Rodgers, L., McCombie, R., Bigner, S.H., Giovanella, B.C., Ittmann, M., Tycko, B., Hibshoosh, H., Wigler, M.H. & Parsons, R. (1997). PTEN, a putative protein tyrosine phosphatase gene mutated in human brain, breast, and prostate cancer. *Science,* Vol.275, No.5308, (March 1997), pp. 1943-1947, ISSN 0036-8075.

Lindor, N.M. & Greene, M.H. (1998). The concise handbook of family cancer syndromes. Mayo Familial Cancer Program. Journal of the National Cancer Institute, Vol.90, No.14, (July 1998), pp. 1039–1071, ISSN 0027-8874.

Liu, Z., Hou, P., Ji, M., Guan, H., Studeman, K., Jensen, K., Vasko, V., El-Naggar, A.K. & Xing, M. (2008). Highly prevalent genetic alterations in receptor tyrosine kinases and phosphatidylinositol 3-kinase/akt and mitogen-activated protein kinase pathways in anaplastic and follicular thyroid cancers. *The Journal of clinical endocrinology and metabolism,* Vol.93, No.8, (August 2008), pp. 3106-3116, ISSN 0021-972X.

Manning, B.D. & Cantley, L.C. (2007). AKT/PKB signaling: navigating downstream. Cell, *Vol.*129, No.7, (June 2007), pp. 1261-74, ISSN 0092-8674.

Máximo, V., Botelho, T., Capela, J., Soares, P., Lima, J., Taveira, A., Amaro, T., Barbosa, A.P., Preto, A., Harach, H.R., Williams, D. & Sobrinho-Simões, M. (2005). Somatic and germline mutation in GRIM-19, a dual function gene involved in mitochondrial metabolism and cell death, is linked to mitochondrion-rich (Hurthle cell) tumours of the thyroid. *British Journal of Cancer,* Vol.92, No.10, (May 2005), pp. 1892–1898, ISSN 0007-0920.

Medina, D.L. & P. Santisteban. (2000). Thyrotropin-dependent proliferation of in vitro rat thyroid cell systems. *European journal of endocrinology,* Vol.143, No.2, (August 2000),161-78, ISSN 0804-4643.

Miller, F.D. & Kaplan, D.R. (2001). On Trk for retrograde signaling. Neuron, Vol.32, No.5, (December 2001), pp. 767-770, ISSN 0896-6273.

Mitsutake, N., Knauf, J.A., Mitsutake, S., Mesa, C.Jr, Zhang, L. & Fagin, J.A. (2005). Conditional BRAFV600E expression induces DNA synthesis, apoptosis, dedifferentiation, and chromosomal instability in thyroid PCCL3 cells. *Cancer Research,* Vol.65, No.6, (March 2005), pp. 2465–2473, ISSN 0008-5472.

Nappi, T.C., Salerno, P., Zitzelsberger, H., Carlomagno, F., Salvatore, G. & Santoro, M. (2009). Identification of Polo-like kinase 1 as a potential therapeutic target in anaplastic thyroid carcinoma. *Cancer Research*, Vol.69, No.5, (March 2009), pp. 1916-1923, ISSN 0008-5472.

Nikiforov, Y.E., Rowland, J.M., Bove, K.E., Monforte-Munoz, H. & Fagin, J.A. (1997). Distinct pattern of ret oncogene rearrangements in morphological variants of radiation-induced and sporadic thyroid papillary carcinomas in children. *Cancer Research*, Vol.57, No.9, (May 1997), pp. 1690-1694, ISSN 0008-5472.

Nikiforova, M.N., Biddinger, P.W., Caudill, C.M., Kroll, T.G. & Nikiforov, Y.E. (2002). PAX8–PPAR□ rearrangement in thyroid tumors: RT-PCR and immunohistochemical analyses. *The American journal of surgical pathology*, Vol.26, No.8, (August 2002), pp. 1016–1023, ISSN 0147-5185.

Nikiforova, M.N., Kimura, E.T., Gandhi, M., Biddinger, P.W., Knauf, J.A., Basolo, F., Zhu, Z., Giannini, R., Salvatore, G., Fusco, A., Santoro, M., Fagin, J.A. & Nikiforov, Y.E. (2003). BRAF mutations in thyroid tumors are restricted to papillary carcinomas and anaplastic or poorly differentiated carcinomas arising from papillary carcinomas *The Journal of clinical endocrinology and metabolism*, Vol.88, No.11, (November 2003), pp. 5399–5404, ISSN 0021-972X.

Nikiforova, M.N. & Nikiforov, Y.E. (2008a). Molecular genetics of thyroid cancer: implications for diagnosis, treatment and prognosis. *Expert Review of Molecular Diagnostic*, Vol.8, No.1, (January 2008), pp. 83-95, ISSN 1473-7159.

Nikiforova, M.N., Tseng, G.C., Steward, D., Diorio, D. & Nikiforov, Y.E. (2008b). MicroRNA expression profiling of thyroid tumors: biological significance and diagnostic utility. *Journal of Clinical Endocrinology and Metabolism*, Vol.93, No.5, (May 2008), pp. 1600–1608, ISSN 0021-972X.

Pallante, P., Visone, R., Ferracin, M., Ferraro, A., Berlingieri, M.T., Troncone, G., Chiappetta, G., Liu, C.G., Santoro, M., Negrini, M., Croce, C.M. & Fusco, A. (2006). MicroRNA deregulation in human thyroid papillary carcinomas. *Endocrine-Related Cancer*, Vol.13, No.2, (June 2006), pp. 497–508, ISSN 1351-0088.

Parma, J., Duprez, L., Van Sande, J., Cochaux, P., Gervy, C., Mockel, J., Dumont, J. &Vassart, G. (1993). Somatic mutations in the thyrotropin receptor gene cause hyperfunctioning thyroid adenomas. *Nature*, Vol.365, No.6447, (October 1993), pp. 649–651, ISSN 0028-0836.

Peyssonnaux, C. & Eychène, A. (2001). The Raf/MEK/ERK pathway: new concepts of activation. Biology of the cell, Vol.93, No.1-2, (September 2001), pp.53-62, ISSN 0248-4900.

Pierotti, M.A. (2001). Chromosomal rearrangements in thyroid carcinomas: a recombination or death dilemma. *Cancer letters*, Vol.166, No.1, (May 2001), pp. 1-7, ISSN 0304-3835.

Polverino, A., Coxon, A., Starnes, C., Diaz, Z., DeMelfi, T., Wang, L., Bready, J., Estrada, J., Cattley, R., Kaufman, S., Chen, D., Gan, Y., Kumar, G., Meyer, J., Neervannan, S., Alva, G., Talvenheimo, J., Montestruque, S., Tasker, A., Patel, V., Radinsky, R. & Kendall. R. (2006). AMG 706, an oral, multikinase inhibitor that selectively targets vascular endothelial growth factor, platelet-derived growth factor, and kit receptors, potently inhibits angiogenesis and induces regression in tumor xenografts. *Cancer Research*, Vol.66, No.17, (September 2006), pp. 8715-8721, ISSN 0008-5472.

Ravaud, A., de la Fouchardière, C., Courbon, F., Asselineau, J., Klein, M., Nicoli-Sire, P., Bournaud, C., Delord, J., Weryha, G. & Catargi, B. (2008). Sunitinib in patients with refractory advanced thyroid cancer: the THYSU phase II trial. *Journal of Clinical Oncology*, Vol.26, No.15S, (May 2008), pp. 6058, ISSN 0732-183X.

Ricarte-Filho, J.C., Ryder, M., Chitale, D.A., Rivera, M., Heguy, A., Ladanyi, M., Janakiraman, M., Solit, D., Knauf, J.A., Tuttle, R.M., Ghossein, R.A. & Fagin, J.A. (2009). Mutational profile of advanced primary and metastatic radioactive iodine-refractory thyroid cancers reveals distinct pathogenetic roles for BRAF, PIK3CA, and AKT1. *Cancer Research,* Vol.69, No.11, (June 2009), pp. 4885-4893, ISSN 0008-5472.

Ringel, M.D., Hayre, N., Saito, J., Saunier, B., Schuppert, F., Burch, H., Bernet, V., Burman, K.D., Kohn, L.D. & Saji, M. (2001). Overexpression and overactivation of Akt in thyroid carcinoma. *Cancer Research,* Vol.61, No.16, (August 2001), pp. 6105-6111, ISSN 0008-5472.

Rocha, A.S., Soares, P., Fonseca, E., Cameselle-Teijeiro, J., Oliveira, M.C. & Sobrinho-Simões, M. (2003). E-cadherin loss rather than □-catenin alterations is a common feature of poorly differentiated thyroid carcinomas. *Histopathology*, Vol.42, No.6, (June 2003), pp. 580–587, ISSN 0309-0167.

Roger, P.P., van Staveren, W.C., Coulonval, K., Dumont, J.E. & Maenhaut, C. (2009). Signal transduction in the human thyrocyte and its perversion in thyroid tumors. *Molecular and Cellular Endocrinology,* Vol.321, No.1, (May 2010), pp. 3-19, ISSN 0303-7207.

Ron, E. Lubin, J.H., Shore, R.E., Ma buchi, K., Modan, B., Pottern, L.M., Schneider, A.B., Tucker, M.A. & Boice, J.D. Jr. (1995). Thyroid cancer after exposure to external radiation: a pooled analysis of seven studies. *Radiation Research,* Vol.141, No.3, (March 1995), pp. 259–277, ISSN 0033-7587.

Rosai, J., Caracangui, M. & DeLellis, R. (1992) Tumors of the thyroid gland, In: *Atlas of Tumor Pathology*, Eds: Rosai,J. & Sobin, L.H., (3rd series, fascicle), Armed Forces Institute of Pathology, ISBN 9781881041146, Washington DC.

Saavedra, H.I., Knauf, J.A., Shirokawa, J.M., Wang, J., Ouyang, B., Elisei, R., Stambrook, P.J. & Fagin, J.A. (2000). The RAS oncogene induces genomic instability in thyroid PCCL3 cells via the MAPK pathway. *Oncogene,* Vol.19, No.34, (August 2000), pp. 3948–3954, ISSN 0950-9232.

Salvatore, G., De Falco, V., Salerno, P., Nappi, T.C., Pepe, S., Troncone, G., Carlomagno, F., Melillo, R.M., Wilhelm, S.M. & Santoro, M. (2006). BRAF is a therapeutic target in aggressive thyroid carcinoma. Clinical cancer research: an official journal of the American Association for Cancer Research, Vol.12, No.5, (March 2006), pp. 1623-1629, ISSN 1078-0432.

Santarpia, L., El-Naggar, A.K., Cote, G.J., Myers, J.N. & Sherman, S.I. (2007). Phosphatidylinositol 3-kinase/akt and ras/raf-mitogen-activated protein kinase pathway mutations in anaplastic thyroid cancer. *The Journal of clinical endocrinology and metabolism,* Vol.93, No.1, (January 2008), pp. 278-284, ISSN 0021-972X.

Santoro, M., Carlomagno, F., Hay, I.D., Herrmann, M.A., Grieco, M., Melillo, R., Pierotti, M.A., Bongarzone, I., Della Porta, G., Berger, N., Peix, J.L., Paulin, C., Fabien, N.,

Vecchio, G., Jenkins, R.B. & Fusco, A. (1992). Ret oncogene activation in human thyroid neoplasms is restricted to the papillary cancer subtype. The Journal of clinical investigation, Vol.89, No.5, (May 1992), pp. 1517-1522, ISSN 0021-9738.

Santoro, M. & Carlomagno, F. (2006). Drug insight: Small-molecule inhibitors of protein kinases in the treatment of thyroid cancer. *Nature clinical practice. Endocrinology & metabolism*, Vol.2, No.1, (January 2006), pp. 42–52, ISSN 1745-8366.

Schlumberger, M., Elisei, R., Bastholt, L., Wirth, L.J., Martins, R.G., Locati, L.D., Jarzab, B., Pacini, F., Daumerie, C., Droz, J.P., Eschenberg, M.J., Sun, Y.N., Juan, T., Stepan, D.E. & Sherman, S.I. (2009). Phase II study of safety and efficacy of motesanib in patients with progressive or symptomatic, advanced or metastatic medullary thyroid cancer. *Journal of Clinical Oncology*, Vol.27, No.23, (August 2009), pp. 3794-3801, ISSN 0732-183X.

Shayesteh, L., Lu, Y., WL Kuo, W.L., Baldocchi, R., Godfrey, T., Collins, C., Pinkel, D., Powell, B., Mills, G.B. & Gray, J.W. (1999). PIK3CA is implicated as an oncogene in ovarian cancer. *Nature Genetics*, Vol.21, No.1, (January 1999), pp. 99-102, ISSN 1061-4036.

Sherman, S.I. (2003). Thyroid carcinoma. *Lancet*, Vol.361, No.9356, (February 2003), pp. 501-511, ISSN 0140-6736.

Sherman, S.I. (2008a). Early clinical studies of novel therapies for thyroid cancers. *Endocrinology and metabolism clinics of North America*, Vol.37, No.2, (June 2008), pp. 511–524, ISSN 0889-8529.

Sherman, S.I., Wirth, L.J., Droz, J.P., Hofmann, M., Bastholt, L., Martins, R.G., Licitra, L., Eschenberg, M.J., Sun, Y.N., Juan, T., Stepan, D.E., Schlumberger, M.J., Motesanib Thyroid Cancer Study Group. (2008b). Motesanib di-phosphate in progressive differentiated thyroid cancer. *New England Journal of Medicine*, Vol.359, No.1, (July 2008b), pp. 31-42, ISSN 0028-4793.

Sherman, S.I. (2009). Advances in chemotherapy of differentiated epithelial and medullary thyroid cancers. *The Journal of clinical endocrinology and metabolism*, Vol.94, No.5, (May 2009), pp. 1493-1499, ISSN 0021-972X.

Shi, Y., Zou, M., Farid, N.R. & al-Sedairy, S.T. (1996). Evidence of gene deletion of p21WAF1/CIP1, a cyclin dependent protein kinase inhibitor, in thyroid carcinomas. *British Journal of Cancer*, Vol.74, No.9, (November 1996), pp. 1336–1341, ISSN 0007-0920.

Shields, J.M., Pruitt, K., McFall, A., Shaub, A. & Der, C.J. (2000). Understanding Ras: 'it ain't over 'til it's over'. *Trends in Cell Biology*, Vol.10, No.4, (April 2000), pp. 147-54, ISSN 0962-8924.

Shirokawa, J.M., Elisei, R., Knauf, J.A., Hara, T., Wang, J., Saavedra, H.I. & Fagin, J.A. (2000) Conditional apoptosis induced by oncogenic ras in thyroid cells. Molecular Endocrinology Vol.14, No.11, (November 2000), pp. 1725–1738, ISSN 0888-8809.

Smallridge, R., Marlow, L. & Copland, J. (2009). Anaplastic thyroid cancer: molecular pathogenesis and emerging therapies. *Endocrine-Related Cancer*, Vol.161, No.6, (December 2009), pp. 17–44, ISSN 1351-0088.

Sorrentino, R., Libertini, S., Pallante, P.L., Troncone, G., Palombini, L., Bavetsias, V., Spalletti-Cernia, D., Laccetti, P., Linardopoulos, S., Chieffi, P., Fusco, A. & Portella, G. (2004). Aurora B overexpression associates with the thyroid carcinoma undifferentiated phenotype and is required for thyroid carcinoma cell proliferation. *The Journal of clinical endocrinology and metabolism*, Vol.90, No.2, (February 2005), pp. 928–935, ISSN 0021-972X.

St Bernard, R., Zheng, L., Liu, W., Winer, D., Asa, S.L. & Ezzat, S. (2004). Fibroblast growth factor receptors as molecular targets in thyroid carcinoma. *Endocrinology*, Vol.146, No.3, (March 2005), pp. 1145-1153, ISSN 0013-7227.

Stambolic, V., Suzuki, A., de la Pompa, J.L., Brothers, G.M., Mirtsos, C., Sasaki, T., Ruland, J., Penninger, J.M., Siderovski, D.P., Mak, T.W. (1998). Negative regulation of PKB/Akt-dependent cell survival by the tumor suppressor PTEN. *Cell*, Vol.95, No.1, (October 1998), pp. 29-39, ISSN 0092-8674.

Stojadinovic, A., Ghossein, R., Hoos, A., Urist, M.J., Spiro, R.H., Shah, J.P., Brennan, M.F., Shaha, A.R. & Singh, B. (2001). Hürthle cell carcinoma: a critical histopathological appraisal. *Journal of Clinical Oncology*, Vol.19, No.10, (May 2001), pp. 2616-2625, ISSN 0732-183X.

Takakura, S., Mitsutake, N., Nakashima, M., Namba, H., Saenko, V.A., Rogounovitch, T.I., Nakazawa, Y., Hayashi, T., Ohtsuru, A. & Yamashita, S. (2008). Oncogenic role of miR-17-92 cluster in anaplastic thyroid cancer cells. *Cancer Science*, Vol.99, No.6, (June 2008), pp. 1147–1154, ISSN 1347-9032.

Tsygankova, O.M., Kupperman, E., Wen, W. & Meinkoth, J.L. (2000). Cyclic AMP activates Ras. *Oncogene*, Vol.19, No.32, (July 2000), pp. 3609–3615, ISSN 0950-9232.

Van der Laan, B.F., Freeman, J.L. & Asa, S.L. (1995). Expression of growth factors and growth factor receptors in normal and tumorous human thyroid tissues. Thyroid Vol.5, No.1, (Febrary 1995), pp. 67–73, ISSN 1050-7256.

Vanhaesebroeck, B. & Waterfield, M.D. (1999). Signaling by distinct classes of phosphoinositide 3-kinases. *Experimental Cell Research*, Vol.253, No.1, (November 1999), pp. 239-254, ISSN 0014-4827.

Vasko, V., Ferrand, M., Di Cristofaro, J., Carayon, P., Henry, J.F. & de Micco, C. (2003). Specific pattern of RAS oncogene mutations in follicular thyroid tumor. *The Journal of clinical endocrinology and metabolism*, Vol.88, No.6, (June 2003), pp. 2745-2752, ISSN 0021-972X.

Vasko, V., Saji, M., Hardy, E., Kruhlak, M., Larin, A., Savchenko, V., Miyakawa, M., Isozaki, O., Murakami, H., Tsushima, T., Burman, K.D., De Micco, C. & Ringel, M.D. (2004). Akt activation and localisation correlate with tumour invasion and oncogene expression in thyroid cancer. *Journal of Medical Genetics*, Vol.41, No.3, (March 2004), pp. 161-170, ISSN 0022-2593.

Vassart, G. & Dumont, J.E. (1992). The thyrotropin receptor and the regulation of thyrocyte function and growth. *Endocrine Reviews*, Vol.13, No.3, (August 1992), pp. 596-611, ISSN 0163-769X.

Visone, R., Russo, L., Pallante, P., De Martino, I., Ferraro, A., Leone, V., Borbone, E., Petrocca, F., Alder, H., Croce, C.M. & Fusco, A. (2007a). MicroRNAs (miR)-221 and miR-222, both overexpressed in human thyroid papillary carcinomas, regulate p27Kip1 protein levels and cell cycle. *Endocrine-Related Cancer,* Vol.14, No.3, (September 2007), pp. 791–798, ISSN 1351-0088.

Visone, R., Pallante, P., Vecchione, A., Cirombella, R., Ferracin, M., Ferraro, A., Volinia, S., Coluzzi, S., Leone, V., Borbone, E., Liu, C.G., Petrocca, F., Troncone, G., Calin, G.A., Scarpa, A., Colato, C.,Tallini, G., Santoro, M., Croce, C.M. & Fusco, A. (2007b). Specific microRNAs are downregulated in human thyroid anaplastic carcinomas. *Oncogene,* Vol.26, No.54, (November 2007), pp. 7590–7595, ISSN 0950-9232.

Vogt, P.K., Kang, S., Elsliger, M.A. & Gymnopoulos, M. (2007). Cancer-specific mutations in phosphatidylinositol 3-kinase. *Trends in biochemical sciences,* Vol.32, No.7, (July 2007), pp. 342-349, ISSN 0968-0004.

Volante, M., Croce, S., Pecchioni, C. & Papotti, M. (2002). E2F-1 transcription factor is overexpressed in oxyphilic thyroid tumors. *Mod Pathol,* Vol.15, No.10, (October 2002), pp. 1038–1043, ISSN 0893-3952.

Wada, N., Yoshida, A., Miyagi, Y., Yamamoto, T., Nakayama, H., Suganuma, N., Matsuzu, K., Masudo, K., Hirakawa, S., Rino, Y., Masuda, M. & Imada, T. (2008). Overexpression of the mitotic spindle assembly checkpoint genes hBUB1, hBUBR1 and hMAD2 in thyroid carcinomas with aggressive nature. *Anticancer Research,* Vol.28, No.1A, (January-February 2008), pp. 139–144, ISSN 0250-7005.

Wang, Y., Hou, P., Yu, H., Wang, W., Ji, M., Zhao, S., Yan, S., Sun, X., Liu, D., Shi, B., Zhu, G., Condouris, S. & Xing, M. (2007). High prevalence and mutual exclusivity of genetic alterations in the phosphatidylinositol-3-kinase/akt pathway in thyroid tumors. *The Journal of clinical endocrinology and metabolism,* Vol.92, No.7, (June 2007), pp. 2387–2390, ISSN 0021-972X.

Weber, F., Teresi, R.E., Broelsch, C.E., Frilling, A. & Eng, C. (2006). A limited set of human microRNA is deregulated in follicular thyroid carcinoma. *Journal of Clinical Endocrinology and Metabolism,* Vol.91, No.9, (September 2006), pp. 3584–3591, ISSN 0021-972X.

Weinstein, I.B. & Joe, A. (2008). Oncogene addiction. *Cancer Research,* Vol.68, No.9, (May 2008), pp. 3077-80, ISSN 0008-5472.

Wilhelm, S.M., Carter, C., Tang, L., Wilkie, D., McNabola, A., Rong, H., Chen, C., Zhang, X., Vincent, P., McHugh, M., Cao, Y., Shujath, J., Gawlak, S., Eveleigh, D., Rowley, B., Liu, L., Adnane, L., Lynch, M., Auclair, D., Taylor, I., Gedrich, R., Voznesensky, A., Riedl, B., Post, L.E., Bollag, G. & Trail, P.A. (2004). BAY 43-9006 exhibits broad spectrum oral antitumor activity and targets the RAF/MEK/ERK pathway and receptor tyrosine kinases involved in tumor progression and angiogenesis. *Cancer Research,* Vol.64, No.19, (October 2004), pp. 7099-7109, ISSN 0008-5472.

Xing, M. (2005). BRAF mutation in thyroid cancer. *Endocrine-related cancer,* Vol.12, No.2, (June 2005), pp. 245–262, ISSN 1351-0088.

Xing, M. (2008). Recent advances in molecular biology of thyroid cancer and their clinical implications. *Otolaryngologic Clinics of North America,* Vol.41, No.6, (December 2008), pp. 1135-1146, ISSN 0030-6665.

Yamashita, H., Noguchi, S., Murakami, N., Kato, R., Adachi, M., Inoue, S., Kato, S. & Nkayama, I. (2008). Effects of dietary iodine on chemical induction of thyroid carcinoma. *Acta Pathologica Japonica,* Vol. 40, No.10, (October 1990), pp. 705–712, ISSN 0001-6632.

Yeh, J.J., Lunetta, K.L., van Orsouw, N.J., Moore, F.D., Mutter, G.L., Vijg, J., Dahia, P.L. & Eng, C. (2000). Somatic mitochondrial DNA (mtDNA) mutations in papillary thyroid carcinomas and differential mtDNA sequence variants in cases with thyroid tumours. *Oncogene,* Vol.19, No.16, (April 2000), pp. 2060–2066, ISSN 0950-9232.

9

Diagnosis and Differential Diagnosis of Medullary Thyroid Cancer

Antongiulio Faggiano, Valeria Ramundo,
Gaetano Lombardi and Annamaria Colao
Department of Molecular and Clinical Endocrinology and Oncology,
"Federico II" University of Naples
Italy

1. Introduction

Medullary thyroid cancer (MTC) occurs in less than 1% of thyroid nodules and accounts for 5-10% of thyroid malignancies. It is a well-differentiated neuroendocrine carcinoma arising from parafollicular calcitonin-producing cells (C-cells) of the thyroid gland and is associated with elevated serum calcitonin levels. Among well-differentiated thyroid carcinomas, MTC is the most aggressive, with survival rates of 40-50% at 10 years (American Thyroid Association [ATA] Guidelines Task Force et al., 2009; Leboulleux et al., 2004). In about 20-25% of cases, MTC can be part of an autosomal dominant inherited cancer syndrome called Multiple Endocrine Neoplasia type 2 (MEN2), caused by activating germline mutations of the *RET* proto-oncogene, where this tumor is isolated (Familial MTC - FMTC) or is associated to other tumors (parathyroid adenoma, pheochromocytoma and cutaneous lichen amyloidosis in MEN2A; pheochromocytoma, mucosal and intestinal ganglioneuromatosis, marfanoid habitus in MEN2B). In the remaining 75-80% of cases MTC is sporadic (ATA Guidelines Task Force et al., 2009; Brandi et al., 2001; Leboulleux et al., 2004). Depending on the type of the genetic syndrome, clinical features, therapeutic approaches and prognosis of MTC are very different (Brandi et al., 2001).
Calcitonin is a small peptide secreted by C-cells. It is the most specific and sensitive marker of MTC in patients with one or more thyroid nodules, useful in the diagnosis and follow-up of this tumor (ATA Guidelines Task Force et al., 2009; Leboulleux et al., 2004). High serum calcitonin levels are physiological in neonates, followed by an age-related decline from birth to about 1 year of age (Leboulleux et al., 2004). Elevated basal serum calcitonin levels are found in subjects with C-cells hyperplasia (CCH) or MTC. Anyway, in some cases it is possible to observe false positive or false negative for serum calcitonin levels in adult individuals.
After excluding conditions that may cause falsely positive high levels of calcitonin, it is necessary to exclude tumors associated to ectopic production of calcitonin, which may represent up to 15% of cases (Pacini et al., 2010; Toledo et al., 2009).
Another tumor marker used in the follow-up of MTC is carcino-embryonic antigen (CEA), a cytosolic enzyme which is not a specific biomarker for MTC being generally expressed by many endocrine and non-endocrine tumors. In MTC, CEA is considered to have lower diagnostic accuracy than calcitonin (Meijer et al., 2010). There is no close relationship

between serum levels of CEA, that are normal in patients with early stage MTC, and calcitonin.

Pentagastrin stimulation test for calcitonin is the most widely used test for calcitonin secretion, useful to distinguish normal C-cells from pathological C-cells (Leboulleux et al., 2004; Milone et al., 2010; Pacini et al., 2010).

CCH and early-stage MTC are often difficult to distinguish on routine biochemical and histological examination. This differentiation is very important for therapy and for prognosis.

If the diagnosis of MTC needs to be always confirmed by histology, by a clinical and biochemical point of view, pentagastrin stimulation test, immunocytochemistry for calcitonin and calcitonin measurement in wash-out fluid from fine-needle aspiration of suspicious thyroid nodules may reliably indicate this diagnosis.

Primary treatment of both hereditary and sporadic MTC is total thyroidectomy with lymph node dissection, with the intention of remove all neoplastic tissue present in the neck (Leboulleux et al., 2004).

The postoperative follow-up of patients with MTC should be performed to early identify recovery or persistence/relapse of MTC in patients with elevated concentrations of biochemical markers after surgery.

1.1 Embryogenesis of C-cells and pathogenesis of MTC

Parafollicular calcitonin-producing cells (C-cells) arise from the neural crest and have a common origin with the adrenal medullary chromaffin cells, enterochromaffin cells, pituitary corticotrophs and melanotrophs, and islet cells. This entire series of cells was included under the descriptive term APUD cells by Pearse (Hazard, 1977). During the embryonic life C-cells migrate forward into the thyroid gland. The thyroid should be looked upon as a double gland with two separate types of peptide-producing cells. C-cells account less than 1% of thyroid cells, are located inside the thyroid follicles and are most numerous at the junction of the upper third and the lower two-thirds of the thyroid lobes (Leboulleux et al., 2004).

Thyroid C-cells differ from solid cell nests (SCN) of the thyroid gland. They are two thyroid specific cell type with a common embryological origin in the ultimobranchial body but with different physiological roles. SCN are found in about 5-60% of human thyroid gland and comprise compact spindle or polygonal cells with a strong and diffuse immunostaining for cytokeratin, galectin-3 (GAL-3) and CEA and rarely for calcitonin. In contrast, normal and hyperplastic C-cells express both calcitonin and CEA but not GAL-3 while malignant C-cells forming MTC are positive for calcitonin, CEA and GAL-3 immunostaining. SCN are often found in both normal and pathological thyroid tissue and they are not related to the presence of thyroid disorder (Faggiano et al., 2003).

GAL-3 is a β-galactoside-binding protein, localized predominantly in the cytoplasm, that plays a role in various processes such as cell adhesion, growth and neoplastic transformation. In epithelial thyroid tumors, GAL-3 immunostaining is positive in malignant tumors but negative in benign lesions. GAL-3 immunostaining is also a reliable marker of malignancy in patients with C-cells disease and its use may have clinically relevant prognostic and therapeutic implications (Faggiano et al., 2002) (Figure 1).

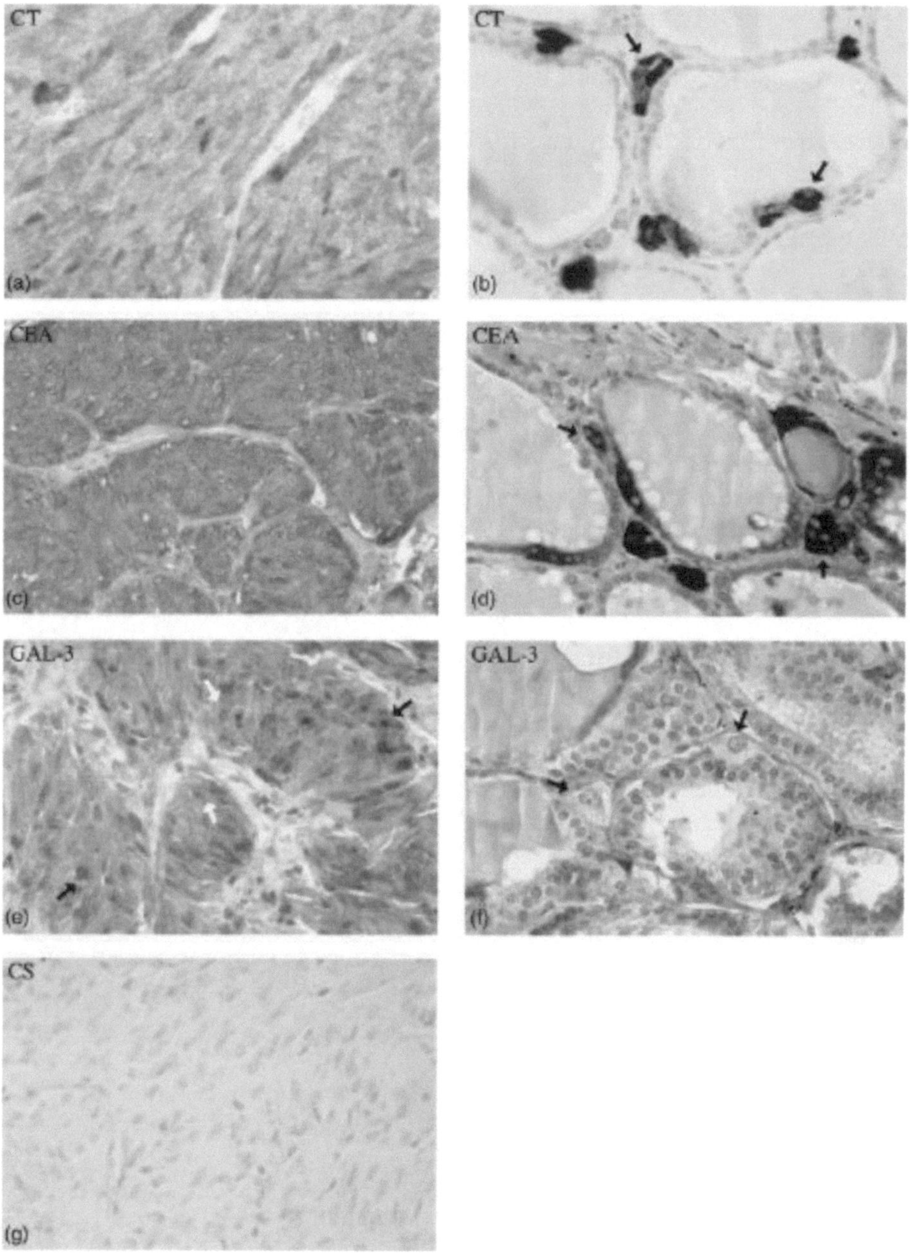

Fig. 1. Expression of calcitonin (CT), CEA and GAL-3 in medullary thyroid cancer (MTC) and C-cells hyperplasia (CCH). Photos a, c, e, g represent a MTC case: CT, CEA and GAL-3 are diffusely expressed in tumor tissue at the cytoplasmatic level. Some tumor cells also display GAL-3 positivity at the nuclear level (black arrows). The specificity of anti-GAL-3 antibodies is demonstrated by negativity in control sections (CS) of the same tumor. Photos b, d, f represent a CCH case: CT and CEA are strongly positive and GAL-3 is negative in large C-cells (from Faggiano et al., 2002).

CCH is defined as the presence of at least three fields containing more than or equal 50 C-cells in a single low-power field (magnification of x 100) (Santesanio et al., 1997). The prototypic histologic features of MTC are sheets, packets or irregular islands of polygonal or plump spindly cells traversed by small fibrovascular septa (Hazard, 1997). MTC is defined by the presence of fibrous and/or amyloid stroma between C-cells, infiltration of interstitial tissue by C-cells and coalescence of hyperplastic C-cells nodules (Faggiano et al., 2002; Faggiano et al., 2003).

MTC cells typically produce an early biochemical signal that consists of hypersecretion of calcitonin. Calcitonin and CEA are expressed in hyperplastic and malignant C-cells (Leboulleux et al., 2004).

In all CCH and MTC there is a positive immunohistochemical staining for calcitonin and CEA. Mixed MTC are uncommon and are characterized by the combination of C-cells and follicular features (Leboulleux et al., 2004).

Sporadic C-cells hyperplasia differs from C-cells hyperplasia associated to hereditary MTC syndromes. While the first one, in fact, is usually benign and associated with much less, is any, malignant potential, the latter is generally considered a precancerous condition in the familial MTC where there is a progression from normal C-cells to CCH, micro-MTC and clinical MTC (Leboulleux et al., 2004; Milone et al., 2010; Perry et al., 1996). Sporadic MTC is usually unifocal and represented by a unique tumor nodule while familial MTC appears bilateral and multicentric, often with multifocal disease in a background of CCH. In fact, all patients with hereditary MTC virtually presented CCH (Leboulleux et al., 2004).

There are two different types of CCH: physiologic or reactive, where the number of follicles with one or more C-cells is increased, associated with inflammatory and metabolic disorders and classically with a chronic lymphocytic thyroiditis, and nodular or neoplastic, characterized by an increased number of C-cells aggregates, frequent in tumors. Physiologic CCH cannot be recognized with certainty on routine histological sections and has to be diagnosed with the help of immunostains. On the other hand, nodular or neoplastic CCH can be identified with conventional histological sections because the C-cells are large, mildly to moderately atypical and cytologically indistinguishable from those of invasive MTC, resulting in a partial or complete replacement of the follicle (Albores-Saavedra & Krueger, 2001; Perry et al., 1996).

1.1.1 Hereditary MTC syndrome

Hereditary MTC syndrome (MEN2 - multiple endocrine neoplasia type 2 or Sipple's syndrome) is an autosomal disorder characterized by activating germline mutations of the *RET* proto-oncogene, with a prevalence of 1:30,000 subjects (Brandi et al., 2001). It is divided in three clinical variants: a) MEN2A (medullary thyroid cancer, mono- or bilateral pheochromocytoma, primary hyperparathyroidism and cutaneous lichen amyloidosis); b) familial medullary thyroid cancer (FMTC); c) MEN2B (medullary thyroid cancer, mono- or bilateral pheochromocytoma, mucosal and intestinal ganglioneuromatosis, marfanoid habitus) (Brandi et al., 2001; Raue & Frank-Raue, 2007). Although these variants have MTC as a common denominator, they differ for the aggressiveness of this cancer, in a decreasing order MEN2B>MEN2A>FMTC (Raue & Frank-Raue, 2007).

In patients with FMTC, MTC is the only clinical manifestation. According to the "International *RET* Mutation Consostium", to make the diagnosis of FMTC is required the onset of MTC in at least four family members (Mulligan et al., 1995).

Patients affected with hereditary MTC syndrome initially develop CCH that then progresses to early invasive medullary microcarcinoma, and eventually develop invasive macroscopic MTC (ATA Guidelines Task Force et al., 2009).
MEN2 has a genotype-phenotype correlation. In fact, an association between specific mutations of the *RET* gene and the age at onset, the aggressiveness of MTC and the presence of other endocrine disorders is well documented. The *RET* mutation screening allows to stratify the risk in three levels, depending on the mutated codon. The specifically mutated *RET* codons correlate with the MEN2 variant, with the age at onset and the aggressiveness of thyroid cancer. MTC generally occurs in the first year of age in subjects with MEN2B, between 5 and 25 years in subjects with MEN2A and later in subjects with FMTC. In patients with MEN2, the therapeutic approach is correlated to the clinical subtype and to the mutation, according to the risk levels (Brandi et al., 2001) (Table 1).

Risk level	Domain	Codons	MEN2 variant
1 (Low)	Extracellular	609	MEN2A
	Intracellular	768, 790, 791, 804	FMTC
	Intracellular	891	MEN2A
2 (High)	Extracellular	611, 618, 620, 630, 634	MEN2A
3 (Very high)	Intracellular	883, 918, 922	MEN2B

Table 1. Risk levels in MEN2 syndrome.

Subjects with the highest risk level (3) have the most aggressive MTC and should have thyroidectomy with a central node dissection within the first six months of life and preferably within the first month of life. In subjects classified as risk 2 level, thyroidectomy with removal of the posterior capsule should be performed before the age of five years. For subjects with the lowest risk level (1) at this moment there are differing opinions on when thyroidectomy should be performed. According to some authors, in fact, total thyroidectomy with lymph node dissection of the central compartment should be practiced within the fifth year of life, according to others such intervention should be performed later, but within the tenth year of life. Other authors finally suggest to periodically perform the pentagastrin stimulation test for calcitonin and to perform the surgery at the first positive test. In all cases, if a pheochromocytoma is present, total thyroidectomy should be performed after surrenectomy to avoid a catecholaminergic crisis during the surgery (Brandi et al., 2001).

1.2 Diagnosis of MTC in patients with the suspicion of MTC

Thyroid tumors are the most common endocrine neoplasms. Most of thyroid nodules are benign but in the 5-10% of cases they are carcinomas. MTC occurs in less than 1% of thyroid nodules and accounts for 5-10% of thyroid malignancies (Schlumberger et al., 2003).
Sporadic MTC can arise clinically at any age but its incidence peaks during the fourth and sixth decades of life (Leboulleux et al., 2004).

The suspicion of MTC arises in a patient with one or more thyroid nodules associated with elevated basal calcitonin levels (> 10 pg/ml), with or without a familial history of MTC.
In the presence of a thyroid nodule, several clinical features may prompt to suspect a MTC: its location in the upper third of the thyroid lobe, pain during the thyroid palpation, a diarrhoeal syndrome and flushing that are more frequent in patients with a large tumor burden. At the ultrasonography, MTC usually appears as a hypoechogenic solid nodule with frequent microcalcifications, with or without lymph node abnormalities (Leboulleux et al., 2004).
High serum calcitonin levels are physiological in neonates, followed by an age-related decline from birth to about 1 year of age (Leboulleux et al., 2004). Elevated basal serum calcitonin levels are found in subjects with CCH or MTC. Anyway, in some cases it is possible to observe false positive for high serum calcitonin levels in adult individuals. Conditions related to high calcitonin levels are: severe chronic renal failure and dialysis, chronic hypercalcemia, therapies with proton-pump inhibitors or other drugs, chronic hypergastrinemia, pernicious anemia, hepatic cirrhosis, auto-immune thyroid disorders or follicular tumor, hyperthyroidism, hyperparathyroidism and pseudo-hypoparathyroidism, systemic inflammatory state, pregnancy and lactation. Furthermore, calcitonin assays can be falsely positive because of interference with circulating heterophilic antibodies binding (Leboulleux et al., 2004; Pacini et al., 2010). Calcitonin levels are also correlated with age and BMI (especially in men) and cigarette smoking can increase the plasma concentration of calcitonin (van Veelen et al., 2009) (Table 2). False negative for calcitonin serum concentrations are also possible and are related to the "hook effect" (Leboeuf et al., 2006).

Non-thyroid diseases	**Thyroid diseases**	**Drugs**	**Physiological conditions**
Hypergastrinemia	Auto-immune thyroiditis	Proton-pump inhibitors	Age
Hyperparathyroidism	Hyperthyroidism	Glucocorticoids	BMI
Pseudohypoparathyroidism	Thyroid carcinoma	Beta-blockers	Sex
Chronic renal failure		Glucagon	Physical activity
Pernicious anemia			Pregnancy
Hepatic cirrhosis		Smoking	Lactation
Inflammatory state			
Neuroendocrine tumors			
Pheochromocytoma			
Paraganglioma			
Breast cancer			
Enteropancreatic tumors			
Small cell lung carcinoma			

Table 2. Conditions associated to high serum calcitonin levels independently of medullary thyroid carcinoma.

MTC may also express a number of genes usually not expressed or expressed at low levels in the normal C-cells. The protein products of these genes include somatostatin, pro-opiomelanocortin, vasointestinal active peptide, serotonin, prostaglandins and others and they can produce clinical syndromes including Cushing's disease, flushing or diarrhoea. Chromogranin-A levels may also be elevated in the presence of large metastases (Leboulleux et al., 2004).

Diagnosis of MTC is based on typical histological characteristics (tumor cells arranged in trabecular, insular or sheet-like patterns with or without stromal amyloid deposits) and immunohistochemical findings (positive staining for calcitonin, CEA and chromogranin and negative staining for thyroglobulin) (Costante et al., 2007). Anyway, pentagastrin stimulation test, immunocytochemistry for calcitonin and calcitonin measurement in wash-out fluid from fine-needle aspiration of thyroid nodules are suggestive.

The primary treatment of both hereditary and sporadic MTC is total thyroidectomy with lymph node dissection, with the intention of remove all neoplastic tissue present in the neck. Surgery should be performed after careful exclusion of pheochromocytoma (Leboulleux et al., 2004). Classification of MTC is based on the pathological tumor node metastases (TNM) system (Table 3).

T (primary tumor)	**Tx:** Primay tumor cannot be assessed **T0:** No evidence of primary tumor **T1:** Tumor size ≤ 2 cm and no growth out of the thyroid **T1a:** Tumor size < 1 cm and no growth out of the thyroid **T1b:** Tumor size between 1 and 2 cm and no growth out of the thyroid **T2:** Tumor size between 2 and 4 cm and no growth out of the thyroid **T3:** Tumor size ≥ 4 cm or small growth out of the thyroid **T4a:** Tumor of any size with extensive growth beyond the thyroid gland into nearby tissues of the neck (Moderately advanced disease) **T4b:** Tumor of any size with either back toward the spine or into nearby large blood vessels (Very advanced disease)
N (regional lymph node metastases)	**Nx:** Regional lymph nodes cannot be assessed **N0:** No evidence of regional lymph nodes **N1:** The cancer has spread to nearby lymph nodes **N1a:** The cancer has spread to lymph nodes around the thyroid **N1b:** The cancer has spread to other lymph nodes in the neck or behind the throat or in the upper chest
M (distant metastases)	**Mx:** Distant metastases cannot be assessed **M0:** No evidence of distant metastases **M1:** Evidence of distant metastases

Table 3. TNM system for medullary thyroid cancer (MTC).

A diagnosis of MTC in an early and therefore potentially surgically eradicable and higher curable stage of disease is essential to improve the prognosis of this tumor (Pacini et al., 1994).

In patients with non-metastatic MTC, survival rates amount about 78-100% at 5-year and 75% at 10-year, respectively. Survival rates strongly decrease in case of metastatic disease and amount about 24% at 5-year and 10% at 10-year respectively (Kapiteijn et al., 2011).

1.3 Usefulness of pentagastrin stimulation test for diagnosis of MTC and differential diagnosis between subjects affected by C-cells proliferation and normal subjects and between CCH and MTC

Pentagastrin stimulation test for calcitonin is the most widely used test for calcitonin secretion, useful to distinguish normal C-cells from pathological C-cells (Leboulleux et al., 2004; Milone et al., 2010; Pacini et al., 2010). This test is performed in case of borderline serum calcitonin levels or in case of high serum calcitonin levels but less than 100 pg/ml. After overnight fasting, basal serum calcitonin is measured and then the patient receives a slow intravenous injection of 0.5 µg pentagastrin per Kg body weight and calcitonin is measured again 3 and 5 minutes after the injection.

Serum calcitonin concentrations are helpful in the early detection of C-cells disease but it is still unclear whether they can be used also for the preoperative differential diagnosis between CCH and MTC on the basis of the calcitonin peak after pentagastrin stimulation test. Few studies have been performed to preoperatively discriminate between CCH and MTC but they show high variability in the calcitonin cut-offs after pentagastrin test to discriminate between CCH and MTC. A calcitonin cut-off after pentagastrin stimulation test corresponding to about 300 pg/ml seems to be highly predictive in preoperatively distinguishing CCH from MTC (Figure 2). In the clinical practice, this finding may need to perform surgery in patients with calcitonin levels higher than these after pentagastrin stimulation test and to submit a periodical re-evaluation with the stimulation test and neck ultrasonography in those patients with calcitonin levels between about 100 and 300 pg/ml (Milone et al., 2010).

The pentagastrin stimulation test is contraindicated during pregnancy and in patients with asthma, coronary disease, severe hypertension or duodenal ulcer. Side-effects include dizziness, tachycardia/bradycardia, nausea and substernal tightness (Leboulleux et al., 2004; Pacini et al., 2010).

1.4 Differential diagnosis between CCH/MTC and ectopic calcitonin secretion

In about 15% of cases high levels of calcitonin are associated to ectopic production by tumors. Neuroendocrine tumors arising from gastro-entero-pancreatic tract (gastrinoma, VIPoma, insulinoma, etc.), respiratory tract (lung, bronchus), breast , medulla of adrenal gland and paraganglia may be associated with elevated serum calcitonin levels, even in cases where there is a negative immunohistochemistry reaction for calcitonin (Pacini et al., 2010; Toledo et al., 2009) (Table 2).

Considering false positive causes of increased serum calcitonin levels and the above mentioned tumors associated with ectopic secretion of this marker, it is not surprising that hypercalcitoninemia could result sometimes in erroneous recommendations of total thyroidectomy. Therefore, in order to avoid misdiagnosis and unnecessary thyroid surgery, it is mandatory to conduct correct investigations in cases with elevated basal serum calcitonin levels in order to rule out possible diagnosis different from MTC (Toledo et al., 2009).

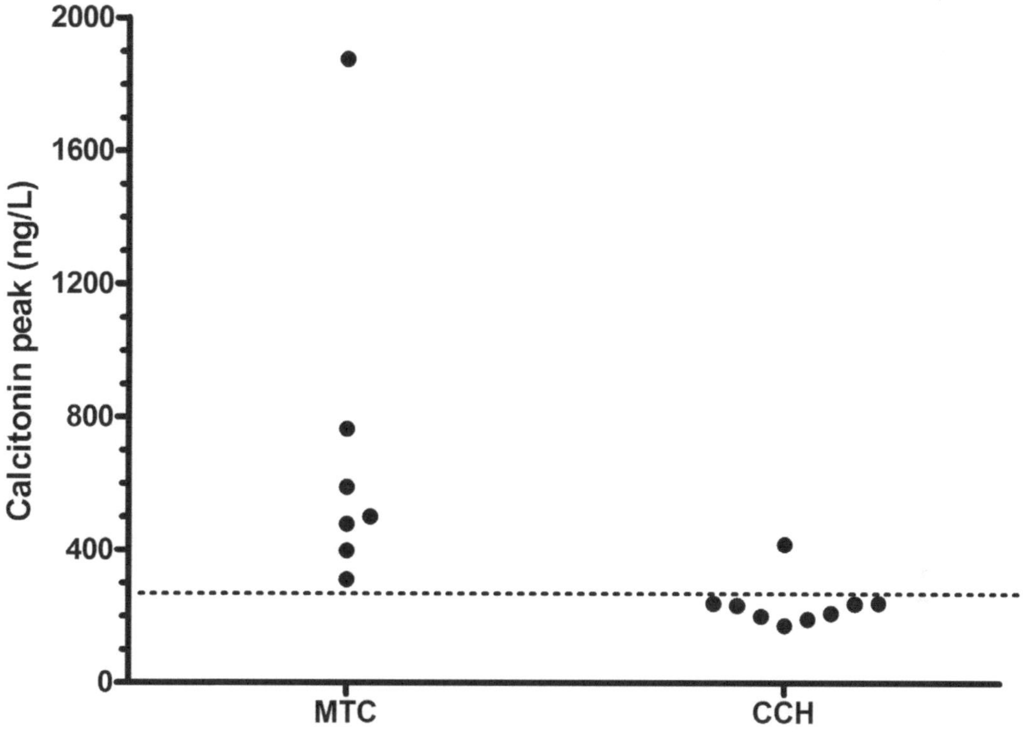

Fig. 2. Calcitonin peak after pentagastrin stimulation test performed before surgery to preoperatively distinguish C cell hyperplasia (CCH) and medullary thyroid cancer (MTC) (from Milone et al., 2010).

1.5 Usefulness of fine-needle cytology (FNC) to preoperatively recognize a MTC

Fine-needle aspiration cytology (FNC) represents the main tool in the diagnostic evaluation of thyroid nodules, but it is not frequently proposed as a routine procedure in patients with high serum calcitonin levels, due to its low specificity and sensitivity (Boi et al., 2007).
Routine measurement of calcitonin in nodular thyroid disease is a specific and sensitive method to improve the early preoperative diagnosis of unsuspected sporadic MTC with better accuracy than routine FNC. Serum calcitonin is also more sensitive than FNC in the pre-operative diagnosis of MTC (Elisei et al., 2004). Serum calcitonin is the most sensitive and accurate diagnostic tool for MTC, but it is not helpful to localize primary tumor in the thyroid and its neck recurrence or metastases in patients submitted to thyroidectomy (Boi et al., 2007). Immunohistochemistry with anti-calcitonin antibodies improves the diagnostic sensitivity of FNC. Anyway, this procedure is only performed when there is a strong suspicion of MTC and not on routine basis. On this basis, serum calcitonin should be measured routinely in the clinical work-up of thyroid nodules, followed by a pentagastrin stimulation test in all cases of detectable basal calcitonin levels (Elisei et al., 2004). Increasing the diagnostic accuracy could help the surgeon to perform more radical treatment of MTC, thus achieving frequent normalization of postoperative serum calcitonin levels. Anyway, whether this results indicates definitive cure remains to be established on the basis of longer follow-up (Pacini et al., 1994).

Assaying calcitonin in the wash-out fluid and immunohistochemistry for calcitonin from FNC under ultrasonographic guidance could be useful in the preoperative diagnosis of MTC.
There are several studies that aimed to evaluate the usefulness of calcitonin assay in the wash-out from FNC, alone or combined with cytology in the pre-surgical evaluation of MTC patients with thyroid nodules. Anyway, although elevated serum calcitonin levels, basal and after pentagastrin stimulation test, strongly suggest the presence of MTC, no study showed a statistical correlation between serum calcitonin levels and calcitonin levels in the wash-out fluid from FNC.
Calcitonin assay in the wash-out from FNC seems to be a highly reliable diagnostic procedure to identify primary tumor and recurrent or metastatic MTC (Boi et al., 2007).

1.6 Diagnosis of MTC persistence/relapse after surgery

The definitive cure of MTC is strongly dependent on the completeness of the first surgical treatment. If tumor tissue is not totally removed, the subsequent surgeries are not as effective as a complete primary surgery in achieving the disease remission. Anyway, the clinical, biochemical and radiological criteria to establish how extended has to be the surgical act to completely abrogate the risk of relapse are not clear.
For node-positive thyroid cancers, compartment-oriented microdissection is the gold standard of care, whereas the concept of prophylactic lymph-node dissection continues to arouse controversy. Most studies agree that routine lymph-node dissection is unnecessary for low-risk well-differentiated thyroid cancer. Because occult lymph-node metastases are frequent in high-risk MTC, compartment-oriented microdissection helps prevent reoperations for recurrences arising from residual nodes, sparing patients the excess morbidity from reoperations in the neck (Dralle & Machens, 2008).
Total thyroidectomy and central neck dissection is recommended for all patients with MTC, but the indication for lateral neck dissection is still controversial and there is not a standard approach to neck surgery. The total number of lymph node metastases is predictive for biological remission after surgery. Because of the same frequency in the ipsilateral, controlateral and central compartments involvement in either sporadic or hereditary MTC, Scollo et al. suggested performing a central and bilateral neck dissection in all patients with MTC. A bilateral neck dissection may be avoided in patients with unilateral tumor involvement of the thyroid only when no involvement of the ipsilateral and central neck compartment is found (Scollo et al., 2003).
Intraoperative calcitonin monitoring seems to be a predictor of the final outcome after surgery in patients with MTC. A calcitonin decrease greater than 50% 30 minutes after surgery is associated with a complete tumor removal while a decrease of calcitonin less than 50% 30 minutes after surgery indicates an incomplete tumor removal and suggests to extend the surgery on other lymph node compartments (Faggiano et al., 2010) (Figure 3).
In comparison to the differentiated thyroid carcinoma, MTC is more difficult to treat and has higher rates of recurrence and mortality. Unlike differentiated carcinoma, there is no known effective systemic therapy since MTC cells do not concentrate radioactive iodine and MTC does not respond well to external radiotherapy or conventional chemotherapy (Czepczyński et al., 2007).
Prognostic factors (relevant) to predict outcome in MTC include: age at diagnosis, gender, initial extent of the disease, such as lymph node and distant metastases, tumor size, extra-

thyroid invasion, vascular invasion, calcitonin immunoreactivity, amyloid staining and Ki-67 score in tumor tissue, postoperative gross residual disease, and postoperative plasma calcitonin levels (Schlumberger et al., 2003) (Table 4).

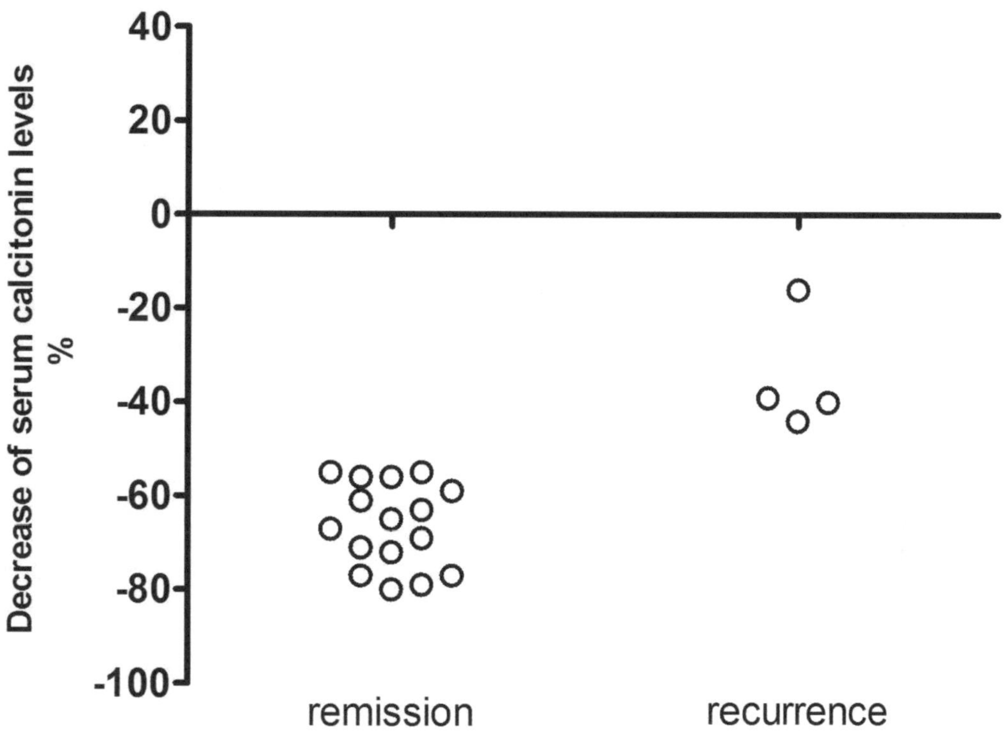

Fig. 3. Correlation between percentage calcitonin decrease 30 minutes after surgery and post-surgical outcome in patients undergone surgery for medullary thyroid cancer (from Faggiano et al., 2010).

Age	Patients aged over 50-60 years fare worse
Sex	The male sex has been associated with a worse prognosis
Stage of MTC	This is the most important prognostic factor. The presence of lymph node and distant metastases at presentation is associated with a worse prognosis with poor survival
Genetics	In a decreasing order, the aggressiveness of hereditary medullary thyroid cancer is MEN2B>MEN2A>FMTC. MTC of the MEN2A variety is associated with a better prognosis than the sporadic variety
Size	Small tumors <1 cm are associated with a better prognosis
Biochemical cure	It predicts a good survival
Histological features	High mitotic count (> 1 per 25 high-power field), high Ki-67%, small-cell variant, necrosis, absence of amyloid are associated with a worse prognosis

Table 4. Prognostic factors to predict outcome in patients with medullary thyroid carcinoma (MTC).

In patients with MTC a long-term biochemical monitoring including serum calcitonin and CEA measurements is mandatory (ATA Guidelines Task Force et al., 2009).
Postoperative unsuppressed calcitonin and CEA concentrations may persist elevated during 2-3 months after surgery due to their long half-life in the blood, while increasing calcitonin and CEA serum levels after this time indicate disease persistence and progression (Leboulleux et al., 2004; Pacini et al., 2010; Faggiano et al., 2009). Undetectable basal serum calcitonin levels, further confirmed after a pentagastrin stimulation test, are a strong predictor of complete remission (Pacini et al., 2010).
In patients with postoperative persistent calcitonin levels the use of imaging techniques is mandatory for diagnostic purposes and therapy decision. Anyway, the detection of tumor foci is often not achieved with conventional imaging techniques (neck ultrasonography, CT-scan, MRI, bone scintigraphy). Postoperative calcitonin concentrations less than 500 pg/ml usually indicate a small residual disease in the neck or mediastinal lymph nodes, not easily detectable. The evaluation of the clinico-biological and immunohistochemical tumor profile may be used in order to select the best imagine technique to be performed in patients with postoperative persistent or relapsing MTC. In particular, FDG-PET seems to correlate to tumor proliferation index Ki-67% and to be able to detect metastases in patients with postoperative persistent MTC when conventional imaging techniques are negative (Faggiano et al., 2009) (Figure 4).

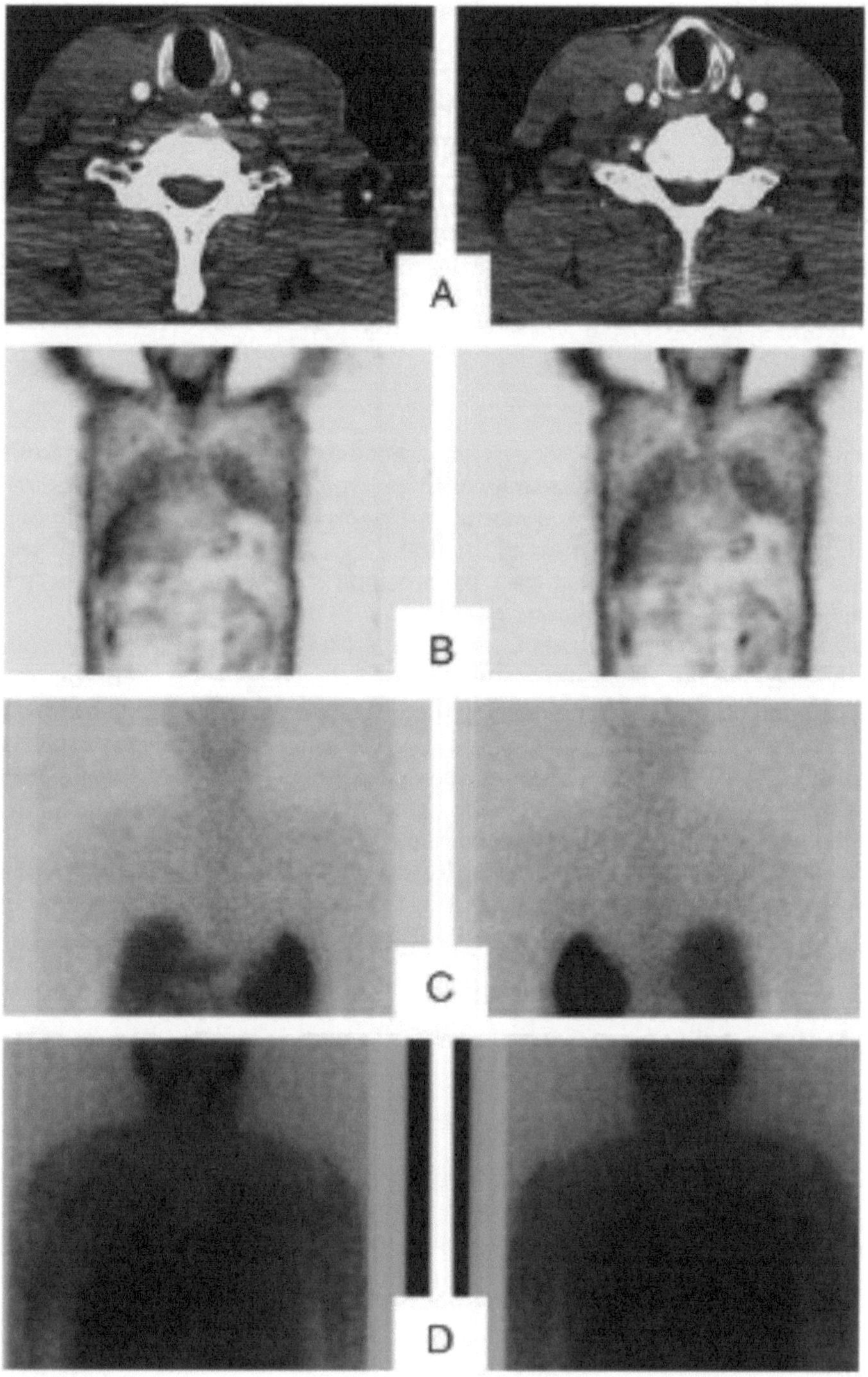

Fig. 4. Lymph node metastases in a patient with postoperative persistence of medullary thyroid carcinoma (MTC) positive at FDG-PET (B) and negative at conventional imaging techniques (CT-scan [A], Octreoscan [C] and MIBG-scintigraphy [D]) (from Faggiano et al., 2009).

For advanced MTC, conventional oncological therapies (radiotherapy and systemic chemotherapy) have scarce effectiveness. For patients with MTC unresponsive to conventional treatments, novel therapies are needed to improve disease outcomes. As a result of the increasing knowledge on the biological basis of MTC, therapeutic agents that target specific molecular pathways have been developed (Kapiteijn et al., 2011). Multiple novel therapies primarily targeting angiogenesis have entered clinical trials for metastatic thyroid carcinoma (including MTC). Partial response rates up to 30% have been reported, but prolonged disease stabilization is more commonly observed. The most successful agents are those targeting the vascular endothelial growth factor receptors (VEGFRs) (Sherman, 2011). Monotarget kinase inhibitors and multikinase inhibitors could represent the best therapeutic option to manage patients with advanced MTC (Kapiteijn et al., 2011).

2. Conclusions

Medullary thyroid carcinoma is a secretive neuroendocrine tumor originating from thyroid C-cells. This tumor is, after the anaplastic carcinoma, the most aggressive thyroid malignancy with high morbidity and mortality. The prognosis of MTC strongly depends on early diagnosis and the completeness of the first surgical treatment. In case of lymph node involvement at the time of the diagnosis, the outcome is poorer because of a very high rate of disease persistence or relapse after surgery.

Treatment for patients with metastatic or advanced MTC has to taken in account novel agents targeting specific molecular pathways and resulting in arrest of tumor growth. Future efforts should be directed to develop diagnostic and therapeutic algorithms to obtain as early as possible the identification of tumor onset and to differentiate MTC from CCH, ensuring high rates of cure and long-time disease free survival. Further studies are required to improve knowledge of CCH and MTC, to detect new hereditary MTC-causing mutations and develop new diagnostic procedures and therapeutic strategies.

Finally, to optimize the management of patients with MTC, a multidisciplinary team of all the different specialists involved in MTC diagnosis and therapy is highly recommended.

3. Acknowledgments

This work was partially supported by a grant from the Italian Minister of Research and University in Rome (no. 2008LFK7J5).

4. References

Albores-Saavedra, J.A. & Krueger, J.E. (2001). C-cell hyperplasia and medullary thyroid microcarcinoma. *Endocrine Pathology*, Vol.12(No.4):365-377.

American Thyroid Association Guidelines Task Force, Kloos, R.T., Eng, C., Evans, D.B., Francis, G.L., Gagel, R.F., Gharib, H., Moley, J.F., Pacini, F., Ringel, M.D., Schlumberger, M. & Wells, S.A. Jr. (2009). Medullary thyroid cancer: management guidelines of the American Thyroid Association. *Thyroid*, Vol.19(No.6):565-612.

Boi, F., Maurelli, I., Pinna, G., Atzeni, F., Piga, M., Lai, M.L. & Mariotti, S. (2007). Calcitonin measurement in wash-out fluid from fine needle aspiration of neck masses in patients with primary and metastatic medullary thyroid carcinoma, *Journal of Clinical Endocrinology and Metabolism*, Vol. 92(No.6):2115-2118

Brandi, M.L., Gagel, R.F., Angeli, A., Bilezikian, J.P., Beck-Peccoz, P., Bordi, C., Conte-Devolx, B., Falchetti, A., Gheri, R.G., Libroia, A., Lips, C.J., Lombardi, G., Mannelli, M., Pacini, F., Ponder, B.A., Raue, F., Skogseid, B., Tamburrano, G., Thakker, R.V., Thompson, N.W., Tomassetti, P., Tonelli, F., Wells, S.A. Jr & Marx, S.J. (2001). Guidelines for diagnosis and therapy of MEN type 1 and type 2. *Journal of Clinical Endocrinology and Metabolism*, Vol.86(No.12):5658-5671

Costante, G., Meringolo, D., Durante, C., Bianchi, D., Nocera, M., Tumino, S., Crocetti, U., Attard, M., Maranghi, M., Torlontano, M. & Filetti, S. (2007). Predictive value of serum calcitonin levels for preoperative diagnosis of medullary thyroid carcinoma in a cohort of 5817 consecutive patients with thyroid nodules. *Journal of Clinical Endocrinology and Metabolism*, Vol.92(No.2):450-455

Czepczyński, R., Parisella, M.G., Kosowicz, J., Mikołajczak, R., Ziemnicka, K., Gryczyńska, M., Sowiński, J. & Signore, A. (2007). Somatostatin receptor scintigraphy using 99mTc-EDDA/HYNIC-TOC in patients with medullary thyroid carcinoma. *European Journal of Nuclear Medicine and Molecular Imaging*, Vol.34(No.10):1635-1645

Dralle, H. & Machens, A. (2008).Surgical approaches in thyroid cancer and lymph-node metastases. *Best Practice and Research. Clinical Endocrinology and Metabolism*, Vol.22(No.6):971-987

Elisei, R., Bottici, V., Luchetti, F., Di Coscio, G., Romei, C., Grasso, L., Miccoli, P., Iacconi, P., Basolo, F., Pinchera, A. & Pacini, F. (2004). Impact of routine measurement of serum calcitonin on the diagnosis and outcome of medullary thyroid cancer: experience in 10,864 patients with nodular thyroid disorders. *Journal of Clinical Endocrinology and Metabolism*, Vol.89(No.1):163-168

Faggiano, A., Grimaldi, F., Pezzullo, L., Chiofalo, M.G., Caracò, C., Mozzillo, N., Angeletti, G., Santeusanio, F., Lombardi, G., Colao, A., Avenia, N. & Ferolla, P. (2009). Secretive and proliferative tumor profile helps to select the best imaging technique to identify postoperative persistent or relapsing medullary thyroid cancer. *Endocrine-Related Cancer*, Vol.16(No.1):225-231

Faggiano, A., Milone, F., Ramundo, V., Chiofalo, M.G., Ventre, I., Giannattasio, R., Severino, R., Lombardi, G., Colao, A. & Pezzullo, L. (2010). A decrease of calcitonin serum concentrations less than 50 percent 30 minutes after thyroid surgery suggests incomplete C-cell tumor tissue removal. *Journal of Clinical Endocrinology and Metabolism*, Vol.95(No.9):E32-6

Faggiano, A., Talbot, M., Baudin, E., Bidart, J.M., Schlumberger, M. & Caillou, B. (2003). Differential expression of galectin 3 in solid cell nests and C cells of human thyroid. *Journal of Clinical Pathology*, Vol.56(No.2):142-143.

Faggiano, A., Talbot, M., Lacroix, L., Bidart, J.M., Baudin, E., Schlumberger, M. & Caillou, B. (2002). Differential expression of galectin-3 in medullary thyroid carcinoma and C-cell hyperplasia. *Clinical Endocrinology*, Vol.57(No.6):813-819

Hazard, J.B. (1977) The C cells (parafollicular cells) of the thyroid gland and medullary thyroid carcinoma. A Review, *American Journal of pathology*, Vol.88 (No.1) :213-250

Kapiteijn, E., Schneider, T.C., Morreau, H., Gelderblom, H., Nortier, J.W., Smit, J.W. (2011) New treatment modalities in advanced thyroid cancer. *Annals of Oncology*, Apr 6. [Epub ahead of print]

Leboeuf, R., Langlois, M.F., Martin, M., Ahnadi, C.E. & Fink, G.D. (2006). "Hook effect" in calcitonin immunoradiometric assay in patients with metastatic medullary thyroid carcinoma: case report and review of the literature. *Journal of Clinical Endocrinology and Metabolism*, Vol.91(No.2):361-364

Leboulleux, S., Baudin, E., Travagli, J.P. & Schlumberger, M. (2004). Medullary thyroid carcinoma. *Clinical Endocrinology*, Vol.61(No.3):299-310

Meijer, J.A., le Cessie, S., van den Hout, W.B., Kievit, J., Schoones, J.W., Romijn, J.A. & Smit, J.W. (2010). Calcitonin and carcinoembryonic antigen doubling times as prognostic factors in medullary thyroid carcinoma: a structured meta-analysis. *Clinical Endocrinology*, Vol.72(No.4):534-542.

Milone, F., Ramundo, V., Chiofalo, M.G., Severino, R., Paciolla, I., Pezzullo, L., Lombardi, G., Colao, A. & Faggiano, A.. (2010). Predictive value of pentagastrin test for preoperative differential diagnosis between C-cell hyperplasia and medullary thyroid carcinoma in patients with moderately elevated basal calcitonin levels. *Clinical Endocrinology*, Vol.73(No.1):85-88

Mulligan, L.M., Marsh, D.J., Robinson, B.G., Schuffenecker, I., Zedenius, J., Lips, C.J., Gagel, R.F., Takai, S.I., Noll, W.W., Fink, M., et al. (1995). Genotype-phenotype correlation in multiple endocrine neoplasia type 2: report of the International RET Mutation Consortium. *Journal of Internal Medicine*, Vol.238(No.4):343-346

Pacini, F., Castagna, M.G., Cipri, C. & Schlumberger, M. (2010). Medullary thyroid carcinoma. *Clinical Oncology*, Vol.22(No.6):475-485

Pacini, F., Fontanelli, M., Fugazzola, L., Elisei, R., Romei, C., Di Coscio, G., Miccoli, P. & Pinchera, A. (1994). Routine measurement of serum calcitonin in nodular thyroid diseases allows the preoperative diagnosis of unsuspected sporadic medullary thyroid carcinoma. *Journal of Clinical Endocrinology and Metabolism*, Vol.78(No.4):826-829

Perry, A., Molberg, K. & Albores-Saavedra, J. (1996). Physiologic versus neoplastic C-cell hyperplasia of the thyroid: separation of distinct histologic and biologic entities. *Cancer*, Vol.77(No.4):750-756

Raue, F. & Frank-Raue, K. (2007). Multiple endocrine neoplasia type 2: 2007 update. *Hormone Research*, Vol.68(Suppl.5):101-114

Santesanio, G., Iafrate, E., Partenzi, A., Mauriello, A., Autelitano, F. & Spagnoli, L.G. (1997) A critical reassessment of the concepì of C-cell hyperplasia of the thyroid: a quantitative immunohistochemical study. *Applied Immunohistochemistry*, Vol.5:160-172

Scollo, C., Baudin, E., Travagli, J.P., Caillou, B., Bellon, N., Leboulleux, S. & Schlumberger, M. (2003). Rationale for central and bilateral lymph node dissection in sporadic and hereditary medullary thyroid cancer. *Journal of Clinical Endocrinology and Metabolism*, Vol.88(No.5):2070-2075.

Schlumberger, M.D., Sebastiano Filetti, S., & Hay I.D. (2003) Nontoxic Goiter and Thyroid Neoplasia, In: *Williams Textbook of Endocrinology*, Elsevier Science (USA)

Sherman, S.I. (2011) Targeted therapies for thyroid tumors. *Modern Pathology*, Vol.24 (Suppl 2):44-52

Toledo, S.P., Lourenço, D.M. Jr, Santos, M.A., Tavares, M.R., Toledo, R.A. & Correia-Deur, J.E. (2009). Hypercalcitoninemia is not pathognomonic of medullary thyroid carcinoma. *Clinics*, Vol.64(No.7):699-706.

van Veelen, W., de Groot, J.W., Acton, D.S., Hofstra, R.M., Höppener, J.W., Links, T.P. & Lips, C.J. (2009). Medullary thyroid carcinoma and biomarkers: past, present and future. *Journal of Internal Medicine*, Vol.266(No.1):126-140

Molecular Diagnostics in Treatment of Medullary Thyroid Carcinoma

Brigitte M. Pützer, Alf Spitschak and David Engelmann
University of Rostock, Department of Vectorology and Experimental Gene Therapy
Germany

1. Introduction

Medullary thyroid carcinoma (MTC) is accounting for 5 - 8% of all thyroid cancers and arises from calcitonin producing parafollicular C cells of the thyroid gland. Mainly MTC is sporadic in nature, but in 20 - 30% of cases it is present in an autosomal dominant inherited pattern with defined phenotype referred as multiple endocrine neoplasia type 2 (MEN 2) and familial medullary thyroid carcinoma (FMTC). The identification of missense germline mutations in the *RET* proto-oncogene between 1993 and 1998 as the cause of MEN 2 and FMTC ushered in the molecular age. Specific mutations in the *RET* gene encoding a transmembrane tyrosine kinase result in "gain-of-function" of the receptor with definite changes in downstream signal transduction pathways. Intriguingly, examination of the mutated codons led to the growing recognition of a striking genotype–phenotype correlation between the transforming activity inherent in these mutations and disease onset and aggressiveness, implicating that manifestation and clinical progression is conditioned by the type of mutation. Detection of the mutant alleles in kindred members predicts disease inheritance and provides the basis for prophylactic thyroidectomy in children. This seminal discovery, enabling predictive testing, paved the way for an evidence-based practice of clinical cancer genetics. In case of novel *RET* mutations it is exceedingly important to clarify whether it represents a harmless polymorphism or a causative pathogenic mutation. For this purpose, we established a molecular diagnosis program that, in conjunction with clinical data, allows individualized risk stratification for patients.

2. RET proto-oncogene and MTC

2.1 RET proto-oncogene – Genotype to phenotype

Transfection studies using DNA from human T cell lymphoma led to the isolation of a transforming gene called *RET* (REarranged during Transfection) that consists of two linked sequences caused by cointegration during transfection (Takahashi et al., 1985). The resulting chimeric gene encodes a fusion protein comprising an N-terminal region with a dimerization motif fused to a tyrosine kinase (TK) domain. Subsequently, the name RET has been retained to designate the gene coding for the tyrosine kinase domain of this fused oncogene. The human *RET* gene is localized on chromosome 10q11.2 (Donghi et al., 1989) and spans 21 exons. Homologues of *RET* have been identified in higher and lower vertebrates as well as in *Drosophila melanogaster* (Hahn and Bishop, 2001). The *RET* proto-oncogene encodes a transmembrane receptor of the tyrosine kinase family with three major isoforms that arise through alternative splicing of the 3´-terminus, leading to expression of proteins that differ by their last 51 (RET51), 43 (RET43) or nine (RET9) amino acids, respectively (Manie et al., 2001). It is expressed primarily in neural crest and urogenital precursor cells, and is implicated in developmental processes, such as maturation of peripheral nervous system lineages, kidney morphogenesis or spermatogonia differentiation (Durbec et al., 1996; Meng et al., 2000; Schuchardt et al., 1994). Among them, RET9 and RET51 are the major isoforms consisting of 1072 and 1114 amino acids, respectively. The signaling complex associated with RET9 markedly differs from RET51-associated factors, which might have an influence on the higher transforming potential of the RET51 isoform (Le Hir et al., 2000; Tsui-Pierchala et al., 2002). The RET protein is composed of three functional domains: The intracellular tyrosine kinase domain, a transmembrane region and a stretch of four extracellular cadherin-like domains that are implicated in ligand binding. The extracellular domain consists of four cadherin-like regions and a cysteine-rich tract, which facilitates receptor dimerization upon ligand stimulation (Iwamoto et al., 1993; Takahashi et al., 1998). This region also contains several glycosylation sites (Takahashi et al., 1991). The fully glycosylated form (170-175 kDa) of RET is found in the plasma membrane, while the 150-155 kDa species is believed to be an immature, partially processed form found only in the endoplasmic reticulum (ER). RET serves as a functional receptor for neurotrophic factors of the glial cell-line derived neurotrophic factor (GDNF) family: GDNF, neurturin, artemin and persephin (Ichihara et al., 2004; Takahashi, 2001). Binding to and activation of RET occurs via glycosylphosphatidylinositol-anchored as well as soluble co-receptors that are designated as GDNF-family receptors (GFRs) α1-4 (Airaksinen and Saarma, 2002; Manie et al., 2001) (**Fig. 1 A**). Ligand stimulation leads to activation of the RET receptor by dimerization and subsequent autophosphorylation of intracellular tyrosine residues. These, in turn, serve as docking sites for a number of interacting molecules activating downstream signal transduction pathways (Chiariello et al., 1998; Hayashi et al., 2001; Murakami et al., 1999). Although tyrosine residues 905, 981, 1015, 1062 and 1096 are all phopshorylated upon ligand binding, it is the phosphorylation of tyr1062 that plays a crucial role in RET signaling as it acts as a multifunctional docking site for many adaptor or effector proteins (Jijiwa et al., 2004).

Autosomal dominant gain of function mutations in the *RET* proto-oncogene have been identified as the key cause for the development of the multiple endocrine neoplasia type 2 (MEN 2) syndrome, which can be further divided into three distinct clinical manifestations MEN 2A, MEN 2B, and familial medullary thyroid carcinoma (FMTC) (Bocciardi et al., 1997; Carlomagno et al., 1997; Hofstra et al., 1994; Mulligan et al., 1993; Santoro et al., 1995). In addition, 30-70% of sporadic medullary thyroid carcinomas harbor a mutation in the *RET* gene. Mutations render the RET receptor constitutively active and display striking genotype-phenotype correlations. Patients with MEN 2A always develop medullary thyroid carcinoma (MTC), but also pheochromocytoma (50%) and parathyroid hyperplasia or adenoma (20-30%). MEN 2B, in contrast, is the most aggressive subtype and is characterized by the same features as MEN 2A, but with earlier onset and developmental abnormalities such as mucosal neuromas, intestinal ganglioneuromas, ocular and skeletal abnormalities (marfanoid habitus). The most indolent subtype FMTC is characterized by the incidence of MTC-only (Brandi et al., 2001). Mutations identified in more than 98% of MEN 2A patients affect one of six cysteine residues in the cysteine-rich region at codons 609, 611, 618, 620 (exon 10), 630 or 634 (exon 11) and cause ligand-independent homodimerization through covalent intermolecular disulphide bonds, resulting in subsequent constitutive activation of the RET kinase which, in turn, leads to permanent downstream signaling (Santoro et al., 1995) **(Fig. 1 C)**. Approximately 87% of MEN 2A mutations affect codon 634 (Eng et al., 1996; Hansford and Mulligan, 2000). In contrast, mutations found in MEN 2B patients affect residues in the tyrosine kinase domain and activate the RET receptor in its monomeric state, thereby changing the substrate specificity towards other cellular substrates and downstream signaling pathways (Borrello et al., 1995; Murakami et al., 1999; Santoro et al., 1999) **(Fig. 1 B)**.

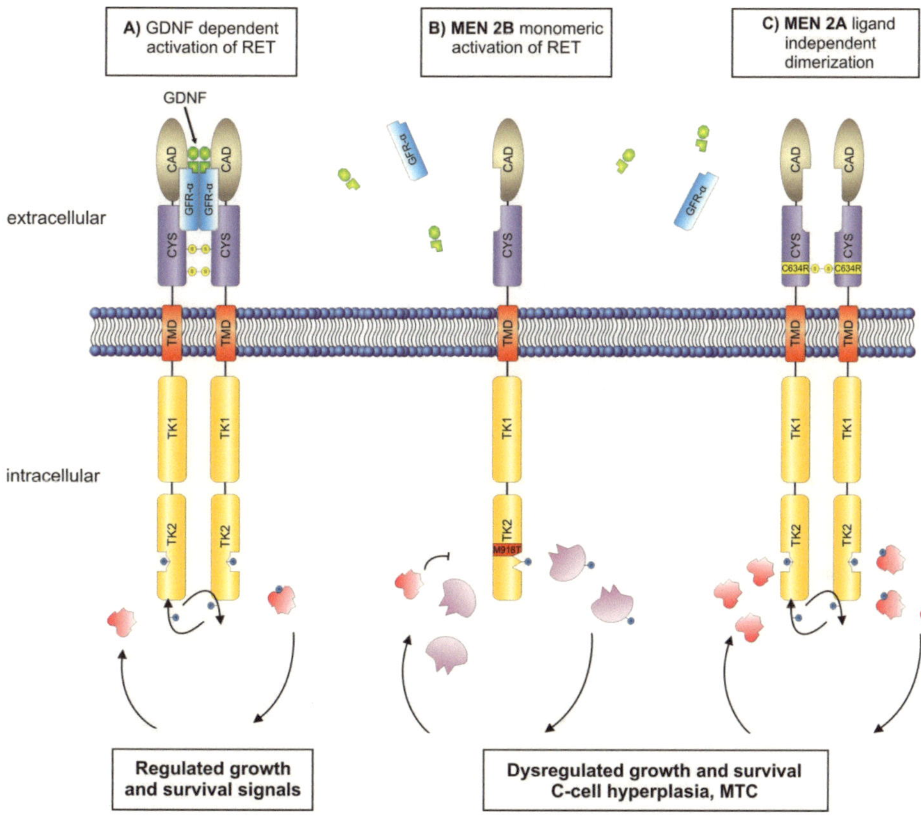

Fig. 1. Schematic mechanisms of RET tyrosine kinase activation in healthy status versus MEN 2B and MEN 2A. A) Normal RET activation by glial cell line-derived neurotrophic factor (GDNF). GDNF binds to GFR α and leads to RET dimerization and autophosphorylation. B) Constitutive RET activation by MEN 2B mutations. C) Ligand independent RET activation by MEN 2A mutations. CAD Cadherin like domain; Cys Cysteine-rich domain; TMD Transmembrane domain; TK Tyrosine kinase domain

Moreover, increased autophosphorylation of tyrosine 1062 has been described (Bocciardi et al., 1997; Salvatore et al., 2001; Santoro et al., 1995). MEN 2B is primarily associated with a single missense mutation of codon 918 (M918T), which is detectable in more than 90% of MEN 2B patients (Carlson et al., 1994; Eng et al., 1996; Hofstra et al., 1994; Mulligan et al., 1993). A smaller number of MEN 2B cases contain mutations at codon 883 (A883F) (Gimm et al., 1997; Smith et al., 1997). Mutations identified in FMTC patients (for example at codons 790, 791 or 844) are found in the cysteine-rich region as well as in the tyrosine kinase domain, and lead to low level activation of the RET kinase corresponding to the indolent penetrance phenotype of FMTC (Arighi et al., 2005; Manie et al., 2001). An overview about mutated codons at specific sites of the RET oncogene and the correlating clinical phenotype is mapped in **Fig. 2.**

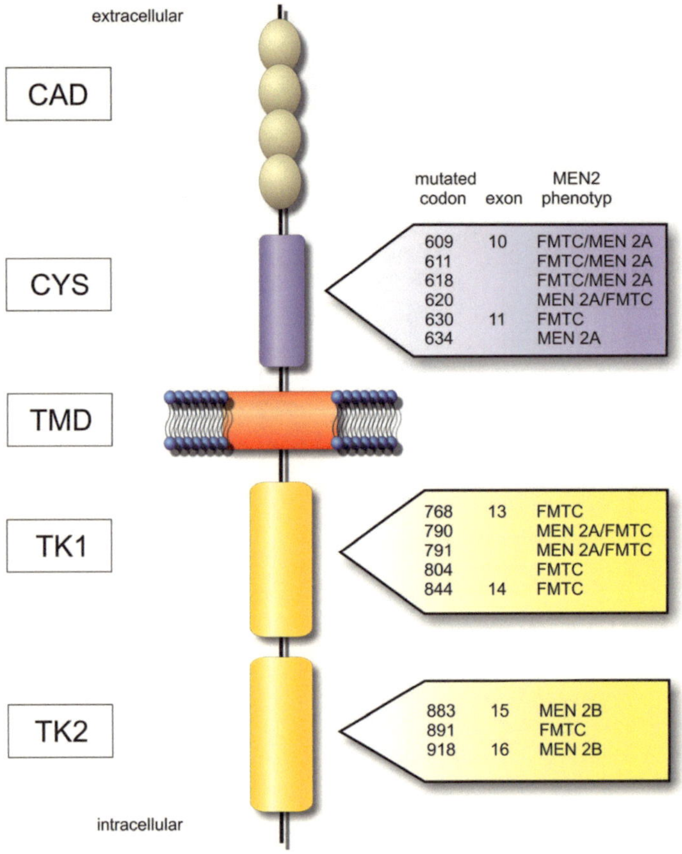

Fig. 2. Domain structure of the RET proto-oncogene: CAD Cadherin like domain; Cys Cysteine-rich domain; TMD Transmembrane domain; TK Tyrosine kinase domain. Arrows point to the affected protein domains and specify the mutated codons and the correlating clinical phenotype.

2.2 Medullary thyroid carcinoma – Standard diagnosis and treatment

In most cases, the prognosis for MTC patients is good after early diagnosis and intervention. Since 1994, genetic screening using DNA from peripheral blood has been available for MEN 2. This method allows diagnosis prior to the onset of symptoms. Moreover, the MEN 2-associated mutations, involving RET exons 8, 10, 11, 13, 14, 15 and 16 are tested routinely. Currently, early genetic screening for *RET* mutations is considered the standard of care for

MEN 2 (Eng, 1999). Preoperative measurement of serum calcitonin is another highly sensitive method to establish the diagnosis of MTC. However, since germline *RET* mutations have been identified as a cause of MEN 2, the use of additional measurement of calcitonin is questionable. Though calcitonin levels can be helpful in determining the extent of disease and the extent of surgery required (Gimm, 2001).

At present treatment of MTC is restricted to surgical removal of neoplastic tissue, and cure is only achieved when the disease is restricted to the thyroid gland. The general recommendation to perform total thyroidectomy seems to be justified since MTC is often multifocal and not susceptible to radioiodine ablation. Overall, *RET* mutations are classified into three groups based on the level of risk (or aggressiveness) for MTC (Sippel et al., 2008). Level 3 mutations (codon 883, 918, and 922) have the most aggressive course, with metastatic disease presenting in the first years of life. Because of the high risk for malignancy at an early age, thyroidectomy is recommended within the first 6 months of life and preferably within the first month of life (Brandi et al., 2001). Level 2 *RET* mutations (codon 611, 618, 620, and 634 mutations) are considered high risk for MTC and the current recommendation is that these patients undergo thyroidectomy before the age of 5 years. Mutations at codon 609, 768, 790, 791, 804 and 891 are classified as level 1. Patients carrying these mutations are still considered high risk for MTC but with the lowest risk of the *RET* mutations. MTC in these patients tends to develop later in life and takes on a more indolent course. Because clinically apparent disease is rarely reported prior to 10 years of age, many recommend waiting until then to perform a thyroidectomy. Based on more detailed research and knowledge the stratification system for *RET* germline mutations was recently reclassified by the Amercian Thyroid Association (ATA) into categories of increasing risk: class A (codons 768, 790, 791, 804, 891), class B (codons 609, 611, 618, 620, 630), C (codon 634), and D (codon 883, 918), with level A representing lowest risk (FMTC) and level D representing the highest risk (MEN 2B) class (Kloos et al., 2009).

Patients with unresectable or metastatic disease display a poor prognosis because radiation and chemotherapy have only a limited role (Cohen and Moley, 2003). Although MTC is less radiosensitive, radiotherapy is used as a palliative for symptomatic bone, central nervous system and mediastinal metastases. Some studies suggested a specific radiotherapy for MTC based on the selective uptake of [^{131}I]MIBG and [^{111}In]pentetreotide (Forssell-Aronsson et al., 1995; Troncone et al., 1991) also concerning their role in diagnosis of neuroendocrine tumors and to some degree localisation of metastases (Kaltsas et al., 2001). Other nuclear approaches using radionuclide-labeled antibodies combined with pretargeting strategies to improve uptake of these antibodies have raised interest in targeted radiotherapy for MTC (Juweid et al., 1996; Juweid et al., 2000; Kraeber-Bodere et al., 1999; Mirallie et al., 2005).

Since activated RET is proven to be causative for the development of MTC, molecular strategies to inhibit its activity or expression in cancer cells are highly promising. Targeting the enzymatic activity of tyrosine kinases by small molecule inhibitors like STI571 (Gleevec® or Imatinib), BAY 43-9006 (Sorafenib), allyl-geldanamycin, or arylidine 2-indolinone (RPI-1) selectively inhibit RET kinase activity and cell growth (Cohen et al., 2002; Lanzi et al., 2000). For example, oral daily RPI-1 treatment reduces the growth of human medullary thyroid carcinoma xenografts in mice by 81% (Cuccuru et al., 2004). Also, two indolocarbazole derivatives, CEP-701 and CEP-751, have been shown to effectively block RET phosphorylation at nanomolar levels and MTC cell growth (Strock et al., 2003), whereas the pyrazolo-pyrimidine PP1 inhibits tumorigenesis induced by RET/PTC oncogenes and causes degradation of activated membrane-bound RET receptors through proteosomal targeting (Carlomagno et al., 2002b; Carniti et al., 2003; Strock et al., 2003). In addition, the pyrazolo-pyrimidine PP2, and the 4-anilinoquinazoline ZD6474 (Vandetanib) displayed a strong inhibitory activity towards constitutively active oncogenic RET kinases (Carlomagno et al., 2003; Carlomagno et al., 2002a). However most of the tyrosine kinase inhibitors are mulitkinase inhibitors and are also active against multiple signaling molecules (Santarpia et al., 2009). Moreover, some *RET* mutations (e.g. valine 804) cause resistance to these drugs (Carlomagno et al., 2004). Finally the efficacy in human patients has to be proven by treatment. Until now first clinical trials with several kinase inhibitors showed no beneficial or only moderate effects of the drugs (**Table 1**). Thus, development and evaluation of novel treatment strategies, including gene therapeutic approaches are further needed.

Kinase inhibitor	**Clinical trial**	**Reference**
Imatinib	Phase II	de Groot et al., 2007
Sorafenib	Phase II	Lam et al., 2010
Vandetanib	Phase III	Wells et al., 2010
Sunitinib	Phase II	De Souza et al., 2010
Motesanib	Phase II	Schlumberger et al., 2009

Table 1. Summary of some tyrosine kinase inhibitors used in clinical trials

Gene therapy is attractive for thyroid cancer treatment because of the possibility to selectively target therapeutic genes by application of tissue-specific promoters, such as the thyroglobulin or the calcitonin promoter. A range of therapeutic strategies were under investigation utilizing various genes: pro-drug activating genes (herpes simplex virus thymidine kinase /ganciclovir and purine nucleoside phosphorylase/fludarabine), the nitric oxide synthase II gene in a direct toxin therapy, gene for IL-12 in an immune stimulation strategy, and the expression of the sodium iodide symporter gene in radiotherapy application (Spitzweg and Morris, 2004). Moreover, molecular mimics (competition) directed toward specific mutations of *RET* by using the mutant EC-RET C634Y that is able to inhibit the membrane bound receptor RETC634Y through interfering with its dimerization (Cerchia et al., 2003).

Another attractive approach is to block oncogenic signal transduction either by reducing RET expression or by interfering with receptor autophosphorylation using dominant-negative RET protein. In this regard, adenovirus (Ad)-mediated expression of RET containing mutations in the N-terminal region of the extracellular domain such as HSCR32 associated with Hirschsprung´s disease or FLAG has been shown to substantially inhibit receptor maturation, thereby preventing its transport to the membrane (Drosten et al., 2002; Drosten et al., 2003). These molecules proved to be highly active against MTC in cultures of human TT cells, which harbour the RETC634W mutation, and after inoculation of *ex vivo* infected tumor cells into nude mice. A second dominant-negative RET protein (RETΔTK), lacking the intracellular tyrosine kinase domain, showed the ability to block oncogenic activated RET autophosphorylation by forming an inactive dimer with the mutated RET receptor. Transduction of TT cells with RETΔTK resulted in decreased cell-cycle progression, but also, more importantly induction of cell death by apoptosis. Activity of RETΔTK against MTC was also demonstrated in RET transgenic mice, which develop orthotopic tumors in the thyroid. Injection of an Ad vector expressing dominant-negative RET protein into MTC of the thyroid glands significantly decreased the tumor size after two weeks (Drosten et al.,

2004). To enhance tumor specificity of anti-RET Ad vectors in order to target systemically spreaded medullary thyroid carcinoma cells, we have recently identified a number of MTC-specific peptides that can be used to efficiently redirect the therapeutic gene to primary MTC, their migrating populations, and potentially tumor metastases under *in vivo* conditions (Böckmann et al., 2005a; Böckmann et al., 2005b; Schmidt et al., 2011).

3. Combining tools – RET molecular diagnostics

RET gene analysis widely used to identify carriers at risk of developing medullary thyroid cancer, occasionally uncovers novel sequence variants of unknown clinical significance. For these newly identified or rare mutations in the *RET* gene, the causative role of the mutation and the genotype-phenotype relationship must be evaluated to define the mutation´s codon-specific risk level. For this purpose, we have implemented a molecular diagnostic approach that allows us to classify *RET* mutations into one of the four clinical risk groups. Based on such molecular diagnosis recommendations for treatments of patients with hitherto undefined *RET* mutations are made. The program established allows direct translation of a genetic event into individualized clinical settings and is critical for treating physicians to decide whether a prophylactic thyroidectomy is necessary or not. Considering the potential risks after thyroidectomy e.g. reduced flexibility of the vocal cord and subsequent restrictions for the patient like hormone replacement therapy, molecular diagnostics in MTC-treatment have a direct impact on affected patients.

3.1 From clinical RET mutation analysis to functional in vitro and in vivo characterization

Clinical classification and DNA based screening

Diagnosis of putative carriers of *RET* genes with novel mutations starts with clinical work up and subsequent *RET* mutation analysis. Therefore preoperatively basal and pentagastrin-stimulated calcitonin levels, as a marker for MTC tumors, are determined by appropriate chemiluminescence assay. By utilizing histology analysis after total thyroidectomy tumor staging is performed according to the International Union Against Cancer tumor-node-metastasis (TNM) classification from 1997. To detect mutations genomic DNA is isolated and five fragments covering the exons 8, 10, 11 and 13 to 16 of the *RET* proto-oncogene are amplified with exon specific PCR primers using high-fidelity PCR systems. The resulting fragments are sequenced to specify the point mutation.

Construction and characterization of mutant RET expressing cell lines in vitro

On the basis of the clinical findings the first goal is to determine whether a particular mutation is capable of converting RET into a dominantly transforming oncogene. At this point wet lab work starts to generate a RET51 mutant with defined specific mutation. pLPCX vectors are used to express the mutated *RET* gene. The pLPCX vector contains elements derived from Moloney murine leukemia virus (MoMuLV) and Moloney murine sarcoma virus (MoMuSV), and is mostly designed for retroviral gene delivery and expression. The cDNA fragment encoding the human tyrosine kinase RET51wt is ligated downstream from the CMV promoter of pLPCX retroviral vector (**Fig. 3 A**). pLPCX expression vectors containing the selected *RET* point mutation are generated by site directed mutagenesis using primers harboring the desired codon and pLPCX RET51wt plasmid as a template. All constructed plasmids are routinely sequenced to confirm the presence of the desired mutations. NIH3T3 fibroblasts were chosen as *in vitro* model because they do not express endogenous RET protein and are generally accepted as a reliable transformation system to study oncogene function. In order to investigate the effects of mutated RET proteins on cellular transformation, NIH3T3 mouse fibroblasts are stably transfected with the pLPCX-RET expression vector. Single puromycine-resistant clones are separated by limited dilution, cultivated and finally checked for RET protein expression (**Fig. 3 B**). After construction of the desired cell line a plethora of assays is applied to determine specific cellular parameters that help to evaluate aggressiveness of the investigated receptor mutant (**Fig. 3 C**).

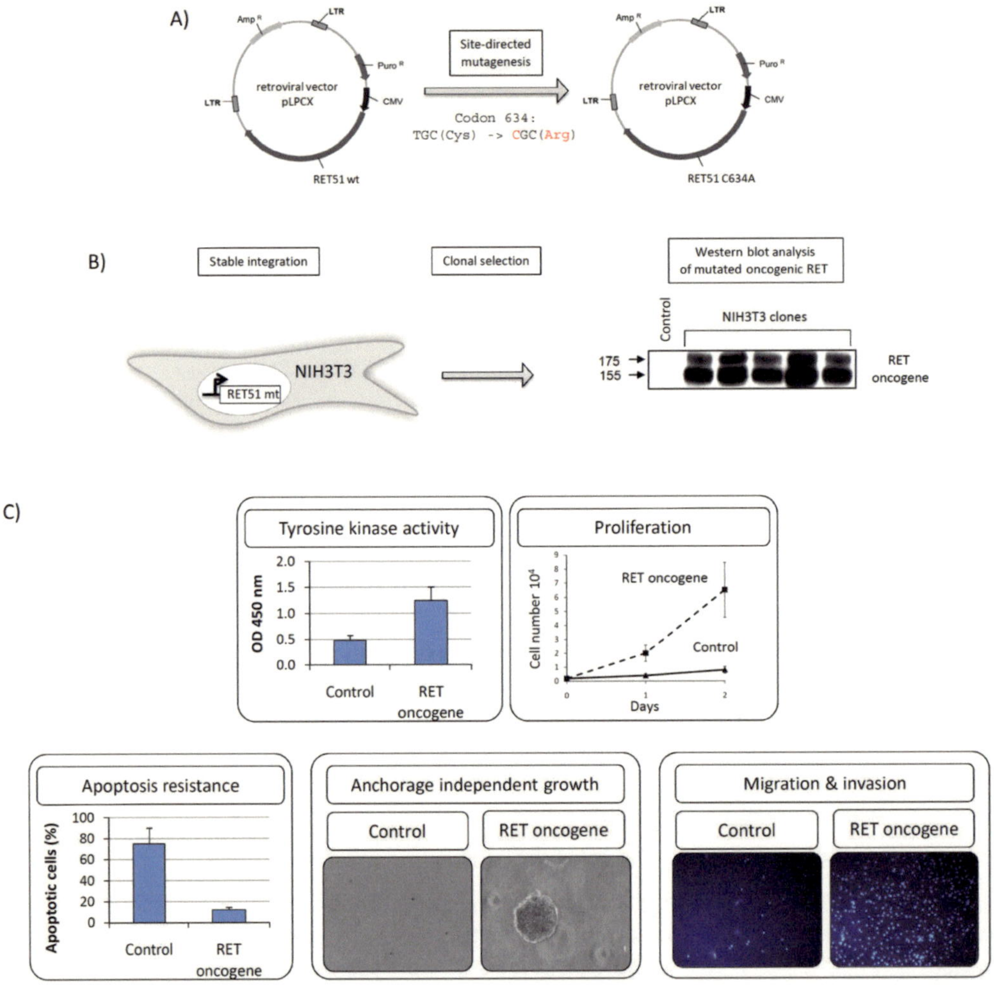

Fig. 3. Schematic workflow for generation and characterization of mutant RET-expressing NIH3T3 stable cell lines and in vitro assays. A) Site directed mutagenesis of RET51 wildtype containing retroviral plasmid to gain oncogenic RET point mutations. B) Transfection of NIH3T3 with mutant RET gene followed by clonal selection and subsequent control of RET protein levels of stably expressing NIH3T3-RET cell lines. C) Established in vitro assays from selected RET clones for evaluation of the transforming potential of single RET mutants.

1. **Tyrosine kinase activity** induced by mutated RET proteins: Protein extracts from NIH3T3 transfectants stably expressing mutated forms of RET are immunoprecipitated with an anti-RET antibody and subjected to a kinase assay.
2. Analysis of growth properties by determining the **proliferation rate** through cell counting or cell viability assays.
3. **Apoptosis resistance**: DNA-Damage induced cell death is activated by chemotherapeutics like doxorubicine or cisplatin. Subsequent killing of cells expressing oncogenic RET mutants is measured by flow cytometry. Here, propidium iodide staining is used to analyze cellular DNA content and look for sub-diploid or apoptotic cell population, respectively.
4. **Anchorage-independent growth** as one of the most important oncogenic properties of cancer cells is determined by soft agar assays. Therefore, stable NIH3T3 transfectants are seeded in semisolid medium and cultured over a period of 30 days. Formed cell colonies are stained and counted under the microscope.
5. **Migration and invasiveness** are major characteristics describing the aggressiveness and metastatic behavior of cancer cells. NIH3T3 fibroblasts expressing distinct mutant RET proteins are tested for their motility by matrigel invasion assays in Boyden chambers. Boyden chamber inserts contain membranes that are permeabilized by small pores coated with Matrigel™-Basement-Matrix. Hereon cells are seeded in serum-free medium. Medium containing a high concentration of fetal calf serum is added as chemoattractant in the lower chamber. Staining of cells enables examination of migrated cells under a fluorescence microscope.

In all experiments established, already characterized NIH3T3 transfectants harboring well known point mutations in the RET gene like Y791F (FMTC), C634R (MEN 2A) and M918T (MEN 2B) with a defined genotype to phenotype correlation (Mise et al., 2006) are carried along as standard to classify new point mutations of as yet unknown oncogenic potential. In addition, short-term cultured parental NIH3T3 cells are employed as untransformed negative control.

Establishing tumor allografts in nude mice through injection of NIH3T3-RET cell lines

To investigate the transforming potential and aggressiveness of a particular RET mutant *in vivo*, experimental research in animal models is needed (**Fig. 4**). As *in vivo* transformation model, athymic nude mice are used. NIH3T3 stable transfectants are subcutaneously injected into the hind flank of 6 to 8 weeks old mice. Parental NIH3T3 cells are used as negative control. After injection tumor formation is monitored over time. To estimate the growth rate, tumor dimensions are measured with calipers every 2 days. Tumor volumes are calculated by the rotational ellipsoid formula: $V=AxB^2/2$ (A-axial diameter; B-rotational diameter). Finally, after sacrificing the animals, tumors are removed, weighted, embedded in paraffin and submitted to immunohistochemistry. In detail, tumor sections carrying *RET* mutations are cut, dewaxed, rehydrated and probed with antibody against Ki-67 nuclear antigen, which recognizes actively proliferating cells. The percentage of proliferating cells can be determined by counting Ki-67 positive cells under a bright-field microscope. At the same time tumors can also be subjected to gene expression analysis. Therefore, tumor tissues are snap frozen in liquid nitrogen and stored at -80°C. RNA and protein extracts from samples are isolated by grinding 1 g of frozen tissue into a fine powder using a cold mortar and pestle by standard procedures for subsequent western blot and/or qPCR analysis.

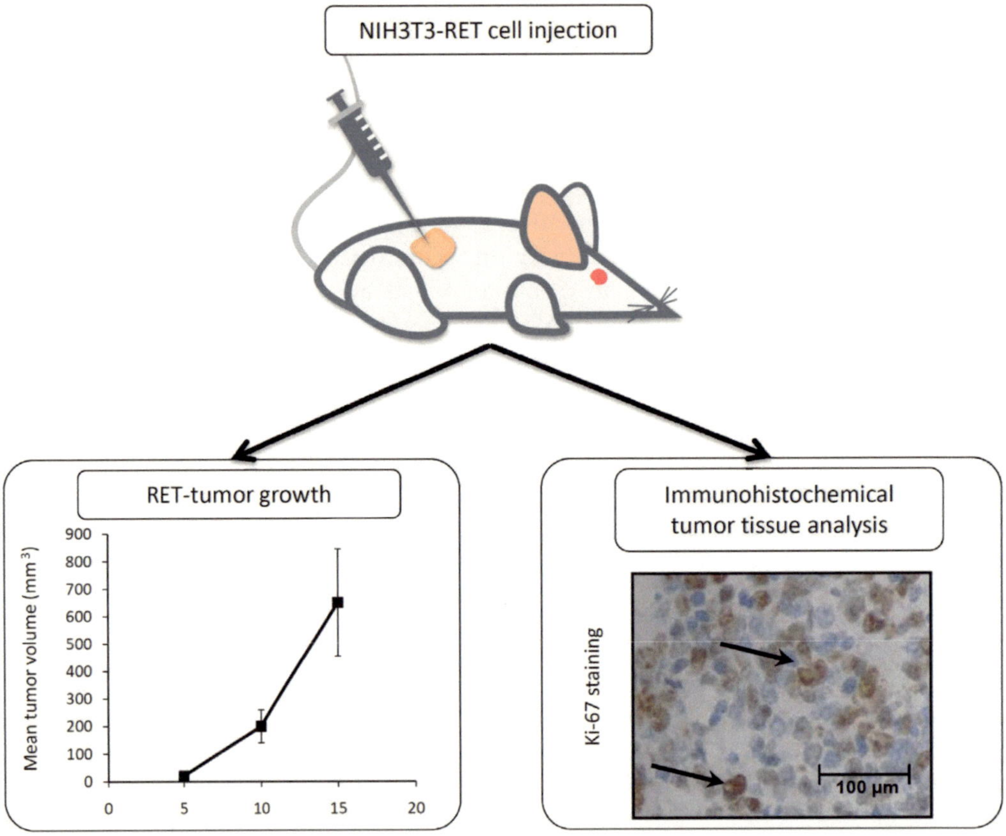

Fig. 4. Induction of RET tumor formation by subcutaneous injection of stable NIH3T3 transfectants. Measurement of tumor volume and immunohistochemical examination of cancer cell proliferation allows estimation of tumor aggressiveness.

3.2 Fingerprinting of RET-derived tumors by microarray analysis

Our main concern is to find genotype-associated molecular signatures that could predict the onset and aggressiveness of MEN 2-RET-related MTCs with a defined point mutation. Therefore, we generated transcriptomic profiles of RET-derived tumors differing in their clinical appearance (FMTC, level 1; MEN 2A, level 2; MEN 2B, level 3). This genetic fingerprint library is compared with the expression profile of a tumor with an unclassified RET-mutation. Consequently a hitherto clinically undefined mutation is classified into the three risk levels.

Identification of the differential gene expression pattern for a specific RET point mutation

First, a GeneChip expression analysis is performed for the investigated RET-derived tumor (**Fig. 5**). Total RNA from frozen tumor tissue is used to prepare biotinylated cRNA targets, which are hybridized to Affymetrix Mouse 430 2.0 GeneChips. Hybridization and washing of gene chips is routinely performed on an Affymetrix GeneChip Hybridization Oven and Fluidics Station. Afterwards microarrays are analyzed by laser scanning (Affymetrix Gene-Chip Scanner). Background-corrected signal intensities are determined and processed using MAS5 function of the R/Bioconductor affy package (www.r-project.org/ www.bioconductor.org). All calculations including normalization of microarray data, statistical tests, clustering, and further filtering methods are accomplished by up to date gene expression analysis software (e.g. GeneSpring GX 9.0 Agilent Technologies). Genes whose transcripts are not detected in any of the investigated mutations are excluded from statistical analysis to reduce the number of false positive genes. To determine differentially expressed genes, expression data are statistically analyzed using t-test and multiple testing correction (Benjamini and Hochberg False Discovery Rate). Cut-offs are set empirically to three fold and $P \leq 0.01$.

Analyzing and classifying the array data

The methods described above generate a gene list and expression profile that is unique for a certain point mutation. The obtained expression profile is normalized and clustered together with our pre-existing RET tumor transcriptomic database. This allows us to estimate the potential outcome of a RET point mutation on the genetic level. Information about biological processes and signaling pathways that participate in RET-induced cellular transformation are from outstanding importance, because this could reveal attractive therapeutic targets such as small molecules inhibitors. To extract therapy relevant information, functional annotation clustering is applied by using the **D**atabase for **A**nnotation, **V**isualization and **I**ntegrated **D**iscovery (DAVID, http://david.abcc.ncifcrf.gov/). This online database provides a comprehensive set of functional annotation tools to understand biological meaning behind large list of genes. In detail, functional annotation clustering condenses an input gene list into smaller, much more organized biological annotation modules in a term-centric manner. It allows investigators to focus on the annotation group level by quickly organizing many redundant/similar/hierarchical terms within the group. Annotation clusters, such as immune response, transcriptional regulation, chemokine activity, cytokine activity, kinase activity, signaling transduction, cell death and so on, could be found on the top of the output as expected for this study. With these results one can quickly focus on the major biology at an annotation cluster level. The enrichment score is to rank the overall importance (enrichment) of annotation term groups. It is the geometric mean of all the enrichment P-values of each annotation term in the group.

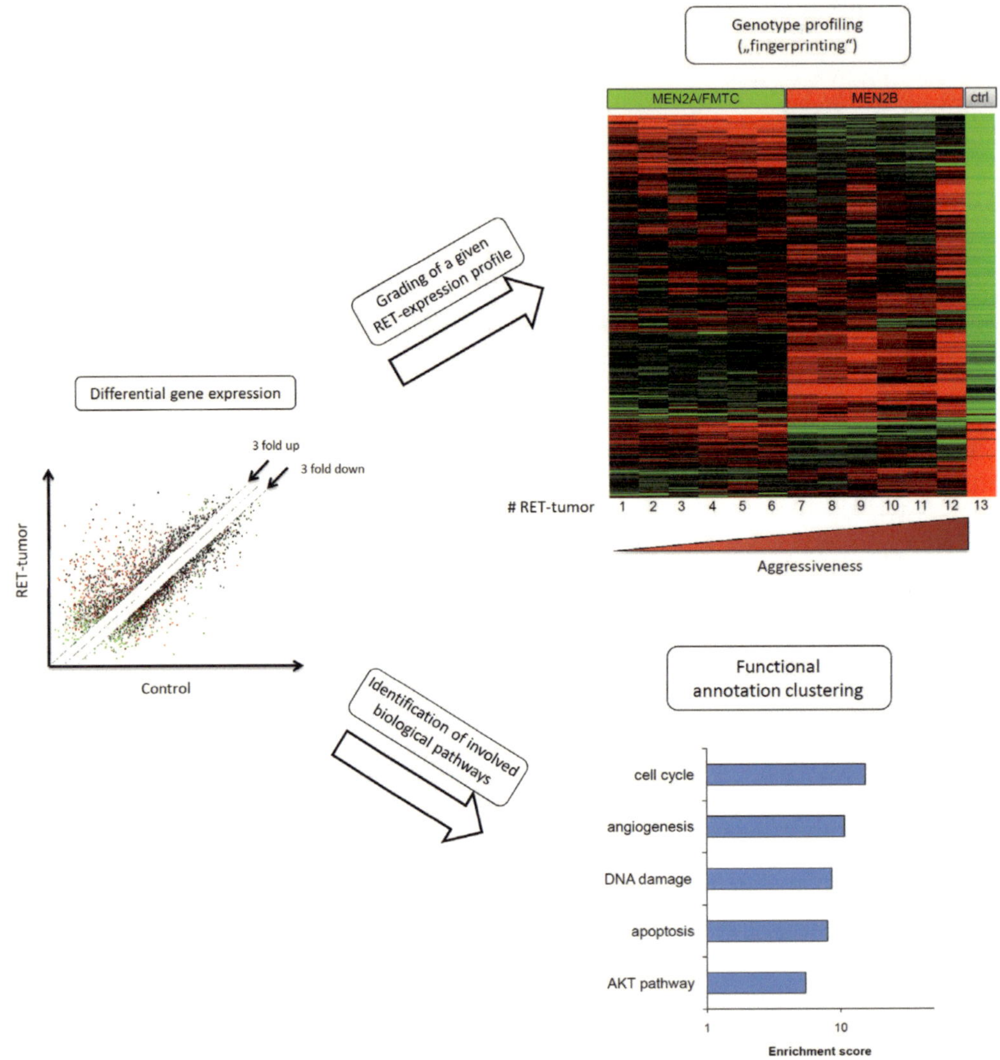

Fig. 5. Microarray data mining and expression analysis strategies to classify RET tumors with uncharacterized point mutations. Functional annotation clustering can be used to identify targets with therapeutic potential.

Expression profiling identified a statistically significant modification of 1494 genes, 628 down- and 866 upregulated in MEN 2B compared with MEN 2A/FMTC tumors. By contrast, no obvious alterations were observed among individual MEN 2B and MEN 2A type mutations, or between MEN 2A and FMTC. Functional clustering of differential genes revealed RET-MEN 2B specific upregulation of genes associated with novel growth and survival pathways. A central finding of this study was the extent of changes in genes whose products affect the immune response. In particular, we observed a remarkable accumulation of genes encoding NK cell receptors, T-lymphocyte antigens, regulators of NK- and T-cell proliferation/attraction, and apoptosis molecules important for the ability of NK cells and cytotoxic T cells to kill their targets in the tumors initiated by RET-MEN 2A/FMTC mutations, while expression of these genes was nearly completely suppressed in RET-MEN 2B related cancers. Quantitative real-time PCR on tumors versus cultured NIH-RET cell lines demonstrated that they are largely attributed to the host innate immune system, whereas expression of CX3CL1 involved in leukocyte recruitment is exclusively RET-MEN 2A/FMTC tumor cell dependent. In correlation, massive inflammatory infiltrates were apparent only in tumors carrying MEN 2A/FMTC mutations, suggesting that RET-MEN 2B receptors specifically counteract immune infiltration by preventing chemokine expression, which may contribute to the different clinical outcome of both subtypes (Engelmann et al., 2009). In summary, our data support a model of *RET* oncogene-specific interference with the host immune system, in which chemokine production by RET-MEN 2A/FMTC cancer cells initiates an antitumor immune attack, while RET-MEN 2B receptors avoid tumor infiltration as a mechanism of evasion that may be critical for the different clinical outcome of both subtypes.

4. Conclusion and future perspectives

In 1993, activating mutations in RET were identified as a cause for the development of MTC. In the following years, extensive research has been dedicated to exploring the mechanisms involved in RET-mediated tumorigenesis. All acquired data emphasize the essential role of mutated RET in the process of MTC development and already indicate a role for RET as an anticancer target. In recent years, many different studies have experimentally verified that RET inhibition might have an adverse effect on MTC progression, and that oncogenic activated RET is indeed a highly promising target for the development of a targeted strategy. Our results obtained from functional investigations of *RET* oncogene mutations imposingly demonstrate how clinical practice is empowered by molecular information that dictates medical management, lending future credence to the concept of gene-informed personalized healthcare. In the molecular age, however, it would be farfetched to believe that focussing on the DNA levels is the entire truth to solve an individual´s prognosis. Downstream of the transcriptional level regulation of mRNA awaits to be the next step in oncogenesis research. At this point small non-coding microRNAs (miRNAs) appear on stage. The discovery of miRNAs and their impact on functions in many biological and physiological processes has opened a new broad area of possible interactions in the regulatory network of cells. Furthermore, in the past few years it became evident that these regulatory RNAs also have an emerging role in development and progression of tumors. Extensive profiling of miRNAs in many cancer types revealed significant differences in their expression patterns, making them an interesting tool for cancer treatment. Until now the expression and functions of miRNAs in thyroid cancers has been described for follicular, anaplastic and papillary thyroid carcinomas. The studies demonstrated that in these cancer types distinct miRNAs are up and down regulated. In turn, these miRNAs regulate several transcription factors and effector molecules that are implicated in proliferation, cell adhesion, apoptosis and finally lead to oncogenesis and de-differentiation. Thus, miRNAs can act as oncogenes or tumor suppressors in thyroid cancers. To date complete miRNA profiles of MTCs harboring distinct *RET* mutations are missing. An opportunity that must be exploited for moving towards individualized medicine in cancer treatment beyond ATA risk stratification or, even more important, for prevention of metastasis. The technical procedure developed in our laboratory to identify MTC-associated miRNAs contributing to the oncogenic potential of the mutated RET receptor are illustrated in **Fig. 6**.

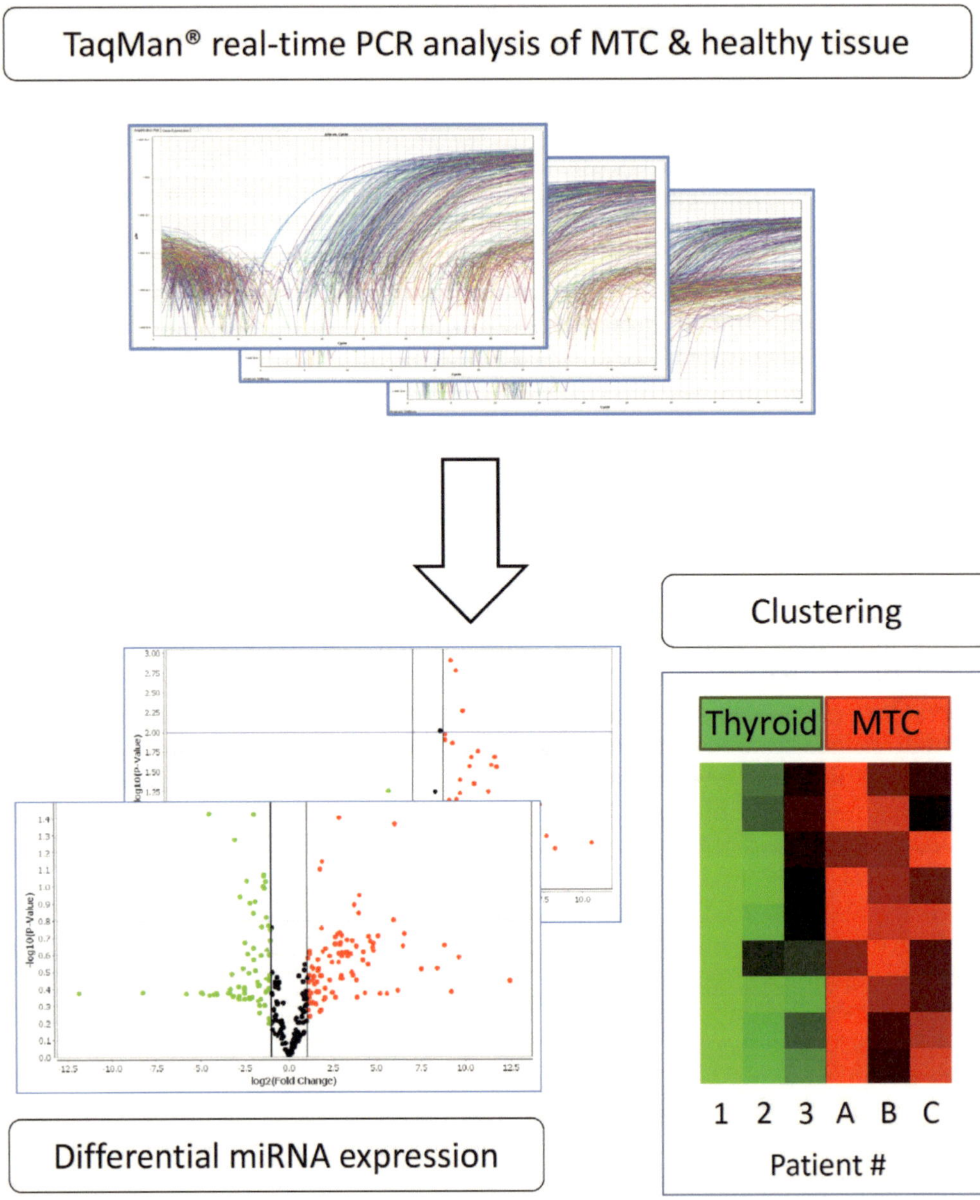

Fig. 6. Real-time PCR based screening for microRNA profiles in various human MTCs harboring RET point mutations. Clustering is used to reveal differential expression patterns of distinct microRNAs in tumors compared to healthy donor tissue.

5. Acknowledgment

We thank all clinical colleagues and the members of our lab who have contributed to these ideas. Our work was funded by Deutsche Forschungsgemeinschaft (DFG) and FORUN program of the Medical Faculty of Rostock University.

6. References

Airaksinen, M.S. & Saarma, M. (2002). The GDNF family: signalling, biological functions and therapeutic value. *Nat Rev Neurosci*, Vol. 3, No. 5, 383-394.

Arighi, E.; Borrello, M.G. & Sariola, H. (2005). RET tyrosine kinase signaling in development and cancer. *Cytokine Growth Factor Rev*, Vol. 16, No. 4-5, 441-467.

Bocciardi, R.; Mograbi, B.; Pasini, B.; Borrello, M.G.; Pierotti, M.A.; Bourget, I.; Fischer, S.; Romeo, G. & Rossi, B. (1997). The multiple endocrine neoplasia type 2B point mutation switches the specificity of the Ret tyrosine kinase towards cellular substrates that are susceptible to interact with Crk and Nck. *Oncogene*, Vol. 15, No. 19, 2257-2265.

Böckmann, M.; Drosten, M. & Pützer, B.M. (2005a). Discovery of targeting peptides for selective therapy of medullary thyroid carcinoma. *J Gene Med*, Vol. 7, No. 2, 179-188.

Böckmann, M.; Hilken, G.; Schmidt, A.; Cranston, A.N.; Tannapfel, A.; Drosten, M.; Frilling, A.; Ponder, B.A. & Pützer, B.M. (2005b). Novel SRESPHP peptide mediates specific binding to primary medullary thyroid carcinoma after systemic injection. *Hum Gene Ther*, Vol. 16, No. 11, 1267-1275.

Borrello, M.G.; Smith, D.P.; Pasini, B.; Bongarzone, I.; Greco, A.; Lorenzo, M.J.; Arighi, E.; Miranda, C.; Eng, C.; Alberti, L. & et al. (1995). RET activation by germline MEN2A and MEN2B mutations. *Oncogene*, Vol. 11, No. 11, 2419-2427.

Brandi, M.L.; Gagel, R.F.; Angeli, A.; Bilezikian, J.P.; Beck-Peccoz, P.; Bordi, C.; Conte-Devolx, B.; Falchetti, A.; Gheri, R.G.; Libroia, A.; Lips, C.J.; Lombardi, G.; Mannelli, M.; Pacini, F.; Ponder, B.A.; Raue, F.; Skogseid, B.; Tamburrano, G.; Thakker, R.V.; Thompson, N.W.; Tomassetti, P.; Tonelli, F.; Wells, S.A., Jr. & Marx, S.J. (2001). Guidelines for diagnosis and therapy of MEN type 1 and type 2. *J Clin Endocrinol Metab*, Vol. 86, No. 12, 5658-5671.

Carlomagno, F.; Guida, T.; Anaganti, S.; Vecchio, G.; Fusco, A.; Ryan, A.J.; Billaud, M. & Santoro, M. (2004). Disease associated mutations at valine 804 in the RET receptor tyrosine kinase confer resistance to selective kinase inhibitors. *Oncogene*, Vol. 23, No. 36, 6056-6063.

Carlomagno, F.; Salvatore, G.; Cirafici, A.M.; De Vita, G.; Melillo, R.M.; de Franciscis, V.; Billaud, M.; Fusco, A. & Santoro, M. (1997). The different RET-activating capability of mutations of cysteine 620 or cysteine 634 correlates with the multiple endocrine neoplasia type 2 disease phenotype. *Cancer Res*, Vol. 57, No. 3, 391-395.

Carlomagno, F.; Vitagliano, D.; Guida, T.; Basolo, F.; Castellone, M.D.; Melillo, R.M.; Fusco, A. & Santoro, M. (2003). Efficient inhibition of RET/papillary thyroid carcinoma oncogenic kinases by 4-amino-5-(4-chloro-phenyl)-7-(t-butyl)pyrazolo[3,4-d]pyrimidine (PP2). *J Clin Endocrinol Metab*, Vol. 88, No. 4, 1897-1902.

Carlomagno, F.; Vitagliano, D.; Guida, T.; Ciardiello, F.; Tortora, G.; Vecchio, G.; Ryan, A.J.; Fontanini, G.; Fusco, A. & Santoro, M. (2002a). ZD6474, an orally available inhibitor of KDR tyrosine kinase activity, efficiently blocks oncogenic RET kinases. *Cancer Res*, Vol. 62, No. 24, 7284-7290.

Carlomagno, F.; Vitagliano, D.; Guida, T.; Napolitano, M.; Vecchio, G.; Fusco, A.; Gazit, A.; Levitzki, A. & Santoro, M. (2002b). The kinase inhibitor PP1 blocks tumorigenesis induced by RET oncogenes. *Cancer Res*, Vol. 62, No. 4, 1077-1082.

Carlson, K.M.; Dou, S.; Chi, D.; Scavarda, N.; Toshima, K.; Jackson, C.E.; Wells, S.A., Jr.; Goodfellow, P.J. & Donis-Keller, H. (1994). Single missense mutation in the tyrosine kinase catalytic domain of the RET protooncogene is associated with multiple endocrine neoplasia type 2B. *Proc Natl Acad Sci U S A*, Vol. 91, No. 4, 1579-1583.

Carniti, C.; Perego, C.; Mondellini, P.; Pierotti, M.A. & Bongarzone, I. (2003). PP1 inhibitor induces degradation of RETMEN2A and RETMEN2B oncoproteins through proteosomal targeting. *Cancer Res*, Vol. 63, No. 9, 2234-2243.

Cerchia, L.; Libri, D.; Carlomagno, M.S. & de Franciscis, V. (2003). The soluble ectodomain of RetC634Y inhibits both the wild-type and the constitutively active Ret. *Biochem J*, Vol. 372, No. Pt 3, 897-903.

Chiariello, M.; Visconti, R.; Carlomagno, F.; Melillo, R.M.; Bucci, C.; de Franciscis, V.; Fox, G.M.; Jing, S.; Coso, O.A.; Gutkind, J.S.; Fusco, A. & Santoro, M. (1998). Signalling of the Ret receptor tyrosine kinase through the c-Jun NH2-terminal protein kinases (JNKS): evidence for a divergence of the ERKs and JNKs pathways induced by Ret. *Oncogene*, Vol. 16, No. 19, 2435-2445.

Cohen, M.S.; Hussain, H.B. & Moley, J.F. (2002). Inhibition of medullary thyroid carcinoma cell proliferation and RET phosphorylation by tyrosine kinase inhibitors. *Surgery*, Vol. 132, No. 6, 960-966; discussion 966-967.

Cohen, M.S. & Moley, J.F. (2003). Surgical treatment of medullary thyroid carcinoma. *J Intern Med*, Vol. 253, No. 6, 616-626.

Cuccuru, G.; Lanzi, C.; Cassinelli, G.; Pratesi, G.; Tortoreto, M.; Petrangolini, G.; Seregni, E.; Martinetti, A.; Laccabue, D.; Zanchi, C. & Zunino, F. (2004). Cellular effects and antitumor activity of RET inhibitor RPI-1 on MEN2A-associated medullary thyroid carcinoma. *J Natl Cancer Inst*, Vol. 96, No. 13, 1006-1014.

de Groot, J.W.; Zonnenberg, B.A.; van Ufford-Mannesse, P.Q.; de Vries, M.M.; Links, T.P.; Lips, C.J. & Voest, E.E. (2007). A phase II trial of imatinib therapy for metastatic medullary thyroid carcinoma. *J Clin Endocrinol Metab*, Vol. 92, No. 9, 3466-3469.

De Souza, J.A.; Busaidy, N.; Zimrin, A.; Seiwert, T.; Villflor, V.M.; Poluru, K.B.; Reddy, P.L.; Nam, J.; Vokes, E.E. & Cohen, E.E. (2010). Phase II trial of sunitinib inmedullary thyroid cancer (MTC). *J Clin Oncol*, Vol. 28, No. 15:5504.

Donghi, R.; Sozzi, G.; Pierotti, M.A.; Biunno, I.; Miozzo, M.; Fusco, A.; Grieco, M.; Santoro, M.; Vecchio, G.; Spurr, N.K. & et al. (1989). The oncogene associated with human papillary thyroid carcinoma (PTC) is assigned to chromosome 10 q11-q12 in the same region as multiple endocrine neoplasia type 2A (MEN2A). *Oncogene*, Vol. 4, No. 4, 521-523.

Drosten, M.; Frilling, A.; Stiewe, T. & Pützer, B.M. (2002). A new therapeutic approach in medullary thyroid cancer treatment: inhibition of oncogenic RET signaling by adenoviral vector-mediated expression of a dominant-negative RET mutant. *Surgery*, Vol. 132, No. 6, 991-997; discussion 997.

Drosten, M.; Hilken, G.; Böckmann, M.; Rodicker, F.; Mise, N.; Cranston, A.N.; Dahmen, U.; Ponder, B.A. & Pützer, B.M. (2004). Role of MEN2A-derived RET in maintenance and proliferation of medullary thyroid carcinoma. *J Natl Cancer Inst*, Vol. 96, No. 16, 1231-1239.

Drosten, M.; Stiewe, T. & Pützer, B.M. (2003). Antitumor capacity of dominant-negative RET proto oncogene mutant in a medullary thyroid carcinoma model. *Hum Gene Ther*, Vol. 14, No. 10, 971-982.

Durbec, P.; Marcos-Gutierrez, C.V.; Kilkenny, C.; Grigoriou, M.; Wartiowaara, K.; Suvanto, P.; Smith, D.; Ponder, B.; Costantini, F.; Saarma, M. & et al. (1996). GDNF signalling through the Ret receptor tyrosine kinase. *Nature*, Vol. 381, No. 6585, 789-793.

Eng, C. (1999). RET proto-oncogene in the development of human cancer. *J Clin Oncol*, Vol. 17, No. 1, 380-393.

Eng, C.; Clayton, D.; Schuffenecker, I.; Lenoir, G.; Cote, G.; Gagel, R.F.; van Amstel, H.K.; Lips, C.J.; Nishisho, I.; Takai, S.I.; Marsh, D.J.; Robinson, B.G.; Frank-Raue, K.; Raue, F.; Xue, F.; Noll, W.W.; Romei, C.; Pacini, F.; Fink, M.; Niederle, B.; Zedenius, J.; Nordenskjold, M.; Komminoth, P.; Hendy, G.N.; Mulligan, L.M. & et al. (1996). The relationship between specific RET proto-oncogene mutations and disease phenotype in multiple endocrine neoplasia type 2. International RET mutation consortium analysis. *Jama*, Vol. 276, No. 19, 1575-1579.

Engelmann, D.; Koczan, D.; Ricken, P.; Rimpler, U.; Pahnke, J.; Li, Z. & Pützer, B.M. (2009). Transcriptome analysis in mouse tumors induced by Ret-MEN2/FMTC mutations reveals subtype-specific role in survival and interference with immune surveillance. *Endocr Relat Cancer*, Vol. 16, No. 1, 211-224.

Forssell-Aronsson, E.; Fjalling, M.; Nilsson, O.; Tisell, L.E.; Wangberg, B. & Ahlman, H. (1995). Indium-111 activity concentration in tissue samples after intravenous injection of indium-111-DTPA-D-Phe-1-octreotide. *J Nucl Med*, Vol. 36, No. 1, 7-12.

Gimm, O. (2001). Multiple endocrine neoplasia type 2: clinical aspects. *Front Horm Res*, Vol. 28, No. 103-130.

Gimm, O.; Marsh, D.J.; Andrew, S.D.; Frilling, A.; Dahia, P.L.; Mulligan, L.M.; Zajac, J.D.; Robinson, B.G. & Eng, C. (1997). Germline dinucleotide mutation in codon 883 of the RET proto-oncogene in multiple endocrine neoplasia type 2B without codon 918 mutation. *J Clin Endocrinol Metab*, Vol. 82, No. 11, 3902-3904.

Hahn, M. & Bishop, J. (2001). Expression pattern of Drosophila ret suggests a common ancestral origin between the metamorphosis precursors in insect endoderm and the vertebrate enteric neurons. *Proc Natl Acad Sci U S A*, Vol. 98, No. 3, 1053-1058.

Hansford, J.R. & Mulligan, L.M. (2000). Multiple endocrine neoplasia type 2 and RET: from neoplasia to neurogenesis. *J Med Genet*, Vol. 37, No. 11, 817-827.

Hayashi, Y.; Iwashita, T.; Murakamai, H.; Kato, Y.; Kawai, K.; Kurokawa, K.; Tohnai, I.; Ueda, M. & Takahashi, M. (2001). Activation of BMK1 via tyrosine 1062 in RET by GDNF and MEN2A mutation. *Biochem Biophys Res Commun*, Vol. 281, No. 3, 682-689.

Hofstra, R.M.; Landsvater, R.M.; Ceccherini, I.; Stulp, R.P.; Stelwagen, T.; Luo, Y.; Pasini, B.; Hoppener, J.W.; van Amstel, H.K.; Romeo, G. & et al. (1994). A mutation in the RET proto-oncogene associated with multiple endocrine neoplasia type 2B and sporadic medullary thyroid carcinoma. *Nature*, Vol. 367, No. 6461, 375-376.

Ichihara, M.; Murakumo, Y. & Takahashi, M. (2004). RET and neuroendocrine tumors. *Cancer Lett*, Vol. 204, No. 2, 197-211.

Iwamoto, T.; Taniguchi, M.; Asai, N.; Ohkusu, K.; Nakashima, I. & Takahashi, M. (1993). cDNA cloning of mouse ret proto-oncogene and its sequence similarity to the cadherin superfamily. *Oncogene*, Vol. 8, No. 4, 1087-1091.

Jijiwa, M.; Fukuda, T.; Kawai, K.; Nakamura, A.; Kurokawa, K.; Murakumo, Y.; Ichihara, M. & Takahashi, M. (2004). A targeting mutation of tyrosine 1062 in Ret causes a marked decrease of enteric neurons and renal hypoplasia. *Mol Cell Biol*, Vol. 24, No. 18, 8026-8036.

Juweid, M.; Sharkey, R.M.; Behr, T.; Swayne, L.C.; Herskovic, T.; Pereira, M.; Rubin, A.D.; Hanley, D.; Dunn, R.; Siegel, J. & Goldenberg, D.M. (1996). Radioimmunotherapy of medullary thyroid cancer with iodine-131-labeled anti-CEA antibodies. *J Nucl Med*, Vol. 37, No. 6, 905-911.

Juweid, M.E.; Hajjar, G.; Stein, R.; Sharkey, R.M.; Herskovic, T.; Swayne, L.C.; Suleiman, S.; Pereira, M.; Rubin, A.D. & Goldenberg, D.M. (2000). Initial experience with high-dose radioimmunotherapy of metastatic medullary thyroid cancer using 131I-MN-

14 F(ab)2 anti-carcinoembryonic antigen MAb and AHSCR. *J Nucl Med*, Vol. 41, No. 1, 93-103.

Kaltsas, G.; Korbonits, M.; Heintz, E.; Mukherjee, J.J.; Jenkins, P.J.; Chew, S.L.; Reznek, R.; Monson, J.P.; Besser, G.M.; Foley, R.; Britton, K.E. & Grossman, A.B. (2001). Comparison of somatostatin analog and meta-iodobenzylguanidine radionuclides in the diagnosis and localization of advanced neuroendocrine tumors. *J Clin Endocrinol Metab*, Vol. 86, No. 2, 895-902.

Kloos, R.T.; Eng, C.; Evans, D.B.; Francis, G.L.; Gagel, R.F.; Gharib, H.; Moley, J.F.; Pacini, F.; Ringel, M.D.; Schlumberger, M. & Wells, S.A., Jr. (2009). Medullary thyroid cancer: management guidelines of the American Thyroid Association. *Thyroid*, Vol. 19, No. 6, 565-612.

Kraeber-Bodere, F.; Faibre-Chauvet, A.; Sai-Maurel, C.; Gautherot, E.; Fiche, M.; Campion, L.; Le Boterff, J.; Barbet, J.; Chatal, J.F. & Thedrez, P. (1999). Bispecific antibody and bivalent hapten radioimmunotherapy in CEA-producing medullary thyroid cancer xenograft. *J Nucl Med*, Vol. 40, No. 1, 198-204.

Lam, E.T.; Ringel, M.D.; Kloos, R.T.; Prior, T.W.; Knopp, M.V.; Liang, J.; Sammet, S.; Hall, N.C.; Wakely, P.E., Jr.; Vasko, V.V.; Saji, M.; Snyder, P.J.; Wei, L.; Arbogast, D.; Collamore, M.; Wright, J.J.; Moley, J.F.; Villalona-Calero, M.A. & Shah, M.H. (2010). Phase II clinical trial of sorafenib in metastatic medullary thyroid cancer. *J Clin Oncol*, Vol. 28, No. 14, 2323-2330.

Lanzi, C.; Cassinelli, G.; Pensa, T.; Cassinis, M.; Gambetta, R.A.; Borrello, M.G.; Menta, E.; Pierotti, M.A. & Zunino, F. (2000). Inhibition of transforming activity of the ret/ptc1 oncoprotein by a 2-indolinone derivative. *Int J Cancer*, Vol. 85, No. 3, 384-390.

Le Hir, H.; Charlet-Berguerand, N.; Gimenez-Roqueplo, A.; Mannelli, M.; Plouin, P.; de Franciscis, V. & Thermes, C. (2000). Relative expression of the RET9 and RET51 isoforms in human pheochromocytomas. *Oncology*, Vol. 58, No. 4, 311-318.

Manie, S.; Santoro, M.; Fusco, A. & Billaud, M. (2001). The RET receptor: function in development and dysfunction in congenital malformation. *Trends Genet*, Vol. 17, No. 10, 580-589.

Meng, X.; Lindahl, M.; Hyvonen, M.E.; Parvinen, M.; de Rooij, D.G.; Hess, M.W.; Raatikainen-Ahokas, A.; Sainio, K.; Rauvala, H.; Lakso, M.; Pichel, J.G.; Westphal, H.; Saarma, M. & Sariola, H. (2000). Regulation of cell fate decision of undifferentiated spermatogonia by GDNF. *Science*, Vol. 287, No. 5457, 1489-1493.

Mirallie, E.; Sai-Maurel, C.; Faivre-Chauvet, A.; Regenet, N.; Chang, C.H.; Goldenberg, D.M.; Chatal, J.F.; Barbet, J. & Thedrez, P. (2005). Improved pretargeted delivery of radiolabelled hapten to human tumour xenograft in mice by avidin chase of circulating bispecific antibody. *Eur J Nucl Med Mol Imaging*, Vol. 32, No. 8, 901-909.

Mise, N.; Drosten, M.; Racek, T.; Tannapfel, A. & Pützer, B.M. (2006). Evaluation of potential mechanisms underlying genotype-phenotype correlations in multiple endocrine neoplasia type 2. *Oncogene*, Vol. 25, No. 50, 6637-6647.

Mulligan, L.M.; Kwok, J.B.; Healey, C.S.; Elsdon, M.J.; Eng, C.; Gardner, E.; Love, D.R.; Mole, S.E.; Moore, J.K.; Papi, L. & et al. (1993). Germ-line mutations of the RET proto-oncogene in multiple endocrine neoplasia type 2A. *Nature*, Vol. 363, No. 6428, 458-460.

Murakami, H.; Iwashita, T.; Asai, N.; Shimono, Y.; Iwata, Y.; Kawai, K. & Takahashi, M. (1999). Enhanced phosphatidylinositol 3-kinase activity and high phosphorylation state of its downstream signalling molecules mediated by ret with the MEN 2B mutation. *Biochem Biophys Res Commun*, Vol. 262, No. 1, 68-75.

Salvatore, D.; Melillo, R.M.; Monaco, C.; Visconti, R.; Fenzi, G.; Vecchio, G.; Fusco, A. & Santoro, M. (2001). Increased in vivo phosphorylation of ret tyrosine 1062 is a potential pathogenetic mechanism of multiple endocrine neoplasia type 2B. *Cancer Res*, Vol. 61, No. 4, 1426-1431.

Santarpia, L.; Ye, L. & Gagel, R.F. (2009). Beyond RET: potential therapeutic approaches for advanced and metastatic medullary thyroid carcinoma. *J Intern Med*, Vol. 266, No. 1, 99-113.

Santoro, M.; Carlomagno, F.; Melillo, R.M.; Billaud, M.; Vecchio, G. & Fusco, A., Molecular mechanisms of RET activation in human neoplasia. *J Endocrinol Invest* (1999), pp. 811-819.

Santoro, M.; Carlomagno, F.; Romano, A.; Bottaro, D.P.; Dathan, N.A.; Grieco, M.; Fusco, A.; Vecchio, G.; Matoskova, B.; Kraus, M.H. & et al. (1995). Activation of RET as a dominant transforming gene by germline mutations of MEN2A and MEN2B. *Science*, Vol. 267, No. 5196, 381-383.

Schlumberger, M.J.; Elisei, R.; Bastholt, L.; Wirth, L.J.; Martins, R.G.; Locati, L.D.; Jarzab, B.; Pacini, F.; Daumerie, C.; Droz, J.P.; Eschenberg, M.J.; Sun, Y.N.; Juan, T.; Stepan, D.E. & Sherman, S.I. (2009). Phase II study of safety and efficacy of motesanib in patients with progressive or symptomatic, advanced or metastatic medullary thyroid cancer. *J Clin Oncol*, Vol. 27, No. 23, 3794-3801.

Schmidt, A.; Eipel, C.; Furst, K.; Sommer, N.; Pahnke, J. & Pützer, B.M. (2011). Evaluation of systemic targeting of RET oncogene-based MTC with tumor-selective peptide-tagged Ad vectors in clinical mouse models. *Gene Ther*, Vol. 18, No. 4, 418-423.

Schuchardt, A.; D'Agati, V.; Larsson-Blomberg, L.; Costantini, F. & Pachnis, V. (1994). Defects in the kidney and enteric nervous system of mice lacking the tyrosine kinase receptor Ret. *Nature*, Vol. 367, No. 6461, 380-383.

Sippel, R.S.; Kunnimalaiyaan, M. & Chen, H. (2008). Current management of medullary thyroid cancer. *Oncologist*, Vol. 13, No. 5, 539-547.

Smith, D.P.; Houghton, C. & Ponder, B.A. (1997). Germline mutation of RET codon 883 in two cases of de novo MEN 2B. *Oncogene*, Vol. 15, No. 10, 1213-1217.

Spitzweg, C. & Morris, J.C. (2004). Gene therapy for thyroid cancer: current status and future prospects. *Thyroid*, Vol. 14, No. 6, 424-434.

Strock, C.J.; Park, J.I.; Rosen, M.; Dionne, C.; Ruggeri, B.; Jones-Bolin, S.; Denmeade, S.R.; Ball, D.W. & Nelkin, B.D. (2003). CEP-701 and CEP-751 inhibit constitutively activated RET tyrosine kinase activity and block medullary thyroid carcinoma cell growth. *Cancer Res*, Vol. 63, No. 17, 5559-5563.

Takahashi, M. (2001). The GDNF/RET signaling pathway and human diseases. *Cytokine Growth Factor Rev*, Vol. 12, No. 4, 361-373.

Takahashi, M.; Asai, N.; Iwashita, T.; Murakami, H. & Ito, S. (1998). Molecular mechanisms of development of multiple endocrine neoplasia 2 by RET mutations. *J Intern Med*, Vol. 243, No. 6, 509-513.

Takahashi, M.; Buma, Y. & Taniguchi, M. (1991). Identification of the ret proto-oncogene products in neuroblastoma and leukemia cells. *Oncogene*, Vol. 6, No. 2, 297-301.

Takahashi, M.; Ritz, J. & Cooper, G.M. (1985). Activation of a novel human transforming gene, ret, by DNA rearrangement. *Cell*, Vol. 42, No. 2, 581-588.

Troncone, L.; Rufini, V.; Maussier, M.L.; Valenza, V.; Daidone, M.S.; Luzi, S. & De Santis, M. (1991). The role of [131I]metaiodobenzylguanidine in the treatment of medullary thyroid carcinoma: results in five cases. *J Nucl Biol Med*, Vol. 35, No. 4, 327-331.

Tsui-Pierchala, B.A.; Milbrandt, J. & Johnson, E.M., Jr. (2002). NGF utilizes c-Ret via a novel GFL-independent, inter-RTK signaling mechanism to maintain the trophic status of mature sympathetic neurons. *Neuron*, Vol. 33, No. 2, 261-273.

Wells, S.A.; Robinson, B.G.; Gagel, R.F.; Dralle, H.; Fagin, J.A.; Santoro, M.; Baudin, E.; Vasselli, J.R.; Read, J. & Schlumberger, M. (2010). Vandetanib (VAN) in locally advanced or metastatic medullary thyroid cancer (MTC): A randomized, double-blind phase III trial (ZETA). *J Clin Oncol* Vol. 28, No. 15:5503.

11

Medullary Thyroid Carcinoma Associated with *RET* Mutations Located in Exon 8

Melpomeni Peppa[1] and Sotirios A. Raptis[2,3]
[1]*Endocrine Unit, Second Dept of Internal Medicine-Propaedeutic, Research Institute and Diabetes Center, Athens University Medical School, Attikon University Hospital, Athens*
[2]*Second Dept of Internal Medicine-Propaedeutic, Research Institute and Diabetes Center, Athens University Medical School, Attikon University Hospital, Athens*
[3]*Hellenic National Diabetes Center for the Prevention, Research and Treatment of Diabetes Mellitus and its Complications (H.N.D.C), Athens*
Greece

1. Introduction

Medullary thyroid carcinoma is a neuroendocrine tumor which accounts for 5-10% of all thyroid cancers, with a various clinical course, being either an extremely benign tumor or an aggressive variant with a high mortality rate. Medullary thyroid carcinoma is sporadic in 80% of cases while in 20% of cases it follows a hereditary pattern, known as isolated familial MTC or multiple endocrine neoplasia type 2 syndromes, transmitted in an autosomal-dominant manner. Genetic analysis of the RET protooncogene constitutes an excellent powerful diagnostic tool for medullary thyroid carcinoma, especially for the hereditary form. Somatic, germline but also *de novo* mutations have all been associated with sporadic and hereditary forms of the disease and exons 10,11,13-16 of the RET gene locus are mainly involved. However, accumulating data support the association of other exons, including exon 8, with MTC but more studies need to be done, in order to provide more information about its role on the disease start, progression, potential and penetrance. At present, a "complete" germline *RET* testing should be performed in all MTC patients, independently of the family history and especially in the case of a negative testing, should include "non classical" exons, including exon 8.

2. Medullary thyroid carcinoma

Medullary thyroid carcinoma (MTC) is a neuroendocrine tumor which originates from the parafolicular C-cells of the thyroid gland, accounting for 5-10% of all thyroid cancers. (Pacini, 2010, Alevizaki 2006, Leboulleux 2004) Nowadays, the rate of MTC diagnosis gradually increases due to high awareness and thus careful investigation. MTC is a multifacet disease being either an extremely benign tumor or an aggressive variant which is associated with a high mortality rate because of lack of appropriate therapeutic regimens. (Pacini, 2010, Alevizaki 2006, Leboulleux 2004, Roman 2006)

MTC, is sporadic in 80% of cases (SMTC), presenting as an asymptomatic, accidentally found neck mass in the middle age, which spreads to regional lymph nodes in up to 50% of cases, as well as to distant sites (mediastinum, liver, lungs,bone). (Moo-Young 2009, Raue 2010, Alevizaki 2009) However, in 7% of individuals with apparently sporadic tumors, genetic screening revealed germline mutations of the RET (REarranged during Transfection) protooncogene (*RET*), indicating an overdiagnosis of SMTC in the absence of genetic screening. (Elisei 2007, Romei 2011).

In 20% of cases, MTC follows a hereditary pattern (HMTC), known as isolated familial (FMTC) or multiple endocrine neoplasia type 2 (MEN2) syndromes, transmitted in an autosomal-dominant manner. (Moo-Young 2009, Raue 2010, Alevizaki 2009) In opposite to the sporadic form, HMTC is characterized by small, frequently multifocal and bilateral nodules. (Moo-Young 2009, Raue 2010, Alevizaki 2009) The earlier identification of kindreds at risk of HMTC and the earlier selection of affected members for prophylactic thyroidectomy (14.9 versus 36.4 years), has resulted in a decrease in primary tumor size from 0.8 to 0.2 cm, a reduction in the percentage of bilateral neoplasms from 100% to 13%, a fall in the rate of lymph node metastases from 58% to 0%, all of them associated with less morbidity and mortality from HMTC. (Wells 1994, Graze 1978, Lips 1994)

FMTC, accounts for 35-40% of HMTC, exhibits variable expressivity and penetrance and follows a more indolent course compared to MEN syndromes, with a late onset or no clinically manifest disease and relative good prognosis. (Moo-Young 2009, Raue 2010, Alevizaki 2009) However, the diagnosis of MTC as FMTC is not sometimes correct. MTC is often the first manifestation of MEN2A, misclassified as FMTC with pheochromocytomas diagnosed later while a significant overlap in the genetic mutations between FMTC and MEN2A is observed. (Moo-Young 2009, Raue 2010, Alevizaki 2009) Thus, the definition of FMTC is strict and needs multiple members affected after the age of 50 years and the absence of either pheochromocytoma or hyperparathyroidism in more than 10 carriers. (Brandi 2001) Nowadays, FMTC is considered as a phenotypic mildest variant of MEN2A, in which there is a strong predisposition to MTC and decreased penetrance of pheochromocytoma and primary hyperparathyroidism. In practical terms, especially in smaller kindreds, it is suggested that it is safer to label a family as MEN2A than FMTC, which ensures that patients are screened and monitored for the development of pheochromocytomas. (Moo-Young 2009, Raue 2010, Alevizaki 2009, Brandi 2001)

MEN2, is a rare cancer syndrome, transmitted in an autosomal dominant manner. The estimated prevalence is 2.5 per 100,000 cases in the general population. More than 1,000 kindreds have been described while many others have never been reported. MEN2 syndromes, involve MTC, following by pheochromocytoma in 50% of cases, primary hyperparathyroidism in 30% of cases and less commonly other clinical manifestations such as cutaneous lichen amyloidosis or Hirschsprung's disease. (Moo-Young 2009, Raue 2010, Alevizaki 2009)

MEN2A, accounts for 55% of all cases with MEN2, consisting of MTC in 75% -90% of cases, in combination with pheochromocytoma and primary hyperparathyroidism. MTC is typically multifocal and bilateral, starts in early adulthood and is responsible for most of the mortality associated with MEN2A, indicating the need for early recognition and treatment. (Moo-Young 2009, Raue 2010, Alevizaki 2009)

MEN2B syndrome, accounts for 5-10% of cases with MEN2, consisting of MTC, pheochromocytoma (50%), ganglioneuromatosis, Marfanoid habitus and less often clinical manifestations (megacolon, skeletal abnormalities, markedly enlarged peripheral nerves). MTC has its onset at a very young age (infancy), is most commonly aggressive and the patients are rarely cured of their disease, due to delayed diagnosis. (Moo-Young 2009, Raue 2010, Alevizaki 2009)

3. Diagnosis of medullary thyroid carcinoma

Since MTC is a multifacet thyroid cancer with a benign or aggressive course, the early recognition and treatment, even at the preclinical stage, is of crucial importance, leading in a higher cure rate of affected patients and a much better prognosis. (Roman 2006, Wells 1994, Graze 1978).

During the last decade, a great progress in the diagnostic identification of MTC has been made. Although questionable, calcitonin screening in patients with thyroid nodules has led to an increased rate of MTC diagnosis. Traditionally, calcitonin levels either basal or after provocative testing, constitute important diagnostic tools, in the identification of patients harbouring MTC. (Lips 1994) However, since the late 1990s, with the advent of molecular biology, genetic analysis of the *RET*, has been proved as a powerful diagnostic tool for MTC, especially HMTC . (Brandi 2001, Kouvaraki 2005)

4. Genetics of medullary thyroid carcinoma

MTC has been associated with mutations in the *RET*, a 21 exons gene, mapped to chromosome 10q11.2. (Brandi 2001, Kouvaraki 2005, Arighi 2005, Plaza-Menacho 2006) *RET* is a receptor tyrosine kinase, which exhibits trans-autophosphorylation of intracellular tyrosine residues and activation of downstream signaling pathways (Ras/ERK, phosphotidylinositol-3-kinase/AKT, beta-catenin/WNT, phospholipase, C gamma, Src), in tissues that express the receptor. The *RET* protein consists of a N terminal signal peptide, an extracellular region with 4 cadherin-like repeats, a calcium- binding site and a cysteine-rich domain, a transmembrane region, and an intracellular portion with two tyrosine kinase domains.(Kouvaraki 2005, Arighi 2005, Plaza-Menacho 2006) Activating point mutations in *RET* lead to constitutive activity of the receptor, C-cell hyperplasia (CCH) and MTC. The scenario of the "two hits" is now supported, including an inherited "first hit" leading to C-cell hyperplasia and a secondary somatic "second hit" in activated C cells, leading to HMTC. (Roman 2006) Genetic analysis of *RET* diagnoses MTC in about 98% of known families. (Brandi 2001) Since the distinction between sporadic and hereditary forms of MTC is not often clear, nowadays, *RET* molecular testing has solved a lot of diagnostic problems in patients with MTC, ensuring a better management of patients and their families and less MTC associated morbidity and mortality. (Wells 1994, Graze 1978, Lips 1994)

4.1 *RET* mutations

Since 1993, that the first germline mutation of the *RET* was identified, an accumulating number of *RET* mutations has been isolated, linked to MTC. (Brandi 2001, Kouvaraki 2005, Arighi 2005, Plaza-Menacho2006) Based on the *RET* molecular testing, 1-7% of cases with apparently sporadic tumors were found to have *RET* mutations. (Elisei 2007, Romei 2011, Wohllk 1996, Blaugrund 1994, Elisei 2008)

Genetic testing of the *RET* is performed by PCR amplification of the patient's germline DNA obtained from white blood cells or thyroid tissue. Initially, exons 10, 11, 13, 14, 15, and 16 are carefully screened and if no mutations are detected, the remaining 15 exons of the RET gene should be sequenced. It has been estimated that mutations are found in over 95% of cases of HMTC. Otherwords, the predicted risk of HMTC in a patient with a negative genetic testing is estimated to be only 0.18%. (Kouvaraki 2005)
The *RET* mutations might occur: in the substrate recognition pocket of the catalytic core (mutations in codon 918), leading to receptor dimerization and cross-phosphorylation; in the extracellular domain (exons 8, 10, 11) leading to ligand-independent homodimerization, cross-phosphorylation and receptor activation; in the intracellular domain (exons 13, 14, 15, 16), leading to alteration in the substrate recognition pocket of the catalytic core with constitutive activation of the RET kinase enzyme catalytic site and autophosphorylation. *RET* mutations in MEN2 are typically missense mutations that lead to ligand independent receptor activation, a model that is well known for a variety of human cancers, but is uncommon for a hereditary cancer gene. (Kouvaraki 2005, Arighi 2005, Plaza-Menacho2006)
The identified *RET* mutations exhibit a strong genotype-phenotype correlation and they are classified into 3 groups with a 14-fold incremental increase from mutations in level 1 to level 3. (Kouvaraki 2005, Donis-Keller 1993, Eng 1996, Alevizaki 1997, Yip 2003, Marx 2005, Mulligan 1993, Machens 2003) Recent guidelines from the American Thyroid Association (ATA) propose a classification of *RET* mutations in 4 levels (A–D), with level D mutations denoting the highest risk for early onset or aggressive MTC and level A mutations carrying the lowest risk. (Kloos 2009).

4.2 *RET* mutations and sporadic medullary thyroid cancer

Approximately 50-60% of specimens from patients with SMTC, contain somatic but not germline *RET* mutations. (Wohllk 1996, Blaugrund 1994, Elisei 2008) The most common somatic mutations occur in codons 918 and 833 (exons 15 and 16) while less commonly somatic mutations in exons 10 and 11 are found which are associated with poor prognosis (Wohllk 1996, Blaugrund 1994, Elisei 2008) Murra et al, has demonstrated somatic mutations in 64.7% of MTC tumours. Exon 16 was the most frequently affected (60.6%), followed by exon 15, while exons 5,8,10-14, were less affected. Mutations in exons 15 and 16, were associated with higher prevalence of persistent, multifocal MTC with a spread in regional lymph nodes, while mutations in exons 5,8,10-14, were associated with the most indolent course of MTC. (Moura 2009) Schilling et al, examined multiple lymph nodes from patients with SMTC and demonstrated that 76% of patients with SMTC had concordant codon-918 mutation in all lymph nodes tested (43% all positive, 33% all negative). Moreover, patients with somatic codon-918 mutations had an increased rate of metastases to distant sites (lung, bone, liver) and an overall worst prognosis. (Schilling 2001 A single nucleotide polymorphism (SNP) of *RET*, G961S, has been shown to be more frequent in patients with SMTC compared with healthy subjects, associated with an earlier age of MTC, and with higher calcitonin levels. (Cardot-Bauters 2008, Robledo 2003, Elisei 2004). The real significance of the observed mutations is not clear. The coexistence of mutation positive and negative regions in MTC tumors, suggests that these mutations may not always be initiating or essential. (Eng 1996)
At present, genetic testing for tumor mutations of the *RET* is not part of the routine practice in patients with SMTC, as the clinical utility is still undefined. However, screening of individuals with apparently sporadic MTC may uncover germline *RET* mutations in approximately 7% of

cases, which in about 2-9% are *de novo* mutations, suggesting that these cases had actually HMTC and not SMTC. (Elisei 2007, Romei 2011, Wohllk 1996, Blaugrund 1994, Elisei 2008) In addition, the existing clinical data suggest a correlation of the *RET* mutations with the course of the disease and possibly the response to treatment which is going to be further evaluated by clinical trials which are in progress. Thus, it might be useful to perform *RET* genetic testing in all patients with MTC, even in those with apparently SMTC.

4.3 *RET* mutations and hereditary medullary thyroid cancer

To date, 98% of affected families with HMTC apparently exhibit genetic linkage to the *RET* gene locus and only a small percentage of MEN2 families have had no *RET* mutation detected. (Kouvaraki 2005, Donis-Keller 1993, Eng 1996, Alevizaki 1997, Yip 2003, Marx 2005, Mulligan 1993)

Isolated FMTC has been traditionally associated with germline-activating mutations of the extracellular region of *RET*, mainly at cysteine codons 609, 611, 618, 620, 630, 634 in exons 10 and 11, in the extracellular domain which is associated with the three-dimensional ligand-binding pocket. These mutations lead to ligand-independent dimerization and receptor activation. Noncysteine mutations of the intracellular region of *RET* in exons 13–16 are less commonly linked to FMTC while mutations in other exons have been rarely reported in isolated families. Some mutations (particularly codons 532, 533, 630, 769, V804M, 844, 912) are thought to be relatively specific for FMTC. However, codon 533 is also associated with MEN2A, indicating that only time and observation in large numbers of families can confirm this specificity. (Kouvaraki 2005, Peppa 2008, Kamakari 2008) Nowadays, FMTC constitutes a challenging form of MTC, which is considered as a phenotypic mildest variant of MEN2A. A number of FMTC patients finally have MEN2A while a significant overlap in the observed *RET* mutations, is commonly found.

Different *RET* mutations lead to the distinct clinical syndromes of MEN2A, MEN2B, and FMTC while a significant overlap exists between *RET* mutations associated with FMTC or MEN2A. The great majority of patients with MEN2A have mutations of *RET* in exons 10,11,13-16 while patients with MEN2B exhibit a single mutation at codon 918 of exon 16. (Kouvaraki 2005, Donis-Keller 1993, Eng 1996, Alevizaki 1997, Yip 2003, Marx 2005, Mulligan 1993, Hofstra 1994)

Due to a strong genotype-phenotype correlation in MTC, the genetic analysis and the identification of specific germline *RET* mutations offer important information regarding the penetrance of MTC and associated lesions. For example, mutations at codon 634 in exon 11 accounts for approximately 60% of all MEN2 families rather than FMTC, with hyperparathyroidism occurring in 20% of patients, a manifestation which is uncommon with other *RET* mutations. (Schuffenecker 1998, Karga 1998) In addition, the same mutations are associated with significantly earlier progression from C-cell hyperplasia to MTC and earlier lymph node involvement than patients with most other mutations related to MEN2A and FMTC. (Peppa 2008, Hofstra 1994) According to the International RET Exon 10 Consortium, codon-associated penetrance by age 50, ranged from 60% (codon 611) to 86% (620) while more advanced stage and increasing risk of metastases correlated with mutation in codon position (609→620) near the juxtamembrane domain. (Frank-Raue 2011) A large European consortium study reported by Machens et al, offer detailed clinical penetrance data, analyzed according to individual mutations. (Machens 2003)

4.4 *De novo RET* mutations and hereditary medullary thyroid carcinoma

A small percentage (3-6%), of patients with MTC, have a negative family history and germline *RET* mutations which arise *de novo*. Such *de novo* mutations are noted at a much higher frequency in the allele inherited from the patient's father. (Wohllk 1996, Donis-Keller 1993, Eng 1996, Alevizaki 1997, Carlson 1994) Unlike MEN2A, MEN2B is commonly associated with *de novo* germline mutations and the diagnosis is most often based on the characteristic clinical features (elongated facies, oral ganglioneuromas of the lips and tongue). Such *de novo* mutation at codon 883 in exon 15, has been found in a small number of MEN2B families. (Gimm 1997) Because of frequent *de novo* mutations, patients with MEN2B should be suspected on the basis of the characteristic features and not on the family history. *De novo RET* mutations, tend to be disproportionately clustered in the intracellular domain (exons 13–15), linked with reduced MTC penetrance, compared to the more classic familial patterns associated with extracellular mutations in exons 10 and 11.

4.5 *RET* mutations in exon 8 and hereditary medullary thyroid carcinoma

In addition to the classical *RET* mutations observed in exons 10,11,13-16, accumulating data support the association of *RET* mutations in other exons associated with HMTC, including exon 8. The first report by Pigny et al. described a 9 bp duplication of exon 8 in a family with FMTC. (Pigny 1999) Da Silva et al, in a study of 76 patients with FMTC from a 6-generation Brazilian family with 229 subjects, demonstrated a new missense point *RET* mutation in exon 8 (1597G-->T) corresponding to a Gly(533)Cys substitution in the cysteine-rich domain. (Da Silva 2003) Kaldrymides et al, detected the same mutation in all seven FMTC Greek patients and in 13 heterozygotes and 1 homozygote asymptomatic relatives, with a wide clinical heterogenecity. (Kaldrymides 2006) Fazioli et al, found 4 novel *RET* variants, located in the extracellular domain (p.A510V, p.E511K and p.C531R) coded by exon 8 on the leukocyte DNA from apparently sporadic cases, in addition to the intracellular juxtamembrane region (p.K666N) coded by exon 11, suggesting that these variants are associated with FMTC. (Fazioli 2008) Peppa et al, found the same mutation, in 2 index patients with MEN2A, consisting of pheochromocytoma and MTC and in 6 out of 12 (50%) family members. Additionally, one of the index patients was asymptomatic, the pheochromocytoma being accidentally found, while the second patient had hypertension but negative testing for pheochromocytoma despite repeated measurements. Furthermore, the MTC was least aggressive as it was not clinically apparent, while none of the family members died from MTC-related causes. (Peppa 2008) Moreover, Kamakari et al, have identified the same G533C mutation in 11 unrelated families with FMTC and 4 with MEN2A, explaining the 'RET-negative' FMTC/MEN2A patients. (Kamakari 2008). The above observations are considered quite interesting points in the characterization of the MEN2A phenotype associated with the G533C point mutation in exon 8 of the RET which seems to be less aggressive. The existing data, reveal an oncogenic potential for all the novel germline *RET* variants, including exon 8 genomic variations, which seem to have a higher oncogenic potential than previously thought. (Muzza 2010)

The above findings indicate that patients with MTC should be screened for other components of MEN and also should be evaluated through a complete genetic screening including exon 8, especially if the classical *RET* screening is negative.

5. Conclusion

RET molecular testing has offered tremendous help on the early identification of patients with MTC, the distinction between the sporadic and hereditary forms of MTC, the prognosis of the natural course of the disease and the response to treatment. To date, the identified *RET* mutations exhibit a strong genotype-phenotype correlation, which has been the basis for establishing the clinical risk levels depending on the nature of the mutations. A "complete" germline *RET* testing should be performed in all MTC patients, independently of the family history, including 10, 11, 13–16 and other " non classical" exons including exon 8, especially in the case of a negative testing. At present, the risk profiles and the penetrance estimations cannot be done in patients with MTC of all causes, caused by *RET* mutations in exon 8, due to the deteriorated data. More studies need to be done, in order to provide more information about the role of exon 8 genomic variations, on the disease start, progression, potential and penetrance.

6. References

[1] Alevizaki M. Medullary thyroid carcinoma: clinical presentation and diagnosis. In Thyroid Cancer, Thessaloniki,2006; pp 395–411. Ed.Hercules Vainas.

[2] Alevizaki M, Stratakis CA. Multiple endocrine neoplasias: advances and challenges for the future. J Intern Med. 2009;266(1):1-4.

[3] Alevizaki M, Sarika H, Koutras DA, Souvatzoglou A. Genetic screening for RET mutations in families with multiple endocrine neoplasia 2 syndromes. Ann N Y Acad Sci. 1997;816:383-8.

[4] Arighi E, Borrello MG, Sariola H. RET tyrosine kinase signaling in development and cancer. Cytok Growth Factor Rev 2005; 16(4–5):441–467

[5] Blaugrund JE, Johns MM Jr, Eby YJ, et al. RET proto-oncogene mutations in inherited and sporadic medullary thyroid cancer. Hum Mol Genet 1994; 3:1895–1897.

[6] Brandi ML, Gagel RF, Angeli A, et al. Guidelines for diagnosis and therapy of MEN type 1 and type 2. J Clin Endocrinol Metab 2001; 86:5658–5671.

[7] Cardot-Bauters C, Leteurtre E, Leclerc L, et al. Does the RET variant G691S influence the features of sporadic medullary thyroid carcinoma? Clin Endocrinol (Oxf) 2008; 69(3):506–510

[8] Carlson KM, Bracamontes J, Jackson CE, et al. Parent-of-origin effects in multiple endocrine neoplasia type 2B. Am J Hum Genet 1994; 5:1076–1082.

[9] Da Silva AM, Maciel RM, Da Silva MR, Toledo SR, De Carvalho MB, Cerutti JM. A novel germ-line point mutation in RET exon 8 (Gly(533)Cys) in a large kindred with familial medullary thyroid carcinoma. J Clin Endocrinol Metab. 2003; 88(11):5438-43.37.

[10] Donis-Keller H, Dou S, Chi D, et al. Mutations in the RET protooncogene are associated with MEN 2A and FMTC. Human Molecular Genetics 1993;2 851–856.

[11] Elisei R, Romei C, Cosci B, et al. RET genetic screening in patients with medullary thyroid cancer and their relatives: experience with 807 individuals at one center. J Clin Endocrinol Metab 2007; 92(12):4725–4729

[12] Elisei R, Cosci B, Romei C, et al. Prognostic significance of somatic RET oncogene mutations in sporadic medullary thyroid cancer: a 10-year follow-up study. J Clin Endocrinol Metab 2008; 93(3):682–687
[13] Elisei R, Cosci B, Romei C, et al. RET exon 11 (G691S) polymorphism is significantly more frequent in sporadic medullary thyroid carcinoma than in the general population. J Clin Endocrinol Metab 2004; 89(7):3579–3584
[14] Eng C, Clayton D, Schuffenecker I, et al. The relationship between specific RET proto-oncogene mutations and disease phenotype in multiple endocrine neoplasia type 2: International RET Mutation Consortium analysis. J Am Med Assoc 1996; 276:1575–1579.
[15] Eng C, Mulligan LM, Healey CS, et al. Heterogeneous mutation of the RET proto-oncogene in subpopulations of medullary thyroid carcinoma. Cancer Res 1996; 56:2167–2170.
[16] Fazioli F, Piccinini G, Appolloni G, et al. A new germline point mutation in Ret exon 8 (cys515ser) in a family with medullary thyroid carcinoma. Thyroid. 2008;18(7):775-82.
[17] Frank-Raue K, Rybicki LA, Erlic Z, et al. International RET Exon 10 Consortium. Risk profiles and penetrance estimations in multiple endocrine neoplasia type 2A caused by germline RET mutations located in exon 10.Hum Mutat. 2011;32(1):51-8.
[18] Gimm O, Marsh DJ, Andrew SD, et al. Germline dinucleotide mutation in codon 883 of the RET proto-oncogene in multiple endocrine neoplasia type 2B without codon 918 mutation. J Clin Endocrinol Metab 1997; 82:3902–3904.
[19] Graze K, Spiler IJ, Tashjian AH, et al. Natural history of familial medullary thyroid carcinoma. Effect of a program for early diagnosis. N Engl J Med 1978; 299:980–985.
[20] Hofstra RM, Landsvater RM, Ceccherini I, et al. A mutation in the RET proto-oncogene associated with multiple endocrine neoplasia type 2B and sporadic medullary thyroid carcinoma. Nature 1994;367:375–376.
[21] Kaldrymides P, Mytakidis N, Anagnostopoulos T, et al. A rare RET gene exon 8 mutation is found in two Greek kindreds with familial medullary thyroid carcinoma: implications for screening. Clin Endocrinol (Oxf). 2006 ; 64(5):561-6.
[22] Kamakari S, Alevizaki M, Bei T, et al. The rare mutation of RET gene G533C is found in 15 unrelated Greek families explaining the 'RET-negative' patients FMTC/MEN2A.(Abstract). Hormones 2008;7 (Suppl 2):70.
[23] Karga HJ, Karayianni MK, Linos DA, Tseleni SC, Karaiskos KD, Papapetrou PD. Germ line mutation analysis in families with multiple endocrine neoplasia type 2A or familial medullary thyroid carcinoma. Eur J Endocrinol. 1998;139(4):410-5. 25.26. 30.31.
[24] Kloos RT, Eng C, Evans DB, et al. Medullary thyroid cancer: management guidelines of the American Thyroid Association. Thyroid 2009; 19(6):565–612
[25] Kouvaraki MA, Shapiro SE, Perrier ND, et al. RET proto-oncogene: A review and update of genotype-phenotype correlations in hereditary medullary thyroid cancer and associated endocrine tumors. Thyroid 2005; 15:531−544.
[26] Leboulleux S, Baudin E, Travagli JP, Schlumberger M. Medullary thyroid carcinoma. Clin Endocrinol (Oxf). 2004;61:299–310.

[27] Lips CJM, Landsvater RM, Hoppener JWM, et al. Clinical screening as compared with DNA analysis in families with multiple endocrine neoplasia type 2A. N Engl J Med 1994;331:828–835.

[28] Machens A, Niccoli-Sire P, Hoegel J, et al. Early malignant progression of hereditary medullary thyroid cancer. N Engl J Med. 2003; 349: 1517–1525.

[29] Marx SJ. Molecular genetics of multiple endocrine neoplasia types 1 and 2. Nat Rev Cancer 2005; 5(5):367–375

[30] Moo-Young TA, Traugott AL, Moley JF. Sporadic and familial medullary thyroid carcinoma: state of the art. Surg Clin North Am. 2009;89(5):1193-204.

[31] Moura MM, Cavaco BM, Pinto AE, et al. Correlation of RET somatic mutations with clinicopathological features in sporadic medullary thyroid carcinomas. Br J Cancer 2009; 100(11):1777–1783

[32] Mulligan LM, Kwok JB, Healey CS, et al. Germ-line mutations of the RET protooncogene in multiple endocrine neoplasia type 2A. Nature 1993; 363 458–460.

[33] Muzza M, Cordella D, Bombled J, et al. Four novel RET germline variants in exons 8 and 11 display an oncogenic potential in vitro. Eur J Endocrinol. 2010; 162(4):771-7.

[34] Pacini F, Castagna MG, Cipri C, Schlumberger M. Medullary thyroid carcinoma. Clin Oncol (R Coll Radiol). 2010; 22(6):475-85.

[35] Peppa M, Boutati E, Kamakari S, et al. Multiple endocrine neoplasia type 2A in two families with the familial medullary thyroid carcinoma associated G533C mutation of the RET proto-oncogene. Eur J Endocrinol. 2008;159(6):767-71.

[36] Pigny P, Bauters C, Wemeau JL, et al. A novel 9-base pair duplication in RET exon 8 in familial medullary thyroid carcinoma. J Clin Endocrinol Metab 1999; 84:1700–1704

[37] Plaza-Menacho I, Burzynski GM, de Groot JW, Eggen BJ & Hofstra RM. Current concepts in RET-related genetics, signaling and therapeutics. Trends in Genetics 2006; 22 627–636.

[38] Raue F, Frank-Raue K. Update multiple endocrine neoplasia type 2. Familial Cancer 2010; 9:449–457

[39] Robledo M, Gil L, Pollán M, et al. Polymorphisms G691S/S904S of RET as genetic modifiers of MEN 2A. 2003; Cancer Res 63(8):1814–1817

[40] Roman S, Lin R, Sosa JA. Prognosis of medullary thyroid carcinoma: demographic, clinical, and pathologic predictors of survival in 1252 cases. Cancer. 2006;107(9):2134–42.

[41] Romei C, Cosci B, Renzini G, et al. RET genetic screening of sporadic medullary thyroid cancer (MTC) allows the preclinical diagnosis of unsuspected gene carriers and the identification of a relevant percentage of hidden familial MTC (FMTC). Clin Endocrinol (Oxf). 2011;74(2):241-7.

[42] Schilling T, Bürck J, Sinn HP, et al. Prognostic value of codon 918 (ATG-->ACG) RET proto-oncogene mutations in sporadic medullary thyroid carcinoma. Int J Cancer. 2001; 95(1):62-6.

[43] Schuffenecker I, Virally-Monod M, Brohet R, et al. Risk and penetrance of primary hyperparathyroidism in multiple endocrine neoplasia type 2A families with mutations at codon 634 of the RET proto-oncogene. J Clin Endocrinol Metab 1998; 83:487–491.

[44] Wells SA, Chi DD, Toshima K, et al. Predictive DNA testing and prophylactic thyroidectomy in patients at risk for multiple endocrine neoplasia type 2A. Ann Surg 1994;220:237–250.

[45] Wohllk N, Cote GJ, Bugalho MM, et al. Relevance of RET protooncogene mutations in sporadic medullary thyroid carcinoma. J Clin Endocrinol Metab 1996; 81:3740–3745.

[46] Yip L, Cote GJ, Shapiro SE, et al. Multiple endocrine neoplasia type 2: evaluation of the genotype-phenotype relationship. Arch Surg 2003; 138 (4):409–416

12

Status for Congenital Hypothyroidism at Advanced Ages

Sevil Ari Yuca
Deparment of Pediatric Endocrinology, Selcuk University, Meram Medical Faculty, Turkey

1. Introduction

Congenital hypothyroidism is one of the most frequent causes of growth and developmental delay and preventable mental retardation. It's incidence of approximately 1 in 4,000 births (Fisher, 2008). Recently in some countries higher incidences were 1/1800, 1/2759 reported (Skordis e*t al., 2005; Henry et al., 2002*).

2. Classification and etiology

Congenital hypothyroidism is usually classifiated as primary, secondary and tertiary or as permanently and transient hypothyroidism. Primary congenital hypothyroidism accounts for 90% of all cases. Approximately 85% of cases are sporadic, while 15% are hereditary. Besides dietary iodine deficiency, the causing reasons of permanently congenital hypothyroidism are embryologic and anatomical defect of the thyroid gland, biosyntetic defect in the production of thyroid hormones in sporadic cases. The most common causes are thyroid gland dysgenesis associated with ectopic, hypoplastic and absent gland (athyreosis). The next most common cause of permanent congenital hypothyroidism is dyshormonogenesis (MacGillivray, 2004). Affected patients have normally located and normally shaped thyroid gland but are enlarged due to thyroid-stimulating hormone chronic and hyperstimulation

The pathogenesis of dysgenesis is largely unknown, some cases are now discovered to be the result of mutations in the transcription factors PAX-8 and TTF-2. Loss of function mutations in the thyrotropin (TSH) receptor have been demonstrated to cause some familial forms of athyreosis. The most common hereditary etiology is the inborn errors of thyroxine (T4) synthesis. Recent mutations have been described in the genes coding for the sodium/iodide symporter, thyroid peroxidase (TPO), and thyroglobulin. Transplacental passage of a maternal thyrotropin receptor blocking antibody (TRB-Ab) causes a transient form of familial congenital hypothyroidism (Brown, 2009).

3. Actions of thyroid hormone and clinical findings in congenital hypothyroid

Thyroid hormone has multiple effects in cells, including stimulation of thermogenesis, water and ion transport and acceleration of substrate turnover and amino acid and lipid metabolism. Thyroid hormone also potentiates the action of catecholamine's (Brown, 2009).

Whereas thyroid hormone-mediated effects in the pituitary, brain and bone can be detected prenatally, thyroid hormone-dependent action in brown adipose tissue, liver, heart, skin and carcass are apparent only postnatally.

The most prominent finding in view of the rough face of delayed diagnosis. In some cases, depending on the TSH stimulation can be found enlarged thyroid gland (fig 1a-1b). During the perinatal period, brown adipose tissue is essential for non-shivering thermogenesis. Thyroid hormone stimulates transcription of thermogenin that protein that uncouples nucleotide phosphorylation and the storage of energy as ATP. As the child matures, shivering thermogenesis assumes greater importance and brown adipose tissue disappears (Brown, 2009). In children with thyroid hormone deficiency is impaired temperature regulation. Thus the skin is rough and cold skin, and is evidence " cutis marmorata " signs. Hypertrichosis in children with delayed diagnosis and treatment of hypothyroidism can be seen in the back (fig 2).

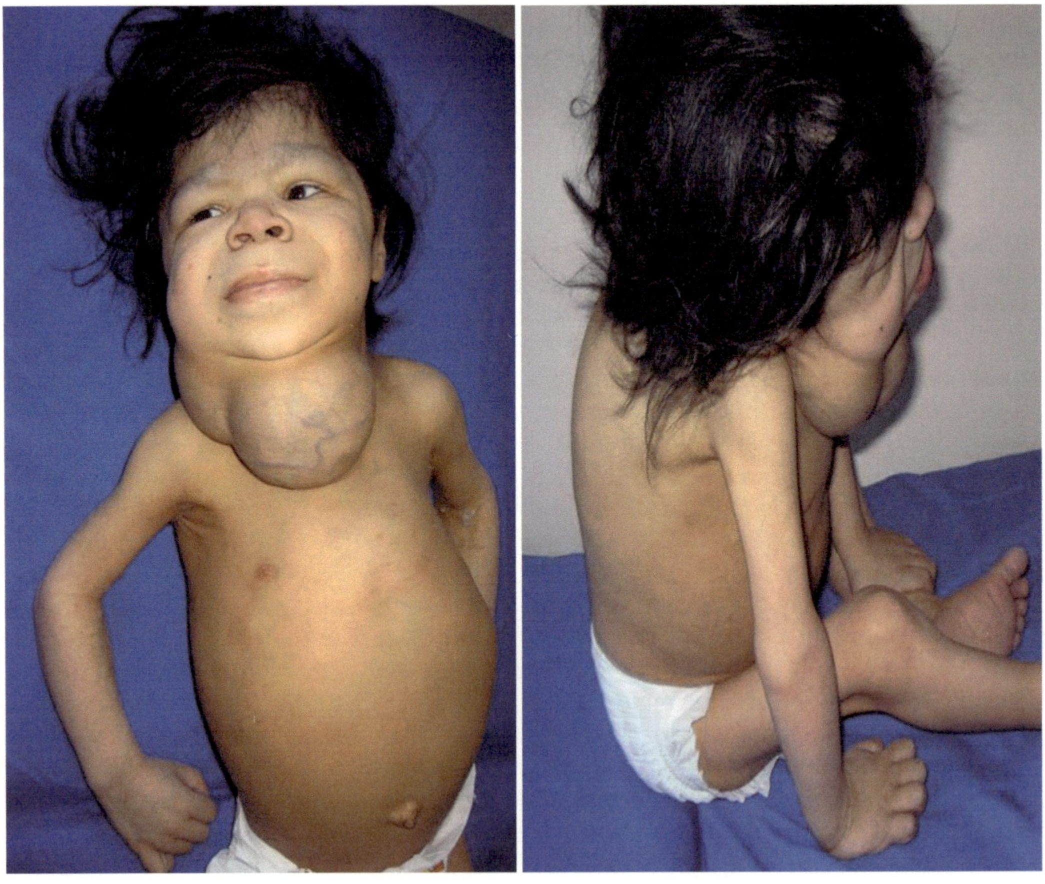

Fig. 1a, 1b. A 19-year-old girl with congenital primary hypothyroidism. Enlarged thyroid gland, coarse facial, umbilical hernia, thick hair, outpouring of the medial parts of the eyebrows, abdominal distantion and delayed pubertal findings are seen (*Nobel Med,* 2010; 6(1):74-77).

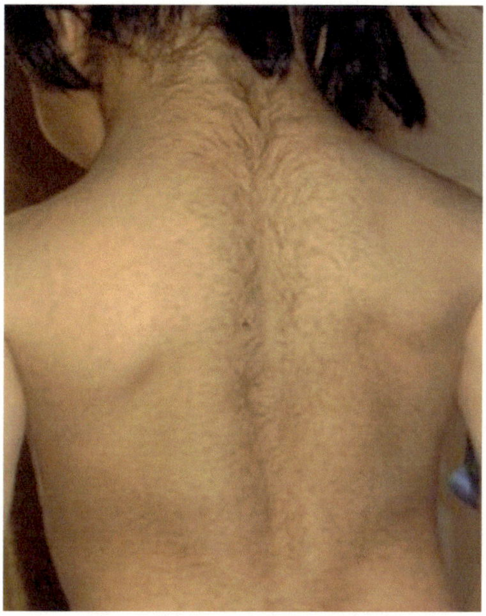

Fig. 2. A 6-year-old girl with congenital primary hypothyroidism. Dark and thick hairs on her back are seen.

Other important thyroid hormone target in the perinatal period is bone, as evidenced by the striking growth retardation, decreased growth velocity and delayed ossification of the epiphyseal growth plate characteristic of long-standing untreated hypothyroidism in infancy and childhood. Thyroid hormone-mediated bone maturation involves both direct and indirect actions. The indirect action mediated by regulation of growth hormone gene expression and the IGF system (Robson et al., 2000, 2002). T3 regulates endochondral ossification and controls chondrocyte differentiation in the growth plate both in vitro and in vivo as a direct (Robson et al., 2000; Ball et al., 1997). Osteoblasts and growth plate chondrocytes both express TRs and several T3-specific target genes have been identified in bone (Stevens et al., 2003). T3 also stimulates closure of the skull sutures in vivo, the basis for the enlarged anterior and posterior fontanelle characteristic of infants with congenital hypothyroidism (Akita et al., 1994). Due to delayed bone maturation, there were skeletal deformed, kyphoscoliosis, on thoraco lumbar vertebrae in a 21 year old female with delayed diagnosis of hypothyroidism (fig 3). Bone age is retarded in hypothyroidism almost always exceeds the retardation in linear growth. Tooth eruption may be delayed, and in rare cases stippled epiphyses are evident radiograpically.

In the brain, thyroid hormone provides the induction signal for the differentiation and maturation of neural system, and a critical window of brain development. These processes include neurogenesis and neural cell migration (occurring predominantly between 5 and 24 weeks), neuronal differentiation, dendritic and axonal growth, synaptogenesis, gliogenesis (late fetal to 6 months postpartum), myelination (second trimester to 24 months postpartum) and neurotransmitter enzyme synthesis. The thyroid hormone- deficient patient usually exhibits slowing of the deep tendon reflexes, with a delayed relaxation phase. (Brown, 2009). The sella turcica may be enlarged (Oatridge, 2002).

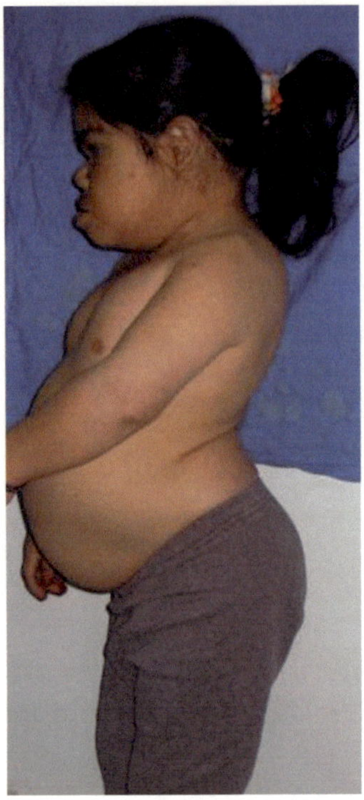

Fig. 3. A 21-year-old female with congenital primary hypothyroidism. Short stature, coarse facial, kyphoscolyosis on her back and absent of pubertal findings are seen (Nobel Med, 2010; 6(1):74-77).

The absence of thyroid hormone appears to delay rather than eliminate the timing of critical morphological events or gene products, resulting in a disorganization of intercellular communication. TRs are found in highest concentration in developing neurons and in multiple areas of the fetal brain, including the cerebrum, cerebellum, auditory and visual cortex. Consistent with a nuclear receptor-mediated mode of action, thyroid hormone stimulates numerous developmentally regulated genes, including genes for myelin, neurotropins and their receptors, cytoskeletal components, transcription factors, extracellular matrix proteins and adhesion molecules, intracellular signaling molecules, as well as mitochondrial and cerebellar genes. In addition, thyroid hormones regulate some genes at the level of mRNA stability or mRNA splicing (Brown, 2009).

Sexual development of most hypothyroid children is delayed in approximate proportion to the retardation of skeletal maturation (fig 1a-3). However, rare children with severe hypothyroidism present with signs of precocious puberty, the Van Wyk-Grumbach syndrome, (Van Wyk & Grumbach, 1960; Hemady et al., 1978; Chattopadhyay et al., 2003). Girls manifest precocious menstruation, breast development, and galactorrhea. In boys, this syndrome is associated with excessive enlargement of the penis and testes. Most of these patients lack pubic hair, and bone age is retarded in keeping with the duration of the hypothyroid state. Serum prolactin and TSH levels are elevated in some children, but the molecular mechanism of precocious puberty is not clear. The increased serum prolactin levels are probably explained by the fact that TRH stimulates TSH and prolactin release from the pituitary. A paracrine action of the hyperstimulated thyrotropic cells on gonadotrope cells may explain the increased gonadotropin secretion. It is also possible that these patients have genetic variants of the gonadotropin receptors that can be stimulated by the increased TSH levels (Anasti et al., 1995). Similar findings have been reported for TSH and FSH receptor variants stimulated by HCG (Rodien et al., 1998; Montanelli et al, 2004). When the hypothyroid state is alleviated, the manifestations of sexual precocity regress— and normal puberty ensues when the general level of maturity has progressed appropriately.

4. Newborn screening for congenital hypothyroidism

The morbidity of congenital hypothyroidism can be reduced to a minimum by early diagnosis and therapy. Thus mental retardation in affected infants is eliminated completely with treatment. Unfortunately, usually the disease may become evident after many symptoms of the condition leads to an irreversible brain damage. It was reported that, during the first month of birth, only 10% of the congenital hypothyroidism cases were diagnosed by clinical findings while 35% were diagnosed within 3 months after labor and 70% within a year and 100% only within 3-4 years of age, before screening for hypothyroid (Klein, 1972). Diagnosis of hypothyroidism has been delayed in the countries not applied national newborn screening yet (Malik & But, 2008; Tahirović & Toromanović, 2005).

The process involves measurement of T_4 and/or TSH on dried blood spots obtained from skin puncture done in first days after birth. In most center, only TSH is used to screen newborn infant, because of primary hypothyroidism is most common causes of congenital hypothyroidism. The cutoff for reporting an elevated TSH is a level above 20-25 U/L in most screening programs.

4.1 Diagnostic criteria

Diagnosis of congenital hypothyroidism has essentially based levels of serum TSH and frees T_4. In affected infants presenting with very low serum free T_4 and very high TSH levels. Rarely, some infants have only a moderate elevation of serum TSH and normal T_4 levels.

Congenital hypothyroidism is usually diagnosed during the neonatal period or early infancy. Sometimes, the diagnosis may be delayed in families with low level of socio-economic, and if the birth at home is frequent in population (Yuca et al. 2010). The newborn screening programs for early diagnosis and treatment is vital in congenital hypothyroidism.

5. Treatment

The primary aim of treatment for congenital hypothyroidism is begin adequate thyroid hormone replacement as early as possible to optimize the prognosis for intellectual development. L-thyroxin is preferred to triiodothyronine, because T_4 to T_3 convert locally in brain and peripheral tissues.

The starting oral dose of L-thyroxin is 10 to 12 µg/kg/day. The target range for serum is T_4 to 10-16 µg/dl. The clinical responses vary among infants even on the standardized dose regimen. Adjustment dose is based on the serum T_4 levels and the clinical examination. The patient should be follow at regular intervals.

6. Prognosis in delayed diagnosis and treatment

At 2-year-old and over children may refer to hospital due to uncertain growth and developmental retardation. Untreated congenital hypothyroidism cases may display different levels of mental retardation and delayed linear growth and bone maturation. Infants with delayed treatment may demonstrate neurological disorders such as spasticity and corrupted walking patterns, dysarthia or mutism and autistic behavior (Delong, 1996).

Patients receiving treatment with delayed diagnosis is under an obvious target height, but can show some physical growth. These are may gain the skill and awareness of their daily functions, and if they does not speak, will be start talking or improve of talking. If they not walking, are start walk, and have more active movements. It returns to the findings of thermogenesis and skin disorders. The findings of the skeleton will have been better by support therapies such as vitamin D_3 and calcium. In the patients had goiter with pressure symptoms, in fact the thyroid gland is nonfunctional, must be thyroidectomy.

Eventually, puberty is developed in the patients with congenital hypothyroid, and they may be fertile. But they cannot reach the mental development accordance with their own age, which is easy for patient with early diagnose and treatment (Oerbeck et al., 2003; Kempers et al., 2006; Josef et al., 2008).

7. Conclusion

Today, there is sensitive radioimmunoassay to measure serum T_4 and TSH using a blood spot made it possible to initiate newborn thyroid screening programs. Affected patients have get out of permanent mental retardation by early diagnosis and treatment with adequate dose of L-thyroxine.

Hypothyroidism not only the brain but also the other tissues affect and lead to functional and developmental abnormalities there. Some of these functions are recovered a small amount with long-term treatment. Unfortunately, in the patients diagnosed after the completion of the development of the brain, mental retardation is severe and irreversible despite appropriate therapy.

8. References

Akita S, Nakamura T, Hirano A, Fujii T, Yamashita S (1994). Thyroid hormone action on rat calvarial sutures. *Thyroid*, 4, 99–106, 1050-7256.

Anasti JN, Flack MR, Frochlich J, et al. (1995). A potential novel mechanism for precocious puberty in juvenile hypothyroidism. *J Clin Endocrinol Metab* 80:276, 0021-972X.

Ball SG, Ikeda M, Chin WW (1997). Deletion of the thyroid hormone beta1 receptor increases basal and triiodothyronine-induced growth hormone messenger ribonucleic acid in GH3 cells. *Endocrinology*, 138, 3125–3132, 1355-008X.

Brown GS (2009). The Thyroid. In: *Brook's Clinical Pediatric Endocrinology*, 6th ed. Brook C, Clayton C and Brown R, eds. 250-282. Willey-Blackwell, ISBN 978-1-4051-8080-1, Singapore.

Chattopadhyay A, Kumar V, Marulaiah M (2003). Polycystic ovaries, precocious puberty and acquired hypothyroidism: The Van Wyk and Grumbach syndrome. *J Ped Surg*, 38,1390, 0022-3468.

DeLong GR (1996). The neuromuscular system and brain in hypothyroidism. In: *Werner & Ingbar's the Thyroid: A Fundamental and Clinical Text* (7th Ed), 826–836. Lippincott Williams & Wilkins, Philadelphia, USA.

Fisher DA (2008). Disorders of the thyroid in the newborn and infant. In: *Pediatric Endocrinology*, 3rd ed. sperling MA,ed. 198-226. WB Saunders, ISBN: 978-1-4160-4090-3, Philadelphia, USA.

Hemady ZS, Siler-Khodr TM, Najjar S (1978). Precocious puberty in juvenile hypothyrodism. *Pediatrics*, 92,55, 0031-4005 .

Henry G, Sobki SH, Othman JM. Screening for congenital hypothyroidism (2002). *Saudi Med* ; 23: 529–535, 0379-5284.

Joseph R (2008). Neuro-developmental deficits in early-treated congenital hypothyroidism. *Ann Acad Med Singapore*, 37(12), 42-3, 0304-4602. Review.

Kempers MJ, van der Sluijs Veer L, Nijhuis-van der Sanden MW, Kooistra L, Wiedijk BM, Faber I, Last BF, de Vijlder JJ, Grootenhuis MA, Vulsma T (2006). Intellectual and motor development of young adults with congenital hypothyroidism diagnosed by neonatal screening. *J Clin Endocrinol Metab.* 91(2), 418-24, 0021-972X.

MacGillivray MH (2004). Congenital Hypothyroidism. In: *Pediatric Endocrinology*, Pescovitz OH and Eugster EA, eds., Lippincott Willims & Wilkins, 490-507, IBN 0-7817-4059-2, Philadelphia, USA.

Malik BA, Butt MA (2008). Is delayed diagnosis of hypothyroidism still a problem in Faisalabad, Pakistan. *J Pak Med Assoc*, 58(10), 545-9, 0030-9982.

Montanelli L, Delbaere A, Di Carlo C, Nappi C, Smits G, Vassart G, Costagliola S. (2004). A mutation in the follicle-stimulating hormone receptor as a cause of familial spontaneous ovarian hyperstimulation syndrome. *J Clin Endocrinol Metab* 89, 1255, 0021-972X.

Oatridge A, Barnard ML, Puri BK, Taylor SD, Hajnal JV, Saeed N and Bydder GM (2002). Changes in Brain Size with Treatment in Patients with Hyper- or Hypothyroidism. *AJNR*, 23, 1539–1544, 0195-6108.

Oerbeck B, Sundet K, Kase BF, Heyerdahl S (2003). Congenital hypothyroidism: influence of disease severity and L-thyroxine treatment on intellectual, motor, and school-associated outcomes in young adults. *Pediatrics*, 112(4), 923-30, 0031-4005 .

Robson H, Siebler T, Stevens DA, Shalet SM, Williams GR (2000). Thyroid hormone acts directly on growth plate chondrocytes to promote hypertrophic differentiation and inhibit clonal expansion and cell proliferation. *Endocrinology*, 141, 3887–3897, 1355-008X.

Robson H, Siebler T, Shalet SM, Williams GR (2002). Interactions between GH, IGF-I, glucocorticoids and thyroid hormones during skeletal growth. *Pediatr Res*, 52, 137–147, 0031-3998 .

Rodien P, Brémont C, Sanson ML, Parma J, Van Sande J, Costagliola S, Luton JP, Vassart G, Duprez L (1998). Familial gestational hyperthyroidism caused by a mutant thyrotropin receptor hypersensitive to human chorionic gonadotropin. *N Engl J Med*, 17, 339, 0028-4793.

Skordis N, Toumba M, Savva SC, Erakleous E, Topouzi M, Vogazianos M, Argyriou A. (2005). High prevalence of congenital hypothyroidism in the Greek Cypriot population: results of the neonatal screening program 1990–2000. *J Pediatr Endocrinol Metab*; 18, 453–461, 0021-972X.

Stevens DA, Harvey CB, Scott AJ, O'Shea PJ, Barnard JC, Williams AJ, Brady G, Samarut J, Chassande O, Williams GR (2003). Thyroid hormone activates fibroblast growth factor receptor-1 in bone. *Mol Endocrinol,* 17(9):1751-66, 0888-8809.

Tahirović H, Toromanović A (2005). Clinical presentation of primary congenital hypothyroidism: experience before mass screening. *Bosn J Basic Med Sci,*5(4), 26-29, 1512-8601.

Van Wyk JJ, Grumbach MM (1960). Syndrome of precocious menstruation and galacorrhea in juvenile hypothyroidism: An example of hormonal overlap in pituitary feedback. *J Pediatr,* 57, 416, 00223476 .

Yuca SA, Cesur Y, Yılmaz C (2010). Congenital Primary Hypothyroidism Diagnosed at Advanced Ages. *Nobel Med,* 6(1), 74-77, .

Part 4

Adrenal Glands

13

Adrenal Incidentaloma and Adrenocortical Carcinoma: A Clinical Guideline on Treating the Unexpected and a Plea for Specialized Care

S.H.A. Brouns, T.M.A. Kerkhofs, I.G.C. Hermsen and H.R. Haak
Máxima Medical Center, Eindhoven
The Netherlands

1. Introduction

An adrenal incidentaloma is an important clinical finding that is often considered harmless, but can be the tip of the iceberg. The term incidentaloma indicates an adrenal mass larger than 1 cm, incidentally discovered during imaging studies performed for reasons other than suspicion of adrenal pathology. Lesions identified during staging procedure or work-up for patients with a known extra-adrenal malignancy are not considered to be an incidentaloma (Young, Jr. 2000; Grumbach et al. 2003; Young, Jr. 2007; Singh & Buch 2008; Terzolo et al. 2009; Androulakis et al. 2011).

The entity incidentaloma is not a new finding and has been reported for many years (Grumbach et al. 2003; Young, Jr. 2007; Singh & Buch 2008; Terzolo et al. 2009; Androulakis et al. 2011). Because of the increased use of imaging techniques and improvement in abdominal imaging, the frequency of incidentaloma findings is increasing as well. Recent studies using high-resolution computed tomography (CT) have reported an estimated prevalence of 4% (Young, Jr. 2007; Singh & Buch 2008). In autopsy studies the prevalence ranged 0.2%-8.7%, depending on definitions used and age group, as there is an age-dependent occurrence of adrenal incidentalomas (Young, Jr. 2000; Grumbach et al. 2003; Young, Jr. 2007; Singh & Buch 2008; Terzolo et al. 2009; Androulakis et al. 2011). The estimated prevalence in patients younger than 30 years is < 1%, in contrast to a 7% frequency in patients 70 years of age or older (Young, Jr. 2007). With an aging population and advanced radiological techniques becoming more widely available, the increasing frequency of adrenal incidentalomas is of growing importance.

When an incidentaloma is found, it is of vital importance to make an early and reliable differentiation between benign and (potentially) malignant lesions, but also to assess tumor functionality. The mass can originate from either the adrenal medulla or cortex (Androulakis et al. 2011). Consequently, a spectrum of different pathological conditions may underlie an incidentaloma, all requiring a different therapeutic approach. As much as 38 different diagnoses have been reported in patients with a serendipitous discovered adrenal tumor (Young, Jr. 2000). Most adrenal incidentalomas are clinically nonhypersecretory benign adenomas, with an estimated frequency of 70-80%, which cause no health problems. However, in 5-20% of patients who have no endocrinological signs or symptoms, analysis reveals subclinical hypercortisolism (Grumbach et al. 2003; Young, Jr. 2007; Singh & Buch

2008; Terzolo et al. 2009). Other frequently reported diagnoses besides a nonfunctioning adenoma include adrenocortical carcinoma (ACC), pheochromocytoma, metastasis and aldosterone-producing adenoma. Although malignancy is rare, it is of great clinical concern because of the poor prognosis (Grumbach et al. 2003; Terzolo et al. 2009).

After recognition of an incidentaloma both patient and physician are faced with uncertainties regarding the course, likelihood of a malignancy and treatment of the adrenal mass. Unfortunately, no diagnostic or therapeutic strategy has been validated in prospective clinical trials. Thus, the diagnostic work-up as well as management of an incidentaloma is a growing public health challenge (Young, Jr. 2007; Singh & Buch 2008; Terzolo et al. 2009).

The goal of this chapter is to provide a diagnostic guideline, which contains information about clinical presentation, biochemical work-up and radiological imaging. In addition, this chapter offers practical recommendations for the management of adrenal incidentaloma, including surgery and follow-up. Also, therapeutic options for adrenal carcinoma are discussed. Furthermore, we present organisational recommendations concerning the management of adrenal incidentaloma and emphasize the need for centralization of adrenal disease-research and patient care. This will provide patients with an opportunity to receive optimal care, as the beneficial effects of specialization have been proven multiple times in other rare diseases.

2. Diagnostics of incidentaloma

The first step in the evaluation of adrenal incidentalomas is establishing the definition of the tumor type, beginning with a thorough history taking and extensive physical examination, with attention to signs or symptoms of hormonal overproduction, a malignancy or pheochromocytoma. Furthermore, hormonal work-up and radiological imaging is required in the diagnostic evaluation of the adrenal mass.

2.1 History and physical examination

2.1.1 History

Signs suggestive of hormonal overproduction may include Cushing's characteristics, symptoms of hyperaldosteronism or sex hormone excess. Cushing's syndrome may be asymptomatic in the event of subclinical disease or present with weight gain and central obesity, flushes, proximal muscle weakness, and polydipsia. Furthermore, cognitive changes, such as irritability, depression or restlessness, may also be present. Hirsutism, acne, gynaecomastia and oligomenorrhoe may be symptoms of hypercortisolism or sex hormone overproduction. Features of primary hyperaldosteronism are nocturia, muscle cramps and polyuria in case of hypokalaemia and palpitations (Young, Jr. 2007; Singh & Buch 2008; Androulakis et al. 2011).

The classic triad of symptoms associated with a pheochromocytoma includes episodic headaches of variable duration, tachycardia and generalized sweating. However, this combination of symptoms is present in only a small percentage of patients (10%) (Nieman 2010). Characteristics less commonly present are pallor, dyspnea and anxiety and secondary, complaints of hyperglycemia, unintentional weight loss, arrhythmias and cardiomyopathy (Young, Jr. 2007; Androulakis et al. 2011).

An adrenocortical carcinoma may either present with signs of adrenal hypersecretion as mentioned above or symptoms related to mass effect, such as abdominal fullness or abdominal pain. Cancer-related signs (e.g. fever, unintentional weight loss) are less frequently present (Young, Jr. 2007; Singh & Buch 2008; Terzolo et al. 2009; Androulakis et al. 2011).

2.1.2 Physical examination

Clinical features of Cushing's syndrome detected during physical examination are hypertension, central obesity, striae, facial rounding ('moon face'), supraclavicular and dorsocervical fat pads ('buffalo hump'), proximal muscle weakness, clitoris hypertrophy, acne and hirsutism. Primary aldosteronism is characterized by hypertension. In rare cases, female patients can present with signs of virilization (e.g. acne, hirsutism) as a result of testosterone excess. In contrast, an estrogen secreting adrenal lesion can produce signs of feminization, such as gynaecomasty in the male patient. A pheochromocytoma may present with hypertension (paroxysmal or sustained), orthostatic hypotension, pallor and sweating on physical examination. Adrenocortical carcinoma may as well present signs of hormonal overproduction mentioned above. In addition, a palpable mass may be present at abdominal examination (Young, Jr. 2007; Singh & Buch 2008; Terzolo et al. 2009; Androulakis et al. 2011).

Causes	Estimated prevalence	Clinical presentation
Adenoma		
Subclinical Cushing's Syndrome	9 %	Weight gain with central obesity, flushes, proximal muscle weakness, polydipsia, cognitive changes
Primary aldosteronism	1.2 %	Nocturia, muscle cramps, polyuria, palpitations
Androgen overproduction	Rare	Hirsutism, acne, oligomenorrhoe
Nonfunctioning	73.9 %	-
Pheochromocytoma	4.7 %	Episodic headaches, tachycardia, generalized sweating, pallor, dyspnea, anxiety
Malignancy		
Adrenocortical carcinoma	4.8 %	Symptoms of functioning mass (see above), abdominal pain or fullness
Metastasis	2.3 %	Cancer-related symptoms (fever, unintentional weight loss)

Table 1. Prevalence and clinical presentation of the most frequent types of adrenal incidentaloma (Young, Jr. 2007, Singh and Buch 2008)

2.2 Hormonal evaluation

Additional hormonal work-up is necessary in the evaluation of tumor functionality. Although an adrenal mass may appear clinically nonhypersecretory, up to 20% of patients with an incidentaloma may have hormonal dysfunction, which might be associated with a higher risk of morbidity, such as metabolic disorders and cardiovascular disease (Singh & Buch 2008; Androulakis et al. 2011).

2.2.1 Subclinical Cushing's Syndrome

The most frequently diagnosed endocrine alteration in patients with an incidentaloma is Subclinical Cushing's Syndrome (SCS), which refers to autonomous and dysregulated cortisol secretion by the tumor, which may cause mild cortisol excess without typical signs and symptoms of hypercortisolism (Young, Jr. 2007; Singh & Buch 2008; Androulakis et al. 2011). It is also known as subclinical autonomous glucocorticoid hypersecretion (Grumbach et al. 2003). The average prevalence is 9% (range 1-29%, depending on criteria used)(Singh and Buch 2008). It is difficult to characterize, since clinical Cushing's syndrome is not present and patients may have normal 24-hour urinary free cortisol secretion (Terzolo et al. 2009). Therefore, late-night salivary cortisol and/or overnight dexamethasone (1 mg) suppression test is recommended to detect subclinical hypercortisolism (Grumbach et al. 2003; Nieman 2010). The optimal cut-off value is much discussed. A cortisol value greater than 138 nmol per liter (5 microg/dL) in response to 1mg dexamethasone overnight is associated with glucocorticoid overproduction and has an estimated sensitivity of 98% and specificity of 80-98% (Singh and Buch 2008). When a level between 50-70 nmol/L (1.8-2.5 microg/dL) is used as cut-off value, confirmatory testing is indicated, such as midnight plasma cortisol or serum ACTH level (Grumbach et al. 2003; Young, Jr. 2007; Singh & Buch 2008; Terzolo et al. 2009).

Recent studies and own observations identify urinary steroid profiling as a very promising screening instrument for early differentiation between benign and malignant tumors. A quantitative analysis of steroid precursors by gas chromatography and mass spectrometry reveals steroid patterns associated with particular clinical problems. A recently designed algorithm screens for nine metabolites in a 24-hour urine sample and has impressive test characteristics with high sensitivity and specificity (Taylor A & Arlt 2010).

2.2.2 Primary aldosteronism

Primary aldosteronism (Conn's syndrome) is present in approximately 1.2% of patients with an adrenal incidentaloma (Androulakis et al. 2011). The textbook presentation comprises hypertension and hypokalaemia, however almost 40% of patients are normokalaemic (Young, Jr. 2000; Singh & Buch 2008). Therefore, serum potassium level is not considered a reliable screening method. Hormonal work-up includes routine measurement of ambulatory morning plasma aldosterone concentration to plasma renin activity ratio (PAC/PRA ratio) in hypertensive patients. This can be performed during treatment with antihypertensive drugs with the exception of beta blockers and aldosterone antagonists. A PAC/PRA ratio ≥ 30 and plasma aldosterone concentration greater than 0.5 nmol/L is indicative of autonomous aldosterone secretion. Since the PAC/PRA ratio is influenced by time of sampling and posture of the patient, the diagnosis needs to be confirmed by additional measurement of mineralocorticoid secretory autonomy (e.g. saline infusion test) (Young, Jr. 2000; Grumbach et al. 2003; Young, Jr. 2007; Singh & Buch 2008; Nieman 2010).

2.2.3 Sex hormone overproduction

Sex hormone-secreting adrenal tumors rarely present as an incidentaloma, since they are usually symptomatic (e.g. hirsutism, virilization, gynaecomasty). Androgen overproduction may be a feature of ACC, but measurement of androgens and their precursors in serum has a low diagnostic accuracy in differentiating malignant from benign adrenal masses. Routine measurement of androgen or estrogen production is not necessary in patients with an incidentaloma (Young, Jr. 2000; Young, Jr. 2007)

Nonclassical congenital adrenal hyperplasia may cause unilateral or bilateral adrenal lesions and is an uncommon cause (< 1%) of incidentalomas. Routine cosyntropin-stimulation testing with measurement of cortisol precursors is not warranted, unless the diagnosis is suspected based on clinical manifestation (hirsutism, acne, menstrual irregularities) or the presence of bilateral adrenal masses (Young, Jr. 2000; Young, Jr. 2007; Nieman 2010).

2.2.4 Silent pheochromocytoma

The estimated prevalence of a pheochromocytoma among patients with an adrenal incidentaloma is 4-7% Although it is mostly a benign condition, it may cause significant morbidity and mortality. Hypertension is constantly present in only half of the patients and paroxysmal in approximately 30%. It is essential to diagnose a catecholamine-secreting pheochromocytoma, since it has the potential to cause cardiac arrhythmias and hemodynamic instability even in asymptomatic patients. Therefore, routine measurement of fractionated metanephrines and catecholamines in 24-hour urine specimen is indicated in all patients presenting with an incidentaloma. Recent research reported the superiority of determination of fractionated plasma free metanaphrines, with a diagnostic sensitivity of 99% and specificity of 89%. However, this method is not widely available (Grumbach et al. 2003; Young, Jr. 2007; Singh & Buch 2008; Terzolo et al. 2009; Nieman 2010; Androulakis et al. 2011).

2.3 Radiologic evaluation

Imaging studies that brought the incidentaloma to light should be reviewed with a focus on the adrenal glands, but will often be insufficient. The goal is to distinguish adenomas from malignant masses. Several imaging characteristics are used to assess the malignant potential and to provide information concerning appropriate management.

2.3.1 Computed Tomography

It is advised to perform an unenhanced CT-scan to help distinguish adenomas from nonadenomas, followed by a delayed contrast-enhanced sequence and computed wash-out percentage (Hamrahian et al. 2005). Attenuation of adrenal masses is measured in Hounsfield Units. A low attenuation on CT before contrast administration indicates high lipid content and is found in adenomas. However, around 30% (range 10-40%) of adenomas do not have a large lipid content and consequently may be difficult to discriminate from nonadenomas.

Furthermore, size and appearance of the adrenal lesion may as well help to differentiate between benign and malignant tumors. The probability of an incidentaloma being an ACC is directly related to size of the lesion. A diameter greater than 4 cm is reported to have 90% sensitivity for identifying ACC, but a low specificity, since only approximately 25% of lesions greater than 4 cm are malignant. In addition, calcifications, necrosis and hemorrhage are indicative of a malignancy (Young, Jr. 2000; Terzolo et al. 2009; Nieman 2010).

CT-characteristic	**Adenoma**	**Pheochromocytoma**	**Adrenocortical carcinoma**	**Metastasis**
Size	Usually < 4 cm	Large, usually > 3 cm	Large, usually > 3 cm	Variable, usually < 3 cm
Shape	Round, smooth margins	Round, smooth margins	Irregular, unclear margins	Oval, irregular margins
Attenuation on unenhanced CT	< 10 HU	> 10 HU	> 10 HU	> 10 HU
Washout (in 10 minutes)	Rapid, > 50%	Delayed, < 50%	Delayed, < 50%	Delayed, < 50%
Growth rate	Stable	Slow (usually)	Rapid (usually)	Variable
Other features	Rarely necrosis, hemorrhage or calcification	Hemorrhage, cystic necrotic areas	Necrosis, hemorrhage, calcification	Hemorrhage, cystic necrotic areas

HU = Hounsfield Units

Table 2. CT characteristics of the most frequent types of an incidentaloma (Young, Jr. 2000; Young, Jr. 2007; Terzolo et al. 2009)

2.3.2 Magnetic Resonance Imaging

Magnetic Resonance Imaging (MRI) is equally effective as CT in differentiating benign from malignant adrenal masses (Grumbach et al. 2003). A normal adrenal gland is characterized by an equal or slightly lower intensity than that of the liver on T1 and T2. In contrast, malignant lesions are hyperintense on T2-weighted images (Young, Jr. 2000; Androulakis et al. 2011).

2.3.3 Positron Emission Tomography

Additional advanced radiological testing is generally not indicated. 18-Fluoro-2-deoxy-D-glucose positron emission tomography (PET) is highly sensitive in identifying malignant lesions. However, it is of limited use regarding the evaluation of adrenal incidentaloma (in patients without a prior history of malignancy) (Young, Jr. 2007; Singh & Buch 2008; Boland 2011)

2.4 Fine-Needle Aspiration

There is no evidence to support the routine use of computed tomography-guided fine-needle aspiration (FNA) in the diagnostic evaluation of an incidentaloma. It is rarely informative, since it has a high-false negative rate, and there is a risk of complications, such as hemorrhage, abdominal pain, pancreatitis and pneumothorax. Moreover, its added value over radiological imaging has not been established. In case of a suspected pheochromocytoma FNA is contraindicated, since manipulation of the tumor can potentially cause a hypertensive crisis. Furthermore, biopsy of an adrenocortical carcinoma may lead to tumourspill and consequently tumor recurrence along the needle track. The only role of FNA in the evaluation of an incidentaloma is in confirming metastatic disease in patients with a known extra-adrenal malignancy without other signs of metastases (Young,

Jr. 2000; Grumbach et al. 2003; Young, Jr. 2007; Quayle et al. 2007; Singh & Buch 2008; Terzolo et al. 2009; Nieman 2010).

3. Diagnostic evaluation

The work-up leads to a preliminary conclusion which determines further management. The spectrum varies from benign adenoma to the presumption of malignancy or a pheochromocytoma.

3.1 Suspect adenoma

As noted before, the first step in evaluation of an adrenal incidentaloma is discrimination between a benign or malignant adrenal mass, in which radiological imaging by CT-scan has a fundamental role. Most adrenal incidentalomas exhibit characteristic features of adrenocortical adenoma (ACA). Adenomas typically present as small (< 4 cm) lesions, with clear margins and high lipid content, which is characterized by low attenuation (< 10 HU) on unenhanced CT. Furthermore, they display rapid washout of contrast medium (e.g. more than 50% after 10 minutes) (see figure 1) (Androulakis et al. 2011).

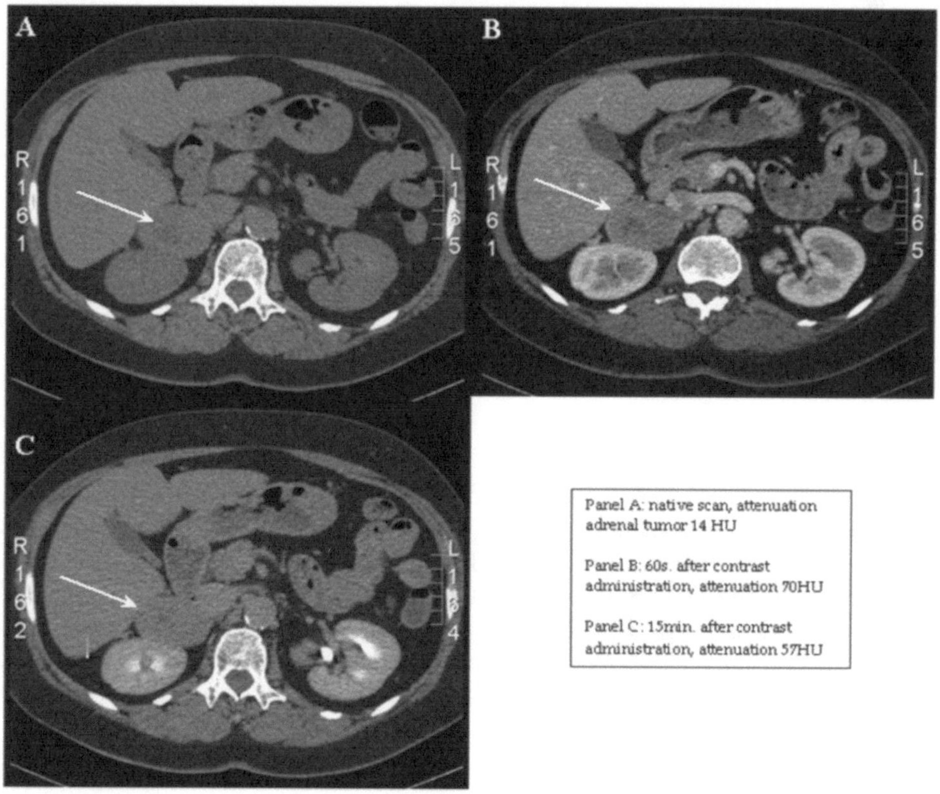

Fig. 1. Washout sequence of an adrenocortical adenoma

In patients with non-functioning ACA, size of the adrenal mass is the major determinant in choice of management (Nieman 2010; Androulakis et al. 2011). Over 60% of incidentalomas less than 4 cm in diameter are ACA, in contrast only 2% are malignant. For a small non-functioning adenoma surgical resection is not necessary, follow-up through CT-imaging and biochemical screening will suffice. In lesions larger than 6 cm the prevalence of ACC increases to approximately 25% and surgery is indicated (Singh & Buch 2008). Management of adrenal masses with a diameter between 4 to 6 cm is less well defined. Because of a higher risk of malignancy in this subgroup of patients, surgical approach is recommended in most cases.

In about 20% of adrenal adenomas hormonal work-up reveals overproduction of aldosterone (0.5-1%) or cortisol (5-20%), which may have a negative influence on patient's health. Primary hyperaldosteronism is associated with increased risk of cardiovascular events. Additionally, patients with SCS may be at risk for potential morbidity attributable to cortisol overproduction. However, progression to clinical overt Cushing's syndrome is uncommon. Surgical resection is considered the treatment of choice when biochemical overproduction is confirmed.

3.2 Suspect pheochromocytoma

It is essential to exclude a pheochromocytoma in patients presenting with an adrenal incidentaloma, because they are potentially lethal even when clinically asymptomatic (Young, Jr. 2007). Increased metanephrines and catecholamines in 24-hour urine specimen or fractionated plasma free metanaphrines in combination with features on CT, such as increased attenuation on unenhanced CT (>10 HU), prominent vascularity of the mass and delayed washout of contrast (<50% after 10 minutes), are highly suggestive of a pheochromocytoma (Terzolo et al. 2009). Characteristics indicative of pheochromocytoma on MRI include hyperintensity on T2-weighted imaging, with approximately 92% sensitivity and 88% specificity (Androulakis et al. 2011). When a pheochromocytoma is suspected, surgical treatment is indicated. Patients should be adequately prepared pre-operatively by adrenergic blockade, to prevent a perioperative hypertensive crisis caused by manipulation of the tumor and subsequent catecholamine-release.

3.3 Suspect malignancy

3.3.1 Adrenocortical carcinoma

The risk of a malignancy is the main concern in patients with an incidentaloma. The prevalence of ACC in these patients without a history of malignancy is estimated at 4.8%, which makes it the most commonly identified adrenal malignancy (Terzolo et al. 2009). It is an aggressive malignancy with a median survival of 19 months (range 8-29 months), as calculated from data of 191 patients diagnosed between 2000 and 2010 in The Netherlands. Prognosis of ACC is still mainly dependent on stage at diagnosis (Fassnacht & Allolio 2009). For that reason it is vital to make accurate decisions regarding the necessary diagnostic and therapeutic measurements.

A smaller tumor size corresponds with a lower tumor stage and consequently better prognosis. The risk of ACC is, as mentioned, associated with mass size. However, because the prevalence of adrenal adenoma is age-dependent, the presence of small adrenal masses in young patients should raise major concern of a potential malignancy. A malignant adrenal lesion typically presents as a larger mass (> 6 cm) and is characterized by an irregular border,

high attenuation on unenhanced CT (> 10 HU) and slow washout after contrast administration (see figure 2) (Terzolo et al. 2009). Own observations from the authors show that although an ACC may appear clinically non-functioning, in about 80-95% additional hormonal work-up and urinary steroid profiling reveals presence of hormone excess.
When an adrenal malignancy is suspected, further investigation concerning cancer staging is warranted before directing the patient to surgery.

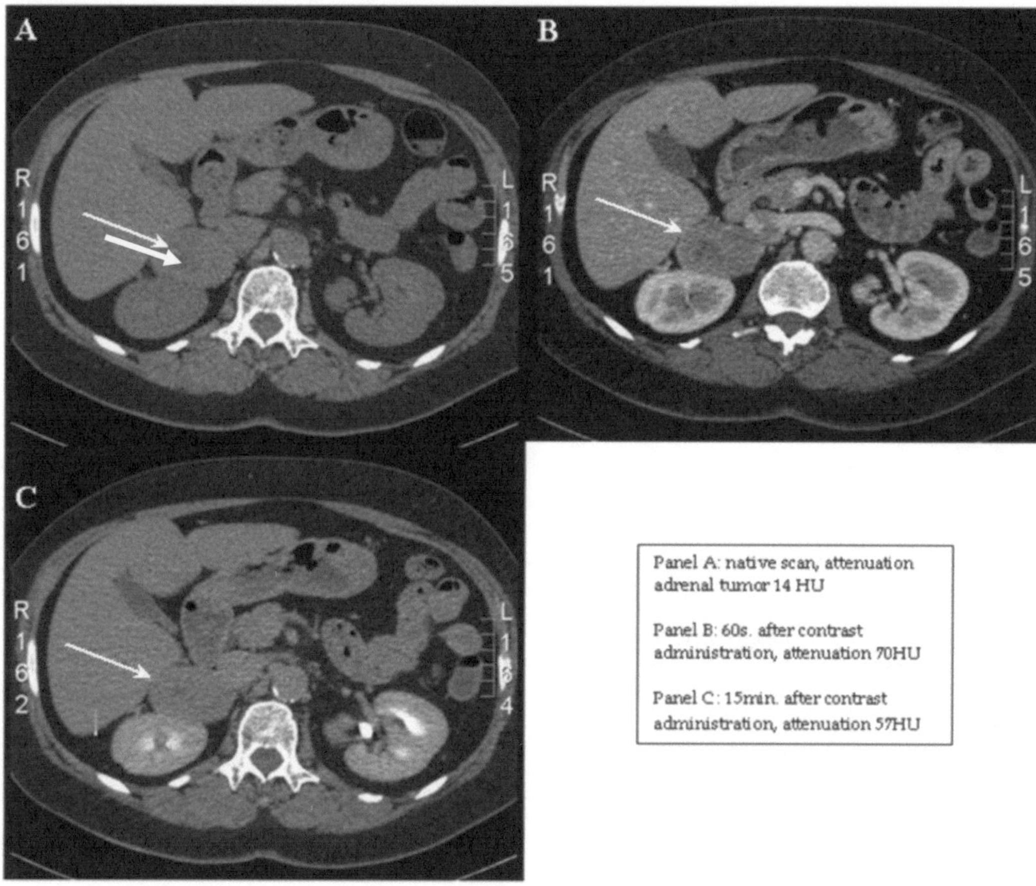

Fig. 2. Washout sequence of an adrenocortical carcinoma

3.3.2 Metastasis

Tumors that frequently metastasize to adrenal glands include carcinomas of lungs, esophagus, kidney, colon, breast, liver, pancreas and stomach (Young, Jr. 2007). Metastases frequently occur bilateral and are variable in size, mostly smaller than 3 cm. Abdominal imaging may also reveal the presence of necrosis, hemorrhage or calcifications (Young, Jr. 2000). Adrenal metastasis may cause beginning adrenal insufficiency. The suspicion of metastasis in an incidentaloma has clinical implications for prognosis and management and the search for a primary neoplasm is indicated. Resection of an isolated adrenal metastasis is associated with improved (disease-free and overall) survival. However, only in a limited number of cases adequate treatment of adrenal metastasis is possible (Terzolo et al. 2009).

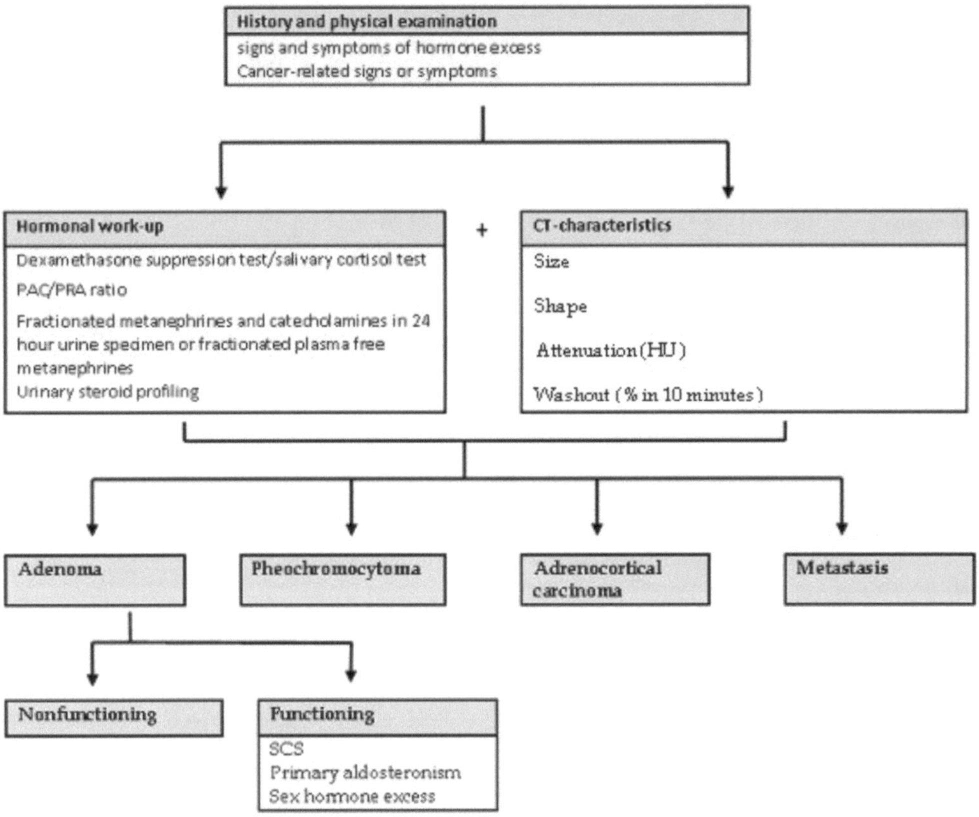

PPAC/PRA ratio = plasma aldosterone concentration to plasma renin activity ratio.
HU = Hounsfield Units. SCS = Subclinical Cushing's Syndrome.

Fig. 3. Algorithm for diagnostic evaluation of adrenal incidentaloma

4. Surgical treatment of incidentaloma

Based on results of the diagnostic evaluation of the adrenal incidentaloma, decisions are made regarding the required therapeutic approach. However, a prospective randomized comparison of laparoscopic versus open adrenalectomy has not yet been performed. Recommendations are made based on little known evidence and pragmatism.

4.1 Adenoma

When an adrenocortical adenoma is suspected, subsequent management is founded on size of the mass and functionality. As mentioned, in case of overproduction of cortisol, aldosterone or sex hormones, surgical resection of the mass is the treatment of choice. Mortality associated with adrenalectomy is estimated at less than 2% (Grumbach et al. 2003). Laparoscopic approach allows for a minimal invasive procedure associated with less morbidity in the patient and shorter period of hospitalization, while surgical results are comparable if performed by an experienced surgical team (Gill 2001). An important issue in resection of functioning adrenal masses is steroid suppletion peri- and postoperatively, because of the risk of adrenal insufficiency, hemodynamic crisis and death. In most cases this can be tapered over time.

It is common practice to perform a surgical resection of incidentalomas larger then 6 cm, even if they are non-functioning and there are no signs of malignancy. It is unclear whether this is a good indication for a surgical resection, as follow-up might be sufficient as well. In lesions smaller than 4 cm, surgical resection is deemed not necessary and follow-up is generally accepted as the correct management. For lesions between 4 cm and 6 cm in diameter, a clear recommendation is lacking. In this group, surgery might be the safest option regarding the increasing risk of malignancy, however the number needed to treat with respect to curing a carcinoma will be large. The other option is to repeat medical imaging on a shorter term, for example 3 months. We expect urinary steroid profiling to become a valuable instrument in differentiating between benign and malignant lesions in this particular subgroup.

4.2 Pheochromocytoma

In patients with an adrenal incidentaloma and suspicion of a pheochromocytoma, rapid surgical resection is the standard curative option, associated with an excellent prognosis (Terzolo et al. 2009). Due to potential perioperative catecholamine excess, removal of a pheochromocytoma is accompanied with unusual hemodynamic and technical conditions, which require thorough preoperative medical preparation and adrenergic blockade to minimize perioperative cardiovascular morbidity. Furthermore, close perioperative monitoring is mandatory (Gill 2001; Ichikawa et al. 2002). Catecholamine release is suggested to be lower during laparoscopy than open adrenalectomy. Therefore, and because of the other benefits of laparoscopic surgery mentioned earlier, a laparoscopic approach is recommended in patients with an incidentaloma suspected for a pheochromocytoma (Cheah et al. 2002; Matsuda et al. 2002).

4.3 Adrenocortical carcinoma

A radical surgical resection is the only chance of cure for patients with an adrenocortical carcinoma, so an aggressive surgical approach is warranted (Dackiw et al. 2001; Miller et al. 2010). A complete resection is possible in most cases when the diagnosis is suspected preoperatively. Success rates drop significantly in cases where a carcinoma is not recognized before or during surgery, as follows from own observations from the authors. This emphasizes the need of a complete diagnostic work-up before the patient is directed for a surgical resection of an incidentaloma. The surgeon has to be prepared to perform an extensive resection and to keep the tumour capsule intact, as tumour spill is strongly associated with the occurrence of peritoneal carcinomatosis and a poor prognosis (Dackiw et al. 2001; Schteingart et al. 2005). Therefore, several authors recommend an open surgical approach instead of a laparoscopic technique, which is being used increasingly in adrenal surgery (Gonzalez et al. 2005; Zografos et al. 2009; Leboulleux et al. 2010; Miller et al. 2010). This topic is controversial, as prospective studies are lacking and retrospective studies show contradictory results. It is our belief that in general, a laparotomy is the safest option with respect to achieving a complete resection, although an expert surgeon in laparoscopic adrenalectomies might achieve better results than a less experienced surgeon can achieve performing a laparotomy.

We therefore recommend that these patients should be treated by a multidisciplinary team with at least an endocrinologist, a surgeon, an oncologist, a pathologist and an experienced radiologist. The team should evaluate all patients with a suspect adrenal incidentaloma and decide on which patients will be treated surgically. Peri-operative hydrocortisone suppletion is recommended in all patients. The surgical technique should be determined with respect to the preference and specific qualities of the surgeon. The pathological examination of the tumour requires special attention, as carcinomas might be difficult to recognize. Rating systems as the Weiss-score and the Van Slooten score should be applied to all adrenal tumours. Close follow-up using medical imaging is strongly recommended as the risk of recurrence is high, even after complete resection. The debate regarding adjuvant therapy with mitotane is still ongoing, but it is the opinion of the authors that this is recommended if the tumor has a ki-67 index >10% (Terzolo et al. 2007).

5. Follow-up of nonfunctioning adenoma

A much discussed matter in the management of patients with an non-functioning adrenal adenoma is the frequency and duration of follow-up evaluation. Recommendations regarding follow-up are aimed at identifying changes in size or functionality of the adrenal adenoma and to recognize lesions with malignant potential that have escaped detection on primary analysis. Research suggests that approximately 8% of non-functional adrenal incidentalomas increase in size by at least 1 cm during follow-up, whereas 3-4% decrease in size (Singh and Buch 2008, Young, Jr. 2000). The majority of adrenal adenomas remain stable. In contrast, adrenocortical carcinomas usually display rapid growth. It is recommended to repeat adrenal imaging by CT-scan in patients with nonfunctioning adenomas smaller than 4 cm within 6-12 months after the initial discovery to detect size changes (Grumbach et al. 2003).

Approximately 20% of adrenal adenomas which displayed no excess hormone secretion at time of discovery, become autonomous during subsequent period of 4 years. Lesions of at least 3 cm in diameter are more likely to develop subclinical hyperfunction in contrast to smaller tumors (Androulakis et al. 2011). It is reported that the risk seems to disappear after 3-4 years follow-up. Hyperaldosteronism or catecholamine hypersecretion occurs rarely during follow-up (Grumbach et al. 2003). Cortisol overproduction is more likely to occur. Hence, annual repetition of hormonal work-up, including late-night salivary cortisol and/or overnight dexamethasone (1 mg) suppression test is recommended during 4 years of follow-

up. Whether measurement of PAC/PRA ratio and determination of fractionated metanephrines and catecholamines in 24-hour urine specimen or fractionated plasma free metanephrines should be repeated, is left to the discretion of the clinician as the indication may vary per patient.
Further follow-up is not indicated in patients with an adrenal mass that remains stable on two imaging studies, done at least 6 months apart and do not demonstrate hormonal overproduction during 4 years of follow-up (Grumbach et al. 2003). Recommendations regarding follow-up of patients with a functional adenoma who are surgically treated, have not been developed.

Suspicion	Management	Considerations
Adenoma		
Functioning	Laparoscopic resection	Post-operative steroid hormone suppletion
Nonfunctioning		
< 4 cm	Follow-up - CT-scan within 6-12 months - Hormonal work-up annually during 4 years	
4-6 cm	Risk group: - Repeat CT-scan within 6 months - Consider surgical resection - Urinary steroid profiling - Consider referral to specialized centre	Suspicious imaging phenotype: open adrenalectomy
> 6 cm	Laparoscopic resection	
Pheochromocytoma	Laparoscopic resection	Pre-operative preparation
Adrenocortical carcinoma	Referral to specialized centre Open adrenalectomy by specialized surgical team	Post-operative steroid hormone suppletion Additional treatment depending on stage

Fig. 4. Recommendations for management of adrenal incidentaloma

6. Treatment in advanced stages

6.1 Introduction

The occurrence of metastatic disease in patients with adrenocortical carcinoma is not rare, as 35% of patients present with stage 4 disease. 50% of patients who initially have had a curative resection, ultimately suffer a recurrence (Pommier & Brennan 1992; Stojadinovic et al. 2002). Even in advanced stages, a surgical debulking should be considered as our own observations indicate this might give a survival benefit. The backbone of treatment in advanced stages is formed by drug therapy with mitotane. Cytotoxic chemotherapy may be added, but response percentages vary. The role of radiation therapy remains disputed. Current experimental treatments include IGF-R blockers (OSI-906) and sunitinib.

6.2 Surgery

In their recent review article, Fassnacht and Allolio provide a flowchart for management of ACC, which advocates at least consideration of surgery in every stage of disease (Fassnacht & Allolio 2009). Surgery including metastasectomy should at least be considered in stage IV patients and should be pursued if technically feasible and if the patient is motivated and in appropriate physical condition. On the other hand, the absolute survival gain might not weigh up against morbidity after surgery in certain (older) patients. This implies that the decision to perform surgery should be tailored to individual cases and should be discussed in a multidisciplinary team including an experienced surgeon. An additional benefit in cases of hormonal overproduction is that surgery might help controlling hormonal excess (Fassnacht & Allolio 2009).

Repeat surgery should be considered individually, results indicate that this could be beneficial with regard to survival, especially if the interval between the two operations is more than 6 months (Allolio & Fassnacht 2006; Veytsman et al. 2009).

6.3 Mitotane

Mitotane is the only adrenal-specific agent available for the treatment of ACC (Haak et al. 1994). The exact mechanism of action is not known, but it is proposed and generally accepted that mitotane is metabolized in adrenal mitochondria and causes cytotoxicity by oxidative damage through the production of free radicals (Veytsman et al. 2009). Whatever the exact pathway may be, the main effect is focal degeneration of the fascicular and (particularly) the reticular zone, which clinically leads to adrenal insufficiency for which glucocorticoid substitution is needed. (Hahner & Fassnacht 2005).

When describing results of mitotane, one should differentiate between antitumor- and antihormonal effects. Regarding antitumor activity, mitotane has been assessed in several clinical studies, with variable results. Most studies were retrospective and comprised only small numbers of patients. Results show that mitotane does have activity against ACC. Percentages vary, but most investigators report total or partial tumor responses in about 25% to 30% of cases.

Concerning hormone excess, therapy with mitotane is sufficient in the majority of patients. However, the onset of mitotane is slow due to its lipophilic properties and the resulting accumulation in adipose tissues. It can take up to three months before therapeutic levels are established, so in patients with severe hypercortisolism another agent must be used concurrently to treat this condition while mitotane levels are being built up. The recommended treatment in this situation would be ketoconazol, which is generally well tolerated. Other options, dependent on the case at hand, could be etomidate, mifeprestone or metyrapone (Igaz et al. 2008; Veytsman et al. 2009).

Mitotane treatment with a plasma concentration >14mg/L is associated with prolonged survival (Haak et al. 1994). Adverse effects occur in over 80% of patients and involve mainly the gastro-intestinal tract: anorexia, nausea, vomiting and diarrhea are frequently observed (Hahner & Fassnacht 2005). Reported symptoms caused by effects on the central nervous system are ataxia, speed disturbances, confusion and somnolence. Typically, all adverse effects are reversible after mitotane withdrawal (Lanser et al. 1992).

It is important to bear in mind that mitotane not only has adrenolytic effects, impairing adrenal steroidogenesis and thus inducing a need for replacement hydrocortisone, but also stimulates peripheral cortisol metabolism, so that hydrocortisone should be administered in higher doses. A second issue in managing patients on mitotane is monitoring thyroid

hormone and thyroid stimulating hormone levels, as mitotane can decrease thyroid hormone as well. A third and possibly favorable interaction is the supposedly increased efficacy of cytotoxic chemotherapy when combined with mitotane. However, evidence on this topic is not conclusive. The proposed mechanism for this synergistic effect is the possible negative effect of mitotane on multidrug resistance proteins, as investigated in vitro, which could decrease the resistance of adrenocortical cancer cells to cytotoxic agents (Hahner & Fassnacht 2005; Igaz et al. 2008).
Given the rarity of the indication and use of mitotane, it is recommended to leave treatment with mitotane to experienced doctors who are familiar with possible adverse events and are able to manage them.

6.4 Cytotoxic chemotherapy

Regarding cytotoxic chemotherapy, several combinations of agents have been tried so far. The highest response rates have been found in a trial with a treatment regimen combining mitotane with etoposide, doxorubicine and cisplatin (response rate 49%) and another trial with a treatment regimen combining mitotane and streptozotocine (response rate 36%) (Berruti et al. 2005), (Khan et al. 2000). Recently, these two regimens were compared in the First International Trial in Locally Advanced and Metastatic Adrenocortical Cancer (FIRM-ACT). Results of this trial are expected in 2011.

6.5 Radiation therapy

Whether there is a place for radiation therapy in the treatment of adrenocortical carcinoma, is not yet clear according to the literature. Some authors claim to have accomplished favorable results, like prevention of local recurrence and adequate pain relief in metastatic disease, whereas toxicity was low (Fassnacht et al. 2006; Polat et al. 2009; Hermsen et al. 2010).
Other investigators recommend a more conservative approach, seeing that re-operations in a post-radiation tumor bed would be more difficult and that the favorable results are not all too convincing, given the retrospective character of research so far (Veytsman et al. 2009). One could argue that radiation therapy can be of use in a palliative setting, especially in alleviating pain or neurologic complaints caused by metastatic disease in bone or brain and that a prospective trial is needed to determine the efficacy in an adjuvant setting.

6.6 Future therapeutic agents

The insulin-like growth factor receptor (IGF-R) in adrenocortical carcinoma is regarded as a possible target for treatment. Both antibody and tyrosine kinase inhibitor trials targeted against IGF-R are in progress. A trial using sunitinib as therapeutic agent produced disappointing results, but a better understanding of the metabolic complexity of the disease might lead to better trials in the future. Other areas of interest are VEGFR inhibitors and FGFR inhibitors, but these have not been translated into clinical trials yet.

7. Limitations

Due to limited evidence and guidelines, there are still multiple unresolved issues regarding management of incidentalomas, mainly concerning the duration of follow-up. The most important health risk in patients with an incidentaloma is related to several characteristics of the adrenal mass associated with a malignant mass or pheochromocytoma (Kievit & Haak 2000). The rate of growth of a benign adrenal lesion remains unclear. Besides this, the percentage of patients that will develop hormonal overproduction when initial analysis was negative is uncertain as well. Furthermore, there is some concern regarding the side effects of repeated CT imaging. One report estimated the risk of fatal cancer due to exposure to ionising radiation during CT-imaging to be one in 430-2170 (Androulakis et al. 2011). This is comparable to the chance of developing an adrenocortical carcinoma during 3-year follow-up of an incidentaloma. Additionally, a long follow-up period with repeated extensive hormonal work-up and radiological imaging is associated with high costs. Since the frequency of discovered adrenal incidentalomas is expected to increase and the use of abdominal imaging is also increasing, the cost-effectiveness of repeated hormonal work-up and imaging becomes an important issue in health care. However, in practice, choices of follow-up or treatment are also based on psychological or social mechanisms, such as anxiety, doubt and risk aversion as well as cost-effectiveness. To elucidate these uncertainties prospective trials are warranted to evaluate the optimal diagnostic approach and management of an incidentaloma and provide an answer for unresolved questions.

8. Organization of care

The rarity of a number of adrenal disorders, such as ACC or pheochromocytoma, and the dismal prognosis associated with an adrenal malignancy, requires a multidisciplinary approach of each patient. In the event of an ACC, physicians often are not familiar with the disorder and its few available treatment options, resulting in inferior patient care. Given that a large part of diagnostics and management is based on pragmatism and expert opinion instead of prospective trials, additional studies concerning treatment and follow-up of adrenal tumors are necessary. In order to improve care in patients with adrenal disorders and stimulate scientific research, national and international collaboration is vital. In a number of European countries (France, Germany, Italy, The Netherlands), national networks have been set up to coordinate adrenal diseases-research and - patient care. (Koschker et al. 2006; van Ditzhuijsen et al. 2007)

In the southern region of The Netherlands, our hospital acts as a tertiary referral center for patients with adrenal tumors. We have provided local hospitals with a guideline for diagnostics and patient referral similar to the procedure described in this chapter. The subsequent centralization of these patients facilitates reliable pre-operative diagnostics and specialized surgery, of which the importance cannot be overemphasized. Too many patients each year see their chance of survival be ruined because an adrenal malignancy is not recognized before, during or even after surgery. Irradical resection and/or rupture of the tumor capsule in adrenocortical carcinoma is fatal without exception, but can often be prevented if treated by experienced doctors.

Therefore, we strongly support initiatives of centralization being deployed in other regions and countries, as the beneficial effects of specialization have been proven multiple times in other rare diseases (Sosa et al. 1998; Kumar et al. 2001). Centralization and multidisciplinary approach is associated with more complete resections, improved survival and enhanced patient care. A secondary benefit is the facilitation of scientific research and participation in clinical trials in centralized populations of patients with a rare disease.

9. Conclusion

Due to the increasing discovery of adrenal incidentalomas, the diagnostic work-up as well as the management of incidentalomas is a growing public health challenge. Hormonal functionality and malignant potential of the lesion need to be evaluated. Incidentalomas are mostly benign nonhypersecretory adrenal adenomas, however important diagnoses to exclude are (subclinical) Cushing's Syndrome, primary aldosteronism, sex hormone overproduction, pheochromocytoma or malignancy (e.g. adrenocortical carcinoma, metastasis). Surgical treatment is recommended in all patients with a hormonally active tumor or a tumor larger than 6 cm. Furthermore, surgery may be indicated in individual cases depending on radiological characteristics. In patients with nonfunctioning adrenal adenomas smaller than 4 cm follow-up with CT-scan after 6-12 months and annual hormonal work-up for 4 years is recommended. An adrenocortical carcinoma is rare, but often lethal. Surgery is the cornerstone of initial treatment, whereas drug therapy with mitotane is inevitable in advanced stages. It is recommended that patients with adrenal disorders are treated in a multidisciplinary setting by experienced physicians. Centralization of care is strongly encouraged in order to improve patient outcome and to stimulate research and trial participation.

10. References

Allolio,B. & Fassnacht,M. 2006. Clinical review: Adrenocortical carcinoma: clinical update. J Clin Endocrinol. Metab, 91, 2027-2037.

Androulakis,I.I., Kaltsas,G., Piaditis,G. & Grossman,A.B. 2011. The clinical significance of adrenal incidentalomas. Eur J Clin Invest, 41, 552-560.

Berruti,A., Terzolo,M., Sperone,P., Pia,A., Casa,S.D., Gross,D.J., Carnaghi,C., Casali,P., Porpiglia,F., Mantero,F., Reimondo,G., Angeli,A. & Dogliotti,L. 2005. Etoposide, doxorubicin and cisplatin plus mitotane in the treatment of advanced adrenocortical carcinoma: a large prospective phase II trial. Endocr. Relat Cancer, 12, 657-666.

Boland,G.W. 2011. Adrenal imaging: why, when, what, and how? Part 3. The algorithmic approach to definitive characterization of the adrenal incidentaloma. AJR Am J Roentgenol., 196, W109-W111.

Cheah,W.K., Clark,O.H., Horn,J.K., Siperstein,A.E. & Duh,Q.Y. 2002. Laparoscopic adrenalectomy for pheochromocytoma. World J Surg, 26, 1048-1051.

Dackiw,A.P., Lee,J.E., Gagel,R.F. & Evans,D.B. 2001. Adrenal cortical carcinoma. World J Surg, 25, 914-926.

Fassnacht,M. & Allolio,B. 2009. Clinical management of adrenocortical carcinoma. Best. Pract. Res. Clin Endocrinol. Metab, 23, 273-289.

Fassnacht,M., Hahner,S., Polat,B., Koschker,A.C., Kenn,W., Flentje,M. & Allolio,B. 2006. Efficacy of adjuvant radiotherapy of the tumor bed on local recurrence of adrenocortical carcinoma. J Clin Endocrinol. Metab, 91, 4501-4504.

Gill,I.S. 2001. The case for laparoscopic adrenalectomy. J Urol., 166, 429-436.

Gonzalez,R.J., Shapiro,S., Sarlis,N., Vassilopoulou-Sellin,R., Perrier,N.D., Evans,D.B. & Lee,J.E. 2005. Laparoscopic resection of adrenal cortical carcinoma: a cautionary note. Surgery, 138, 1078-1085.

Grumbach,M.M., Biller,B.M., Braunstein,G.D., Campbell,K.K., Carney,J.A., Godley,P.A., Harris,E.L., Lee,J.K., Oertel,Y.C., Posner,M.C., Schlechte,J.A. & Wieand,H.S. 2003. Management of the clinically inapparent adrenal mass ("incidentaloma"). Ann Intern Med, 138, 424-429.

Haak,H.R., Hermans,J., van de Velde,C.J., Lentjes,E.G., Goslings,B.M., Fleuren,G.J. & Krans,H.M. 1994. Optimal treatment of adrenocortical carcinoma with mitotane: results in a consecutive series of 96 patients. Br J Cancer, 69, 947-951.

Hahner,S. & Fassnacht,M. 2005. Mitotane for adrenocortical carcinoma treatment. Curr. Opin. Investig. Drugs, 6, 386-394.

Hamrahian,A.H., Ioachimescu,A.G., Remer,E.M., Motta-Ramirez,G., Bogabathina,H., Levin,H.S., Reddy,S., Gill,I.S., Siperstein,A. & Bravo,E.L. 2005. Clinical utility of noncontrast computed tomography attenuation value (hounsfield units) to differentiate adrenal adenomas/hyperplasias from nonadenomas: Cleveland Clinic experience. J Clin Endocrinol. Metab, 90, 871-877.

Hermsen,I.G., Groenen,Y.E., Dercksen,M.W., Theuws,J. & Haak,H.R. 2010. Response to Radiation Therapy in Adrenocortical Carcinoma. J Endocrinol. Invest.

Ichikawa,T., Mikami,K., Suzuki,H., Imamoto,T., Yamazaki,T., Naya,Y., Ueda,T., Igarashi,T. & Ito,H. 2002. Laparoscopic adrenalectomy for pheochromocytoma. Biomed. Pharmacother., 56 Suppl 1, 149s-153s.

Igaz,P., Tombol,Z., Szabo,P.M., Liko,I. & Racz,K. 2008. Steroid biosynthesis inhibitors in the therapy of hypercortisolism: theory and practice. Curr Med Chem., 15, 2734-2747.

Khan,T.S., Imam,H., Juhlin,C., Skogseid,B., Grondal,S., Tibblin,S., Wilander,E., Oberg,K. & Eriksson,B. 2000. Streptozocin and o,p'DDD in the treatment of adrenocortical cancer patients: long-term survival in its adjuvant use. Ann Oncol, 11, 1281-1287.

Kievit,J. & Haak,H.R. 2000. Diagnosis and treatment of adrenal incidentaloma. A cost-effectiveness analysis. Endocrinol. Metab Clin North Am, 29, 69-ix.

Koschker,A.C., Fassnacht,M., Hahner,S., Weismann,D. & Allolio,B. 2006. Adrenocortical carcinoma -- improving patient care by establishing new structures. Exp. Clin Endocrinol. Diabetes, 114, 45-51.

Kumar,H., Daykin,J., Holder,R., Watkinson,J.C., Sheppard,M.C. & Franklyn,J.A. 2001. An audit of management of differentiated thyroid cancer in specialist and non-specialist clinic settings. Clin Endocrinol. (Oxf), 54, 719-723.

Lanser,J.B., van Seters,A.P., Moolenaar,A.J., Haak,H.R. & Bollen,E.L. 1992. Neuropsychologic and neurologic side effects of mitotane and reversibility of symptoms. J Clin Oncol, 10, 1504.

Leboulleux,S., Deandreis,D., Al,G.A., Auperin,A., Goere,D., Dromain,C., Elias,D., Caillou,B., Travagli,J.P., De,B.T., Lumbroso,J., Young,J., Schlumberger,M. & Baudin,E. 2010. Adrenocortical carcinoma: is the surgical approach a risk factor of peritoneal carcinomatosis? Eur J Endocrinol..

Matsuda,T., Murota,T., Oguchi,N., Kawa,G. & Muguruma,K. 2002. Laparoscopic adrenalectomy for pheochromocytoma: a literature review. Biomed. Pharmacother., 56 Suppl 1, 132s-138s.

Miller,B.S., Ammori,J.B., Gauger,P.G., Broome,J.T., Hammer,G.D. & Doherty,G.M. 2010. Laparoscopic Resection is Inappropriate in Patients with Known or Suspected Adrenocortical Carcinoma. World J Surg.

Nieman,L.K. 2010. Approach to the patient with an adrenal incidentaloma. J Clin Endocrinol. Metab, 95, 4106-4113.

Polat,B., Fassnacht,M., Pfreundner,L., Guckenberger,M., Bratengeier,K., Johanssen,S., Kenn,W., Hahner,S., Allolio,B. & Flentje,M. 2009. Radiotherapy in adrenocortical carcinoma. Cancer, 115, 2816-2823.

Pommier,R.F. & Brennan,M.F. 1992. An eleven-year experience with adrenocortical carcinoma. Surgery, 112, 963-970.

Quayle,F.J., Spitler,J.A., Pierce,R.A., Lairmore,T.C., Moley,J.F. & Brunt,L.M. 2007. Needle biopsy of incidentally discovered adrenal masses is rarely informative and potentially hazardous. Surgery, 142, 497-502.

Schteingart,D.E., Doherty,G.M., Gauger,P.G., Giordano,T.J., Hammer,G.D., Korobkin,M. & Worden,F.P. 2005. Management of patients with adrenal cancer: recommendations of an international consensus conference. Endocr. Relat Cancer, 12, 667-680.

Singh,P.K. & Buch,H.N. 2008. Adrenal incidentaloma: evaluation and management. J Clin Pathol, 61, 1168-1173.

Sosa,J.A., Bowman,H.M., Tielsch,J.M., Powe,N.R., Gordon,T.A. & Udelsman,R. 1998. The importance of surgeon experience for clinical and economic outcomes from thyroidectomy. Ann Surg, 228, 320-330.

Stojadinovic,A., Ghossein,R.A., Hoos,A., Nissan,A., Marshall,D., Dudas,M., Cordon-Cardo,C., Jaques,D.P. & Brennan,M.F. 2002. Adrenocortical carcinoma: clinical, morphologic, and molecular characterization. J Clin Oncol, 20, 941-950.

Taylor A & Arlt,W. Urinary Steroid Profiling as a High-Throughput Screening Tool for the Detection of Malignancy in Patients with Adrenal Tumors. Society for Endocrinology BES 2010 Abstract, 3-72. 2010.

Terzolo,M., Angeli,A., Fassnacht,M., Daffara,F., Tauchmanova,L., Conton,P.A., Rossetto,R., Buci,L., Sperone,P., Grossrubatscher,E., Reimondo,G., Bollito,E., Papotti,M., Saeger,W., Hahner,S., Koschker,A.C., Arvat,E., Ambrosi,B., Loli,P., Lombardi,G., Mannelli,M., Bruzzi,P., Mantero,F., Allolio,B., Dogliotti,L. & Berruti,A. 2007. Adjuvant mitotane treatment for adrenocortical carcinoma. N Engl J Med, 356, 2372-2380.

Terzolo,M., Bovio,S., Pia,A., Reimondo,G. & Angeli,A. 2009. Management of adrenal incidentaloma. Best. Pract. Res Clin Endocrinol. Metab, 23, 233-243.

van Ditzhuijsen,C.I., van de,W.R. & Haak,H.R. 2007. Adrenocortical carcinoma. Neth. J Med, 65, 55-60.

Veytsman,I., Nieman,L. & Fojo,T. 2009. Management of Endocrine Manifestations and the Use of Mitotane as a Chemotherapeutic Agent for Adrenocortical Carcinoma. J Clin Oncol.

Young,W.F., Jr. 2000. Management approaches to adrenal incidentalomas. A view from Rochester, Minnesota. Endocrinol. Metab Clin North Am., 29, 159-85, x.

Young,W.F., Jr. 2007. Clinical practice. The incidentally discovered adrenal mass. N. Engl. J Med, 356, 601-610.

Zografos,G.N., Vasiliadis,G., Farfaras,A.N., Aggeli,C. & Digalakis,M. 2009. Laparoscopic surgery for malignant adrenal tumors. JSLS., 13, 196-202.

14

Adrenal Cortex Tumors and Hyperplasias

Duarte Pignatelli[1,2,3]
[1]Endocrinology, Hospital S. João, Porto
[2]Faculty of Medicine of the University of Porto
[3]IPATIMUP, University of Porto
Portugal

1. Introduction

The adrenal cortex tumors include both malignant adrenal cortex cancers (ACC) and benign masses (ACT) that can be either secreting, of one of the hormones normally produced in the adrenal cortex (Cushing's syndrome if the hypersecretion is of cortisol or Conn's syndrome if it is aldosterone) or non-secretory (Incidentalomas).

The outer part of the adrenal glands, the adrenal cortex, is responsible for regulating important body functions including blood sugar levels, body water and salt levels, and consequently blood pressure and kidney functions, the immune system, the inflammatory response, the physiological response to stress, and, finally, sexual and reproductive functions.

The three different parts of the adrenal cortex, *zona glomerulosa, zona fasciculata* and *zona reticularis*, are responsible for producing different hormones namely mineralocorticoids, glucocorticoids, and androgens (and eventually also estrogens). The *glomerulosa* secretes aldosterone, and gives rise to Primary Aldosteronism (PA)/Hyperaldosteronism that can result either from an adenoma (Conn's syndrome) or from bilateral hyperplasia (BAH). The *zona fasciculata* secretes cortisol and adenomas that produce this hormone are associated to a distinct syndrome called Cushing's syndrome. Finally the adrenal cortex *reticularis* zone is supposed to produce adrenal androgens (namely dehydroepiandrosterone - DHEA and dehydroepiandrosterone sulfate - DHEA-s) that can in turn be either converted into testosterone or aromatized to estrogen in peripheral organs like the adipose tissue. In spite of the fact that normally this peripheral conversion is more important than the local production, there are adrenal cortex tumors that can produce testosterone directly, the Androgen-secreting tumors as well as adrenocortical carcinomas expressing aromatase and producing estrogens, the Estrogen-secreting tumors.

The majority of adrenocortical tumors (ACT) are benign and silent (non-secreting adenomas or incidentalomas) since they do not ever result in hormone secretion. Its true incidence is still unknown because it is probable that many of these cases still go undiagnosed. However, it is estimated that they are present in at least 3% of the adult population (especially over 50 years of age) (National Institutes of Health, 2002; Grumbach et al., 2003). Most of these tumors are discovered incidentally due to the widespread availability of imaging studies for intra-abdominal diseases. This is the reason why they are designated as Incidentalomas.

In summary, only a minority of the adrenocortical benign tumors (about 15%) are hormone-secreting adenomas, responsible for Cushing's syndrome, primary aldosteronism (Conn's syndrome) or even sometimes virilization.
Adrenocortical carcinoma is a rare, highly malignant tumor usually associated with a poor prognosis which may occur either in children or adults. This is a malignancy with an heterogeneous presentation and despite probably still underestimated it has an expected incidence of about 1-2 cases per 1 million population per year (Wajchenberg et al., 2000; Dackiw et al., 2001; Kebebew et al., 2006). Although the adrenocortical carcinomas may occur and develop at any age, two different disease peaks were identified, one before the age of five and the other in the fifth decade of life (Wajchenberg et al., 2000; Ng & Libertino, 2003).

2. Adrenal cortex cancer

The evaluation and categorization of adrenocortical neoplasms remain among the most challenging areas in adrenal pathology (Lau & Weiss, 2009), since the pathological diagnosis of ACC, which is based on gross and microscopic criteria, is still full of areas of subjectivity. Moreover, in the absence of the gold standards that constitute the appearance of metastases, local invasion or recurrence, the diagnosis of malignancy may represent a great difficulty for both clinicians and pathologists.
Several multiparametric systems have been developed to assess this malignancy (Aubert, 2005). Among them, the Weiss system (Weiss, 1984), first introduced 25 years ago, and based on nine microscopic criteria, appears to be the most employed scoring methodology, because of its simplicity and reliability.
This system provides specific guidelines for differentiating adrenocortical adenoma from adrenocortical carcinoma and is considered the standard for determining malignancy in tumors of the adrenal cortex. However, considerable advances in the understanding of the pathology of adrenocortical neoplasias have occurred since delineation of the Weiss system, offering alternative approaches in the contemporary assessment of adrenocortical tumors (Lau & Weiss, 2009). In a recent study based on whole genome gene analysis the authors proposed a molecular assay for the classification and prognosis of adrenocortical tumors (Giordano et al., 2009). There were many genetic expression differences between ACC and ACT and normal adrenals. There were in fact 879 genes over expressed and 1011 under expressed in ACC that could differentiate ACC from ACT and normal adrenals. The most significant ones were related to cell proliferation, as would be expected. But the reality is that such systems are still very expensive and add very little to the diagnostic power of the morphological analyses. Therefore, in most adrenocortical tumors, the morphological approach considering the probability of malignancy in adrenal masses > 6 cm and that of being benign in tumors < 4 cm, together with the postoperative assessment by the Weiss system, brings sufficient elements to establish the differential diagnosis between a benign and a malignant tumor (Tissier, 2010).
The Weiss system, which, as previously was said, is currently the most popular scoring system, combines nine morphological parameters, of which three are structural ("dark" cytoplasm, diffuse architecture, necrosis), three are cytological (atypia, mitotic count, atypical mitotic figures) and three are related to invasion (of sinusoids, veins and tumor capsule) (Volante et al., 2008). The nine histological criteria are:

- High nuclear grade (grades 3 or 4) (High Nuclear/Cytoplasm ratio; marked variation of nuclear characteristics; giant cells with hyperchromatic nuclei; visible nucleoli)
  1. Small roundish nuclei; without nucleoli
  2. Larger nuclei, more irregular in shape and with visible nucleoli (at 400x magnification)
  3. Irregular nuclei, with larger size, with visible nucleoli (at 100x)
  4. enormous cells with polylobulated nuclei
- Mitoses (>5 per 50 HPF vs. <6)
- Abnormal mitoses (absent vs. present)
- Clear cells (≤25% vs. >25%)
- Diffuse architecture (>33% vs. ≤33% of the area) (cells unorganized in trabecular or alveolar structures)
- Necrosis (present vs. absent)
- Venous invasion (present vs. absent)
- Sinusoidal invasion (present vs. absent)
- Capsular invasion (present vs. absent)

1. Nuclear grade: nuclear grade III and IV based on criteria of Fuhrman (Fuhrman et al., 1982).
2. Mitotic rate: greater than 5/50 HPF (x400 objective). According to Weiss, "mitosis was evaluated by counting 10 random high-power-fields in the area of the greatest numbers of mitotic figures on the five slides with greatest number of mitoses. If less than five slides were available for a case, a correspondingly greater number of fields per slide were used to make fifty high power-fields."
3. Atypical mitotic figures: "mitosis was regarded as atypical when it definitely showed an abnormal distribution of chromosomes or an excessive number of mitotic spindles."
4. Cytoplasm: presence of ≤25% "clear or vacuolated cells resembling the normal *zona fasciculata*."
5. Diffuse architecture: diffuse architecture was present "if greater than one-third of the tumor formed patternless sheets of cells." Trabecular, columnar, alveolar or nesting organizations were regarded as non-diffuse patterns.
6. Necrosis: necrosis was "regarded as present when occurring in at least confluent nests of cells."
7. Venous invasion: Weiss defined a vein as an "endothelial-lined vessel with smooth muscle as a component of the wall."
8. Sinusoid invasion: a sinusoid was defined as "endothelial-lined vessel in the adrenal gland with little supportive tissues." Only sinusoids located within the tumor were considered.
9. Invasion of tumor capsule: "invasion of the capsule was accepted as present when nests or cords of tumor extended into or through the capsule, with a corresponding stroma reaction."

Fig. 1. Weiss classification

Tumors are classified as malignant when they meet 4 or more of these histological criteria. However, it must be stated that there are still some difficulties and subjectivity in the application of this system. Also, whether the presence of 3 criteria represents malignancy, is still controversial (Aubert et al., 2005). But, despite the referred limitations and subjectivity the Weiss classification is still the most reliable and most used criteria system.

Other markers not included in the Weiss scores are now perfectly identified as being associated with the risk of recurrence and lower survival. Ki67 expression ≥ 10% for instance is associated with much less chances of survival at 5 years. The same can be said about a high expression of SF-1. The immuno-histochemistry of these two factors is now routine in most pathology labs. (Fassnacht et al., 2011; Sbiera et al., 2010; Terzolo et al., 2001)

2.1 Adrenal cortex cancer pathogenesis

Molecular studies support the fact that uncontrolled cell proliferation is probably the most important factor in the development of cancers and ACC is no exception. ACC consist of monoclonal populations of cells (Beuschlein et al., 1994) while for instance adrenocortical macronodular hyperplasias are usually polyclonal. It is a basic rule that the mutations that give rise to cancer development are deletions of tumor suppressor genes or amplifications of oncogenes. The increase in cell proliferation induced by growth factors like the IGFs, bFGF or TGF β1 (Feige et al., 1991; Mesiano et al., 1991; Mesiano et al., 1993) leads to the development of polyclonal tumors but also renders the cells more susceptible to mutations in tumor suppressor genes or in oncogenes and if these mutations give those cells a genetic advantage, cancer development may ensue. Genomic instability is the basis of gross chromosomal alterations and aneuploidy (Giordano et al., 2009).

Most cases of adrenocortical cancers appear to be sporadic and only a small percentage of patients present ACC as a component of one of the known hereditary cancer syndromes, such as the Li-Fraumeni's syndrome, the Beckwith-Wiedemann syndrome or the Multiple Endocrine Neoplasia type 1 (Koch et al., 2002; Sidhu et al., 2004; Libé & Bertherat, 2005; Kjellman et al., 1999; Schulte et al., 2000; Heppner et al., 1999).

One important difference between these two forms of adrenocortical carcinomas (either sporadic or part of an hereditary syndrome) is the current degree of knowledge about its tumorigenesis (Soon et al., 2008). For sporadic adrenocortical malignant tumors the molecular mechanisms underlying its development are still far from completely understood (Sidhu et al, 2002). One hypothesis refers the possible evolution of adrenocortical cancers from adrenal adenomas (Bernard et al., 2003); however long-term follow-up data of incidentally discovered adrenal neoplasms do not support that hypothesis (Barzon et al., 2003; Bernini et al., 2005).

The study and investigation of the pathophysiology of ACC is not only crucial for the understanding of these malignant tumors but also for the development of more sensitive means of diagnosis and better ways of treatment. And despite the fact that knowledge of these tumors has greatly evolved in the last decades, the understanding of the genes and pathways underlying the development of adrenal cortex cancers has been slow. Many genes and pathways are thought to play an important role in their development but frequently their biological plausibility is still missing.

Hereditary tumor syndrome	Gene (*locus*)	Prevalence of ACT
Li-Fraumeni syndrome (LFS)	*TP53* (17p13), HIC-1 (17p13), *hCHK2* (22q12.1)	ACC 3%-4%
Beckwith-Wiedemann syndrome (BWS)	*IGF-II, H19, CDKN1C (p57kip2), KCNQ1* (11p15)	ACC 5%
Multiple Endocrine Neoplasia 1 (MEN-1)	*Menin gene* (11q13)	ACT 25-50%; ACC rare
Congenital Adrenal Hyperplasia (CAH)	*Mostly CYP21B* (6p21.3)	ACT in up to 82%; ACC (rare) vs Hyperplasia (usual)

- In LFS there is a germline mutation of the tumor suppressor gene TP53 in more than 70% of the families. Tumors associated with this syndrome include breast carcinoma; soft tissue sarcoma; brain tumors; osteosarcoma; leukemia and ACC. Mutations in Checkpoint Kinase 2 gene (hCHK2) encoding a kinase that phosphorylates TP53 were identified in some of these tumors but not in ACC (Libé & Bertherat, 2005).
- In BWS there is, on the contrary, deregulation of the imprinted IGF-II locus at 11p15. The IGF-II gene is maternally imprinted and so it's expressed only from the paternal allele. H19 and p57kip2 are paternally imprinted. In cases of paternal isodisomy, IGF-II is over-expressed and H19 and p57kip2 are under-expressed! BWS is a syndrome of "overgrowth" that includes many tumors like the renal' Wilms tumor, ACC, neuroblastoma and hepatoblastoma (Libé & Bertherat, 2005).
- In MEN-1 the germline mutation is in the Menin gene (90% of the families). This gene is also a tumor suppressor gene and it is located in chromosome 11 (11q13). LOH at 11q13 exist in more than 90% of ACC (Kjellman et al., 1999; Schulte et al., 2000; Heppner et al., 1999)

Adapted from Soon P. et al., (2008). Molecular markers and the pathogenesis of adrenocortical cancer. The Oncologist 13: 548-561

Table 1. Hereditary tumor syndromes, responsible genes and associated ACT prevalence

In **sporadic ACC** it has been reported that hyper-expression of the insulin-like growth factor II (**IGF-II**) is observed in the vast majority of cases (Boulle et al., 1998; Gicquel et al., 1994; Gicquel et al., 1997; Gicquel et al., 2001; Ilvesmaki et al., 1993). Together with the increase of this growth factor there is also an increased expression of its receptor (IGF-IR) in most ACC (Weber et al., 1997). The over-expression of IGF-II is probably related to adrenal cancer cell proliferation, through the IGF-I receptor (Fottner et al., 2001 and Logié et al., 1999).
The IGF-II overexpression is the result of changes at the 11p15 locus (Gicquel et al., 1994; Gicquel et al., 1997). LOH at 11p15 is much more frequent in ACC (78,5%) than in ACT (9,5%) (Gicquel et al., 2001). It is associated with a higher risk of tumor recurrence, and correlates with Weiss score. Thus, according to Gicquel and colleagues, 11p15 alterations could be used as a biological marker for confirming ACC malignancy after surgical removal of the tumor (Gicquel et al., 2001).

The 11p15 region is organized in a telomeric domain containing the IGF-II gene and H19 and a centromeric domain including the CDKN1C (p57kip2) (DeChiara et al., 1991; Hao et al., 1993; Lee et al., 1995; Matsuoka et al., 1995). Genetic and epigenetic changes in the imprinted 11p15 region resulting in low p57kip2 and H19 and elevated IGF2 mRNA expression levels have been reported in sporadic ACCs (Gicquel et al., 1994; Gicquel et al., 1997). The IGF-II system, in the adrenal gland, is responsible for growth-promoting and differentiating functions during the fetal period (Mesiano et al., 1993), but its role has been largely documented in adrenocortical malignant tumors, also in adult patients (Gicquel et al., 2001). In fact, several studies have been successful in showing the strong overexpression of IGF-II in malignant adrenocortical tumors (in approximately 90%of the cases) (Boulle et al., 1998; Gicquel et al., 1994; Gicquel et al., 1997; Gicquel et al., 2001; Ilvesmaki et al., 1993a).

Inactivating mutations of the **TP53 gene** located at the 17p13 locus are another genetic alteration that is frequently encountered in ACC. TP53 is one of the most relevant tumor suppressor genes, frequently mutated in human cancers. The TP53 mutations are thought to happen late in the evolution of sporadic malignant adrenocortical tumors. Mutations in the exons 5-8 are found more frequently in ACC than in ACT (Hollstein et al., 1991; Reincke et al., 1994). The germline mutations in TP53 have been observed in 50-80% of children diagnosed with sporadic ACC (Libé & Bertherat, 2005; Wagner et al., 1994; Varley et al., 1999). In southern Brazil where the prevalence of ACC in children is 10 times greater than in the rest of the world, there is a particular mutation at exon 10 of TP53 (Arginine 337 Histidine) in most of the cases (Ribeiro et al., 2001; Latronico et al., 2001).

Considering TP 53 gene mutations in sporadic ACC in adults, its frequency has been reported in different proportions in diverse studies ranging from 25% to 70%. (Ohgaki et al., 1993; Reincke et al., 1994; Barzon et al., 2001; Lin et al., 1994) Loss of Heterozigoty (LOH) at 17p13 was reported in 95% of ACC and only in 30% of ACT (Gicquel et al., 2001) and therefore this can also be used as a marker of malignancy.

Other reported molecular studies have suggested that genetic alterations of the **Wnt signaling pathway** may also be associated with the development of adrenocortical tumors. In fact the activation of the Wnt signaling pathway is the most prevalent defect in adrenocortical tumorigenesis particularly due to the fact that it is not only present in malignant lesions but in benign adrenocortical adenomas as well (Tissier et al., 2005).

The Wnt family includes a group of growth factors involved in developmental and homeostatic processes. Some regulatory genes in this pathway (including the down regulators of β-catenin, GSK3, Axin and APC, and β-catenin itself) can be mutated in primary human cancers (Polakis et al., 2000). In all of them the common denominator is the activation of gene transcription by β-catenin (via the transcription factors TCF and LEF).

β-catenin has a dual function in the cell: cell-adhesion (conjugated with E-cadherin) and transcriptional regulation. When the regulators of β-catenin are down-regulated the transcriptional function is increased and the adhesion is reduced and both of these alterations lead to the progression of malignancies (Brembeck et al., 2006).

Genetic alterations in the Wnt pathway conducting to β-catenin accumulation in the cytoplasm have been correlated with the pathogenesis of different types of cancer

(Gordon & Nusse, 2006). Curiously, in adrenocortical tumors, the accumulation of β-catenin has been found in both benign and malignant situations although with a slightly higher prevalence in adrenal cortex cancer (Tissier et al., 2005). It is a fact that β-catenin mutations are the most frequent genetic defects reported in adrenocortical adenomas and in these benign ACT it is mostly the non-secretory adenomas that have these mutations (Tissier et al., 2005). According to that study, abnormal cytoplasmic and/or nuclear accumulation of β-catenin was found in 38% of the adrenocortical adenomas (ACA) and in 77% of the ACC, but mutations in the β-catenin gene were found with similar frequencies of in both ACA and ACC (27% *vs.* 31%) (Tissier et al., 2005). These somewhat opposite results suggest that other components of the Wnt signaling pathway, such as the adenomatous polyposis coli (APC) or axin, may be contributing to the pathogenesis of ACC (Tissier et al., 2005).

2.2 Adrenal cortex cancer – Diagnosis and clinical presentation

Adrenocortical tumors can be classified as functional, when their hormonal secretions result in clinical consequences, or nonfunctional tumors, when they do not secrete hormones in a sufficient level to produce clinical consequences. About 50 to 60% of the adrenocortical carcinomas are functional, therefore, associated with hormonal secretion (Ng & Libertino, 2003; Allolio & Fassnacht, 2006). The most frequent presentation among adults is the Cushing's syndrome alone (45%) or the association of Cushing's syndrome with a virilization syndrome, with over-production of both glucocorticoids and androgens (25%) (Ng & Libertino, 2003; Wajchenberg et al., 2000). Other forms of functional tumors include the virilization syndrome alone and the feminization syndrome. Thus, signs and symptoms of adrenocortical tumors may vary significantly according to their origin and depending on the type of hormones that are released. Cortisol excess can be associated to symptoms such as centripetal obesity, protein wasting with skin thinning and striae, muscle atrophy (myopathy), osteoporosis, psychiatric disturbances, impaired defense against infections, diabetes, hypertension and gonadal dysfunction in men and women. In the case of aggressive malignant ACC weight loss may be observed. Androgen over-secretion is associated with various manifestations in women like hirsutism, menstrual abnormalities, infertility and eventually virilization, while excess of estrogen, although not so common, can present as gynecomastia in men. It is most important to characterize the adrenocortical carcinoma's secretory profile in order to establish its origin and better guide its treatment and follow-up (Libé et al., 2007).

Due to the elevated possibility of non-specific symptoms, both symptomatic and apparently asymptomatic patients should be evaluated.

According to the European Network for the Study of Adrenal Tumors (ENSAT), both should be studied with the following laboratory tests to determine the secretory activity of the tumor (Fassnacht & Allolio, 2009):

- fasting blood glucose and HbA1c;
- serum potassium;
- adrenal androgens (DHEA-s, androstenedione, testosterone, 17-OH progesterone);
- serum estradiol in men and postmenopausal women;
- cortisol and adrenocorticotropic hormone (ACTH) both fasting and around midnight (in the serum or in the saliva);

- fasting serum cortisol at 8 AM following a 1 mg dose of dexamethasone on the previous day at bedtime;
- 24-hour urinary free cortisol.

After careful hormonal assessment, imaging studies, by means of computerized tomography (CT), magnetic resonance imaging (MRI) or 18 F-fluorodeoxyglucose positron emission tomography (FDG-PET), are the next essential exams both to localize and delimitate the tumor and to distinguish benign adenomas from adrenocortical carcinomas (Boland et al., 1998; Hamrahian et al., 2005; Szolaret al., 2005; Caoili et al., 2002; Groussin et al., 2009; Minn et al., 2004; Metser et al., 2006 Wajchenberg et al., 2000). Despite sometimes being considered a controversial position, several studies have shown that the size and the appearance of the tumor remains one of the best indicators of malignancy (most molecular studies add only a little to the accuracy of malignancy identification by the mere determination of tumor size). In a study from the National Italian Study Group on Adrenal Tumors including 887 patients with adrenal incidentalomas, adrenocortical carcinomas were significantly associated with mass size, with 90% being more than 4 cm in diameter when discovered (Angeli et al., 1997). According, to a study by Sturgeon and colleagues at the University of California (San Francisco) including 457 ACC cases, a size of ≥4 cm makes the likelihood of malignancy double (to 10%) while in tumors ≥8 cm it gets more than ninefold higher (47%) (Sturgeon et al., 2006).

However, because of the growing evidence of adrenocortical cancers diagnosed with a diameter between 4 and 6 cm (Sturgeon et al., 2006; Grumbach et al., 2003; Herrera et al., 1991; Mantero et al., 2000) and since it seems evident that during their early stages of development, carcinomas have to be small, it becomes clear that surgical intervention would be most beneficial the smaller and more localized the tumor would be.

Overall, prognosis does improve for patients with smaller adrenocortical tumors at the time of diagnosis. In a retrospective review of 62 ACC cases (Henley et al., 1983) patients with stages I to III lesions who underwent curative resections had significantly longer survival rates. In another study done by Fassnacht and colleagues, the five year survival significantly improved (82% *vs* 18%) for patients with smaller tumors (stages I and II, confined to the adrenal gland) vs. metastatic disease, stage IV (Fassnacht et al., 2009).

As general rules, one could say that the prognosis is better in the case of young children, in smaller and localized tumors specially if nonfunctioning and in which a complete resection can be achieved.

Despite the importance of evaluating an adrenal mass size and appearance, this should not be the only parameter guiding diagnosis and posterior treatment, since radiographic features are often of strong predictive value (Dunnick et al., 1996). MRI and CT images may in fact be useful in helping to define what will be the histological type of the adrenal tumor:

On unenhanced CT scanning, the measurements of Hounsfield units (HU) are of great value in differentiating malignant from benign adrenocortical tumors. The Hounsfield scale is a semi-quantitative method of measuring x-ray attenuation. Despite the fact that around 30% of adenomas do not contain large amounts of lipid, being indistinguishable from non-adenomas, adrenal masses with < 10 HU on unenhanced CT are almost certainly benign tumors (Grumbach et al., 2003). Therefore, this seems to be the consensus cut-off for distinguishing adrenocortical carcinomas from benign adrenal tumors, according to several studies (Boland et al., 1998; Hamrahian et al., 2005). However, in those cases of benign tumors with poor intracytoplasmatic lipid concentration a better discrimination can be obtained by searching for a delayed contrast clearance in contrast-enhanced CT. In this case, tumors measuring > 10HU in a unenhanced CT, that show a contrast washout of less than 50% after 10- to 15-min of contrast-enhanced CT and also a delayed attenuation of more than 35HU, are suspicious for malignancy (Szolar et al., 2005; Caoili et al., 2002).

The use of MRI for differentiating benign and malignant adrenocortical tumors is equally effective to CT scan. But since MRI is more expensive and less standardized, CT scan remains the primary adrenal imaging procedure,

The utilization of the PET scanning with fluorodeoxyglucose (FDG) has been successful in identifying unilateral adrenal tumors with higher suspicion for malignancy, due to the greater reported uptake of FDG by malignant tumors compared to the benign adrenocortical tumors (Groussin et al., 2009; Maurea et al. 2001; Minn et al., 2004). The use of integrated PET-CT can further improve the capacity to distinguish between malignant and benign tumors by increasing the quality of the image. This improvement is also due to the combination of CT attenuation measurements with the intensity of FDG uptake, as described by the standardized uptake value (SUV) for the adrenal lesion (Metser et al., 2006; Caoili et al., 2007).

In what concerns **fine-needle aspiration biopsy** (FNA) one must stress that usually it is not successful in distinguishing between malignant and benign tumors and there are doubts about the risk of disseminating a carcinoma through the abdominal cavity; it can however be of some utility in differentiating an adrenal tumor from a metastasis to the adrenal and in evaluating staging for a known cancer (Jhala et al., 2004; Kocijancic et al., 2004).

2.3 Adrenal cortex cancer staging

The first staging system published by the World Health Organization (WHO) dates from in 2004 (DeLellis, 2004), and was based on different staging systems, such as the Sullivan modification of the Macfarlane system (Sullivan, 1978). The AJCC (American Joint Committee on Cancer)/UICC (International Union Against Cancer) developed a TNM staging system with the same definitions for the first time in 2009, being published on the AJCC/UICC Cancer Staging Manual, Seventh Edition. A simplified classification system was recently proposed by the European network ENSAT in which stage III includes cases with lymph nodes metastasis, infiltration of surrounding tissues and venous tumor thrombosis and stage IV only cases with distant metastases (Fassnacht et al., 2009).

Tumor clinical staging is most dependent of clinical examination and radiographic imaging in order to evaluate the size of the primary tumor and the extent of local and distant disease. Since disease-free and overall survival rates seem to be strongly related with tumor staging, resection of the primary tumor and examination of local extension of the disease and regional lymph nodes involvement should be performed for a better pathologic tumor staging.

The following table describes the AJCC/UICC anatomic stages and prognostic groups:

Stage	T	N	M	Description
Stage I	T1	N0	M0	Tumor 5 cm or less in greatest dimension, no extra-adrenal invasion.
Stage II	T2	N0	M0	Tumor greater than 5 cm, no extra-adrenal invasion.
Stage III	T1	N1	M0	Tumor 5 cm or less in greatest dimension, no extra-adrenal invasion but with metastasis in regional lymph node(s).
	T2	N1	M0	Tumor greater than 5 cm, no extra-adrenal invasion but with metastasis in regional lymph node(s).
	T3	N0	M0	Tumor of any size with local invasion, but not invading adjacent organs*.
Stage IV	T3	N1	M0	Tumor of any size with local invasion, but not invading adjacent organs* plus metastasis in regional lymph node(s).
	T4	N0	M0	Tumor of any size with invasion of adjacent organs*.
	T4	N1	M0	Tumor of any size with invasion of adjacent organs* plus metastasis in regional lymph node(s).
	Any T	Any N	M1	Tumor of any size and with or without invasion of adjacent organs and lymph nodes, but with distant metastases.

Adapted from Edge, SB., Byrd, DR., Compton, CC., Fritz, AG., Greene, FL., Trotti, A. (Eds.). (2010). AJCC Cancer Staging Manual, 7th Ed. Springer, Chicago.
*Adjacent organs include kidney, diaphragm, great vessels, pancreas, spleen and liver.

Table 2. AJCC/UICC anatomic stages and prognostic groups

2.4 Adrenal cortex cancer treatment

For being a very rare and aggressive carcinoma the prognosis for patients with adrenocortical cancer is poor, also due to usually not being diagnosed in the early stages of the disease (Ng & Libertino, 2003; Harrison et al., 1999). Its rarity is one of the main reasons for the lack of robust clinical studies on the most efficacious treatments (Decker et al., 1991; Bukowski et al., 1993; Khan et al., 2000). Several studies and clinical trials, however, have shown that this trend in prognosis is changing and in fact patients with this type of carcinoma are living longer as progresses are being made in its treatment (Berruti et al., 2005; Adam et al., 2006; Allolio et al., 2004; Terzolo et al., 2007; van Ditzhuijsen et al, 2007; Fassnacht et al., 2011).
Currently, the only potentially curative treatment for adrenal cortex carcinomas is total resection of the tumor at the time of initial evaluation (Allolio et al., 2006; Dackiw et al., 2001). However, in a study of Haak and colleagues with 96 patients, the overall five-year survival rate after total resection was only 49% (Haak et al., 1994). This happens probably due to the presence of hidden micrometastases that will only become apparent some months to years later (Allolio & Fassnacht, 2006; Stojadinovic et al., 2002). In fact, many patients may develop distant metastases two or more years after the diagnosis date (Abiven et al., 2006).

Therefore, surgery in these patients must be as extensive as possible, with lymphadenectomy associated. One should be very careful to avoid capsular damage and the spill of malignant cells that may result in the development of metastasis (Terzolo et al., 2007; van Ditzhuijsen et al., 2007). Nowadays, open adrenalectomy is the most consensual operation type, since laparoscopy is associated with greater risk of malignant cells spread and therefore higher risk of recurrence or dissemination (Schteingart et al., 2005; Gonzalez et al., 2005; Cobb et al., 2005). Studies have also shown that whenever total resection is not possible, maximal debulking is associated with a decrease in excess of hormone production and with better overall survival when compared with non-surgical treatments (Ng & Libertino, 2003; Luton, et al., 1990).

Whenever surgery is not feasible or is unable to completely remove the tumor, mitotane (Lysodren), an adrenocorticolytic drug, was shown to be effective, either as a primary therapy or as an adjuvant therapy (Henley et al., 1983; Dackiw et al., 2001; Berruti et al., 2005; Terzolo et al., 2007; Luton et al 1990; Hahner & Fassnacht, 2005). Mitotane has a specific effect on adrenal cells resulting in their lysis (Hahner & Fassnacht, 2005).

As a primary treatment for unresectable tumors, mitotane is especially beneficial in improvement of symptoms associated with hypercortisolism. However this benefit tends to last for short periods of time, and is associated to inconsistent survival rates (Henley et al., 1983; Baudin et al., 2001).

In what concerns the adjuvant use of mitotane therapy, its benefits have been questioned mainly due to the lack of data from controlled clinical trials and even from large prospective studies with consistent assessments of dosing and tumor variability (Kendrick et al., 2001; Kopf et al., 2001). Despite the lack of robust data, several retrospective analyses have reported higher recurrence-free survival when compared to control groups and tumor regression rates of around 30% also being associated with a better control of hormone excess (Allolio & Fassnacht, 2006; Terzolo et al., 2007). Treatment with mitotane has especially good results in patients previously submitted to tumor resection, who begun therapy right after surgery and who are submitted to regular monitoring of mitotane plasma levels (Daffara et al., 2008).

When considering recurrent or advanced adrenocortical cancer, aggressive resection of local or distant disease is still considered to be an effective therapy method capable of increasing overall survival (Schteingart et al., 1982; Meyer et al., 2004). However, in these cases the use of cytotoxic drugs such as mitotane alone or in combination with other chemotherapeutic agents has to be utilized (Allolio & Fassnacht, 2006).

Mitotane is recommended even in patients with unresectable advanced disease, since several studies have reported the effectiveness of this drug in producing objective improvements in the majority of treated patients, despite its low impact on survival. Moreover, it has been demonstrated that cytotoxic activity of chemotherapeutic agents is increased when combined with mitotane in human adrenal carcinoma cells in vitro (Bukowski et al., 1993; Abraham et al., 2002). Despite the modest results found in the few prospective trials published until now, the combination of mitotane with different chemotherapeutic regimens resulted in overall response rates varying between 14 to 49% (Berruti et al., 2005; Khan et al., 2000; Abraham et al., 2002; Bonacci et al., 1998).

Other regimens of chemotherapy without mitotane have been also evaluated in a few clinical trials but showed modest response rates, revealing the need for the development of more and better drugs and well-designed prospective trials (Schlumberger et al., 1988; Quinkler et al., 2008; Khan et al., 2004).

One must be conscious that progresses in this cancer treatment are limited and slow. More clinical trials and large prospective studies are necessary to better support physicians' choices of treatment. An example of those trials was the recently concluded "First International Randomized trial in locally advanced and Metastatic Adrenocortical Carcinoma Treatment" (FIRM-ACT), an international clinical study comparing the efficacy of etoposide, doxorubicin and cisplatin (EDP) plus mitotane versus streptozotocin plus mitotane in patients with metastatic adrenocortical cancer. This sufficiently large prospective study gave support to the use of the first therapeutic combination (EDP+mitotane) in these conditions (Fassnacht et al., 2011).
The use of radiation therapy or radiofrequency ablation are the least studied hypothesis. They are mainly beneficial in patients with unresectable local tumors with local symptoms or symptomatic metastasis (Schteingart et al., 2005; Polat et al., 2009; Magee et al., 1987). Their impact in patients' survival is still unknown and needs further investigation (Wood et al., 2003; Mayo-Smith et al., 2004).
In the future one may expect that the understanding of the specific molecular alterations in these malignant cells can identify suitable therapeutical targets that may significantly improve the prognosis for these patients.

3. Primary hyperaldosteronism/Conn's syndrome

The synthesis of aldosterone by the adrenal glands occurs in the *zona glomerulosa*. The major conditions for the production of this hormone such as the low concentration of 17-alpha-hydroxylase and the ability to add an hydroxyl group at the 18-carbon position and its subsequent oxidation to an aldehyde, only occur in the *zona glomerulosa* and this processing is mediated by a single multifunctional cytochrome P450 - CYP11B2 or Aldo Synthase (White et al., 1987; White, 1994; Ulick et al., 1992; Holland & Carr, 1993).
The aldosterone-producing adenoma was first described by Conn in 1954 (Conn, 1955; Young, 2007a), who also established for the first time the relationship between adrenal aldosterone-producing tumors, hypertension, and hypokalemia (Gittler & Fajans, 1995). In addition to the aldosterone-producing adenoma (APA), other subtypes of primary aldosteronism (PA) have been described over the subsequent four decades (Conn, 1955; Conn, 1964; Gitler & Fajans, 1995; Young, 2007a; Stowasser, 2009). The most common is the bilateral idiopathic hyperaldosteronism (IHA) which represent approximately 70% of all PA cases (while APA, approximately 30%). Other forms include unilateral hyperplasia or primary adrenal hyperplasia (caused by hyperplasia of the *zona glomerulosa* of only one adrenal gland), familial hyperaldosteronism type I (glucocorticoid-remediable aldosteronism - GRA) caused by the existence of an hybrid gene composed of the CYP11B1 promoter and CYP11B2 gene in which aldosterone is produced in response to ACTH and hence responds to glucocorticoid mediated suppression of ACTH, familial hyperaldosteronism type II (the familial occurrence of aldosterone-producing adenoma or bilateral idiopathic hyperplasia or both), and also the familial or sporadic occurrence of APA due to a mutation in the gene of the K^+ channel (KCNJ5) (Choi et al., 2011).
Finally, in spite of being very rare, pure aldosterone-producing adrenocortical carcinomas and ectopic aldosterone-secreting tumors (e.g. neoplasms in the ovary or kidney) may also occur.
The screening of PA is done by the demonstration of an elevated aldosterone level (> 15 ng/dl) together with the suppression of Plasma Renin Activity (PRA), translated in an

increased Aldosterone (*in ng/dl*)/PRA (*in ng/ml/h*) ratio above 20 or 40 (accordingly to the desired sensitivity).
Then a confirmatory test is needed and this can be done by one of the following tests:

- fludrocortisone suppression test
- oral salt load
- saline infusion test
- Captopril test

Since these tumors are generally very small, CT scan has a low sensitivity to localize them, and the fact that in people above 40 to 50 years of age, the prevalence of incidentalomas is high makes its specificity also decrease. Therefore the gold standard for a correct diagnosis of APA is Adrenal Venous Sampling in spite of the fact that it is an invasive method with a good success rate only in the hands of experienced radiologists.
During the past two decades it has become increasingly recognized that primary aldosteronism is much more common than previously thought. It is currently acknowledged that primary aldosteronism accounts for up to 5-10% of hypertensive patients, correlating with the severity of hypertension and going up to 20% in cases of resistant hypertension (i.e one that does not respond to 3-drug-regimen).
The clinical features of PA are mostly determined by the renal actions of aldosterone. Its diagnosis is more frequently made in patients who are in the third to sixth decades of life, with resistant hypertension, accompanied by marked hypokalemia, possibly muscle weakness and cramping, headaches, palpitations, polydipsia, polyuria, nocturia, or a combination of these. There is, however, generally a characteristic lack of edema!
Hypokalemia, once the most important "screening" method for PA is observed less and less frequently both due to the sodium restriction that most doctors recommend to their patients with high blood pressure and also to the higher prevalence of BAH *vs* APA observed in the more recent series.
Patients' elevated blood pressure is a major clinical finding in PA (Mattsson & Young, 2006; Young, 2007a). However, PA is rarely associated with malignant hypertension (Zarifis et al., 1996). In a study of Blumenfeld and colleagues, the mean blood pressure was 184/112 mmHg in patients with an adrenal adenoma and 161/105 mmHg in patients diagnosed with bilateral hyperplasia (Blumenfeld et al., 1994). One important and special feature associated with PA hypertension is the failure to achieve the goal blood pressure (BP) despite a complete adherence to a multi-drug regimen of treatment.
It was also clearly demonstrated that aldosterone excess has direct adverse cardiovascular consequences that go well beyond the risks associated with this type of hypertension (Stowasser, 2009). Aldosterone is responsible for the development of myocardial fibrosis aggravating the prognosis post myocardial infarct (MI) and in congestive heart failure (CHF).
Cardiovascular risk factors seem to be more severe with PA, since when matched for age, blood pressure and the duration of hypertension, these patients have greater left ventricular mass measurements when compared to patients with other types of hypertension, including essential hypertension, pheochromocytoma, and Cushing's syndrome (Milliez et al., 2005; Tanabe et al., 1997). Also, in a case-control study of 124 patients with PA and 465 patients with essential hypertension, matched for age, sex, and systolic and diastolic blood pressure, it was found that patients presenting with either APA or bilateral hyperplasia had a significantly higher rate of cardiovascular events (e.g. stroke, atrial fibrillation and myocardial infarction) than the matched essential hypertension patients (Milliez et al., 2005).

Furthermore, some particular renal effects may be also experienced by PA patients, independently of their systemic hypertension. Several reports have shown that glomerular filtration rate (GFR) and urinary albumin excretion may be increased in these patients; however these changes appear to be largely reversible after appropriate treatment. Adrenalectomy increased the serum creatinine and decreased the mean GFR. Treatment with spironolactone resulted in a similar decline in GFR. Thus, surgical cure or mineralocorticoid receptor blockade reverse the hyperfiltration state and unmask the underlying renal insufficiency (Stowasser, 2009).
One final point to be stressed in relation to PA is that generally APA should be treated surgically while bilateral adrenal hyperplasias are better treated medically with mineralocorticoid inhibition by means of spironolactone, eplerenone or amiloride. Nevertheless, even APAs, specially the small ones, may also be treated appropriately with these drugs and hence, the choice should always be given to the patients.

4. Androgen-secreting adrenal cortex tumors

Androgen-secreting adrenal cortex tumors are rare tumors, accounting for only 0.2% of the causes of androgen excess (Azziz et al., 2004; Carmina et al., 2006). Androgen over-secretion results in the development of androgenic features in affected women, with the development of hirsutism, androgenic alopecia, acne, ovulatory dysfunction, and, if the oversecretion is extreme or prolonged, even virilization may ensue (Wajchenberg et al., 2000; Azziz et al., 2004).
Despite the fact that benign androgen-secreting adrenal tumors have been described, the finding of androgen secretion by an ACT is considered to be highly suggestive of malignancy. The presence of a virilizing adrenocortical carcinoma can be suggested by very high testosterone levels and the failure of androgen suppression in response to glucocorticoid administration (Kaltsas et al., 2003; Waggoner et al., 1999; Derksen et al., 1994). In a report of 21 women with androgen-secreting tumors, serum testosterone levels were 2.6-fold higher in the women with malignant tumors (n=10) than in women with benign tumors (n=11) (Moreno et al., 2004).
Benign cortisol-secreting adenomas can also produce small amounts of androgens, but the serum androgen levels are usually not elevated (Kamenicky et al., 2007).
Considering its elevated probability of malignancy it is of great importance to identify patients with this type of rare carcinomas among women with androgen excess, due to its life-threatening potential (Wajchenberg et al., 2000). Despite several authors having considered that a clinical presentation with rapidly progressive virilization was sufficient to identify patients requiring a more extensive investigation (Kettel, 1989), it is consensual that some androgen-secreting adrenocortical tumors may produce only moderate levels of androgens and have a rather indolent presentation (Rosenfield , 2005; Kaltsas et al., 2003).
It should also be noticed that androgen-secreting tumors in men same as estrogen secreting tumors in women, may not result in clinically significant syndromes, and both can be erroneously considered as non-functioning, delaying their treatment. If one doesn't apply an extensive analytical protocol to nonfunctioning adrenocortical tumors, only the development of mass effects or the occurrence of metastases would lead to their recognition as malignant.

5. Estrogen-secreting adrenal cortex tumors

Estrogen-secreting adrenal cortex tumors correspond to a very rare type of tumors characterized by the over-production of estrogens (estrone or estradiol). The over- secretion of these hormones may cause precocious puberty with very early menarche in girls and more often sex-reversal characteristics in men (feminizing symptoms) (Advani et al., 2010). The feminizing symptoms, such as the characteristic gynecomastia, are associated with the expression of the cytochrome P450 aromatase (aromatase) in adrenocortical cells. Normally, aromatase catalyses the conversion of C19 steroids into estrogens in tissues such as the ovarian follicles' granulosa layer and the adipose tissue, whereas normal adrenal tissues have no detectable aromatase activity (Watanabe & Nakajin, 2004).

6. Cushing's syndrome

The Cushing's syndrome was first described by Harvey Cushing in 1932, and can be caused by several mechanisms associated with increased levels of cortisol in the blood. The diagnosis of Cushing's syndrome is determined through biochemical tests, since the presence of suggestive symptoms and signs are not enough to sustain it. In fact none of its symptoms is pathognomonic and most of them are non-specific such as obesity, hypertension and increased cardiovascular risk, menstrual irregularity and infertility, osteoporosis and glucose intolerance. It can also cause some form of psychological distress, going from impaired quality of life to depression and even psychosis. It should always be borne in mind, however, that if left untreated, Cushing's syndrome has a 5 fold excess mortality.

The high levels of cortisol in the blood can be caused not only by adrenocortical tumors but also by adrenocorticotropic hormone (ACTH) or corticotropin-releasing hormone (CRH) hyperproduction, as well as by the excessive intake of glucocorticoid drugs. This is even one of the most frequent causes of Cushing's syndrome (Iatrogenic Cushing's). In the study of a Cushing's syndrome case these situations need to be excluded (Weber SL., 1997; Hughes et al., 1996; Quddusi et al., 1998). Moreover, special attention is also required for other disorders causing hypercortisolism-related symptoms and sometimes also exhibiting mild to moderate elevations of plasma cortisol, known as pseudo-Cushing's syndrome. The pseudo-Cushing's syndromes may include:

- Patients who are physically stressed (e.g. severe bacterial infections) (Liddle, 1960);
- Patients with severe obesity, especially visceral obesity or polycystic ovary syndrome (Liddle, 1960);
- Patients with psychological stress (major depressive disorder and severe melancholic syndromes) (Gold et al., 1986);
- Rarely, also patients with chronic alcoholism (Kirkman & Nelson, 1988).

The difficulties normally met in Cushing's syndrome diagnostic process are well translated by the fact that patients normally express some signs and symptoms of the syndrome, 2 years before a confirmation of diagnosis can be reached. After raising the suspicion by the observation of a patient with central (truncal) obesity plus hypertension, in many cases accompanied by a typical cushingoid facies (round, plethoric face), the most specific signs are the presence of thin skin, easy bruising and proximal myopathy. However, to avoid mistakes in diagnosing Cushing's syndrome due to all of the different conditions that might imitate its signs and symptoms, initial diagnostic tests for hypercortisolism must be highly sensitive. According to the evidence-based 2008 Endocrine Society Clinical Guidelines the *first-line tests* for this syndrome should be the late night salivary cortisol, the 24h urinary cortisol, or the low-dose dexamethasone suppression test (either the 1 mg, overnight or the 2mg/day, 48h dexamethasone suppression tests). To establish the diagnosis of Cushing's syndrome the following criteria should be met (Nieman et al., 2008):

- At least two of the first-line tests must be abnormal and conservative criteria should be used to interpret it to maximize sensitivity; for instance, in a patient with a symptomatic Cushing's syndrome, the cortisol cutoff level to be considered as un-suppressed after the Dexamethasone test should be >1.8 µg/dl (while in the case of incidentalomas studied to exclude subclinical Cushing's syndrome, specificity should be the main criterion and so the cutoff level should be >5 µg /dl).
- Urinary and salivary cortisol measurements should be obtained at least twice;
- The urinary cortisol excretion should be unequivocally increased (threefold above the upper limit of normal for the assay), or the diagnosis of Cushing's syndrome is uncertain and other tests should be performed;
- The patient should undergo additional evaluation if the test results are discordant or only slightly abnormal;
- If test results are normal, the patient does not have Cushing's syndrome unless it is extremely mild or cyclic. Additional evaluations are not suggested unless symptoms progress or cyclic Cushing's syndrome is suspected.

Cushing's syndrome is rare (it has an incidence of up to 3:1.000.000 persons per year) (Lindholm et al., 2001). It's also an intriguing condition both because of its complex diagnostic protocol and the demand for a correct treatment to avoid its devastating complications that can even conduct to death if left untreated. After diagnosing the hypercortisolism, it is important to determine its cause (Table 3) to better chose the appropriate treatment. It is a disease whose patients should be sent to a major hospital where multidisciplinary and well experienced teams will be available.

Diagnosis	Percentage of Patients (%)
ACTH-dependent Cushing's syndrome	
Cushing's disease	68
Ectopic ACTH syndrome	12
Ectopic CRH syndrome	< 1
ACTH-independent Cushing's syndrome	
Adrenal adenoma	10
Adrenal carcinoma	8
Micronodular hyperplasia	1
Macronodular hyperplasia	< 1
Pseudo-Cushing's syndrome	
Major depressive disorder	1
Alcoholism	< 1

Table 3. Frequency of causes of Cushing's syndrome

One of the most important, and therefore the initial, phase of determining Cushing's syndrome's etiology is to determine if the hypercortisolism is ACTH-dependent or ACTH independent. The ACTH-dependent hypercortisolism is normally due to a pituitary (or less frequently non-pituitary) ACTH secreting tumor, while ACTH-independent hypercortisolism is usually due to an adrenal tumor or hyperplasia. The preferred test is naturally the measurement of plasma ACTH. Usually a low plasma ACTH concentration of <5 pg/mL (1.1 pmol/L) in a hypercortisolemic patient is evidence of ACTH-independent disease (Invitti et al., 1999), while if the plasma ACTH concentration is above 15 pg/mL (3.3 pmol/L) it can be assumed that cortisol secretion is ACTH-dependent. Despite values between 5 and 15 pg/mL (1.1 to 3.3 pmol/L) being less definitive they normally indicate the hypercortisolism is ACTH-dependent. However, it is recommendable to perform a CRH stimulation test in these patients to confirm that hypothesis.

In the presence of an ACTH-independent Cushing's syndrome, it is important to proceed with a thin-section CT imaging of the adrenal glands, to determine its cause. When CT imaging suggests a suspicious lesion (for instance with large size) further investigation will be required to distinguish between the malignant ACC and benign ACT. The presence of bilateral disease on the other hand implies the distinction between, for instance, a bilateral tumor and bilateral macronodular adrenal hyperplasia.

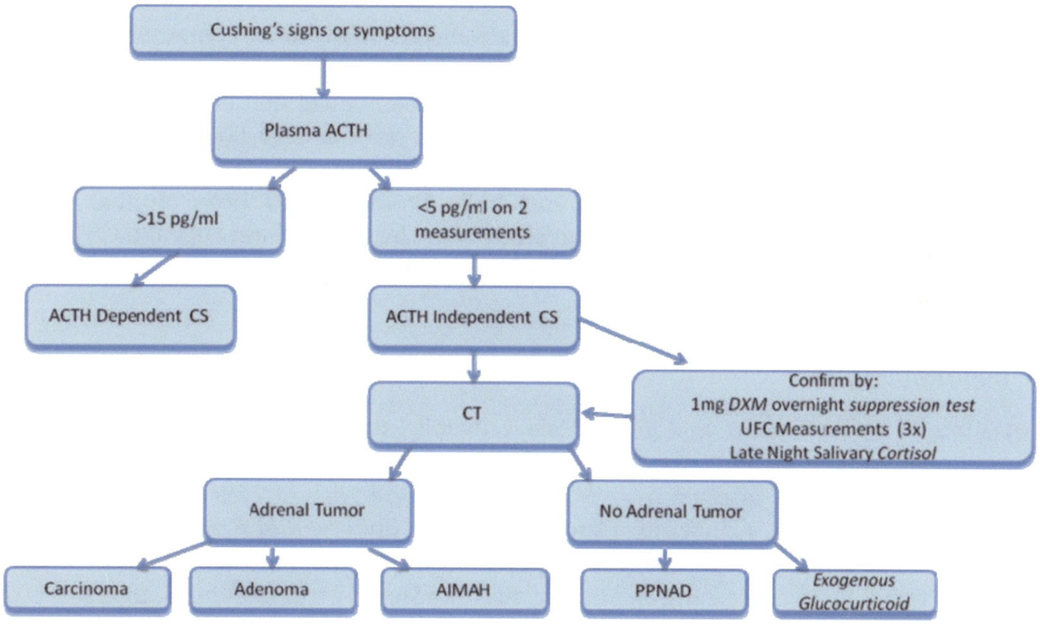

Fig. 2. Cushing syndrome

Unilateral adenomas causing Cushing's syndrome should be surgically removed as they imply a very significant increase in morbidity and mortality, which is due to cardiovascular diseases or infections.

For the great majority of ACTH-dependent Cushing's syndrome patients, the cause of the hypercortisolism is a pituitary corticotroph adenoma (Cushing's disease). Even so, patients with ACTH-dependent disease should undergo non-invasive tests such as the high-dose dexamethasone suppression test and the CRH stimulation test, to confirm the presence of Cushing's disease. It is also important to exclude extrapituitary (ectopic) sources of ACTH.

7. Subclinical Cushing's syndrome

The "subclinical" Cushing's syndrome (SCS) refers to autonomous cortisol production that is insufficient to generate the typical, clinically recognizable, combination of symptoms. The prevalence of overt Cushing's syndrome caused by an adrenal adenoma in the general population is lower than the prevalence of subclinical Cushing's syndrome in patients with clinically non-functioning adrenal adenoma (Ross, 1994).

Patients with SCS have an adrenal mass usually detected incidentally (an incidentaloma) and normally do not show any of the clinical manifestation of the Cushing's syndrome (Terzolo et al., 2005a). Still, they have some endocrine alterations that allows their recognition (Urinary free cortisol > 70 µg /24h; serum cortisol levels after a dexamethasone suppression test >5 µg/dl; morning ACTH levels < 10 pg/ml). According to the Italian National survey on 1,004 adrenal incidentalomas (Mantero et al., 2000), of which 92 were classified as SCS, the hormonal evaluation showed low baseline secretion of ACTH in 79% of the SCS patients, lack of suppressibility of cortisol secretion after 1 mg dexamethasone in 73%, supra-normal 24-hour urinary cortisol excretion in 75% or disturbed cortisol circadian rhythm in 43%. Subclinical Cushing's syndrome is the most commonly detected abnormality in patients with adrenal incidentalomas.

Most patients with SCS may show one or more of the clinical manifestation of cortisol over-secretion, such as arterial hypertension, obesity or diabetes (Terzolo et al., 2000; Angeli & Terzolo, 2002). The association between a clinically silent adrenal adenoma and some of clinical manifestations of the metabolic syndrome has been studied and is considered well proven. In a retrospective study done by Terzolo and colleagues (Terzolo et al., 2005b), of 210 such patients, 53.8% had hypertension, 21.4% were obese and 22.4% had hyperglycemia.

8. Incidentalomas

An adrenal incidentaloma is a mass lesion, usually with 1cm or more in diameter, discovered incidentally by radiologic examination (Young, 2007b). In recent years these incidentally discovered adrenal masses have been found with increasing frequency due to the widespread use of imaging techniques of the abdomen and their prevalence is estimated to be around 4% in the general population (Bovio et al., 2006). Several studies have been published concerning the prevalence of adrenal incidentalomas. In a series of 739 autopsies, Hedeland and colleagues (Hedeland et al., 1968) reported the presence of adrenal masses in 9% of normotensive patients versus 12% in patients with hypertension. In another review including 25 studies (Kloos et al., 1995), the calculated prevalence of adrenal incidentaloma was of 6%. The prevalence of adrenal adenomas increases with age from 0.2%in a patient between 20 and 29 years of age to 7% in a patient over 70 years of age (Young, 2007; Kloos et al., 1995). It is noteworthy that they are rare under the age of 40.

Despite the fact that the majority of adrenal incidentalomas are clinically non-hypersecreting and benign adrenocortical adenomas (Mansmann et al., 2004), frequently, incidentalomas' series include cases that are cortisol secreting adrenocortical adenomas (5 to 9%) (Mantero et al., 2000; Young 2007) or pheochromocytomas (3 to 5%) (Young, 2007; Cawood et al., 2009). Of these pheochromocytomas, 50% are normotensive (Motta Ramirez et al., 2005). Incidentalomas can also be adrenocortical carcinomas and metastatic carcinomas. In a group of 2005 patients with adrenal incidentalomas, almost 5% were adrenocortical carcinomas and 2.5% corresponded to other primary carcinomas'metastases (Young, 2000).

The approach to the evaluation and management of adrenal incidentalomas usually begins with taking patients' clinical history and performing a physical examination, testing for signs or symptoms of adrenal hyperfunction or malignant disease, and performing a complete hormonal evaluation (Young, 2007; Kudva et al., 2003; Terzolo et al., 2005).

The probability to find a primary adrenal carcinoma in these cases has to be considered as rare, in spite of being dependant on the size of the tumor (above 4 cm the probability of an incidentaloma being malignant is 24% (Angeli et al., 1997); however, due to the importance of such a situation the initial major concern in evaluating an adrenal incidentaloma is the possibility of malignancy, followed by the evaluation of the possibility of metastatic cancer. In fact, one should also remember that several types of carcinomas may metastasize to the adrenal glands (e.g. lung, kidney, colon, breast, pancreas, liver and stomach).

Adrenal incidentalomas are bilateral in 10-to 15% of the cases. In these cases the etiology will be one of the following: metastases; congenital adrenal hyperplasia; bilateral adenomas, bilateral adrenocortical macronodular hyperplasia; bilateral pheochromocytomas; hemorrhage, lymphoma; infectious or infiltrative diseases.

As a main conclusion we would like to stress that it is of crucial importance to evaluate all patients with adrenal incidentalomas for the possibility of either subclinical hormonal hyper-function, including SCS and pheochromocytoma, as well as cancer. Table 4 describes major evaluations and clinical features for differential diagnosis of adrenal incidentalomas.

9. Pediatric adrenal cortex tumors

The presence and diagnosis of adrenal cortex tumors in children is rare and may occur sporadically or as a component of certain hereditary tumour syndromes, such as the Li-Fraumeni syndrome, the multiple endocrine neoplasia-1 (MEN1), the Beckwith-Wiedemann syndrome, the Carney complex, and even in some rare cases of congenital adrenal hyperplasia. Its incidence is around 1 to 3 in 10.000.000 except in the southern regions of Brazil where it reaches 1 to 3 :1.000.000 (Agrons et al., 1999; Ribeiro et al., 2000, Wasserman et al., 2011).).

In southern Brazil, these carcinomas are frequently associated with a particular mutation of TP53 (namely Arg337His) (Ribeiro et al., 1990).

Clinical and biological characteristics of adrenocortical tumours are different from those observed in other paediatric carcinomas. About 65% of them are diagnosed in children younger than 5 years of age (Ribeiro et al., 1990). This age distribution has been demonstrated in several reports, including a study of Zerbini and colleagues, with 32 pediatric patients with adrenocortical neoplasms, in which the age at diagnosis ranged from 6 months to 19 years (median age, 5 years), with a predominant number of patients being 5 years of age and younger (Zerbini et al., 1992). In another study of Lefebvre and colleagues, with 42 children with adrenocortical neoplasms, two-thirds were younger than 5 years of age (Lefevre et al., 1983).

Diagnosis	Suggestive Clinical Features	Imaging Characteristics
Adrenocortical Adenoma	May have symptoms related to excess glucocorticoid, mineralocorticoid, androgen, or estrogen secretion	• Round or oval, with smooth margins • Homogeneous • Rare tumor calcification, necrosis or hemorrhage • Small, usually ≤ 3 cm in diameter • Usually solitary, unilateral • CT unenhanced attenuation values ≤10 HU (25% may have low lipid content and hence have attenuation values >10%) • Not highly vascular • Isointense in relation to liver onT1- and T2-weighted images in MRI • No delay in contrast medium washout (ten minutes after administration of contrast, an absolute contrast medium washout of 50 % or more)
Adrenocortical carcinoma	Mass effect symptoms, symptoms related to excess glucocorticoid, mineralocorticoid, androgen, or estrogen secretion. The size (>4/6 cm) and the evolution are the most important signs to raise the suspicion	• Irregular shape • Inhomogeneous density because of central areas of low attenuation due to tumor necrosis • Common tumor calcification • Diameter usually >4 cm • Unilateral location • High unenhanced CT attenuation values (>20 HU) • Inhomogeneous enhancement on CT with intravenous contrast • Delay in contrast medium washout (ten minutes after administration of contrast, an absolute contrast medium washout of less than 50 %) • Hypo-intensity compared with liver on T-1 weighted MRI and high to intermediate signal intensity on T-2 weighted MRI • High standardized uptake value (SUV) on FDG-PET-CT study • Evidence of local invasion or metastases.

Diagnosis	Suggestive Clinical Features	Imaging Characteristics
Pheochromocytoma	Hypertension, Paroxysmal Symptoms (e.g. palpitation, diaphoresis, headache, pallor, tremor). Half of the cases will remain undiagnosed! Plasma metanephrines and 24h urine metanephrines are the initial screening tests	• Round or oval, with clear margins • Heterogeneous, with cystic areas • Usually large • Usually solitary, unilateral • High unenhanced CT attenuation values (>10 HU) (usually >25) • Usually vascular • Delay in contrast medium washout (ten minutes after administration of contrast, an absolute contrast medium washout of less than 50 percent) but may be normal, mimicking the adenomas • Markedly hyper intense in relation to the liver on T2-weighted images, in MRI • Chemical-shift imaging: Pheos and ACC don't loose signal intensity on out-of phase images in comparison with in-phase ones, whereas adenomas do • Hemorrhage and cystic areas common
Metastatic Cancer	Cancer-specific signs. The identification of a primary extra-adrenal cancer favors this possibility	• Irregular shape and inhomogeneous nature • Tendency to be bilateral • High unenhanced CT attenuation values (>20 HU) and enhancement with intravenous contrast on CT • Delay in contrast medium washout (ten minutes after administration of contrast, an absolute contrast medium washout of less than 50 percent) • Isointense or slightly less intense than the liver on T-1 weighted MRI and high to intermediate signal intensity on T-2 weighted MRI (representing an increased water content)

Adapted from Young WF, Jr. Clinical practice. The incidentally discovered adrenal mass. N Engl J Med 2007a; 356: 601-10

Table 4. Clinical features and imaging characteristics of adrenal incidentalomas

About half of the adrenocortical tumours in children have predisposing constitutional genetic factors, and are usually associated with the Li-Fraumeni syndrome or the Beckwith-Wiedemann syndrome (Li & Fraumeni, 1969a; Wiedemann, 1983; Lynch et al., 1978).
The Li-Fraumeni syndrome is a cancer-predisposing syndrome that includes breast cancer, brain carcinoma, sarcomas, leukaemia and adrenocortical carcinoma (Li & Fraumeni, 1969a; Lynch et al., 1978). This syndrome is a rare autosomal dominant condition associated with germline mutations of the tumour suppressor gene TP53 on the chromosome 17 (17p13) (Li & Fraumeni, 1969b; Li et al., 1998;). The patient and the affected family members may develop different types of tumours (Birch, 1994; Srivastava et al., 1990; Sandrini et al., 1997; Hisada et al., 1998).
On the other side the Beckwith-Wiedemann syndrome, associated with abnormalities involving chromosome 11p15, and defined as a growth disorder is sometimes referred to as the EMG [exomphalos-macroglossia-gigantism] syndrome. This syndrome is associated with an increased risk of benign and malignant tumors of multiple organs (Fraumeni & Miller et al., 1967; Wiedemann, 1983), particularly the Wilms tumor of the kidneys and adrenocortical carcinoma (Lack, 1997).
The incidence of adrenocortical carcinomas in children is higher in girls. These pediatric carcinomas are hormone secreting tumors more frequently than in adults (90% vs 50%) (Michalkiewicz et al., 2004; Patil et al., 2002; Bonfig et al., 2003). The classic endocrine syndromes (namely the virilising and the Cushing's syndromes) represent the most common presentations of adrenocortical carcinomas in this age group (Wilkins, 1948 and Ribeiro et al., 2000).
However in spite of being pathologically malignant these carcinomas have a much better prognosis, with many of them becoming cured by the first surgical intervention (Michalkiewicz et al., 2004; Sutter et al., 2006; Wieneke et al., 2003; 27: Sabbaga et al., 1993)

10. ACTH-independent adrenal cortex hyperplasias

ACTH-independent hypercortisolism is always of adrenocortical origin and an adrenocortical adenoma or carcinoma are by far its most common aetiologies (in up to 95% of patients). The remaining cases will be adrenocortical hyperplasias.
Even in these cases it's important to distinguish adrenocorticotropin (ACTH)-dependent forms like Cushing's disease or CAH (due to 21-hydroxylase deficiency) from ACTH-independent ones as a primary step in the differential diagnosis of Cushing's syndrome due to adrenocortical bilateral hyperplasias (Doppman et al., 2000).
Among the adrenal causes of Cushing's syndrome about 10-15% are due to bilateral adrenal lesions that include micronodular (particularly its most common variant the *Primary Pigmented Nodular Adrenocortical Disease – PPNAD*) and macronodular adrenal hyperplasias (*ACTH-Independent Macronodular Adrenocortical Hyperplasia - AIMAH*) and, more rarely, bilateral adenomas or carcinomas (Christopoulos et al., 2005; Stratakis & Boikos, 2007).
The hyperplasias can be sporadic or familial as is the case of PPNAD that can occur isolated or as part of an autosomal dominant disease including other tumors, endocrine and non-endocrine, called the Carney Complex.
Many adrenal cortex hyperplasia cases are thought to be the consequence of genetic changes in several key components of the cyclic AMP (cAMP) pathway (Libé & Betherat, 2005; Groussin et al., 2002a; Stratakis et al., 2007). Activating germline mutations of the ACTH receptor (MC2R) gene, making it display high levels of basal activity, have been reported

(Swords et al., 2002). The same occurred with GNAS activating mutations resulting in constitutive activation of the cAMP pathway that were shown to cause ACTH-independent macronodular adrenocortical hyperplasia (AIMAH) in McCune-Albright syndrome (Weinstein, 1991). On the other hand PRKAR1A-inactivating mutations resulting in a permanent activation of PKA may be associated to the development of PPNAD either isolated or as part of the Carney complex (Kirschner et al., 2000; Groussin et al., 2002b). More recently, inactivating mutations of the phosphodiesterase 11A gene, a gene coding for an enzyme that normally regulates cyclic nucleotide levels was reported both in cases of PPNAD and other bilateral hyperplasias (e.g. macronodular) (Libé et al., 2008).

11. ACTH-independent macronodular hyperplasias

The ACTH-independent macronodular adrenocortical hyperplasias (AIMAH) constitute a rare condition that consists of multiple bilateral adrenocortical macronodules causing a striking enlargement of the adrenal glands (Doppman et al., 1991; Malchoff et al., 1989; Swain et al., 1998). The great majority of AIMAH cases is sporadic. AIMAH is responsible for less than 1% of all the endogenous cases of Cushing's syndrome (Christopoulos et al., 2005). Usually patients present in the fifth and sixth decades of life, a significantly latter age of onset compared to other cortisol producing adenomas (Swain et al., 1998).

11.1 AIMAH pathogenesis

Increased cortisol levels in AIMAH result from the fact that hormones other than ACTH become able to activate cortisol secretion through receptors aberrantly located in the adrenal cortex cells and coupled to cAMP activation. Hormones like GIP, catecholamines, vasopressin, serotonin, LH among others can activate PKA signaling, via cAMP production, leading to a situation of Cushing's syndrome.

In fact a great number of patients with AIMAH have that ectopic expression of and/or increased responsiveness to one of several possible receptors like the gastric inhibitory polypeptide (GIP) receptors (food-dependent hypercortisolism) (Resnik et al., 1992; N'diaye et al., 1998), vasopressin receptors (Horiba et al., 1995), the β-adrenergic receptors (Lacroix et al., 1997), the LH receptors, the serotonin receptors, the leptin receptors and angiotensin II receptors (Lacroix et al., 1997; Lacroix et al., 2001; Lacroix et al., 1992).

In the example of GIP-activated-cortisol-production, k cells from the duodenum and small intestine release, after food ingestion, a gastro-intestinal hormone named GIP (Gastric Inhibiting Peptide or Glucose-dependent Insulinotropic Peptide) in physiological concentrations (Lacroix et al., 2001). The expression of GIP receptors in the cells of the *zona fasciculata*, where they normally don't exist, can then be activated by the GIP secreted in response to meals, causing what is known as "food-dependent" cortisol production. The presence of this receptor can be confirmed *in vivo* by clinical testing or by adrenal imaging following the injection of [^{123}I]-GIP (Lacroix et al., 1992).

To date, more than 30 cases were reported where the adrenal hormonal hypersecretion was associated to GIP stimulation. In the majority of cases patients presented with AIMAH (Lacroix et al., 2004; Groussin et al., 2002c). Besides that, other receptors were identified, some ectopically expressed and some being eutopic but showing an over-expression in the adrenocortical cells, as being the cause of cases of AIMAH and recently also demonstrated in cases of unilateral adenomas (Lacroix, 2009).

The majority of cases of AIMAH is sporadic. Some cases however are familial and in most an autosomal dominant hereditarity has been described (Lacroix, 2009). Nevertheless, the genetic cause for these cases hasn't yet been identified. In addition to those familiar reports, AIMAH has been described in MEN-1 with a frequency between 6% (Burgess et al., 1996) and 21% (Skogseid et al., 1992), and in rare cases of Gs alpha subunit mutations (Weinstein et al., 1991; Fragoso et al., 2003) or activating mutations of the ACTH receptor (MC2R) (Swords et al., 2002):

- **Gs alpha-subunit mutations** — an activating mutation in the gene of the Gsa subunit of G-protein coupled receptors (stimulatory guanine nucleotide-binding protein, Gs) leads to constitutive activation of cAMP. These mutations may be responsible not only for increased production of cortisol but also for increased proliferation and consequently the formation of adrenal nodules (Weinstein et al., 1991; Fragoso et al., 2003).
- **MEN1** - In patients with multiple endocrine neoplasia syndrome type 1 (MEN1) caused by mutations in the the tumor suppressor gene *menin*, together with the more frequent endocrine tumors that are characteristic of the syndrome, adrenocortical adenomas or macronodular bilateral hyperplasias may also occur (Burgess et al., 1996; Skogseid et al., 1992).
- **Other genes** - There were some rare reports of activating mutations of the ACTH receptor (MC2R) gene in adrenal tumors and AIMAH (Swords et al., 2002). Moreover, AIMAH has also been reported in patients with: familial polyposis coli and a mutation in the adenomatous polyposis coli (APC) gene (Kartheuser et al., 1999); in patients with mutations in the fumarate hydratase gene (FH) (Matyakhina et al., 2005) on chromosome 1 (1q42.3-43); and in patients with germline mutations in phosphodiesterase 11A isoform 4 gene (PDE11A) (Libé et al., 2008) located on chromosome 2 (2q31-35).

11.2 AIMAH diagnosis and clinical presentation

Usually AIMAH cases can be discovered after an incidental radiological finding or following the investigation of an adrenal hypersecretion syndrome and can be distinguished from ACTH-dependent macronodular hyperplasia by a suppressed plasma ACTH (<5 pg/mL *vs.* ≥15 pg/mL).

The most common laboratory findings associated with AIMAH are the following:

- Increased serum and urinary cortisol and undetectable plasma ACTH in the basal state (Doppman et al., 2000; Swain et al., 1998; Kirschner et al., 1964; Bourdeau et al., 2001, Lieberman et al., 1994).
- As in any cause of adrenal cortisol hypersecretion, dexamethasone suppression test fails to suppress cortisol production (Christopoulos et al., 2005).

An exception to this general pattern occurs in patients with GIP-dependent Cushing's syndrome in whom cortisol hypersecretion occurs in response to meals and serum cortisol may be low in the fasting state (Resnik et al., 1992; Lacroix et al., 1992).

- Steroid hormone synthesis is relatively inefficient in AIMAH as a consequence of decreased steroidogenic enzymatic activity resulting frequently in elevated 17-hydroxyprogesterone levels after stimulation with ACTH (Bourdeau et al., 2001).
- Serum 18-hydroxycorticosterone, corticosterone and estrone may cause hypertension or feminization in the patients in whom they are increased (Wada et al., 2002).

The diagnosis of AIMAH is usually suspected after typical imaging studies, which can be variable. At the computed tomography (CT) the adrenal glands in patients with AIMAH are greatly enlarged with multiple macronodules up to 5 cm in diameter. These adrenals' weight may vary between 24 to 500g (Doppman et al., 2000; Malchoff et al., 1989).

The asymmetric appearance of the adrenal macronodules in AIMAH has been described (Liebermann et al., 1994; Lacroix et al., 2001) and also, according to a study including patients with surgically proven AIMAH, adrenal masses measuring up to 5 cm of soft tissue density can distort and obscure the adrenal glands (Doppman et al., 1991). This may conduct to the erroneous diagnosis of a unilateral adenoma.
Therefore, other clinical and molecular features must be used in diagnosing AIMAH.
One important suggestion consist of evaluating **all** patients with AIMAH and clinical and sub-clinical Cushing's syndrome for the presence of aberrant receptors, that are very frequently present in AIMAH (Lacroix et al., 2001; Mircescu et al., 2000).
In this scenario, tests that modulate the levels of ligands for those receptors may be useful determining cortisol and other steroid changes. These tests include physiological tests, such as upright posture and mixed meals, and pharmacological tests including gonadotropin-releasing hormone, thyrotropin-releasing hormone, vasopressin, glucagon and metoclopramide (Lacroix et al., 2001; Mircescu et al., 2000). Cortisol increases ≥25% are considered as significant, provided there is no increase in ACTH. If necessary, these tests should be carried out under Dexamethasone suppression. Responses between 25% and 49% are considered partial responses and if ≥50% complete responses. Any positive change should prompt the continuation of the study to identify all the receptors that may be involved (Lacroix et al., 2001)
The importance of identifying these aberrant receptors is the possibility to have specific therapeutical weapons that may permit avoiding bilateral adrenalectomy:

RECEPTOR	IN VIVO SCREENING	MEDICAL TREATMENT
GIP	Mixed meal (Food-dependent Cushing) Stimulation by GIP infusion	Octreotide GIPR antagonist
Vasopressin	Upright posture Inhibition by water load Stimulation by saline infusion Administration of Arginine Vasopressin Administration of DDAVP (- =V1R; + =V2R)	Vasopressin receptor antagonist DDAVP antagonist (V2)
B-adrenergic	Upright posture Stimulation by insulin-induced hypoglycemia Isoproterenol infusion Propranolol suppression	B-blocker (Propranolol)
LH / βHCG	GnRH test hCG Recombinant LH Pregnancy or Menopausal related cortisol elevation Sometimes also androgen secreting	Long acting GnRH agonist GnRH antagonist
5HT-4	Administration of 5HT-4 agonists Metoclopramide/Cisapride/Tegaserod test	5HT-4 receptor antagonist
Angiotensin	Upright posture Angiotensin infusion (?) Angiotensin antagonist	Angiotensin receptor antagonist

(Adapted from Lacroix et al., 2009 ACTH independent macronodular hyperplasia. Best Practice and Research Clinical Endocrinology and Metabolism. Vol 23. Pp 245-259)

Table 5. Receptors involved in AIMAH, in vivo screening tests and possible medical treatments

12. ACTH-independent micronodular hyperplasias

ACTH-independent micronodular hyperplasias are characterized by the presence of multiple cortical micronodules, with less than 1 cm in diameter (Louiset et al., 2010). These micronodular hyperplasias can be divided in two different subtypes, depending on the presence or absence of nodular pigment and internodular atrophy. The most common and predominant type of ACTH-independent micronodular adrenal hyperplasia is the primary pigmented nodular adrenocortical disease (PPNAD), characterized by multiple pigmented micronodules usually surrounded by internodular cortical atrophy. The pigmented nodules are observed in the zone between the cortex and the medulla and the cells have hybrid characteristics between cortical and medullar (for instance the high expression of synaptophysin). The pigment has been identified as lipofuscin (Louiset et al., 2010).

PPNAD is one of the possible causes of Cushing's syndrome. However, it must be stressed that it is a rare disease representing less than 1% of the cases of Cushing's syndrome. It may be sporadic or familial, and in this case it's one of the components of the Carney complex (Carney & Young, 1992; Stratakis et al., 2001).

12.1 ACTH-independent micronodular hyperplasia- pathogenesis

A few genes were already identified as causal for the development of ACTH-independent micronodular hyperplasia:

- **PRKAR1A** - Most patients with PPNAD, especially when the disease is a component of Carney complex, have germline-inactivating mutations of the PRKAR1A [protein kinase A (PKA) regulatory subunit type 1α] gene (Kirschner et al., 2000; Groussin et al., 2002a; Groussin et al., 2002b). These mutations code for a truncated protein that is not produced, and the loss of this protein leads to an increased activation of protein kinase A (PKA) by cyclic AMP (Nadella & Kirschner, 2005). In several different studies of patients with PPNAD associated with Carney complex, 65-82% had PRKAR1A mutations (Groussin et al., 2002; Veugelers et al., 2004; Bertherat et al 2009).
- **Phosphodiesterase 11A (PDE11A)** - PDE11A is a dual-specificity PDE with affinity both to cAMP and cGMP, expressed in several endocrine tissues (D'Andrea et al., 2005). Decreased expression of PDE11A has been correlated to increased adrenocortical levels of cAMP and cAMP-responsive element (CREB) phosphorylation presumably being the cause of adrenal hyperplasia. Besides having been identified in PPNAD and non-pigmented micronodular bilateral adrenocortical hyperplasias, in a study of Libé and colleagues, the PDE11A missense germline variants were also found in 18.8% of adrenocortical tumors (adrenocortical carcinomas, adenomas and bilateral macronodular adrenal hyperplasias) (Libé et al., 2008).
- **Other genes** - PDE8B gene mutations have also been described in patients with PPNAD or nonpigmented variants of the disease (Horvath et al., 2008).

Moreover, in addition to germline PRKAR1A mutations, somatic beta-catenin mutations have been found in the larger nodules of patients with PPNAD, suggesting that secondary events in the Wnt/beta-catenin signaling pathway can contribute to tumorigenesis in PPNAD (Tadjine et al., 2008; Gaujoux et al., 2008).

12.2 ACTH-independent micronodular hyperplasia – Diagnosis and clinical presentation

Most commonly patients with PPNAD present signs and symptoms of hypercortisolism such as weight gain, obesity, hypertension, and menstrual cycle disorders. However, in many of them these symptoms are subtle and slowly progressive. Besides, sometimes the cortisol hypersecretion can be cyclical rendering these cases difficult to diagnose. On the other hand, there are several characteristics that are unique to this type of micronodular hyperplasia (Carney & Young, 1992; Larsen et al., 1986; Stratakis et al., 2001).

- The majority of patients with PPNAD are diagnosed at a young age, usually before turning 30 years, and many cases occur in patients under 15 years of age.
- Another hallmark is the paradoxical cortisol response to Dexamethasone suppression test, meaning that cortisol raises in response to dexamethasone instead of being reduced (Stratakis et al., 1999).
- At surgery the characteristic pigmentation can be observed.
- Most of the nodules found in these patients are less than 4 mm, and reasonably well demarcated from the adjacent atrophic cortex.

As already mentioned, in some patients with this pathology the development of hypercortisolism symptoms can be cyclic and irregular what causes some typical Cushing's syndrome symptoms to be variable or discrete, therefore complicating its diagnosis. On the other hand, in patients with PPNAD, due to the presence of elevated cortisol levels, osteoporosis and avascular hip necrosis have been reported (Ruder et al., 1974; Carney & Young, 1992).

12.3 Carney complex

PPNAD occurs as part of Carney complex in more than 60% of the cases (Bertherat et al., 2009).

This syndrome is an autosomal dominant form of multiple neoplasia. The main signs that characterize this condition are the presence of spotty skin pigmentation (lentiginosis), the presence of endocrine tumors, including PPNAD (the most common endocrine finding in Carney's complex), testicular large cell calcifying Sertoli cells tumors, GH secreting pituitary adenomas and thyroid adenomas and carcinomas, and non-endocrine tumors, including atrial myxomas, cutaneous myxomas, breast ductal adenomas, psammomatous melanotic schwannomas, and osteochondromyxomas (Stratakis et al., 2001; Carney et al., 1985; Stratakis et al., 1997). Cushing's syndrome caused by PPNAD occurs in many of the cases of Carney Complex. However, if one considers also the subclinical cases of Cushing's syndrome, the percentage will surely be higher (Bertherat et al., 2009; Stratakis et al., 2001).

Three genetic loci were associated with the Carney Complex: 2p16, 17q22-24 and 17p12-13. More than 70% Carney Complex cases have a PRKAR1A mutation (Bertherat et al., 2009).

For being a heterogeneous disease that can present with different signs and symptoms, its diagnosis is usually difficult (Carson et al., 1988; Gunther et al., 2004), especially if it shows unusual clinical manifestations and if it is not present in other family members.

The most important steps for its diagnosis can be the same as for the diagnosis of Cushing's syndrome. Therefore initial phases must include confirming hypercortisolism, determining whether the hypercortisolism is ACTH-dependent or ACTH-independent, and whether there is paradoxical response to Dexamethasone suppression test. Then it will be necessary to identify the cause of that hypercortisolism. When investigating family members of patients affected by PPNAD or other forms of micronodular disease, the dexamethasone suppression tests should be used to identify subclinical adrenal disease, since for these patients, even subtle changes of cortisol secretion should be considered abnormal (plasma cortisol >1.8 μg/dL [50 nmol/L] following Liddle's test). ACTH suppression is also significant in this context. After that, the computerized tomography of the adrenals will help to distinguish unilateral from bilateral nodular disease or hyperplasia and so it must be performed next (Rockal et al., 2004). It must be stressed however that the adrenals are not very enlarged and so the interpretation of the images can be difficult (Bertherat et al., 2009). Treatment of PPNAD is often bilateral adrenalectomy, sometimes in two surgical timings years-apart, related to the fact that the development of this bilateral disease is frequently asymmetrical.

13. References

Abiven, G., Coste, J., Groussin, L., Anract, P., Tissier, F., Legmann, P., Dousset, B., Bertagna, X. & Bertherat, J. (2006). Clinical and biological features in the prognosis of adrenocortical cancer: poor outcome of cortisol-secreting tumors in a series of 202 consecutive patients. *J Clin Endocrinol Metab*, Vol. 91, pp. (2650-5), ISSN.

Abraham, J., Bakke, S., Rutt, A., Meadows, B., Merino, M., Alexander, R., Schrump, D., Bartlett, D., Choyke, P., Robey, R., Hung, E., Steinberg, SM., Bates, S. & Fojo, T. (2002). A phase II trial of combination chemotherapy and surgical resection for the treatment of metastatic adrenocortical carcinoma: continuous infusion doxorubicin, vincristine, and etoposide with daily mitotane as a P-glycoprotein antagonist. *Cancer*, Vol. 94, pp. (2333-43), ISSN.

Adam, R., Chiche, L., Aloia, T., Elias, D., Salmon, R., Rivoire, M., Jaeck, D., Saric, J., Le Treut, YP., Belghiti, J., Mantion, G. & Mentha, G., Association Française de Chirurgie. (2006). Hepatic resection for noncolorectal nonendocrine liver metastases: analysis of 1,452 patients and development of a prognostic model. *Ann Surg*, Vol. 244, No. 4, pp. (524-35), ISSN.

Advani, A., Johnson, SJ., Nicol, MR., Papacleovoulou, G., Evans, DB., Vaikkakara, S., Mason, JI. & Quinton, R. (2010). Adult-onset hypogonadotropic hypogonadism caused by aberrant expression of aromatase in an adrenocortical adenocarcinoma. *Endocr J*, Vol. 57, No. 7, pp. (651-6), ISSN.

Agrons, GA., Lonergan, GJ., Dickey, GE. & Perez-Monte, JE. (1999). Adrenocortical neoplasms in children: radiologic-pathologic correlation. *Radiographics*, Vol. 19, No. 4, pp. (989-1008), ISSN.

Allolio, B. & Fassnacht, M. (2006). Clinical review: Adrenocortical carcinoma: clinical update. *J Clin Endocrinol Metab*, Vol. 91, pp. (2027-37), ISSN.

Allolio, B., Hahner, S., Weismann, D. & Fassnacht, M. (2004). Management of adrenocortical carcinoma. *Clin Endocrinol (Oxf)*, Vol. 60, pp. (273-87), ISSN.

Angeli, A., Osella, G., Alì, A. & Terzolo, M. (1997). Adrenal incidentaloma: an overview of clinical and epidemiological data from the National Italian Study Group. *Horm Res*, Vol. 47, pp. (279-83), ISSN.

Angeli, A. & Terzolo, M. (2002). Adrenal incidentaloma – a modern disease with old complications. *J Clin Endocrinol Metab*, Vol. 87, pp. (4869-71), ISSN.

Aubert, S., Buob, D., Leroy, X., Devos, P., Carnaille, B., Do Cao, C., Wemeau, JL. & Leteurtre, E. (2005). Weiss system: a still in-use diagnostic tool for the assessment of adrenocortical malignancy. *Ann* Pathol, Vol. 25, No. 6, pp. (545-54), ISSN.

Azziz, R., Sanchez, LA., Knochenhauer, ES., Moran, C., Lazenby, J., Stephens, KC., Taylor, K. & Boots, LR. (2004). Androgen excess in women: experience with over 1000 consecutive patients. *J Clin Endocrinol Metab*, Vol. 89, pp. (453–62), ISSN.

Barzon, L., Chilosi, M., Fallo, F., Martignoni, G., Montagna, L., Palù, G. & Boscaro, M. (2001). Molecular analysis of CDKN1C and TP53 in sporadic adrenal tumors. *Eur J Endocrinol* , Vol. 145, pp. (207–12), ISSN.

Barzon, L., Sonino, N., Fallo, F., Palu, G. & Boscarom M. (2003). Prevalence and natural history of adrenal incidentalomas. *Eur J Endocrinol*, Vol. 149, pp. (273–85), ISSN.

Baudin, E., Pellegriti, G., Bonnay, M., Penfornis, A., Laplanche, A., Vassal, G. & Schlumberger, M. (2001). Impact of monitoring plasma 1,1-dichlorodiphenildichloroethane (o,p'DDD) levels on the treatment of patients with adrenocortical carcinoma. *Cancer*, Vol. 92, pp. (1385-92), ISSN.

Bernard, MH., Sidhu, S., Berger, N., Peix, JL., Marsh, DJ., Robinson, BG., Gaston, V., Le Bouc, Y. & Gicquel, C. (2003). A case report in favor of a multistep adrenocortical tumorigenesis. *J Clin Endocrinol Metab*, Vol. 88, pp. (998–1001), ISSN.

Bernini, GP., Moretti, A., Oriandini, C., Bardini, M., Taurino, C. & Salvetti. A. (2005). Long-term morphological and hormonal follow-up in a single unit on 115 patients with adrenal incidentalomas. *Br J Cancer*, Vol. 92, pp. (1104 - 9), ISSN.

Berruti, A., Terzolo, M., Sperone, P., Pia, A., Casa, SD., Gross, DJ., Carnaghi, C., Casali, P., Porpiglia, F., Mantero, F., Reimondo, G., Angeli, A. & Dogliotti, L. (2005). Etoposide, doxorubicin and cisplatin plus mitotane in the treatment of advanced adrenocortical carcinoma: a large prospective phase II trial. *Endocr Relat Cancer*, Vol. 12, pp. (657-66), ISSN.

Bertherat, J., Horvath, A., Groussin, L., Grabar, S., Boikos, S., Cazabat, L., Libe, R., René-Corail, F., Stergiopoulos, S., Bourdeau, I., Bei, T., Clauser, E., Calender, A., Kirschner, LS., Bertagna, X., Carney, JA. & Stratakis, CA. (2009). Mutations in regulatory subunit type 1A of cyclic adenosine 5'-monophosphate-dependent protein kinase (PRKAR1A): phenotype analysis in 353 patients and 80 different genotypes. *J Clin Endocrinol Metab*, Vol. 94, No. 6, pp. (2085-91), ISSN.

Beuschlein, F., Reincke, M., Karl, M., Travis, WD., Jaursch-Hancke, C., Abdelhamid, S., Chrousos, GP. & Allolio, B. (1944). Clonal composition of human adrenocortical neoplasms. *Cancer Research*, Vol. 54, pp. (4927–32), ISSN.

Birch, JM. (1994). Li-Fraumeni syndrome. *Eur J Cancer*, Vol. 30A, pp. (1935-41), ISSN.

Blumenfeld, JD., Sealey, JE., Schlussel, Y., Vaughan, ED., Sos, TA., Atlas, SA., Muller, FB., Acevedo, R., Ulick, S. & Laragh, JH. (1994). Diagnosis and treatment of primary hyperaldosteronism. *Ann Intern Med*, Vol. 121, pp. (877-85), ISSN.

Boland, GW., Lee, MJ., Gazelle, GS., Halpern, EF., McNicholas, MM. & Mueller, PR. (1998). Characterization of adrenal masses using unenhanced CT: an analysis of the CT literature. *AJR Am J Roentgenol*, Vol.171, pp. (201–4), ISSN.

Bonacci, R., Gigliotti, A., Baudin, E., Wion-Barbot, N., Emy, P., Bonnay, M., Cailleux, AF., Nakib, I. & Schlumberger, M. Réseau Comète. (1998). Cytotoxic therapy with etoposide and cisplatin in advanced adrenocortical carcinoma. *Br J Cancer*, Vol. 78, pp. (546-9), ISSN.

Bonfig, W., Bittmann, I., Bechtold, S., Kammer, B., Noelle, V., Arleth, S., Raile, K. & Schwarz, HP. (2003). Virilising adrenocortical tumours in children. *Eur J Pediatr*, Vol. 162, No. 9, pp. (623-8), ISSN.

Boulle, N., Logié, A., Gicquel, C., Perin, L. & Le Bouc, Y. (1998). Increased levels of insulin-like growth factor II (IGF-II) and IGF-binding protein-2 are associated with malignancy in sporadic adrenocortical tumors. *J Clin Endocrinol Metab*, Vol. 83, No. 5, pp. (1713-20), ISSN.

Bourdeau, I., D'Amour, P., Hamet, P., Boutin, JM. & Lacroix, A. (2001). Aberrant membrane hormone receptors in incidentally discovered bilateral macronodular adrenal hyperplasia with subclinical Cushing's syndrome. *J Clin Endocrinol Metab*, Vol. 86, pp. (5534-40), ISSN.

Bovio, S., Cataldi, A., Reimondo, G., Sperone, P., Novello, S., Berruti, A., Borasio, P., Fava, C., Dogliotti, L., Scagliotti, GV., Angeli, A. & Terzolo, M. (2006). Prevalence of adrenal incidentaloma in a contemporary computerized tomography series. *J Endocrinol Invest*, Vol. 29, pp. (298–302), ISSN.

Brembeck, FH., Rosário, M. & Birchmeier, W. (2006). Balancing cell adhesion and Wnt signaling, the key role of beta-catenin. *Curr Opin Genet Dev*, Vol. 16, No. 1, pp. (51-9), ISSN.

Bukowski, RM., Wolfe, M., Levine, HS., Crawford, DE., Stephens, RL., Gaynor, E. & Harker, WG. (1993). Phase II trial of mitotane and cisplatin in patients with adrenal carcinoma: a Southwest Oncology Group study. *J Clin Oncol*, Vol. 11, No. 1, pp. (161-5), ISSN.

Burgess, JR., Harle, RA., Tucker, P., Parameswaran, V., Davies, P., Greenaway, TM. & Shepherd, JJ. (1996). Adrenal lesions in a large kindred with multiple endocrine neoplasia type 1. *Arch Surg*, Vol. 131, No. 7, pp. (699-702), ISSN.

Caoili, EM., Korobkin, M., Brown, RK., Mackie, G. & Shulkin, BL. (2007). Differentiating adrenal adenomas from nonadenomas using (18)F-FDG PET/CT: quantitative and qualitative evaluation. *Acad Radiol*, Vol. 14, No. 4, pp. (468-75), ISSN.

Caoili, EM., Korobkin, M., Francis, IR., Cohan, RH., Platt, JF., Dunnick, NR. & Raghupathi, KI. (2002). Adrenal masses: characterization with combined unenhanced and delayed enhanced CT. *Radiology*, Vol. 222, No. 3, pp. (629–33), ISSN.

Carmina, E., Rosato, F., Janni, A., Rizzo, M. & Longo, RA. (2006). Extensive clinical experience: relative prevalence of different androgen excess disorders in 950 women referred because of clinical hyperandrogenism. *J Clin Endocrinol Metab*, Vol. 9, pp. (12–6), ISSN.

Carney, JA., Gordon, H., Carpenter, PC., Shenoy, BV. & Go, VL.. (1985). The complex of myxomas, spotty pigmentation, and endocrine overactivity. *Medicine (Baltimore)*, Vol. 64, No. 4, pp. (270-83), ISSN.

Carney, JA. & Young, WF Jr. (1992). Primary pigmented nodular adrenocortical disease and its associated conditions. *Endocrinologist*, Vol. 2, pp. (6), ISSN.

Carson, DJ., Sloan, JM., Cleland, J., Russell, CF., Atkinson, AB. & Sheridan, B. (1988). Cyclical Cushing's syndrome presenting as short stature in a boy with recurrent atrial myxomas and freckled skin pigmentation. *Clin Endocrinol (Oxf)*, Vol. 28, No. 2, pp. (173-80), ISSN.

Cawood, TJ., Hunt, PJ., O'Shea, D., Cole, D. & Soule, S. (2009). Recommended evaluation of adrenal incidentalomas is costly, has high false-positive rates and confers a risk of fatal cancer that is similar to the risk of the adrenal lesion becoming malignant; time for a rethink? *Eur J Endocrinol*, Vol. 161, No. 4, pp. (513-27), ISSN.

Choi, M., Scholl, UI., Yue, P., Björklund, P., Zhao, B., Nelson-Williams, C., Ji, W., Cho, Y., Patel, A., Men, CJ., Lolis, E., Wisgerhof, MV., Geller, DS., Mane, S., Hellman, P., Westin, G., Åkerström, G., Wang, W., Carling, T. & Lifton, RP. (2011). K+ channel mutations in adrenal aldosterone-producing adenomas and hereditary hypertension. *Science*, Vol. 331, No. 6018, pp. (768-72), ISSN.

Christopoulos, S., Bourdeau, I. & Lacroix, A. (2005). Clinical and subclinical ACTH-independent macronodular adrenal hyperplasia and aberrant hormone receptors. *Horm Res*, Vol. 64, pp. (119–31), ISSN.

Cobb, WS., Kercher, KW., Sing, RF. & Heniford, BT. (2005). Laparoscopic adrenalectomy for malignancy. *Am J Surg*, Vol. 189, pp. (405–11), ISSN.

Conn JW. (1964). Plasma renin activity in primary aldosteronism. Importance in differential diagnosis and in research of essential hypertension. *J Am Med Ass*, Vol. 190, pp. (222–5), ISSN.

Conn, JW. (1955). Presidential address. Part I. Painting the background. Part II. Primary aldosteronism, a new clinical syndrome. *J Lab Clin Med*, Vol. 45, pp. (3–17), ISSN.

Dackiw, AP., Lee, JE., Gagel, RF. & Evans, DB. (2001). Adrenal cortical carcinoma. *World J Surg*, Vol. 25, pp. (914–26), ISSN.

Daffara, F., De Francia, S., Reimondo, G., Zaggia, B., Aroasio, E., Porpiglia, F., Volante, M., Termine, A., Di Carlo, F., Dogliotti, L., Angeli, A., Berruti, A. & Terzolo, M. (2008). Prospective evaluation of mitotane toxicity in adrenocortical cancer patients treated adjuvantly. *Endocr Relat Cancer*, Vol. 15, No. 4, pp. (1043-53), ISSN.

D'Andrea, MR., Qiu, Y., Haynes-Johnson, D., Bhattacharjee, S., Kraft, P. & Lundeen, S. (2005). Expression of PDE11A in normal and malignant human tissues. *J Histochem Cytochem*, Vol. 53, No. 7, pp. (895-903), ISSN.

DeChiara, TM., Robertson, EJ. & Efstratiadis A. (1991). Parental imprinting of the mouse insulin-like growth factor II gene. *Cell*, Vol. 64, pp. (849–59), ISSN.

Decker, RA., Elson, P., Hogan, TF., Citrin, DL., Westring, DW., Banerjee, TK., Gilchrist, KW. & Horton, J. (1991). Eastern Cooperative Oncology Group study 1879: mitotane and adriamycin in patients with advanced adrenocortical carcinoma. *Surgery*, Vol. 110, No. 6, pp. (1006-13), ISSN.

DeLellis, RA., Lloyd, RV., Heitz, PU. & Eng, C. (2004). *Pathology and Genetics of Tumours of Endocrine Organs*, World Health Organization, ISBN, Lyon, France.

Derksen, J., Nagesser, SK., Meinders, AE., Haak, HR. & van de Velde, CJ. (1994). Identification of virilizing adrenal tumors in hirsute women. *N Engl J Med*, Vol. 331, pp. (968–73), ISSN.

Doppman, JL., Chrousos, GP., Papanicolaou, DA., Stratakis, CA., Alexander, HR. & Nieman, LK. (2000). Adrenocorticotropin-independent macronodular adrenal hyperplasia: an uncommon cause of primary adrenal hypercortisolism. *Radiology*, Vol. 216, No. 3, pp. (797-802), ISSN.

Doppman, JL., Nieman, LK., Travis, WD., Miller, DL., Cutler, GB Jr., Chrousos, GP. & Norton, JA. (1991). CT and MR imaging of massive macronodular adrenocortical disease: a rare cause of autonomous primary adrenal hypercortisolism. *J Comput Assist Tomogr*, Vol. 15, No. 5, pp. (773–9), ISSN.

Dunnick, NR., Korobkin, M. & Francis, I. (1996). Adrenal radiology: distinguishing benign from malignant adrenal masses. *AJR Am J Roentgenol*, Vol. 167, pp. (861-7), ISSN.

Edge, SB., Byrd, DR., Compton, CC., Fritz, AG., Greene, FL., Trotti, A. (Eds.). (2010). AJCC Cancer Staging Manual, 7th Ed. Springer, Chicago.

Fassnacht, M. & Allolio, B. (2009). Clinical management of adrenocortical carcinoma. *Best Pract Res Clin Endocrinol Metab*, Vol. 23, No. 2, pp. (273-89); ISSN.

Fassnacht, M., Johanssen, S., Quinkler, M., Bucsky, P., Willenberg, HS., Beuschlein, F., Terzolo, M., Mueller, HH., Hahner, S. & Allolio, B., German Adrenocortical Carcinoma Registry Group, European Network for the Study of Adrenal Tumors. (2009). Limited prognostic value of the 2004 International Union Against Cancer staging classification for adrenocortical carcinoma: proposal for a Revised TNM Classification. *Cancer*, Vol. 115, No. 2, pp. (243-50), ISSN.

Fassnacht, M., Libé R, Kroiss M, Allolio B. (2011). Adrenocortical carcinoma: a clinician's update. Nat Rev Endocrinol. Vol. 7, No 6, pp. (323-35).

Feige, JJ., Cochet, C., Savona, C., Shi, DL., Keramidas, M., Defaye, G. & Chambaz, EM. (1991). Transforming growth factor beta 1: an autocrine regulator of adrenocortical steroid genesis. *Endocr Res*, Vol. 17, pp. (267–79), ISSN.

Fottner, C., Hoeflich, A., Wolf, E. & Weber, MM. (2004). Role of the insulin-like growth factor system in adrenocortical growth control and carcinogenesis. *Horm Metab Res*, Vol. 36, pp. (397–405), ISSN.

Fragoso, MC., Domenice, S., Latronico, AC., Martin, RM., Pereira, MA., Zerbini, MC., Lucon, AM. & Mendonca, BB. (2003). Cushing's syndrome secondary to adrenocorticotropin-independent macronodular adrenocortical hyperplasia due to activating mutations of GNAS1 gene. *J Clin Endocrinol Metab*, Vol. 88, No. 5, pp. (2147), ISSN.

Fraumeni, JF Jr. & Miller, RW. (1967). Adrenocortical neoplasms with hemihypertrophy, brain tumors, and other disorders. *J Pediatr*, Vol. 70, pp. (129-38) ISSN.

Fuhrman, SA., Lasky, LC. & Limas, C. (1982). Prognostic significance of morphologic parameters in renal cell carcinoma. *Am J Surg Patho*, Vol. 6, No. 7, pp. (655-63), ISSN.

Gaujoux, S., Tissier, F., Groussin, L., Libé, R., Ragazzon, B., Launay, P., Audebourg, A., Dousset, B., Bertagna, X. & Bertherat, J. (2008). Wnt/beta-catenin and 3',5'-cyclic adenosine 5'-monophosphate/protein kinase A signaling pathways alterations and somatic beta-catenin gene mutations in the progression of adrenocortical tumors. *J Clin Endocrinol Metab*, Vol. 93, No. 10, pp. (4135-40), ISSN.

Gicquel, C., Bertagna, X., Gaston, V., Coste, J., Louvel, A., Baudin, E., Bertherat, J., Chapuis, Y., Duclos, JM., Schlumberger, M., Plouin, PF., Luton, JP. & Le Bouc, Y. (2001). Molecular markers and long-term recurrences in a large cohort of patients with sporadic adrenocortical tumors. *Cancer Res*, Vol. 61, No. 18, pp. (6762–7), ISSN.

Gicquel, C., Bertagna, X., Schneid, H., Francillard-Leblond, M., Luton, JP., Girard, F. & Le Bouc, Y. (1994). Rearrangements at the 11p15 locus and overexpression of insulin-like growth factor-II gene in sporadic adrenocortical tumors. *J Clin Endocrinol Metab*, Vol. 78, No. 6, pp. (1444–53), ISSN.

Gicquel, C., Raffin-Sanson, ML., Gaston, V., Bertagna, X., Plouin, PF., Schlumberger, M., Louvel, A., Luton, JP. & Le Bouc, Y. (1997). Structural and functional abnormalities at 11p15 are associated with the malignant phenotype in sporadic adrenocortical tumors: Study on a series of 82 tumors. *J Clin Endocrinol Metab*, Vol. 82, No. 8, pp. (2559–65), ISSN.

Giordano, TJ., Kuick, R., Else, T., Gauger, PG., Vinco, M., Bauersfeld, J., Sanders, D., Thomas, DG., Doherty, G. & Hammer, G. (2009). Molecular classification and prognostication of adrenocortical tumors by transcriptome profiling. *Clin Cancer Res*, Vol. 15, No. 2, pp. (668-76), ISSN.

Gittler, RD. & Fajans, SS. (1995). Primary aldosteronism (Conn's syndrome). *J Clin Endocrinol Metab*, Vol. 80, pp. (3438–41), ISSN.

Gold, PW., Loriaux, DL., Roy, A., Kling, MA., Calabrese, JR., Kellner, CH., Nieman, LK., Post, RM., Pickar, D. & Gallucci, W. (1986). Responses to corticotropin-releasing hormone in the hypercortisolism of depression and Cushing's disease. Pathophysiologic and diagnostic implications. *N Engl J Med*, Vol. 314, No. 21, pp. (1329-35), ISSN.

Gonzalez, RJ., Shapiro, S., Sarlis, N., Vassilopoulou-Sellin, R., Perrier, ND., Evans, DB. & Lee, JE. (2005). Laparoscopic resection of adrenal cortical carcinoma: a cautionary note. *Surgery*, Vol. 138, No. 6, pp. (1078–85), ISSN.

Gordon, MD. & Nusse, R (2006). Wnt signaling: Multiple pathways, multiple receptors, and multiple transcription factors. *J Biol Chem*, Vol. 281, pp. (22429–33), ISSN.

Groussin, L., Jullian, E., Perlemoine, K., Louvel, A., Leheup, B., Luton, JP., Bertagna, X. & Bertherat, J. (2002a). Mutations of the PRKAR1A gene in Cushing's syndrome due to sporadic primary pigmented nodular adrenocortical disease. *J Clin Endocrinol Metab*, Vol. 87, No. 9, pp. (4324-9), ISSN.

Groussin, L., Kirschner, LS., Vincent-Dejean, C., Perlemoine, K., Jullian, E., Delemer, B., Zacharieva, S., Pignatelli, D., Carney, JA., Luton, JP., Bertagna, X., Stratakis, CA. & Bertherat, J. (2002b). Molecular analysis of the cyclic AMP-dependent protein kinaseA (PKA) regulatory subunit1A (PRKAR1A) gene in patients with Carney complex and primary pigmented nodular adrenocortical disease (PPNAD) reveals novel mutations and clues for pathophysiology: augmented PKA signaling is associated with adrenal tumorigenesis in PPNAD. *Am J Hum Genet*, Vol. 71, No. 6, pp. (1433-42), ISSN.

Groussin, L., Perlemoine, K., Contesse, V., Lefebvre, H., Tabarin, A., Thieblot, P., Schlienger, JL., Luton, JP., Bertagna, X. & Bertherat, J. (2002c). The ectopic expression of the gastric inhibitory polypeptide receptor is frequent in adrenocorticotropin-independent bilateral macronodular adrenal hyperplasia, but rare in unilateral tumors. *J Clin Endocrinol Metab*, Vol. 87, No. 5, pp. (1980-5), ISSN.

Groussin, L., Bonardel, G., Silvéra, S., Tissier, F., Coste, J., Abiven, G., Libé, R., Bienvenu, M., Alberini, JL., Salenave, S., Bouchard, P., Bertherat, J., Dousset, B., Legmann, P., Richard, B., Foehrenbach, H., Bertagna, X. & Tenenbaum, F. (2009). 18F-Fluorodeoxyglucose positron emission tomography for the diagnosis of adrenocortical tumors: a prospective study in 77 operated patients. *J Clin Endocrinol Metab*, Vol. 94, No. 5, pp. (1713-22), ISSN.

Grumbach, MM., Biller, BM., Braunstein, GD., Campbell, KK., Carney, JA., Godley, PA., Harris, EL., Lee, JK., Oertel, YC., Posner, MC., Schlechte, JA. & Wieand, HS. (2003). Management of the clinically inapparent adrenal mass ("incidentaloma"). *Ann Intern Med*, Vol. 138, No. 5, pp. (424–9), ISSN.

Gunther, DF., Bourdeau, I., Matyakhina, L., Cassarino, D., Kleiner, DE., Griffin, K., Courkoutsakis, N., Abu-Asab, M., Tsokos, M., Keil, M., Carney, JA. & Stratakis, CA. (2004). Cyclical Cushing syndrome presenting in infancy: an early form of primary pigmented nodular adrenocortical disease, or a new entity? *J Clin Endocrinol Metab*, Vol. 89, no. 7, pp. (3173-82), ISSN.

Haak HR, Hermans J, van de Velde CJ, Lentjes EG, Goslings BM, Fleuren GJ, Krans HM. Optimal treatment of adrenocortical carcinoma with mitotane: results in a consecutive series of 96 patients. Br J Cancer. 1994 May;69(5):947-51

Hahner, S. & Fassnacht, M. (2005). Mitotane for adrenocortical carcinoma treatment. *Curr Opin Investig Drugs*, Vol. 6, pp. (386–94), ISSN.

Hamrahian, AH., Ioachimescu, AG., Remer, EM., Motta-Ramirez, G., Bogabathina, H., Levin, HS., Reddy, S., Gill, IS., Siperstein, A. & Bravo, EL. (2005). Clinical utility of noncontrast computed tomography attenuation value (hounsfield units) to differentiate adrenal adenomas/hyperplasias from nonadenomas: Cleveland Clinic experience. *J Clin Endocrinol Metab*, Vol. 90, No. 2, pp. (871-7), ISSN.

Harrison, LE., Gaudin, PB. & Brennan, MF. (1999). Pathologic features of prognostic significance for adrenocortical carcinoma after curative resection. *Arch Surg*, Vol. 134, pp. (181-5), ISSN.

Hedeland, H., Ostberg, G. & Hökfelt, B. (1968). On the prevalence of adrenocortical adenomas in an autopsy material in relation to hypertension and diabetes. *Acta Med Scand*, Vol. 184, pp. (211-4), ISSN.

Henley, DJ., van Heerden, JA., Grant, CS., Carney, JA. & Carpenter, PC. (1983). Adrenal cortical carcinoma--a continuing challenge. *Surgery*, Vol. 94, No. 6, pp. (926-31), ISSN.

Heppner, C., Reincke, M., Agarwal, SK., Mora, P., Allolio, B., Burns, AL., Spiegel, AM. & Marx, SJ. (1999). MEN1 gene analysis in sporadic adrenocortical neoplasms. *J Clin Endocrinol Metab*, Vol. 84, No. 1, pp. (216-9), ISSN.

Herrera, MF., Grant, CS., van Heerden, JA., Sheedy, PF. & Ilstrup, DM. (1991). Incidentally discovered adrenal tumors: an institutional perspective. *Surgery*, Vol. 110, No. 6, pp. (1014-21), ISSN.

Hisada, M., Garber, JE., Fung, CY., Fraumeni, Jr JF. & Li, FP. (1998). Multiple primary cancers in families with Li-Fraumeni syndrome. *J Natl Cancer Inst*, Vol. 90, pp. (606-11), ISSN.

Holland, OB. & Carr, B. (1993). Modulation of aldosterone synthase messenger ribonucleic acid levels by dietary sodium and potassium and by adrenocorticotropin. *Endocrinology*, Vol. 132, pp. (2666-73), ISSN.

Hollstein, M., Sidransky, D., Vogelstein, B. & Harris, CC. (1991). p53 mutations in human cancers. *Science*, Vol. 253, No. 5015, pp. (49–53), ISSN.

Horiba, N., Suda, T., Aiba, M., Naruse, M., Nomura, K., Imamura, M. & Demura, H. (1995). Lysine vasopressin stimulation of cortisol secretion in patients with adrenocorticotropinindependent macronodular adrenal hyperplasia. *J Clin Endocrinol Metab*, Vol. 80, No. 8, pp. (2336–41), ISSN.

Horvath, A., Mericq, V. & Stratakis, CA. (2008). Mutation in PDE8B, a cyclic AMP-specific phosphodiesterase in adrenal hyperplasia. *N Engl J Med*, Vol. 358, pp. (750-2), ISSN.

Hughes, JM., Hichens, M., Booze, GW. & Thorner, MO. (1986). Cushing's syndrome from the therapeutic use of intramuscular dexamethasone acetate. *Arch Intern Med,* Vol. 146, pp. (1848-9), ISSN.

Ilvesmaki, V., Kahri, AI., Miettinen, PJ. & Voutilainen, R. (1993). Insulin-like growth factors (IGFs) and their receptors in adrenal tumors: high IGF-II expression in functional adrenocortical carcinomas. *J Clin Endocrinol Metab,* Vol. 77, No. 3, pp. (852–8), ISSN.

Invitti, C., Pecori Giraldi, F., de Martin, M. & Cavagnini, F. (1999). Diagnosis and management of Cushing's syndrome: results of an Italian multicentre study. Study Group of the Italian Society of Endocrinology on the Pathophysiology of the Hypothalamic-Pituitary-Adrenal Axis. *J Clin Endocrinol Metab,* Vol. 84, pp. (440-8), ISSN.

Jhala, NC., Jhala, D., Eloubeidi, MA., Chhieng, DC., Crowe, DR., Roberson, J. & Eltoum, I. (2004). Endoscopic ultrasound-guided fine-needle aspiration biopsy of the adrenal glands: analysis of 24 patients. *Cancer,* Vol. 102, No. 5, pp. (308-14), ISSN.

Kaltsas, GA., Isidori, AM., Kola, BP., Skelly, RH., Chew, SL., Jenkins, PJ., Monson, JP., Grossman, AB. & Besser, GM. (2003). The value of the low-dose dexamethasone suppression test in the differential diagnosis of hyperandrogenism in women. *J Clin Endocrinol Metab,* Vol. 88, No. 6, pp. (2634–43), ISSN.

Kamenicky, P., Houdoin, L., Ferlicot, S., Salenave, S., Brailly, S., Droupy, S., Meduri, G., Sasano, H., Suzuki, T., Young, J. & Chanson, P. (2007). Benign cortisol-secreting adrenocortical adenomas produce small amounts of androgens. *Clin Endocrinol (Oxf),* Vol. 66, No. 6, pp. (778-88), ISSN.

Kartheuser, A., Walon, C., West, S., Breukel, C., Detry, R., Gribomont, AC., Hamzehloei, T., Hoang, P., Maiter, D., Pringot, J., Rahier, J., Khan, PM., Curtis, A., Burn, J., Fodde, R. & Verellen-Dumoulin, C. (1999). Familial adenomatous polyposis associated with multiple adrenal adenomas in a patient with a rare 3' APC mutation. *J Med Genet,* Vol. 36, No. 1, pp. (65-7), ISSN.

Kebebew, E., Reiff, E., Duh, QY., Clark, OH. & McMillan, A. (2006) Extent of disease at presentation and outcome, for adrenocortical carcinoma: have we made progress? *World J Surgery,* Vol. 30, No. 5, pp. (872-8), ISSN.

Kendrick, ML., Lloyd, R., Erickson, L., Farley, DR., Grant, CS., Thompson, GB., Rowland, C., Young, WF Jr. & van Heerden, JA. (2001). Adrenocortical carcinoma: surgical progress or status quo? *Arch Surg,* Vol. 136, No. 5, pp. (543-9), ISSN.

Kettel, LM. (1989). Management of hirsutism. *Drug Ther Bull,* Vol. 27, pp. (49–51), ISSN.

Khan, TS., Imam, H., Juhlin, C., Skogseid, B., Gröndal, S., Tibblin, S., Wilander, E., Oberg, K. & Eriksson, B. (2000). Streptozocin and o,p'DDD in the treatment of adrenocortical cancer patients: long-term survival in its adjuvant use. *Ann Oncol,* Vol. 11, No. 10, pp. (1281-7), ISSN.

Khan, TS., Sundin, A., Juhlin, C., Wilander, E., Oberg, K. & Eriksson, B. (2004). Vincristine, cisplatin, teniposide, and cyclophosphamide combination in the treatment of recurrent or metastatic adrenocortical cancer. *Med Oncol,* Vol. 21, No. 2, pp. (167-77), ISSN.

Kirkman, S. & Nelson, DH. (1988). Alcohol-induced pseudo-Cushing's disease: a study of prevalence with review of the literature. *Metabolism,* Vol. 37, pp. (390-4), ISSN.

Kirschner, LS., Carney, JA., Pack, SD., Taymans, SE., Giatzakis, C., Cho, YS., Cho-Chung, YS. & Stratakis, CA. (2000). Mutations of the gene encoding the protein kinaseA type Ia regulatory subunit in patients with the Carney complex. *Nat Genet*, Vol. 26, No. 1, pp. (89-92), ISSN.

Kirschner MA, Powell RD Jr, Lipsett MB (1964). Cushing's syndrome: nodular cortical hyperplasia of adrenal glands with clinical and pathological features suggesting adrenocortical tumor. J Clin Endocrinol Metab. Vol.24, pp (947-55).

Kjellman, M., Roshani, L., Teh, BT., Kallioniemi, OP., Höög, A., Gray, S., Farnebo, LO., Holst, M., Bäckdahl, M. & Larsson, C. (1999). Genotyping of adrenocortical tumors: very frequent deletions of the MEN1 locus in 11q13 and of a 1-centimorgan region in 2p16. *J Clin Endocrinol Metab*, Vol. 84. No. 2, pp. (730-5), ISSN.

Kloos, RT., Gross, MD., Francis, IR., Korobkin, M. & Shapiro, B. (1995). Incidentally discovered adrenal masses. *Endocr Rev*, Vol. 16, pp. (460-484), ISSN.

Koch, CA., Pacak, K. & Chrousos, GP. (2002). The molecular pathogenesis of hereditary and sporadic adrenocortical and adrenomedullary tumors. *J Clin Endocrinol Metab*, Vol. 87, pp. (5367-84), ISSN.

Kocijancic, K., Kocijancic, I. & Guna, F. (2004). Role of sonographically guided fine-needle aspiration biopsy of adrenal masses in patients with lung cancer. *J Clin Ultrasound*, Vol. 32, pp. (12-6), ISSN.

Kopf, D., Goretzki, PE. & Lehnert, H. (2001). Clinical management of malignant adrenal tumors. *J Cancer Res Clin Oncol*, Vol. 127, pp. (143-55), ISSN.

Korobkin, M., Francis, IR., Kloos, RT. & Dunnick, NR. (1996). The incidental adrenal mass. *Radiol Clin North Am*, Vol. 34, pp. (1037-54), ISSN.

Kudva, YC., Sawka, AM. & Young, WF. (2003). The laboratory diagnosis of adrenal pheochromocytoma: the Mayo Clinic experience. *J Clin Endocrinol Metab*, Vol. 88, pp. (4533-9), ISSN.

Lack, LEE. (1997). *Atlas of tumor pathology,* Armed Forces Institute of Pathology, ISBN, Washington, DC.

Lacroix, A., Bolte, E., Tremblay, J., Dupré, J., Poitras, P., Fournier, H., Garon, J., Garrel, D., Bayard, F., Taillefer, R., Flanagan & RJ. & Hamet, P.(1992). Gastric inhibitory polypeptide-dependent cortisol hypersecretion — a new cause of Cushing's syndrome. *N Engl J Med*, Vol. 327, No. 14, pp. (974-80), ISSN.

Lacroix, A., Tremblay, J., Rousseau, G., Bouvier, M. & Hamet, P. (1997). Propranolol therapy for ectopic b-adrenergenic receptors in adrenal Cushing's syndrome. *N Engl J Med*, Vol. 337, pp. (429–34), ISSN.

Lacroix, A., N'diaye, N., Tremblay, J. & Hamet, P. (2001). Ectopic and abnormal hormone receptors in adrenal Cushing's syndrome. *Endocr Rev*, Vol. 22, pp. (75-110), ISSN.

Lacroix, A., Baldacchino, V., Bourdeau, I., Hamet, P. & Tremblay, J. (2004). Cushing's syndrome variants secondary to aberrant hormone receptors. *Trends Endocrinol Metab*, Vol. 15, pp. (375-82), ISSN.

Lacroix A. (2009). ACTH-independent macronodular hyperplasia. *Best Practice and Research Clinical Endocrinology and Metabolism*, Vol. 23, pp. (245-259), ISSN.

Larsen, JL., Cathey, WJ. & Odell, WD. (1986). Primary adrenocortical nodular dysplasia, a distinct subtype of Cushing's syndrome. Case report and review of the literature. *Am J Med*, Vol. 80, pp. (976-84), ISSN.

Latronico, AC., Pinto, EM., Domenice, S., Fragoso, MC., Martin, RM., Zerbini, MC., Lucon, AM. & Mendonca, BB. (2001). An inherited mutation outside the highly conserved DNA-binding domain of the p53 tumor suppressor protein in children and adults with sporadic adrenocortical tumors. *J Clin Endocrinol Metab*, Vol. 86, No. 10, pp. (4970-3), ISSN.

Lau, SK. & Weiss, LM. (2009). The Weiss system for evaluating adrenocortical neoplasms: 25 years later. *Hum Pathol*, Vol. 40, No. 6, pp. (757-68), ISSN.

Lee, MH., Reynisdottir, I. & Massague, J. (1995). Cloning of p57kip2, a cyclindependent kinase inhibitor with unique domain structure and tissue distribution. *Genes Dev*, Vol. 9, pp. (639–49), ISSN.

Lefevre, M., Gerard-Marchant, R., Gubler, JP., Chaussain, JL. & Lemerle, J. (1983). *Adrenal and endocrine tumors in children*, Nijhoff, ISBN, Boston.

Li, FP. & Fraumeni, JF Jr. (1969a). Soft-tissue sarcomas, breast cancer, and other neoplasms: a familial syndrome? *Ann Intern Med*, Vol. 71, pp. (747-52), ISSN.

Li, FP. & Fraumeni, Jr JF. (1969b). Rhabdomyosarcoma in children: epidemiologic study and identification of a familial cancer syndrome. *J Natl Cancer Inst*, Vol. 43, pp. (1365-73), ISSN.

Li, FP., Fraumeni, Jr JF., Mulvihil, JJ., Blattner, WA., Dreyfus, MG., Tucker, MA. & Miller, RW. (1998). A cancer family syndrome in twenty-four kindreds. *Cancer Res*, Vol. 48, pp. (5358-62), ISSN.

Libé, R. & Bertherat, J. (2005). Molecular genetics of adrenocortical tumours, from familial to sporadic diseases. *Eur J Endocrinol*, Vol. 153, pp. (477-87), ISSN.

Libé, R., Fratticci, A. & Bertherat, J. (2007). Adrenocortical cancer: pathophysiology and Clinical management. *Endocr Relat Cancer*, Vol. 14, pp. (13–28), ISSN.

Libé, R., Fratticci, A., Coste, J., Tissier, F., Horvath, A., Ragazzon, B., Rene-Corail, F., Groussin, L., Bertagna, X., Raffin-Sanson, ML., Stratakis, CA. & Bertherat, J. (2008). Phosphodiesterase 11A (PDE11A) and genetic predisposition to adrenocortical tumors. *Clin Cancer Res*, Vol. 14, No. 12, pp. (4016-24), ISSN.

Liddle, GW. (1960). Tests of pituitary-adrenal suppressibility in the diagnosis of Cushing's syndrome. *J Clin Endocrinol Metab*, Vol. 20, pp. (1539-60), ISSN.

Lieberman, SA., Eccleshall, TR. & Feldman, D. (1994). ACTH-independent massive bilateral adrenal disease (AIMBAD): A subtype of Cushing's syndrome with major diagnostic and therapeutic implications. *Eur J Endocrinol*, Vol. 131, pp. (67–73), ISSN.

Lin, SR., Lee, YJ. & Tsai, JH. (1994). Mutations of the p53 gene in human functional adrenal neoplasms. *J Clin Endocrinol Metab*, Vol. 78, No. 2, pp. (483-91), ISSN.

Lindholm J, Juul S, Jorgensen JO, Astrup J, Bjerre P, Feldt-Rasmussen U, Hagen C, Jorgensen J, Kosteljanetz M, Kristensen L, Laurberg P, Schmidt K, Weeke J. (2001). Incidence and late prognosis of Cushing's syndrome: a population based study. *J Clin Endocrinol Metab* 86: 117-123

Logie, A., Boulle, N., Gaston, V., Perin, L., Boudou, P., Le Bouc, Y. & Gicquel, C. (1999). Autocrine role of IGF-II in proliferation of human adrenocortical carcinoma NCI H295R cell line. *J Mol Endocrinol*, Vol. 23, pp. (23–32), ISSN.

Louiset, E., Gobet, F., Libé, R., Horvath, A., Renouf, S., Cariou, J., Rothenbuhler, A., Bertherat, J., Clauser, E., Grise, P., Stratakis, CA., Kuhn, JM. & Lefebvre, H. (2010). ACTH-independent Cushing's syndrome with bilateral micronodular adrenal hyperplasia and ectopic adrenocortical adenoma. *J Clin Endocrinol Metab*, Vol. 95, No. 1, pp. (18-24), ISSN

Luton, JP., Cerdas, S., Billaud, L., Thomas, G., Guilhaume, B., Bertagna, X., Laudat, MH., Louvel, A., Chapuis, Y., Blondeau, P., Bonnin, A. & Bricaire, H. (1990). Clinical features of adrenocortical carcinoma, prognostic factors, and the effect of mitotane therapy. *N Engl J Med*, Vol. 322, No. 17, pp. (1195-201), ISSN.

Lynch, HT., Mulcahy, GM., Harris, RE., Guirgis, HA. & Lynch, JF. (1978). Genetic and pathologic findings in kindred with hereditary sarcoma, breast cancer, brain tumors, leukemia, lung, laryngeal, and adrenal cortical carcinoma. *Cancer*, Vol. 41, pp. (2055-64), ISSN.

Magee, BJ., Gattamaneni, HR. & Pearson, D. (1987). Adrenal cortical carcinoma: survival after radiotherapy. *Clin Radiol*, Vol. 38, pp. (587-8), ISSN.

Malchoff, CD., Rosa, J., DeBold, CR., Kozol, RA., Ramsby, GR., Page, DL., Malchoff, DM. & Orth, DN. (1989). Adrenocorticotropin-independent bilateral macronodular adrenal hyperplasia: an unusual cause of Cushing syndrome. *J Clin Endocrinol Metab*, Vol. 68, No. 4, pp. (855–60), ISSN.

Mansmann, G., Lau, J., Balk, E., Rothberg, M., Miyachi, Y. & Bornstein, SR. (2004). The clinically inapparent adrenal mass: update in diagnosis and management. *Endocr Rev*, Vol. 25, pp. (309-40), ISSN.

Mantero, F., Terzolo, M., Arnaldi, G., Osella, G., Masini, AM., Alì, A., Giovagnetti, M., Opocher, G. & Angeli, A. (2000). A survey on adrenal incidentaloma in Italy. Study Group on Adrenal Tumors of the Italian Society of Endocrinology. *J Clin Endocrinol Metab*, Vol. 85, No. 2, pp. (637-44), ISSN.

Matsuoka, S., Edwards, MC., Bai, C., Parker, S., Zhang, P., Baldini, A., Harper, JW. & Elledge, SJ. (1995). P57kip2, a structurally distinct member of the p21CIP1 Cdk inhibitor family, is a candidate tumor suppressor gene. *Genes Dev*, Vol. 9, No. 6, pp. (650–62), ISSN.

Mattsson, C. & Young, WF Jr. (2006). Primary aldosteronism: diagnostic and treatment strategies. *Nat Clin Pract Nephrol*, Vol. 2, pp. (198), ISSN.

Matyakhina, L., Freedman, RJ., Bourdeau, I., Wei, MH., Stergiopoulos, SG., Chidakel, A., Walther, M., Abu-Asab, M., Tsokos, M., Keil, M., Toro, J., Linehan, WM. & Stratakis, CA. (2005). Hereditary leiomyomatosis associated with bilateral, massive, macronodular adrenocortical disease and atypical cushing syndrome: a clinical and molecular genetic investigation. *J Clin Endocrinol Metab*, Vol. 90, No. 6, pp. (3773-9), ISSN.

Maurea, S., Klain, M., Mainolfi, C., Ziviello, M. & Salvatore, M. (2001). The diagnostic role of radionuclide imaging in evaluation of patients with nonhypersecreting adrenal masses. *J Nucl Med*, Vol. 42, No. 6, pp. (884-92), ISSN.

Mayo-Smith, WW. & Dupuy, DE. (2004). Adrenal neoplasms: CT-guided radiofrequency ablation--preliminary results. *Radiology*, Vol. 231, pp. (225-30), ISSN.

Mesiano, S., Mellon, SH., Gospodarowicz, D., Di Blasio, AM. & Jaffe, RB. (1991). Basic fibroblast growth factor expression is regulated by corticotropin in the human fetal adrenal: a model for adrenal growth regulation. *PNAS*, Vol. 88, pp. (5428–32), ISSN.

Mesiano, S., Mellon, SH. & Jaffe, RB. (1993). Mitogenic action, regulation, and localization of insulin-like growth factors in the human fetal adrenal gland. *J Clin Endocrinol Metab*, Vol. 76, pp. (968–76), ISSN.

Metser, U., Miller, E., Lerman, H., Lievshitz, G., Avital, S. & Even-Sapir, E. (2006). 18F-FDG PET/CT in the evaluation of adrenal masses. *J Nucl Med*, Vol. 47, No. 1, pp. (32-7), ISSN.

Meyer, A., Niemann, U. & Behrend, M. (2004). Experience with the surgical treatment of adrenal cortical carcinoma. *Eur J Surg Oncol*, Vol. 30, pp. (444-9), ISSN.

Michalkiewicz, E., Sandrini, R., Figueiredo, B., Miranda, EC., Caran, E., Oliveira-Filho, AG., Marques, R., Pianovski, MA., Lacerda, L., Cristofani, LM., Jenkins, J., Rodriguez-Galindo, C. & Ribeiro, RC. (2004). Clinical and outcome characteristics of children with adrenocortical tumors: a report from the International Pediatric Adrenocortical Tumor Registry. *J Clin Oncol*, Vol. 22, No. 5, pp. (838-45), ISSN.

Milliez, P., Girerd, X., Plouin, PF., Blacher, J., Safar, ME. & Mourad, JJ. (2005). Evidence for an increased rate of cardiovascular events in patients with primary aldosteronism. *J Am Coll Cardiol*, Vol. 45, pp. (1243–8), ISSN.

Minn, H., Salonen, A., Friberg, J., Roivainen, A., Viljanen, T., Långsjö, J., Salmi, J., Välimäki, M., Någren, K. & Nuutila, P. (2004). Imaging of adrenal incidentalomas with PET using (11)C-metomidate and (18)F-FDG. *J Nucl Med*, Vol. 45, No. 6, pp. (972-9), ISSN.

Mircescu, H., Jilwan, J., N'Diaye, N., Bourdeau, I., Tremblay, J., Hamet, P. & Lacroix, A. (2000). Are ectopic or abnormal membrane hormone receptors frequently present in adrenal Cushing's syndrome? *J Clin Endocrinol Metab*, Vol. 85, No. 10, pp. (3531-6), ISSN.

Moreno, S., Montoya, G., Armstrong, J., Leteurtre, E., Aubert, S., Vantyghem, MC., Dewailly, D., Wemeau, JL. & Proye, C. (2004). Profile and outcome of pure androgen-secreting adrenal tumors in women: experience of 21 cases. *Surgery*, Vol. 136, No. 6, pp. (1192-8), ISSN.

Motta Ramirez, G., Remer, E., Herts, B., Gill, I. & Hamrahian, A. (2005). Comparison of CT findings in symptomatic and incidentally discovered pheochromocytomas. *Am J Roentgenol*, Vol. 185, pp. (684-688), ISSN.

N'diaye, N., Tremblay, J., Hamet, P., de Herder, WW. & Lacroix, A. (1998). Adrenocortical overexpression of gastric inhibitory polypeptide receptor underlies food-dependent Cushing's syndrome. *J Clin Endocrinol Metab*, Vol. 83, pp. (2781–5), ISSN.

Nadella, KS. & Kirschner, LS. (2005). Disruption of Protein Kinase A regulation causes immortalization and dysregulation of D-type cyclins. *Cancer Res*, Vol. 65, pp. (10307-15), ISSN.

National Institutes of Health. (2002). NIH state-of-the-science statement on management of the clinically inapparent adrenal mass ("incidentaloma"). *NIH Consensus State-of-the-Science Statements*, Vol. 19, pp. (1–25), ISSN.

Ng, L. & Libertino, JM. (2003). Adrenocortical carcinoma: diagnosis, evaluation and treatment. *J Urol*, Vol. 169, pp. (5-11), ISSN.

Nieman, L., Biller, B., Findling, J., Newell-Price, J., Savage, M., Stewart, P. & Montori, VM. (2008). The diagnosis of Cushing's syndrome: an Endocrine Society Clinical Practice guideline. *J Clin Endocrinol Metab*, Vol. 93, No. 5, pp. (1526-40), ISSN

Ohgaki, H., Kleihues, P. & Heitz, PU. (1993). P53 mutations in sporadic adrenocortical tumors. *Intern J Cancer*, Vol. 54, pp. (408–10), ISSN.

Patil, KK., Ransley, PG., McCullagh, M., Malone, M. & Spitz, L. (2002). Functioning adrenocortical neoplasms in children. *BJU Int*, Vol. 89, No. 6, pp. (562-5), ISSN.

Polakis, P. Wnt signaling and cancer. *Genes Dev*, Vol. 14, No. 15, pp. (1837-51), ISSN.

Polat, B., Fassnacht, M., Pfreundner, L., Guckenberger, M., Bratengeier, K., Johanssen, S., Kenn, W., Hahner, S., Allolio, B. & Flentje, M. (2009). Radiotherapy in adrenocortical carcinoma. *Cancer*, Vol. 115, No. 13, pp. (2816-23), ISSN.

Quddusi, S., Browne, P., Toivola, B. & Hirsch, IB. Cushing syndrome due to surreptitious glucocorticoid administration. *Arch Intern Med*, Vol. 158, pp. (294-6), ISSN.

Quinkler, M., Hahner, S., Wortmann, S., Johanssen, S., Adam, P., Ritter, C., Strasburger, C., Allolio, B. & Fassnacht, M. (2008). Treatment of advanced adrenocortical carcinoma with erlotinib plus gemcitabine. *J Clin Endocrinol Metab*, Vol. 93, No. 6, pp. (2057-62), ISSN.

Reincke, M., Karl, M., Travis, WH., Mastorakos, G., Allolio, B., Linehan, HM. & Chrousos, GP. (1994). P53 mutations in human adrenocortical neoplasms: Immunohistochemical and molecular studies. *J Clin Endocrinol Metab*, Vol. 78, No. 3, pp. (790 –4), ISSN.

Resnik, Y., Allali Zerah, V., Chayvilalle, JA., Leroyer, R., Leymarie, P., Travert, G., Lebrethon, MC., Budi, I., Balliere, AM. & Mahoudeau, J. (1992). Food-dependent Cushing's syndrome mediated by aberrant adrenal sensitivity to gastric inhibitory polypeptide. *N Engl J Med*, Vol. 327, No. 14, pp. (981–6), ISSN.

Ribeiro, RC., Sandrini Neto, RS., Schell, MJ., Lacerda, L., Sambaio, GA. & Cat, I. (1990). Adrenocortical carcinoma in children: A study of 40 cases. *J Clin Oncol*, Vol. 8, pp. (67-74), ISSN.

Ribeiro, RC., Michalkiewicz, EL., Figueiredo, BC., DeLacerda, L., Sandrini, F., Pianovsky, MD., Sampaio, G. & Sandrini, R. (2000). Adrenocortical tumors in children. *Braz J Med Biol Res*, Vol. 33, No. 10, pp. (1225-34), ISSN.

Ribeiro, RC., Sandrini, F., Figueiredo, B., Zambetti, GP., Michalkiewicz, E., Lafferty, AR., DeLacerda, L., Rabin, M., Cadwell, C., Sampaio, G., Cat, I., Stratakis, CA. & Sandrini, R. (2001). An inherited p53 mutation that contributes in a tissue-specific manner to pediatric adrenal cortical carcinoma. *Proc Natl Acad Sci U S A*, Vol. 98, No. 16, pp. (9330-5), ISSN.

Rockall, AG., Babar, SA., Sohaib, SA., Isidori, AM., Diaz-Cano, S., Monson, JP., Grossman, AB. & Reznek, RH. (2004). CT and MR imaging of the adrenal glands in ACTH-independent cushing syndrome. *Radiographics*, Vol. 24, No. 2, pp. (435-52), ISSN.

Rosenfield, RL. Clinical practice. Hirsutism. *N Engl J Med*, Vol. 353, pp. (2578–88), ISSN.

Ross, NS. (1994). Epidemiology of Cushing's syndrome and subclinical disease. *Endocrinol Metab Clin North Am*, Vol. 23, pp (539-46), ISSN.

Ruder, HJ., Loriaux, DL. & Lipsett, MB. (1974). Severe osteopenia in young adults associated with Cushing's syndrome due to micronodular adrenal disease. *J Clin Endocrinol Metab*, Vol. 39, pp. (1138-47), ISSN.

Sabbaga, CC., Avilla, SG., Schulz, C., Garbers, JC. & Blucher, D. (1993). Adrenocortical carcinoma in children: clinical aspects and prognosis. *J Pediatr Surg*, Vol. 28, No. 6, pp. (841-3), ISSN.

Sandrini, R., Ribeiro, R. & DeLacerda, L. (1997). Extensive personal experience: childhood adrenocortical tumors. *J Clin Endocrinol Metab*, Vol. 82, pp. (2027-31), ISSN.

Sbiera S, Schmull S, Assie G, Voelker HU, Kraus L, Beyer M, Ragazzon B, Beuschlein F, Willenberg HS, Hahner S, Saeger W, Bertherat J, Allolio B, Fassnacht M. (2010).

High diagnostic and prognostic value of steroidogenic factor-1 expression in adrenal tumors. J Clin Endocrinol Metab. Vol. 95, No. 10, pp. (161-71).

Schlumberger, M., Ostronoff, M., Bellaiche, M., Rougier, P., Droz, JP. & Parmentier, C. (1988). 5-Fluorouracil, doxorubicin, and cisplatin regimen in adrenal cortical carcinoma. *Cancer*, Vol. 61, No. 8, pp. (1492-4), ISSN.

Schteingart, DE., Motazedi, A., Noonan, RA. & Thompson, NW. (1982). Treatment of adrenal carcinomas. *Arch Surg*, Vol. 117, pp. (1142-6), ISSN.

Schteingart, DE., Doherty, GM., Gauger, PG., Giordano, TJ., Hammer, GD., Korobkin, M. & Worden, FP. (2005). Management of patients with adrenal cancer: recommendations of an international consensus conference. *Endocr Relat Cancer*, Vol. 12, No. 3, pp. (667–80), ISSN.

Schulte, KM., Mengel, M., Heinze, M., Simon, D., Scheuring, S., Köhrer, K. & Röher, HD. (2000). Complete sequencing and messenger ribonucleic acid expression analysis of the MEN I gene in adrenal cancer. *J Clin Endocrinol Metab*, Vol. 85, No. 1, pp. (441-8), ISSN.

Sidhu, S., Marsh, DJ., Theodosopoulos, G., Philips, J., Bambach, CP., Campbell, P., Magarey, CJ., Russell, CF., Schulte, KM., Röher, HD., Delbridge, L. & Robinson, BG. (2002). Comparative genomic hybridization analysis of adrenocortical tumors. *J Clin Endocrinol Metab*, Vol. 87, No. 7, pp. (3467-74), ISSN.

Sidhu, S., Sywak, M., Robinson, B. & Delbridge, L. (2004). Adrenocortical cancer: recent clinical and molecular advances. *Curr Opin Oncol*, Vol. 16, pp. (13-8), ISSN.

Skogseid, B., Larsson, C., Lindgren, PG., Kvanta, E., Rastad, J., Theodorsson, E., Wide, L., Wilander, E. & Oberg, K. (1992). Clinical and genetic features of adrenocortical lesions in multiple endocrine neoplasia type 1. *J Clin Endocrinol Metab*, Vol. 75, No. 1, pp. (76-81), ISSN.

Soon, P., MsDonald, K., Robinson, B. & Sidhu, S. (2008). Molecular markers and the pathogenesis of adrenocortical cancer. *Oncologist*, Vol. 13, pp. (548-61), ISSN.

Srivastava, S., Zou, ZQ., Pirollo, K., Blattner, W. & Chang, EH. (1990). Germ-line transmission of a mutated p53 gene in a cancerprone family with Li-Fraumeni syndrome. *Nature*, Vol. 348, pp. (747-9), ISSN.

Stojadinovic, A., Ghossein, RA., Hoos, A., Nissan, A., Marshall, D., Dudas, M., Cordon-Cardo, C., Jaques, DP. & Brennan, MF. (2002). Adrenocortical carcinoma: clinical, morphologic, and molecular characterization. *J Clin Oncol* , Vol. 20, No. 4, pp. (941-50), ISSN.

Stowasser, M. (2009). Update in primary aldosteronism. *J Clin Endocrinol Metab*, Vol 94, No. 10, pp. (3623-30), ISSN.

Stratakis, CA., Courcoutsakis, NA., Abati, A., Filie, A., Doppman, JL., Carney, JA. & Shawker, T. (1997). Thyroid gland abnormalities in patients with the syndrome of spotty skin pigmentation, myxomas, endocrine overactivity, and schwannomas (Carney complex). *J Clin Endocrinol Metab*, Vol. 82, No. 7, pp. (2037-43), ISSN.

Stratakis CA, Sarlis N, Kirschner LS, Carney JA, Doppman JL, Nieman LK, Chrousos GP, Papanicolaou DA. (1999) Paradoxical response to dexamethasone in the diagnosis of primary pigmented nodular adrenocortical disease. Ann Intern Med. Vol. 131(8), pp (585-91).

Stratakis, CA., Kirschner, LS. & Carney, JA. (2001). Clinical and molecular features of the Carney complex: diagnostic criteria and recommendations for patient evaluation. *J Clin Endocrinol Metab*, Vol. 86, pp. (4041-6), ISSN.

Stratakis, CA. & Boikos, SA. (2007). Genetics of adrenal tumors associated with Cushing's syndrome: a new classification for bilateral adrenocortical hyperplasias. *Nat Clin Pract Endocrinol Metab*, Vol. 3, pp. (748–57), ISSN.

Sturgeon C, Shen WT, Clark OH, Duh QY, Kebebew E. (2006). Risk assessment in 457 adrenal cortical carcinomas: how much does tumor size predict the likelihood of malignancy? J Am Coll Surg. Vol. 202(3), pp (423-30).

Sullivan, M., Boileau, M. & Hodges, CV. (1978). Adrenal cortical carcinoma. *J Urol*, Vol. 120, pp. (660–5), ISSN.

Sutter, JA. & Grimberg, A. (2006). Adrenocortical tumors and hyperplasias in childhood: etiology, genetics, clinical presentation and therapy. *Pediatr Endocrinol Rev*, Vol. 4, No. 1, pp. (32-9), ISSN.

Swain, JM., Grant, CS., Schlinkert, RT., Thompson, GB., vanHeerden, JA., Lloyd, RV. & Young, WF. (1998). Corticotropin-independent macronodular adrenal hyperplasia: a clinicopathologic correlation. *Arch Surg*, Vol. 133, No. 5, pp. (541–6), ISSN.

Swords, FM., Baig, A., Malchoff, DM., Malchoff, CD., Thorner, MO., King, PJ., Hunyady, L. & Clark, AJ. (2002). Impaired desensitization of a mutant adrenocorticotropin receptor associated with apparent constitutive activity. *Mol Endocrinol*, Vol. 16, No. 12, pp. (2746-53), ISSN.

Szolar, DH., Korobkin, M., Reittner, P., Berghold, A., Bauernhofer, T., Trummer, H., Schoellnast, H., Preidler, KW. & Samonigg, H. (2005). Adrenocortical carcinomas and adrenal pheochromocytomas: mass and enhancement loss evaluation at delayed contrast-enhanced CT. *Radiology*, Vol. 234, No. 2, pp. (479–85), ISSN.

Tadjine, M., Lampron, A., Ouadi, L., Horvath, A., Stratakis, CA. & Bourdeau, I. (2008). Detection of somatic beta-catenin mutations in primary pigmented nodular adrenocortical disease (PPNAD). *Clin Endocrinol (Oxf)*, Vol. 69, No. 3, pp. (367-73), ISSN.

Tanabe, A., Naruse, M., Naruse, K., Hase, M., Yoshimoto, T., Tanaka, M., Seki, T., Demura, R. & Demura, H. (1997). Left ventricular hypertrophy is more prominent in patients with primary aldosteronism than in patients with other types of secondary hypertension. *Hypertens Res*, Vol. 20, No. 2, pp. (85–90), ISSN.

Terzolo, M., Osella, G., Alì, A. & Angeli, A. (2000). Adrenal incidentalomas. *In*: De Herder WW (ed). Functional and Morphological Imaging of the Endocrine System. *Boston: Kluwer Academic Publishers*, Vol. 7, pp. (191-211), ISSN.

Terzolo M, Boccuzzi A, Bovio S, Cappia S, De Giuli P, Alì A, Paccotti P, Porpiglia F, Fontana D, Angeli A. (2001). Immunohistochemical assessment of Ki-67 in the differential diagnosis of adrenocortical tumors. Urology. Vol. 57(1), pp (176-82).

Terzolo, M., Bovio, S., Reimondo, G., Pia, A., Osella, G., Borretta, G. & Angeli, A. (2005a). Subclinical Cushing's syndrome in adrenal incidentalomas. *Endocrinol Metab Clin North Am*, Vol. 34, No. 2, pp. (423-39), ISSN.

Terzolo, M., Bovio, S., Pia, A., Conton, PA., Reimondo, G., Dall'Asta, C., Bemporad, D., Angeli, A., Opocher, G., Mannelli, M., Ambrosi, B. & Mantero, F. (2005b). Midnight serum cortisol as a marker of increased cardiovascular risk in patients with a clinically inapparent adrenal adenoma. *Eur J Endocrinol*, Vol. 153, No. 2, pp. (307-15), ISSN.

Terzolo, M., Angeli, A., Fassnacht, M., Daffara, F., Tauchmanova, L., Conton, PA., Rossetto, R., Buci, L., Sperone, P., Grossrubatscher, E., Reimondo, G., Bollito, E., Papotti, M., Saeger, W., Hahner, S., Koschker, AC., Arvat, E., Ambrosi, B., Loli, P., Lombardi, G., Mannelli, M., Bruzzi, P., Mantero, F., Allolio, B., Dogliotti, L. & Berruti, A. (2007). Adjuvant mitotane treatment for adrenocortical carcinoma. *N Engl J Med*, Vol. 356, No. 23, pp. (2372-80), ISSN.

Tissier, F., Cavard, C., Groussin, L., Perlemoine, K., Fumey, G., Hagneré, AM., René-Corail, F., Jullian, E., Gicquel, C., Bertagna, X., Vacher-Lavenu, MC., Perret, C. & Bertherat, J. (2005). Mutations of beta-catenin in adrenocortical tumors: Activation of the Wnt signaling pathway is a frequent event in both benign and malignant adrenocortical tumors. *Cancer Res*, Vol. 65, No. 17, pp. (7622-7), ISSN.

Tissier, F. (2010). Classification of adrenal cortical tumors: what limits for the pathological approach? *Best Pract Res Clin Endocrinol Metab*, Vol. 24, No. 6, pp. (877-85), ISSN.

Ulick, S., Wang, JZ. & Morton, DH. (1992). The biochemical phenotypes of two inborn errors in the biosynthesis of aldosterone. *J Clin Endocrinol Metab*, Vol. 74, pp. (1415-20), ISSN.

van Ditzhuijsen, CI., van de Weijer, R. & Haak, HR. (2007). Adrenocortical carcinoma. *Neth J Med*, Vol. 65, No. 2, pp. (55-60), ISSN.

Varley, JM., McGown, G., Thorncroft, M., James, LA., Margison, GP., Forster, G., Evans, DG., Harris, M., Kelsey, AM. & Birch, JM. (1999). Are there low-penetrance TP53 Alleles? Evidence from childhood adrenocortical tumors. *Am J Hum Genet*, Vol. 65, No. 4, pp. (995-1006), ISSN.

Veugelers, M., Wilkes, D., Burton, K., McDermott, DA., Song, Y., Goldstein, MM., La Perle, K., Vaughan, CJ., O'Hagan, A., Bennett, KR., Meyer, BJ., Legius, E., Karttunen, M., Norio, R., Kaariainen, H., Lavyne, M., Neau, JP., Richter, G., Kirali, K., Farnsworth, A., Stapleton, K., Morelli, P., Takanashi, Y., Bamforth, JS., Eitelberger, F., Noszian, I., Manfroi, W., Powers, J., Mochizuki, Y., Imai, T., Ko, GT., Driscoll, DA., Goldmuntz, E., Edelberg, JM., Collins, A., Eccles, D., Irvine, AD., McKnight, GS. & Basson, CT. (2004). Comparative PRKAR1A genotype-phenotype analyses in humans with Carney complex and PRKAR1a haploinsufficient mice. *Proc Natl Acad Sci U S A*, Vol. 101, No.39, pp. (14222-7), ISSN.

Volante, M., Buttigliero, C., Greco, E., Berruti, A. & Papotti, M. (2008). Pathological and molecular features of adrenocortical carcinoma: an update. *J Clin Pathol*, Vol. 61, No. 7, pp. (787-93), ISSN.

Wada, S., Kitahama, S., Togashi, A., Inoue, K., Iitaka, M. & Katayama, S. (2002). Preclinical Cushing's syndrome due to ACTH-independent bilateral macronodular adrenocortical hyperplasia with excessive secretion of 18-hydroxydeoxycorticosterone and corticosterone. *Intern Med*, Vol. 41, No. 4, pp. (304-8), ISSN.

Waggoner, W., Boots, LR. & Azziz, R. (1999). Total testosterone and DHEAS levels as predictors of androgen-secreting neoplasms: a populational study. *Gynecological Endocrinology*, Vol. 13, pp. (394–400), ISSN.

Wagner, J., Portwine, C., Rabin, K., Leclerc, JM., Narod, SA. & Malkin, D. (1994). High frequency of germline p53 mutations in childhood adrenocortical cancer. *J Natl Cancer Inst*, Vol. 86, No. 22, pp. (1707-10), ISSN.

Wajchenberg, BL., Albergaria Pereira, MA., Medonca, BB., Latronico, AC., Campos Carneiro, P., Alves, VA., Zerbini, MC., Liberman, B., Carlos Gomes, G. & Kirschner,

MA. (2000). Adrenocortical carcinoma: clinical and laboratory observations. *Cancer*, Vol. 88, No. 4, pp. (711-36), ISSN.

Wasserman JD, Zambetti GP, Malkin D. (2011) Towards an understanding of the role of p53 in adrenocortical carcinogenesis. *Mol Cell Endocrinol*. Sep 10. [Epub ahead of print]

Watanabe, M. & Nakajin, S. (2004). Forskolin up-regulates aromatase (CYP19) activity and gene transcripts in the human adrenocortical carcinoma cell line H295R. *J Endocrinol*, Vol. 180, No. 1, pp. (125-33), ISSN.

Weber MM., Auernhammer CJ., Kiess W., and Engelhardt D. (1997) Insulin-like growth factor receptors in normal and timorous adult human adrenocortical glands. European Journal of Endocrinology Vol. 136 pp. (296-303).

Weber, SL. (1997). Cushing's syndrome attributable to topical use of lotrisone. *Endocr Pract*, Vol. 3, pp. (140-4), ISSN.

Weinstein, LS., Shenker, A., Gejman, PV., Merino, MJ., Friedman, E. & Spiegel, AM. (1991). Activating mutations of the stimulatory G protein in the McCune-Albright syndrome. *N Engl J Med*, Vol. 325, pp. (1688-95), ISSN.

Weiss, LM. (1984). Comparative histologic study of 43 metastasizing and nonmetastasizing adrenocortical tumors. *Am J Surg Pathol*, Vol. 8, pp. (163-9), ISSN.

White, PC., New, MI. & Dupont, B. (1987). Congenital adrenal hyperplasia. *N Engl J Med*, Vol. 316, pp. (1519-24), ISSN.

White, PC. (1994). Disorders of aldosterone biosynthesis and action. *N Engl J Med*, Vol. 331, pp. (250-8), ISSN.

Wiedemann, HR. (1983). Tumours and hemihypertrophy associated with Wiedemann-Beckwith syndrome. *Eur J Pediatr*, Vol. 141, pp. (29), ISSN.

Wieneke, JA., Thompson, LD. & Heffess, CS. (2003). Adrenocortical neoplasms in the pediatric population: a clinicopathologic and immunophenotypic analysis of 83 patients. *Am J Surg Pathol*, Vol. 27, No. 7, pp. (867-81), ISSN.

Wilkins, L. (1948). A feminizing adrenal tumor causing gynecomastia in a boy of five years contrasted with a virilizing tumor in a five-year-old girl: classification of seventy cases of adrenal tumor in children according to their hormonal manifestations and a review of eleven cases of feminizing adrenal tumor in adults. *J Clin Endocrinol Metab*, Vol. 8, pp. (111-32), ISSN.

Wood, BJ., Abraham, J., Hvizda, JL., Alexander, HR. & Fojo, T. (2003). Radiofrequency ablation of adrenal tumors and adrenocortical carcinoma metastases. *Cancer*, Vol. 97, pp. (554-60), ISSN.

Young, WF. (2000). Management approaches to adrenal incidentalomas: a view from Rochester, Minnesota. Endocrinol Metab Clin North Am. Vol. 29, pp (159-85).

Young, WF. (2007a). Primary aldosteronism: renaissance of a syndrome. *Clin Endocrinol (Oxf)*, Vol. 66, No. 5, pp. (607-18), ISSN.

Young, WF. (2007b). The incidentally discovered adrenal mass. *N Engl J Med*, Vol. 356, pp. (601-10), ISSN.

Zarifis, J., Lip, GY., Leatherdale, B. & Beevers, G. (1996). Malignant hypertension in association with primary aldosteronism. *Blood Press*, Vol. 5, pp. (250-4), ISSN.

Zerbini, CA., Kozakewich, HP., Weinberg, DS., Mundt, DJ., Edwards, JAI. & Lack, EE. (1992). Adrenocortical neoplasms in childhood and adolescence: analysis of prognostic factors including DNA content. *Endocr Pathol*, Vol. 3, pp. (116-28), ISSN.

15

Autoimmunity to Steroid-Producing Cells

Alberto Falorni and Stefania Marzotti
Department of Internal Medicine, Section of Internal Medicine and Endocrine and Metabolic Sciences, University of Perugia
Italy

1. Introduction

Addison's disease, named after the English physician who provided its full description in 1855, is the result of the destruction or impaired function of adrenocortical cells. Of the 11 cases described by Addison, 10 were likely subsequent to an infiltrative disease (the most common being the secondary localization of *Mycobacterium tuberculosis* to the adrenal gland) and 1 was clinically idiopathic (likely of an autoimmune origin, on the basis of the current knowledge of disease mechanisms). In recent years the ethiologic spectrum of the disease has considerably expanded to include genetic causes not present in the 11 cases described by Thomas Addison. Accordingly, the definition of primary adrenal insufficiency (PAI) appears today more correct. Nevertheless, Autoimmune Addison's Disease (AAD) and post-tuberculosis Addison's disease are still adequate definitions according to the clinical characteristics of the cases described in 1855.

Prevalence of PAI is estimated at 120-160 cases per million in western countries, corresponding to 1 case every 7,000-7,500 individuals (Laureti *et al*, 1999; Løvås *et al*, 2002). The clinical manifestations of the disease result from the glucorticoid, mineralcorticoid and androgen deficiency (Oelkers, 1996). In western countries and Japan, an autoimmune process is responsible for the destruction of the adrenocortical cells and for the clinical manifestations of PAI in around 70-90% of cases (Betterle *et al*, 2002; Nomura *et al*, 1994).

AAD occurs frequently in concomitance with other organ-specific and non-organ-specific autoimmune diseases in the so-called autoimmune polyendocrine syndromes (APS). Since at least two-thirds of patients with AAD have one or more other manifestations of an ongoing autoimmune process against other endocrine glands or different tissues, AAD can be considered a paradigmatic disease for the study of endocrine autoimmunity. On the basis of the type of diseases present in the same patient, different APSs are recognized. APS 1 is caused by mutations of the AIRE (AutoImmune REgulator) gene, which is located on chromosome 21 (The Finnish-German APECED Consortium, 1997). This syndrome is characterized by the concomitant presence of at least two of three diseases: chronic mucocutaneous candidiasis, hypoparathyroidism and AAD. In first-degree relatives of APS1 patients a single disease manifestation is sufficient to formulate the diagnosis. No general agreement exists for the classification of the remaining APSs. Some authors discriminate APS 2, APS 3 and APS 4 according to the different combination of autoimmune diseases present in the same patients. With this classification, APS 2 would identify the association of clinical or pre-clinical AAD with thyroid autoimmune diseases and/or type 1 diabetes mellitus (T1DM). APS 3 would be the association of thyroid autoimmune diseases with other endocrine and non-endocrine autoimmune manifestations (with the exception of AAD) and APS 4 would include all other possible combinations. No sound pathophysiological and/or genetic background, however, supports this classification, as the different endocrine autoimmune diseases tend to share a common genetic background and the same subject that might be initially be classified as APS 3 or APS 4 would be reclassified as APS2 if clinical or subclinical signs of adrenal or thyroid autoimmunity occur at a later stage. Throughout this chapter we will then refer to APS 2 to include all combinations of AAD with other immuno-mediated diseases, different from hypoparathyroidism or chronic mucocutaneous candidiasis.

Most frequently AAD is associated with Hashimoto's thyroiditis or Graves's disease, one or the other being present in over 50% of patients with autoimmune adrenal insufficiency (Betterle *et al*, 2002; Nerup, 1974; Kong *et al*, 1994; Irvine et al, 1967, 1979; McHardy-Young *et al*, 1974; De Rosa *et al*, 1987; Papadopoulos *et al*, 1990; Kasperlik-Zaluska *et al*, 1991; Zelissen *et al*, 1995; Söderbergh *et al*, 1996; Neufeld *et al*, 1981). Atrophic gastritis is present in 20-25% of AAD patients, while type 1 diabetes mellitus (T1DM) has been reported in 1-20% of addisonian patients (Betterle *et al*, 2002; Nerup, 1974; Kong *et al*, 1994; Irvine et al, 1967, 1979; McHardy-Young *et al*, 1974; De Rosa *et al*, 1987; Papadopoulos *et al*, 1990; Kasperlik-Zaluska *et al*, 1991; Zelissen *et al*, 1995; Söderbergh *et al*, 1996; Neufeld *et al*, 1981). Hypergonadotropic hypogonadism is present in 4.5-19% of AAD women. Other autoimmune diseases found associated with AAD at lower frequency include: vitiligo, alopecia, celiac disease, pernicious anemia, multiple sclerosis, inflammatory bowel disease, Sjögren's syndrome, chronic hepatitis and lymphocytic hypophysitis (Betterle *et al*, 2002; Nerup, 1974; Kong *et al*, 1994; Irvine et al, 1967, 1979; McHardy-Young *et al*, 1974; De Rosa *et al*, 1987; Papadopoulos *et al*, 1990; Kasperlik-Zaluska *et al*, 1991; Zelissen *et al*, 1995; Söderbergh *et al*, 1996; Neufeld *et al*, 1981).

2. Adrenal autoimmunity

The human adrenal autoimmune process is made evident by the apperance of circulating autoantibodies directed against the adrenal cortex or its components, which can be detected in the serum of affected individuals.

The first demonstration of adrenal cortex autoantibodies (ACA), detected by a complement-fixation test in the sera from patients with AAD, was provided in 1957 (Anderson *et al*, 1957). The use of the indirect immunofluorescence (IIF) approach, introduced by Blizzard and Kyle, 1963, has subsequently enabled the development of more sensitive assays for the detection of ACA (Blizzard *et al*, 1963, 1967; Goudie *et al*, 1966; Andrada *et al*, 1968; Wuepper *et al*, 1969; Nerup, 1974; Irvine & Barnes, 1974; Sotsiou *et al*, 1980; Elder *et al*, 1981; Papadopoulos *et al*, 1990). ACA have been detected in 40-75% patients with clinically idiopathic Addison's disease (Blizzard *et al*, 1963, 1967; Goudie *et al*, 1966; Andrada *et al*, 1968; Wuepper *et al*, 1969; Nerup, 1974; Irvine & Barnes, 1974; Sotsiou *et al*, 1980; Elder *et al*, 1981; Stechmesser *et al*, 1985; Kosowicz *et al*, 1986; Papadopoulos *et al*, 1990). Differences in the substrate used for detection of autoantibodies (human vs. animal adrenals), in disease duration and in selection of patients are responsible for the high variability in ACA frequency in patients with PAI.

In spite of the very well known technical limitations, because of the relative simplicity of the assay and the high diagnostic sensitivity, ACA-IIF have represented the gold standard for adrenal autoantibody determination until the middle of the '90s. ACA react with cytoplasm autoantigen(s) of cells located in all three layers of the adrenal cortex. More recent studies have detected ACA in approximately 80% of patients with AAD, representing over 90% of patients with recent-onset disease and 79% with long-standing disease (>2 years of disease duration) (Betterle *et al*, 1999). ACA are more frequent in patients with APS1 or APS2 than in patients with isolated Addison's disease (Betterle *et al*, 1999).

Attempts to identify the molecular targets of ACA started during the 1980's, which led to the initial identification of a 55-kDa autoantigen present in human adrenal microsomes (Furmaniak *et al*, 1988). Subsequent studies of the beginning of the 1990's have identified steroid-21-hydroxylase (21OH) as the main autoantigen target of ACA (Winqvist *et al*, 1992; Baumann-Antczak *et al*, 1992; Bednarek *et al*, 1992). Around the same time, steroid-17α-hydroxylase (17OH) (Krohn *et al*, 1992) and P450 side chain cleavage (P450scc) enzyme (Winqvist *et al*, 1993) were identified as additional autoantigens.

The discovery of the molecular targets of ACA led to development of radiobinding assays with radiolabelled human autoantigen. The use of either in vitro translated ^{35}S-21OH (Falorni *et al*, 1995, 1997; Colls *et al*, 1995) or 125 I-21OH (Tanaka *et al*, 1997) has enabled the demonstration that 21OH autoantibodies (21OHAb) have a high diagnostic sensitivity and specificity for AAD, being detected in over 95% of cases with clinically idiopathic adrenal insufficiency. The major epitopes recognised by human 21OHAb are located in the central and COOH-terminal domains of the enzyme. In addition, naturally occurring mutations, associated with the development of congenital adrenal hyperplasia, inhibit the binding of human autoantibodies to recombinant 21OH (Chen *et al*, 1998, Nikoshkov *et al*, 1999). *In vitro* studies (Furmaniak *et al*, 1994) have shown that 21OHAb may inhibit the enzymatic activity of the autoantigen, but this finding has not been confirmed *in vivo*, during the natural history of the disease (Boscaro *et al*, 1996; Laureti *et al*, 2002).

Similarly to other organ-specific autoantibodies, 21OHAb have no major pathogenic role in the development of adrenal insufficiency, as they can be detected in approximately 1/200 healthy subjects who do not necessarily progress towards clinical adrenal insufficiency. During pregnancy, 21OHAb cross the placental barrier, but do not determine any sign of clinical or pre-clinical adrenal insufficiency in the newborn (Betterle *et al*, 2004). Hence, 21OHAb are a highly senstive and specific immunological marker of the ongoing adrenal autoimmune process, but do not act as an effector of the destructive autoimmune process.

Our group has recently shown that 21OHAb are predominantly IgG1, with a minor expression of IgG2 and IgG4, which demonstrates a Th1-oriented type of immune response (Brozzetti *et al*, 2010a). However, approximately 10% of AAD patients express IgG4-21OHAb in the absence of IgG1 (Brozzetti *et al*, 2010a). This type of IgG subclass selection reveals a more Th2-oriented type of activation. At present, it is still unclear whether this distinct subgroup of patients with a more Th2-oriented type of immune response represents a different population of AAD subjects or is the expression of a different stage of the natural history of the disease.

Although 17OHAb and P450sccAb can be detected in a small fraction of patients with AAD, these markers are more frequently present in patients with APS 1 or in women with autoimmune oophoritis which causes autoimmune ovarian insufficiency (*see paragraph on Ovarian Autoimmunity*) (Betterle *et al*, 1999; Perniola *et al*, 2000; Falorni *et al*, 2002a).

Diagnosis of PAI is based on clinical ground and hormonal determination, but the ethiologic diagnosis of AAD requires detection of circulating 21OHAb, by using a radiobinding assay.

Autoantibody titer is also important, because the presence of low titre adrenal autoantibodies does not enable the unequivocal diagnosis of AAD in all cases (Falorni *et al*, 2004). ACA and 21OHAb have sporadically been found also in patients with unequivocal post-tuberculosis Addison's disease (Nomura *et al*, 1994; do Carmo Silva *et al*, 2000). A flow-chart for the etiological classification of PAI, that takes into consideration immunological, biochemical and imaging data, has been developed by the Italian Addison Network (Falorni *et al*, 2004). Published data indicate that the diagnostic accuracy of the 21OHAb assay is higher than that of the ACA-IIF (Falorni *et al*, 2004), and 21OHAb is currently the gold standard for detection of adrenal autoantibodies. In the case of a simultaneous presence of both ACA and 21OHAb, the probability of an accurate diagnosis of AAD is higher than 99% (Falorni *et al*, 2004). All patients with AAD should undergo additional autoantibody analyses, such as thyroid autoantibodies, GAD autoantibodies (GADA), steroid-cell autoantibodies (StCA), 17OHAb, P450sccAb or parietal cell autoantibodies, as approximately two thirds of AAD patients show clinical or pre-clinical signs of another autoimmune disease. Autoimmune AAD can be diagnosed also in the presence of medium-high levels of either 21OHAb or ACA (Falorni *et al*, 2004). In the case of patients positive only for 21OHAb or ACA at low levels, as well as in autoantibody-negative subjects, adrenal imaging should be performed to exclude an infiltrative form of adrenal insufficiency (such as post-tuberculosis, sarcoidosis, mycosis or metastatic localization of non-adrenal tumours) (Falorni *et al*, 2004). In male patients negative for both adrenal autoantibody measurement and adrenal imaging analysis, determination of plasmatic very long chain fatty acids (VLCFA) must be performed to exclude X-linked adrenoleukodystrophy (ALD).

At present, no clear and standardised cut-off is available to discriminate between low and medium-high level autoantibody titers and worskhops for the standardization of adrenal autoantibody assays are strongly needed. In a first international serum exchange to compare the results of 21OHAb determination in four independent laboratories, a good positive-negative concordance was observed, but major discrepancies emerged in quantitation of autoantibody titre (Falorni *et al*, 2011). A European program for the standardization of 21OHAb assay is currently being organised, and is expected to be completed within 2012.

Screening of subjects with endocrine autoimmune diseases for the presence of 21OHAb enables the identification of subjects with so-called *preclinical AAD*, which is characterised by the presence of adrenal autoantibodies in the absence of clinical signs of adrenal insufficiency and in the presence of normal basal cortisol concentrations. In patients with autoimmune diseases, 21OHAb can be detected in around 0.5-1.5% T1DM patients, 0.5-1.5% patients with autoimmune thyroid diseases, 0.5-1.0% patients with vitiligo and in 4-8% women with primary ovarian insufficiency (Betterle *et al*, 2002). 21OHAb-positive individuals exhibit a variable degree of adrenal dysfunction that can be classified in four different stages (Betterle *et al*, 1988).

Stage 0 indicates the apperance of adrenal autoantibodies, as a sign of the ongoing adrenal autoimmune process. 21OHAb appears before ACA, and lasts longer than ACA, during the natural history of the disease.

Often the first dysfunction observed as a consequence of the progression of the autoimmune process is an initial increase of plasmatic renin activity (PRA), at a time when normal ACTH-cortisol axis response is still present (*stage 1*). In *stage 2*, an impaired response to the ACTH stimulation test is documented, while the final *stage 3* represents the pre-clinical stage characterized by increased basal ACTH levels, along with the dysfunctions observed in stage 1 and 2.

No preventative therapy is yet available to delay or block the progressive destruction of adrenocortical cells in pre-clinical AAD. An Italian study has shown that an immunosuppressive therapy with high-dose corticosteroids for the treatment of Graves' ophthalmopathy had been able to revert a stage 2 pre-clinical AAD in a 21OHAb-positive individual (De Bellis *et al*, 1993). As a result of the treatment, disappearance of adrenal autoantibodies and normalization of both ACTH-cortisol and PRA-aldosterone axis function was observed and maintained for over 10 years at follow-up (De Bellis *et al*, 1993). However, the possibility to revert an advanced pre-clinical adrenal insufficiency by high-dose steroid immunosuppression has not yet been confirmed in other independent studies and it is not recommended for the sole purpose of preventing the progression towards clinical AAD.

Among the factors associated with progression towards clinical adrenal insufficiency are adrenal autoantibody levels that tend to increase during the progression of the adrenal dysfunction (Betterle *et al*, 1997).

Approximately 80% of patients with stage 0 and stage 1 do not progress to clinical AAD and may show a spontaneous remission of the pre-clinical dysfunction (Laureti *et al*, 1998). On the other hand, no such spontaneous remission seems to occur in patients with stage 2 and stage 3, in whom progression to clinical AAD is observed in over 95% of cases. A matematical formula that takes into consideration all known factors influencing risk of progression towards clinical AAD has been generated (Coco *et al*, 2006).

In subjects positive for 21OHAb and/or ACA, an ACTH stimulation test discriminates between a potentially reversible and an irreversible stage of the pre-clinical dysfunction. It has been shown that the high-dose 250 μg of synthetic ACTH used in the classical ACTH test (HDT) is supra-maximal and that as little as 1 μg of synthetic ACTH can determine a maximal stimulation of the adrenocortical cells (Arvat *et al*, 2000). The low-dose test with 1 μg of ACTH (LDT) has a high diagnostic sensitivity and specificity for pre-clinical adrenal dysfunction and can substitute the classical high-dose test (Laureti *et al*, 2000, 2002). An ongoing European multicenter study is currently testing the diagnostic accuracy and the predictive value of a 0.5 μg low-dose ACTH test.

Among the factors increasing significantly the risk of progression towards clinical adrenal insufficiency, in subjects with subclinical AAD, the most important are: male gender, presence of other concomitant autoimmune diseases, impaired response to the LDT and a high 21OHAb titer (Coco *et al*, 2006). HLA-DR3-DQ2, DR4-DQ8 and CTLA-4 gene polymorphism are significantly associated with appearance of 21OHAb, but do not influence the natural history of the disease and do not predict future clinical adrenal insufficiency (Coco *et al*, 2006; Falorni *et al*, unpublished data). Homozygosity for MICA5.1 was found to increase significantly the risk of progression towards clinical adrenal insufficiency (Barker *et al*, 2005), but larger, prospective studies are needed to confirm this finding. Because of the high predictive value of 21OHAb for future AAD, which is higher than 30% at 10 years of follow-up, screening of patients with ongoing endocrine autoimmune diseases with this marker is recommended to identify subjects with pre-clinical adrenal insufficiency.

3. Genetics of autoimmune adrenal insufficiency

Autoimmune Regulator (AIRE) is the causative gene for APS1 (The Finnish-German APECED Consortium, 1997). The AIRE gene product, Aire, acts as a strong activator of transcription (Pitkänen *et al*, 2000, 2001; Björses *et al*, 2000). Over 60 disease-associated

mutations of the AIRE gene have been so far identified. Many mutations are located in the homogeneously staining region (HSR) in the N-terminal end of the protein. Other mutations, such as C311Y, P326Q, L397fsX478 are located in the plant homeodomain zinc finger 1 and 2, while only a few mutations, such as G228W or R257X have been identified in the DNA binding motif (Bottomley *et al*, 2001). It has been reported that a kindred carrying the G228W variant presented with an autosomal dominant autoimmune phenotype manifesting predominantly with thyroidits and distinct from APS1 (Cetani *et al*, 2001). The generation of a G228W-knocking mouse model showed that this AIRE variant acts in a dominant-negative manner causing a unique autoimmune syndrome (Su *et al*, 2008).
Disease-associated AIRE mutations are highly conserved within defined geographical areas. The R257X is the most frequently found mutation in Northern Italy and in Finland, while 964del13 is the most common mutation in the UK. In Sardinia, R139X is the typical AIRE mutation found in APS 1 patients.
Outside APS1, AAD shares many predisposing genetic factors with other endocrine autoimmune diseases that are components of APS2, such as thyroid autoimmune diseases and T1DM, the major genetic markers associated with the diseases beeing located in the HLA region on chromosome 6. The disease is strongly and positively associated with both HLA-DRB1*0301-DQA1*0501-DQB1*0201 (DR3-DQ2) and DRB1*04-DQA1*0301-DQB1*0302 (DR4-DQ8) (Falorni *et al*, 2008). The HLA-DRB1*01-DQA1*01-DQB1*0501 and DRB1*13-DQA1*0103-DQB1*0603 haplotypes are negatively associated with genetic risk for AAD. Several studies have shown that the association of HLA class II haplotypes is still highly significant in patients with isolated AAD and does not depend on the coexistence of other autoimmune disorders in the same patient. DRB1-*0404 was more frequent among DRB1*04-positive AAD patients from US (Yu *et al*, 1999) and Norway (Myhre *et al*, 2002) as compared to both DRB1*04-positive healthy control subjects and DRB1*04-positive T1DM patients. The DRB1*0401 subtype was strongly and positively associated with T1DM, but not with AAD (Yu *et al*, 1999; Myhre *et al*, 2002). However, an Italian study from our group (Gambelunghe *et al*, 2005) did not confirm this hypothesis. In that study (Gambelunghe *et al*, 2005), it was observed that no statistically different distribution of DRB1*0401 and DRB1*0404 was detectable among T1DM patients and AAD patients. On the other hand, it was observed that the DRB1*0403 subtype, which was already known to confer strong protection for T1DM, was absent among 56 DRB1*04-positive AAD patients, but present in 27 % DRB1*04-positive healthy control subjects, thus conferring protection also for the development of AAD.
Other HLA genes contribute to the risk for AAD, among which the MHC class I chain-related A (MICA) gene polymorphism. The MICA gene encodes for a ligand for an activating receptor (NKG2D) present on $\gamma\delta$ T cells, CD8+CD28- $\alpha\beta$ T cells, natural killer cells and CD4+CD28- $\alpha\beta$ T cells and is located within the HLA class III region. There are speculations that MICA gene polymorphism might influence affinity for the NKG2D receptor. AAD is strongly associated with the transmembrane MICA 5.1 allele, with odds ratio similar to those observed for HLA class II haplotypes (Gambelunghe *et al*, 1999; Park *et al*, 2002). MICA6 appears to be negatively associated with disease risk for AAD (Gambelunghe *et al*, 1999).
Though the association of MICA with AAD appears to be independent from that with HLA class II haplotypes, the strong *linkage disequilibrium* existing within the DRB1*03-DQA1*0501-DQB1*0201-MICA5.1-HLA-B extended haplotype has so far limited the possibility to discriminate the relative contribution of each gene marker and further studies on large populations are needed to provide an answer to this specific question.

Similarly to T1DM and other autoimmune diseases, the genetic background for AAD includes also other genes believed to modulate the function of the immune system. The CTLA-4 gene polymorphism and the PTPN22 gene polymorphism have been found to modulate genetic risk for AAD (Falorni *et al*, 2008; Skinningsrud *et al*, 2008a). A recent metanalysis of European studies has confirmed that the CTLA-4 Ala 17 polymorphism is strongly associated with genetic risk for AAD, independentenly from the well known association with the polymorphism of HLA class II genes (Brozzetti *et al*, 2010b).
Two independent European studies have shown the association of the class II transactivator (CIITA) (also denominated MHC2TA) gene with AAD (Ghaderi *et al*, 2006; Skinningsrud *et al*, 2008b). Modulation of the expression of HLA class II determinants in antigen-presenting cells may represent a critical factor in the activation and maintenance of the organ-specific autoimmune process and genetic factors that may influence such expression may have an important role on the pathogenesis of autoimmune diseases. The regulatory factor X complex (RFX) and CIITA are essential and specific for activation of class II promoters (Durand *et al*, 1997; Masternak *et al*, 1998; Reith & Mach, 2001; Nekrep *et al*, 2002). More specifically, the class II expression on antigen presenting cells is under the control of CIITA, that exhibits cell-specific, cytokine-inducible and differentiation-specific expression and is expressed in the same cells that express class II molecules, such as B cells, monocytes, dendritic cells and activated T cells. The genetic association of CIITA with AAD appears to be independent from that with HLA gene markers.
Other reported AAD genetic associations include the vitamin D receptor and the CYP27B1 (25-hydroxyvitamin D3-1α-hydroxylase) gene and the NACHT leucine-rich-repeat protein 1 (NALP1) gene (Magitta *et al*, 2009).

4. Pathophysiology of AAD

No model of spontaneous autoimmune primary adrenal insufficiency is yet available. Experimental autoimmune adrenalitis has been induced in mice, guinea pigs, rats and monkeys by injection of adrenal homogenates mixed with adjuvants (Betterle *et al*, 2002), with a resulting delayed type of hypersensitivity to adrenal antigens, rather than the induction of an adrenal autoimmune process. No conclusive data are yet available on the possibility of inducing an autoimmune reaction by injecting the major adrenal autoantigen 21-hydroxylase.
The current unavailability of a reliable animal model of spontaneous adrenal autoimmunity similar to the human disease, has so far limited the studies on the pathophysiology of AAD. Major efforts are being profused to develop an animal model of AAD that may prove useful for the understanding of the molecular mechanisms responsible for the human disease.
The effector cells of the autoimmune-mediated destruction of adrenocortical cells are thought to be T lymphocytes (Hayashi *et al*, 1989; Freeman & Weetman, 1992). Nerup *et al.*, 1969, 1970, showed that patients with autoimmune adrenal insufficiency have T cells reactive against fetal adrenal extracts or adrenal mitochondrial fraction. Subsequently, it was shown that patients with recent-onset AAD have an increased expression of circulating Ia-positive T cells when compared to healthy control subjects (Rabinowe *et al*, 1984). Freeman & Weetman, 1992 were able to demonstrate T cell proliferation in response to stimulation with adrenal proteins fractionated according to molecular weight. Patients with autoimmune polyendocrine syndrome type II, but not individuals with isolated Addison's disease, seem to have $CD4^{+}CD25^{+}$regulatory T cells with defective suppressive capacity (Kriegel *et al*, 2004; Coles *et al*, 2005).

Although several studies support the hypothesis of a major role of cellular immunity in the autoimmune destruction of the adrenocortical cells in Addison's disease, little is known of the individual antigens recognised by autoreactive T cells. Husebye et al. immunized BALB/c and SJL mice with recombinant 21OH and showed a selective significant proliferative response of T cells from lymph nodes against the peptide 342-361 of 21OH that corresponds to the substrate binding site of the enzyme (Husebye *et al*, 2006).

Among Th cell subtypes, two main subtypes, denominated Th1 and Th2, are recognized. AAD is thougth to result from an unbalance of Th1/Th2 responses with a predominance of Th1 activity. Chemokines produced at the site of inflammation participate by recruiting T cells and by sustaining the immune reaction (Rotondi *et al*, 2007). Th1 cells mainly express CXCR3 and are recruited at the site of inflammation by CXCL9, CXCL10 and CXCL11. Th2 cells express different chemokine receptors, such as CCR4 and CCR8, thus being recruited in target tissues by CCL17, CCL22 and CCL1. The existence of an important IFN-γ-mediated pathogenetic loop has been proposed for endocrine autoimmunity, as release of CXCR3-binding chemokines is stimulated by IFN-γ and, in turn, these chemokines recruit Th-1 cells that produce IFN-γ (Rotondi *et al*, 2007).

In one report concerning the role of serum CXCL10 in AAD, serum levels of CXCL10 were significantly increased in patients with either clinically evident or subclinical adrenal insufficiency, as compared to healthy control subjects (Rotondi *et al*, 2005). The absence of a gender-related effect in AAD, either isolated or occurring within APS-2, suggested that autoimmune adrenalitis by itself was responsible for the high circulating levels of CXCL10. In the same study (Rotondi *et al*, 2005), it was also shown that release of CXCL10 by primary cell cultures of human zona fasciculata cells (hZFC) was undetectable basally, but significantly induced by stimulation with IFN-γ or IFN-γ plus TNF-α, while stimulation of hZFC with TNF-α alone was not able to induce chemokine secretion. Interestingly, increasing concentrations of hydrocortisone progressively and significantly inhibited IFN-γ-induced and IFN-γ- plus TNF-α-induced CXCL10 secretion (Rotondi *et al*, 2005).

The inhibitory effect of glucocorticoids on chemokine production is in line with their antiinflammatory and immunosuppressive actions. Glucocorticoids are able to suppress the production of several cytokines and chemokines by inhibiting the nuclear factor-κB and by activating protein-1 transcription factor families (Karin, 1998).

More recently, increased serum levels of Th1-related chemokines CXCL10 and macrophage inflammatory proteins 1alpha (CCL3/MIP-1alpha) and of the Th2- related chemokine macrophage inflammatory proteins 1 beta (CCL4/MIP-1beta) were observed in patients with AAD, which confirms the role of these chemokines in the autoimmune pathology of adrenal gland through the recruitment in loco of Th1 and Th2 cells (Bellastella *et al*, 2011).

Based on the above described body of evidence, we can hypothesize that Th1 cells play a major pathogenetic role, while autoantibody production is a side effect with no pathogenic relevance. The decrease in Treg activity is probably one of the main mechanisms at the basis of the unbalanced activity of Th1 cells. The active role of the adrenocortical cells in modulating the autoimmune inflammation, by producing Th1-attracting chemokines and cortisol, should not be underestimated. Based on knowledge derived from studies on ovarian autoimmunity (Samy *et al*, 2005), it is likely that the continuous drainage of autoantigens to regional lymph nodes be essential to maintain an adequate activity of antiinflammatory Treg cells and that the reduced activity of Tregs and the unbalance Th1/Th2 ratio observed in human endocrine autoimmunity occur at the site of regional lymph nodes.

5. Ovarian autoimmunity

Although it has been proposed that up to 30% of cases of primary ovarian insufficiency (POI) would have an autoimmune origin (Meskhi *et al*, 2006; Calongos *et al*, 2009), a more accurate estimate indicates that a documented ovarian autoimmune reaction is present in not more than 4-5% of women with ovarian insufficiency (Hoek *et al*, 1997; Bakalov *et al*, 2005).

Similarly to the study of adrenal autoimmunity, the unavailability of an animal model of spontaneous autoimmune oophoritis has limited the possibility to define the molecular mechanisms of immune-mediated ovarian insufficiency. The animal model of neonatal thymectomy has proven instrumental to unravel the critical role of $CD4^{+}CD25^{+}$ regulatory T (Treg) cells (Samy *et al*, 2006) in suppressing autoimmune processes in regional lymph nodes, under a continuous stimulation by autologous antigens (Samy *et al*, 2005). The ovarian autoantigen identified in the animal model of neonatal thymectomy is the ooplasm-specific MATER (Maternal Antigen That Embryo Requires) protein.

Immunization of mice with a peptide of inhibin alpha chain induced an initial increase in fertility, mediated by high serum levels of inhibin alpha neutralizing antibodies, that prevented inhibin-mediated downregulation of activin-induced FSH release (Altuntas *et al*, 2006). In a second, delayed phase, the activation of CD4+ T-cells resulted in a lymphocytic infiltration of the ovary that occurred in parallel with a progressive decrease in fertility and ovarian function (Altuntas *et al*, 2006).

However, it is still unclear to what extent these animal models are similar to human autoimmune POI.

Several lines of evidence support the autoimmune origin of a fraction of POI cases. Some autoimmune diseases are more frequent in women with POI than in the general population, and, conversely, POI occurs more frequently in women affected by some autoimmune diseases than in other women. Approximately 15% of women with POI present with autoimmune thyroiditis (Hoek *et al*, 1997) and the frequency of POI is higher in women with T1DM than in the general population (Hoek *et al*, 1997). However, it must be noted that biochemical and/or ultrasound signs of thyroiditis can be detected in 10-15% women in the general population and that the concomitant association of POI and thyroiditis or POI and T1DM in the same woman does not justify *per se* a diagnosis of "autoimmune POI". Surely more relevant is the association between POI and AAD (Betterle *et al*, 2002; Hoek *et al*, 1997; Falorni *et al*, 2002b). Approximately 4-8% of women with POI are positive for circulating adrenal autoantibodies, a frequency significantly higher than that expected in the general population (<0.5%) (Betterle *et al*, 2002; Falorni *et al*, 2002b). On the other hand, 10-20% of women with AAD develop POI before the age of 40 years (Betterle *et al*, 2002).

The existence of ovarian autoantibodies was first shown in the 1960's in studies that used indirect immunofluorescence on cryostatic sections of adrenal, ovary, testis and placenta (Blizzard *et al*, 1967; Irvine & Barnes, 1974). Subsequent studies have repeatedly confirmed the existence of ovarian autoantibodies in women with POI (Sotsiou *et al*, 1980; Elder *et al*, 1981; Ahonen *et al*, 1987; Betterle *et al*, 1993). Ovarian autoantibodies detected by indirect immunofluorescence cross-react with autoantigens expressed in other tissues, mainly the adrenal cortex, the testis and the placenta, which indicates that the autoantigen(s) recognized by these autoantibodies are not restricted to the ovary, but expressed also in other organs. Hence, a more correct definition of these autoantibodies is that of Steroid-Cell Autoantibodies (StCA). Interestingly, although all the tissue components are present in the ovarian cryostatic sections used for the autoantibody assay, the immunofluorescence pattern of StCA is restricted to the theca cells of the growing follicle with no staining of primary follicles or granulosa cells in secondary and tertiary follicles. The same autoantibodies stain specifically Leydig cells of the testis.

Although indirect immunofluorescence is still the most widely used method to detect ovarian autoantibodies in clinical practice, the accuracy of this method has been questioned, mostly because of a low diagnostic specificity (Novosad *et al*, 2003). Some of the autoantigens recognised by StCA have been identified as the steroidogenic enzymes 17α-hydroxylase (17OH) and side-chain cleavage (P450scc) (Chen *et al*, 1996; Perniola *et al*, 2000; Falorni *et al*, 2002b). The development of immunoradiometric assays, using *in vitro* translated recombinant human 35S-radiolabelled autoantigens, have enabled the estimate of the diagnostic sensitivity and specificity of 17OHAb and P450sccAb for autoimmune POI (Chen *et al*, 1996; Perniola *et al*, 2000; Falorni *et al*, 2002b).

17OHAb and P450sccAb are each present in 50 to 80% of women positive for StCA (Chen *et al*, 1996; Perniola *et al*, 2000; Falorni *et al*, 2002b). Over 90% of StCA-positive women are positive for 17OHAb and/or P450sccAb, which is demonstrating that 17OH and P450scc are major targets of StCA, but other autoantigens may also be recognized by a subset of StCA.

StCA, 17OHAb and/or P450sccAb can be detected almost exclusively in women with POI who are also positive for adrenal autoantibodies, most specifically 21OHAb. The association of steroid-cell autoimmunity with adrenal autoimmunity is so strong that 21OHAb appear to be the marker at highest diagnostic sensitivity for autoimmune POI (Perniola *et al*, 2000; Falorni *et al*, 2002b, Bakalov *et al*, 2005). Since only less than 0.5% of women with POI can be found positive for StCA in the absence of 21OHAb, 17OHAb or P450sccAb, we can conclude that unequivocal biochemical signs of ovarian autoimmunity against steroidogenic enzymes are present almost exclusively in women with clinical or pre-clinical AAD.

Several studies have demonstrated that an autoimmune oophoritis can be found at ovarian biopsy only in women positive for ovarian and/or adrenal autoantibodies (Irvine, 1980; Gloor & Hurlimann, 1984; Sedmak *et al*, 1987; Bannatyne et al, 1990; Hoek *et al*, 1997; Bakalov *et al*, 2005), thus confirming that steroidogenic cell autoantibodies identify women with an ongoing ovarian autoimmune process. On the other hand, in the absence of ovarian and adrenal autoantibodies, no histological sign of autoimmune infiltration can typically be detected at ovarian biopsy, even in women who present with other autoimmune diseases, such as thyroiditis, T1DM, inflammatory bowel disease or systemic lupus erithematosus. Accordingly, a classification of autoimmune POI cannot be based only on the presence of other autoimmune manifestations, in the absence of specific autoantibodies in the serum.

Autoimmune oophoritis is characterized by a selective mononuclear cell infiltration into the theca layer of large, antral follicles, with earlier stage follicles consistently free of lymphocytic infiltration (Hoek *et al*, 1997; Bakalov *et al*, 2005). This finding is in line with the selective staining of theca cells at the indirect immunofluorescence assay and confirms that the steroidogenic cell ovarian autoimmune process is mainly directed against theca cells.

The absence of steroidogenic cell autoantibodies does not exclude the possibility that other autoantibodies may be present and other autoimmune mechanisms may be active. Many other potential autoantigens, such as LH receptor (Moncayo *et al*, 1989), FSH receptor (Ryan & Jones, 2004), zona pellucida (Kelkar *et al*, 2005), 82-86 kDa Ags and 52-63 kDa Ags (Wheatcroft *et al*, 1997) have been proposed as markers of ovarian autoimmunity, but the association of these autoantibodies with POI has not been confirmed (Anasti *et al*, 1995;

Tonacchera *et al*, 2004). Only detection of autoantibodies against steroidogenic enzymes can, accordingly, ensure, at present, an accurate identification of women with autoimmune oophoritis. Using these autoantibody markers, autoimmunity accounts for approximately 4-5% of all POI cases.

Along with the decline of serum concentrations of estradiol, POI is typically characterized with a reduction in synthesis and secretion of inhibins (Petraglia *et al*, 1998) and anti-müllerian hormone (AMH) (Méduri *et al*, 2007), as a result of the progressive decline in ovarian function. In an initial study of three women with autoimmune POI (Welt *et al*, 2005) this general paradigma was however questioned, as increased serum concentrations of inhibin B were detected. This initial finding was confirmed in a subsequent larger study (Tsigkou *et al*, 2008) that demonstrated increased levels of serum inhibin B and total inhibin in a group of 22 women with autoimmune POI, as compared to 71 women with idiopathic, non-autoimmune POI and 90 healthy fertile women. The results of these studies (Welt *et al*, 2005; Tsigkou *et al*, 2008) led to the formulation of a novel hypothesis of the pathophysiology of autoimmune POI. Differently from other forms of ovarian insufficiency, in which a general reduction of ovarian function can be observed, autoimmune POI is characterized by the selective autoimmune destruction of theca cells with preservation of granulosa cells that produce low amounts of estradiol because of lack of substrates. The subsequent increase in FSH levels stimulates viable granulosa cells that, in return, produce increased amounts of inhibins.

AMH levels have been found to be normal in women with hypogonadotrophic amenorrhea while they are very low or undetectable in women with physiological menopause or hypergonadotrophic amenorrhea (POI) (Méduri *et al*, 2007; La Marca *et al*, 2006; Knauff *et al*, 2009). AMH is exclusively produced by primary and pre-antral/small antral follicles, and the immunohistochemical findings of the absence of an inflammatory reaction around primary follicles (Hoek *et al*, 1997; Bakalov *et al*, 2005) provided a sound rationale to estimate AMH production in women with autoimmune POI. We recently documented normal serum AMH concentrations in two-thirds of women with recently diagnosed autoimmune POI (La Marca *et al*, 2009), which provides the first demonstration of the existence of a subgroup of women with POI with a preserved ovarian follicle pool for several years. Since AMH is the best biochemical marker of residual follicle pool, the results of our study (La Marca *et al*, 2009) are highly relevant for the future planning of clinical trials of immunotherapy aimed at preserving the residual functional tissue and/or delay the progression of the destructive ovarian autoimmune process in women with autoimmune POI.

6. Conclusions

Autoimmune Addison's disease is made evident by the apperance of circulating 21OHAb, the gold immune marker for the identification of subjects with an ongoing adrenal autoimmune process. The appearance of 21OHAb marks pre-clinical autoimmune Addison's disease, in asymptomatic subjects. In these individuals, the response to the ACTH-stimulation test enables the discrimination of an early, potentially reversible phase, from an irreversible phase of the disease.

POI affects around 1% of women below the age of 40 years and the detection of steroid cell autoantibodies enables the identification of autoimmune cases. At present, only the detection of 21OHAb and 17OHAb or P450sccAb may accurately identify autoimmune cases of POI.

Although autoantibodies are widely used in clinical practice, they have no pathogenic role for either AAD or POI and these diseases are thought to be the consequence of a T-cell mediated autoimmune destruction.

Substitutive therapy of either AAD or POI is not influenced by presence or absence of autoantibodies, but identification of autoimmune forms of these disease is nevertheless important. Approximately two thirds of AAD patients have at least another associated autoimmune disease, either clinical or pre-clinical. Accordingly, screening for other autoimmune disorders is mandatory in autoimmune AAD, but not strictly necessary in other forms of PAI. More importantly, autoimmune POI has a distinct pathophysiology which differs from that of other forms of ovarian insufficiency. Detection of steroid-cell autoantibodies enables the identification of subjects with an initially preserved follicle pool.

No animal models of spontaneous steroid-cell autoimmunity are currently available, and there is strong need for the generation of such models that may enable the improvement of our understanding of the molecular mechanisms of these diseases.

During the next few years large multicentric studies are expected to be performed to identify subjects at high-risk for developing AAD and clinical trials are being planned with the aim of immunomodulate the adrenal autoimmune response and delay progression towards clinical AAD. The availability of novel immunological technologies will prove instrumental in the molecular characterization of the steroid cell autoantigens and peptides recognised by human autoreactive T cells responsible for the adrenocortical cell destruction. In addition, epidemiological studies are needed to provide novel insights on the role of putative environmental factors.

7. References

Ahonen P, Miettinen A, Perheentupa J. Adrenal and steroidal cell antibodies in patients with autoimmune polyglandular disease type I and risk of adrenocortical and ovarian failure. *J Clin Endocrinol Metab* 64:494–500 (1987).

Altuntas CZ, Johnson JM, Tuohy VK. Autoimmune targeted disruption of the pituitary-ovarian axis causes premature ovarian failure. *J Immunol* 177:1988-1996 (2006).

Anasti JN, Flack MR, Froehlich J, Nelson LM. The use of human recombinant gonadotropin receptors to search for immunoglobulin G-mediated premature ovarian failure. *J Clin Endocrinol Metab* 80:824-828 (1995).

Anderson JR, Goudie RB, Gray KG, Timbury GC. Autoantibodies in Addison's disease. *Lancet* 1:1123–1124 (1957).

Andrada JA, Bigazzi PL, Andrada E, Milgrom F, Witebsky E. Serological investigation on Addison's disease. *Clin Sci* 206:1535–1541 (1968).

Arvat E, Di Vito L, Laffranco F *et al*. Stimulatory effect of adrenocorticotropin on cortisol, aldosterone, and dehydroepiandrosterone secretion in normal humans: dose-response study. *J Clin Endocrinol Metab* 88:3141–3146 (2000).

Bakalov VK, Anasti JN, Calis KA, *et al*. Autoimmune oophoritis as a mechanism of follicular dysfunction in women with 46,XX spontaneous premature ovarian failure. *Fertil Steril* 84:958-965 (2005).

Bannatyne P, Russell P, Shearman RP. Autoimmune oöphoritis: a clinicopathologic assessment of 12 cases. *Int J Gynaecol Pathol* 9:191–207 (1990)

Barker JM, Ide A, Hostetler C *et al.* Endocrine and immunogenetic testing in individuals with type 1 diabetes and 21-hydroxylase autoantibodies: Addison's disease in a high-risk population. *J Clin Endocrinol Metab* 90:128-134 (2005).

Baumann-Antczak A, Wedlock N, Bednarek J *et al.* Autoimmune Addison's disease and 21-hydroxylase. *Lancet* 340:429–430 (1992).

Bednarek J, Furmaniak J, Wedlock N, *et al.* Steroid 21-hydroxylase is a major autoantigen involved in adult onset autoimmune Addison's disease. *FEBS Lett* 309:51–55 (1992).

Bellastella G, Rotondi M, Pane E, *et al.* Simultaneous evaluation of the circulating levels of both Th1 and Th2 chemokines in patients with Autoimmune Addison's Disease. *J Endocrinol Invest* (2011), in press

Betterle C, Scalici C, Presotto F, *et al.* The natural history of adrenal function in autoimmune patients with adrenal autoantibodies. *J Endocrinol* 117:467-475 (1988).

Betterle C, Rossi A, Dalla Pria S, et al. Premature ovarian failure: autoimmunity and natural history. *Clin Endocrinol (Oxf)* 39:53-43 (1993).

Betterle C, Volpato M, Rees-Smith B *et al.* I. Adrenal cortex and steroid 21-hydroxylase autoantibodies in adult patients with organ-specific autoimmune diseases: markers of low progression to clinical Addison's disease. *J Clin Endocrinol Metab* 82:932–938 (1997).

Betterle C, Volpato M, Pedini B, Chen S, Rees-Smith B, Furmaniak J.Adrenal-cortex autoantibodies (ACA) and steroid-producing cells autoantibodies (StCA) in patients with Addison's disease: comparison between immunofluorescence and immunoprecipitation assays. *J Clin Endocrinol Metab* 84:618–622 (1999).

Betterle C, Dal Pra C, Mantero F, Zanchetta R. Autoimmune adrenal insufficiency and autoimmune polyendocrine syndromes: autoantibodies, autoantigens, and their applicability in diagnosis and disease prediction. *Endocr Rev* 23:327–364 (2002).

Betterle C, Dal Pra C, Pedini B, *et al.* Assessment of adrenocortical function and autoantibodies in a baby born to a mother with autoimmune polyglandular syndrome Type 2. *J Endocrinol Invest* 27:618-21 (2004).

Björses P, Halonen M, Palvimo JJ *et al.* Mutations in the AIRE gene:effects on subcellular location and transactivation function of the autoimmune polyendocrinopathy-candidiasis-ectodermal dystrophy protein. *Am J Hum Genet* 66:378–392 (2000)

Blizzard RM, Kyle M. Studies of the adrenal antigens and autoantibodies in Addison's disease. *J Clin Invest* 42:1653–1660 (1963).

Blizzard RM, Chee D, Davis W. The incidence of adrenal and other autoantibodies in the sera of patients with idiopathic adrenal insufficiency (Addison's disease). *Clin Exp Immunol* 2:19–30 (1967).

Boscaro M, Betterle C, Volpato M, *et al.* Hormonal responses during various phases of autoimmune adrenal failure: no evidence for 21-hydroxylase enzyme activity block in vivo. *J Clin Endocrinol Metab* 81:2801–2804 (1996).

Bottomley MJ, Collard MW, Huggenvik JI *et al.* The SAND domain structure defines a novel DNA-binding fold in transcriptional regulation. *Nat Struct Biol* 8:626–33 (2001).

Brozzetti A, Marzotti S, La Torre D, *et al.* Autoantibody responses in autoimmune ovarian insufficiency and in Addison disease are IgG1-dominated and suggest a predominant, but not exclusive, Th1 type of response. *Eur. J. Endocrinol* 163:309-317 (2010a).

Brozzetti A, Marzotti S, Tortoioli C, *et al.* Cytotoxic T Lymphocyte Antigen-4 Ala17 polymorphism is a genetic marker of autoimmune adrenal insufficiency: Italian association study and meta-analysis of European studies. *Eur. J.Endocrinology* 162:361-9 (2010b).

Calongos G, Hasegawa A, Komori S, Koyama K. Harmful effects of anti-zona pellucida antibodies in folliculogenesis, oogenesis, and fertilization. *J. Reprod. Immunol.* 79:148-155 (2009).

Cetani F, Barbesino G, Borsari S *et al.* A novel mutation of the autoimmune regulator gene in an Italian kindred with autoimmune polyendocrinopathy-candidiasis ectodermal dystrophy, acting in a dominant fashion and strongly cosegregating with hypothyroid autoimmune thyroiditis. *J. Clin. Endocrinol. Metab.* 86:4747–4752 (2001).

Chen S, Sawicka J, Betterle C, *et al.* Autoantibodies to steroidogenic enzymes in autoimmune polyglandular syndrome, Addison's disease and premature ovarian failure. *J Clin Endocrinol Metab* 81:1871-1876 (1996).

Chen S, Sawicka J, Prentice L, *et al.* Analysis of autoantibody epitopes on steroid 21-hydroxylase (21-OH) using a panel of monoclonal antibodies. *J Clin Endocrinol Metab* 83:2977–2986 (1998).

Coco G, Dal Pra C, Presotto F, *et al.* Estimated risk for developing autoimmune Addison's disease in patients with adrenal cortex autoantibodies. *J Clin Endocrinol Metab* 91:1637-1645 (2006).

Coles AJ, Thompson S, Cox AL, Curran S, Gurnell EM, Chatterjee VK. Dehydroepiandrosterone replacement in patients with Addison's disease has a bimodal effect on regulatory (CD4+CD25hi and CD4+FoxP3+) T cells. *Eur J Immunol.* 35:3694-3703 (2005).

Colls J, Betterle C, Volpato M, Prentice L, Smith BR, Furmaniak J. Immunoprecipitation assay for autoantibodies to steroid 21-hydroxylase in autoimmune adrenal diseases. *Clin Chem* 41:375–380 (1995).

De Bellis A, Bizzarro A, Rossi R, *et al.* Remission of subclinical adrenocortical failure in subjects with adrenal autoantibodies. *J Clin Endocrinol Metab* 76:1002–1007 (1993).

De Rosa G, Corsello SM, Cecchini L, Della Casa S, Testa A. A clinical study of Addison's disease. *Exp Clin Endocrinol* 90:232–242 (1987).

do Carmo Silva R, Kater CE, Dib SA, *et al.* Autoantibodies against recombinant human steroidogenic enzyme 21-hydroxylase, side-chain cleavage and 17α-hydroxylase in Addison's disease and autoimmune polyendocrine syndrome type III. *Eur J Endocrinol* 142:187–194 (2000).

Durand B, Sperisen P, Emery P, Barras E, Zufferey M, Mach B, Reith W. RFXAP, a novel subunit of the RFX DNA binding complex is mutated in MHC class II deficiency. *EMBO J* 16: 1045-1055 (1997).

Elder M, Maclaren N, Riley W. Gonadal autoantibodies in patients with hypogonadism and/or Addison disease. *J Clin Endocrinol Metab* 52:1137–1142 (1981).

Falorni A, Nikoshkov A, Laureti S, *et al.* High diagnostic accuracy for idiopathic Addison's disease with a sensitive radiobinding assay for autoantibodies against recombinat human 21-hydroxylase. *J Clin Endocrinol Metab* 80:2752–2755 (1995).

Falorni A, Laureti S, Nikoshkov A, *et al.* 21-hydroxylase autoantibodies in adult patients with endocrine autoimmune diseases are highly specific for Addison's disease. *Clin. Exper. Immunol.* 107:341-345 (1997).

Falorni A, Laureti S, Candeloro P, *et al.* Steroid-cell autoantibodies are preferentially expressed in women with premature ovarian failure who have adrenal autoimmunity. *Fertility & Sterility* 78:270-279 (2002a).

Falorni A, Laureti S, Santeusanio F. Autoantibodies in autoimmune polyendocrine syndrome type II. *Endocrinol.Metab.Clin.N.Am.* 31:369-389 (2002b).

Falorni A, Laureti S, De Bellis A, *et al.* Italian Addison Network Study: Update of diagnostic criteria for the etiological classification of primary adrenal insufficiency. *J Clin Endocrinol Metab* 89:1598-1604 (2004).

Falorni A, Brozzetti A, La Torre D, Tortoioli C, Gambelunghe G. The association of genetic polymorphisms and autoimmune Addison's disease. *Expert Review of Clinical Immunology* 4:441-456 (2008).

Falorni A, Chen S, Zanchetta R et al. Measuring adrenal autoantibody response: interlaboratory concordance in the first international serum exchange for the determination of 21-hydroxylase autoantibodies. *Clin Immunol* (2011), in press, doi: 10.1016/j.clim.2011.04.012

Freeman M, Weetman AP. T and B cell reactivity to adrenal antigens in autoimmune Addison's disease. *Clin Exp Immunol* 88:275-279 (1992).

Furmaniak J, Talbot D, Reinwein D, Benker G, Creagh FM, Smith B. Immunoprecipitation of human adrenal microsomal antigen. *FEBS Lett* 232:25–28 (1988).

Furmaniak J, Kominami S, Asawa T, Wedlock N, Colls J, Rees-Smith B. Autoimmune Addison's disease. Evidence for a role of steroid 21-hydroxylase autoantibodies in adrenal insufficiency. *J Clin Endocrinol Metab* 79:1517–1521 (1994).

Gambelunghe G, Falorni A, Ghaderi M *et al.* Microsatellite polymorphism of the MHC class I chain-related (MIC-A and MIC-B) genes marks the risk for autoimmune Addison's disease. *J Clin Endocrinol Metab* 84:3701–3707 (1999).

Gambelunghe G, Kockum I, Bini V *et al.* Retrovirus-like long terminal repeat DQ-LTR13 and genetic susceptibility to type 1 diabetes mellitus and autoimmune Addison's disease. *Diabetes* 54:900-905 (2005).

Ghaderi M, Gambelunghe G, Tortoioli C *et al.* MHC2TA single nucleotide polymorphism and genetic risk for autoimmune adrenal insufficiency. *J Clin Endocrinol Metab* 91:4107-4111 (2006).

Gloor E, Hurlimann J. Autoimmune oöphoritis. *Am J Clin Pathol* 81:105–109 (1984).

Goudie RB, Anderson JR, Gray KK, Whyte WG 1966 Autoantibodies in Addison's disease. *Lancet* 1:1173–1176 (1966).

Hayashi Y, Hiyoshi T, Takemura T, Kurashima C, Hirokawa K. Focal lymphocytic infiltration in the adrenal cortex of the elderly: immunohistological analysis of infiltrating lymphocytes. *Clin Exp Immunol* 77:101-105 (1989).

Hoek A, Schoemaker J, Drexhage HA. Premature ovarian failure and ovarian autoimmunity. *Endocr Rev* 18:107-134 (1997).

Husebye ES, Bratland E, Bredholt G, Fridkin M, Dayan M, Mozes E. The substrate-binding domain of 21-hydroxylase, the main autoantigen in autoimmune Addison's disease, is an immunodminant T cell epitope. *Endocrinology* 147:2411-2416 (2006).

Irvine WJ, Stewart AG, Scarth L. A clinical and immunological study of adrenocortical insufficiency (Addison's disease). *Clin Exp Immunol* 2:31–69 (1967).

Irvine WJ, Barnes EW. Addison's disease and associated conditions: with particular references to premature ovarian failure, diabetes mellitus and hypoparathyroidism. In: Gell PH, Coombs RRA, Lachman P, eds. Clinical aspects of immunology. Oxford, UK: Blackwell; 1301–1354 (1974).

Irvine WJ, Toft AD, Feek CM. Addison's disease. In: James VHT, ed. The adrenal gland. New York: Raven Press; 131–164 (1979).

Irvine WJ. Autoimmunity in endocrine disease. *Recent Prog Horm Res* 36:509–556 (1980)

Karin M. New twists in gene regulation by glucocorticoid receptor: is DNA binding dispensable? *Cell* 93:487–490 (1998).

Kasperlik-Zaluska AA, Migdalska B, Czarnocka B, Drac-Kaniewska J, Niegowska E, Czech W. Association of Addison's disease with autoimmune disorders—a long-term observation of 180 patients. Postgrad Med J 67:984–987 (1991).

Kelkar RL, Meherji PK, Kadam SS, Gupta SK, Nandedkar TD. Circulating autoantibodies against the zona pellucida and thyroid microsomal antigen in women with premature ovarian failure. *J Repr Immunol* 66:53-67 (2005).

Knauff EAH, Eijkemans MJC, Lambalk CB, *et al.* Anti-müllerian hormone, inhibin B, and antral follicle count in young women with ovarian failure. *J Clin Endocrinol Metab* 94:786–792 (2009).

Kong MF, Jeffcoate W. Eighty-six cases of Addison's disease. *Clin Endocrinol (Oxf)* 41:757–761 (1994).

Kosowicz J, Gryczynska M, Bottazzo GF. A radioimmunoassay for the detection of adrenal autoantibodies. *Clin Exp Immunol* 63:671–679 (1986).

Kriegel MA, Lohmann T, Gabler C, Blank N, Kalden JR, Lorenz HM. Defective suppressor function of human CD4+ CD25+ regulatory T cells in autoimmune polyglandular syndrome type II. *J Exp Med* 199:1285–1291 (2004).

Krohn K, Uibo R, Aavik E, Peterson P, Savilahti K. Identification by molecular cloning of an autoantigen associated with Addison's disease as steroid 17α-hydroxylase. *Lancet* 339:770–773 (1992).

La Marca A, Pati M, Orvieto R, Stabile G, Carducci Artenisio A, Volpe A. Serum Anti-Mullerian Hormone levels in women with secondary amenorrhea. *Fertil Steril* 85:1547-1549 (2006).

La Marca A, Marzotti S, Brozzetti A, *et al.* Primary ovarian insufficiency due to steroidogenic cell autoimmunity is associated with preserved pool of functioning follicles. *J Clin Endocrinol Metab* 94:3816-3823 (2009).

Laureti S, De Bellis A, Muccitelli VI, *et al.* Levels of adrenocortical autoantibodies correlate with the degree of adrenal dysfunction in subjects with preclinical Addison's disease. *J Clin Endocrinol Metab* 83:3507–3511 (1998).

Laureti S, Vecchi L, Santeusanio F, Falorni A. Is the prevalence of Addison's disease underestimated? *J Clin Endocrinol Metab* 84:1762 (1999)

Laureti S, Arvat E, Candeloro P, *et al.* Low dose (1 μg) ACTH test in the evaluation of adrenal dysfunction in pre-clinical Addison's disease. *Clin Endocrinol (Oxf)* 53:107–115 (2000).

Laureti S, Candeloro P, Aglietti MC, *et al.* Dehydroepiandrosterone, 17α-hydroxyprogesterone and aldosterone responses to the low-dose (1 μg) ACTH test in subjects with preclinical adrenal autoimmunity. *Clin Endocrinol (Oxf)* 57:677-683 (2002).

Løvås K, Husebye ES. High prevalence and increasing incidence of Addison's disease in western Norway. *Clin Endocrinol (Oxf)* 56:787–791 (2002)

Magitta NF, Bøe Wolff AS, Johansson S *et al.* A coding polymorphism in NALP1 confers risk for autoimmune Addison's disease and type 1 diabetes. *Genes Immun.* 10:120-124 (2009).

Masternak K, Barras E, Zufferey M *et al.* A gene encoding a novel RFX-associated transactivator is mutated in the majority of MHC class II deficiency patients. *Nature Gen* 20:273-277 (1998).

McHardy-Young S, Lessof MH, Maisey MN. Serum TSH and thyroid studies in Addison's disease. *Clin Endocrinol (Oxf)* 1:45–56 (1974).

Méduri G, Massin N, Guibourdenche J, *et al.* Serum anti-Müllerian hormone expression in women with premature ovarian failure. Hum Reprod 22:117-123 (2007).

Meskhi A, Seif MW. Premature ovarian failure. *Curr. Opin. Obstet. Gynecol.* 18:418-426 (2006).

Moncayo H, Moncayo R, Benz R, Wolf A, Lauritzen C. Ovarian failure and autoimmunity. Detection of autoantibodies directed against both the unoccupied luteinizing hormone/human chorionic gonadotropin receptor and the hormonereceptor complex of bovine corpus luteum. *J Clin Invest* 84:1857-1865 (1989).

Myhre AG, Undlien DE, Løvås K *et al.* Autoimmune adrenocortical failure in Norway autoantibodies and human leukocyte antigen class II associations related to clinical features. *J Clin Endocrinol Metab* 87:618-623 (2002).

Nekrep N, Jabrane-Ferrat N, Wolf HM, Eibl MM, Geyer M, Peterlin BM. Mutation in a winged-helix DNA-binding motif causes atypical bare lympocyte syndrome. *Nature Immunol.* 3:1075-1081 (2002).

Nerup J, Andersen V, Bendixen G. Anti-adrenal, cellular hypersensitivity in Addison's disease. *Clin Exp Immunol* 4:355-363 (1969).

Nerup J, Andersen V, Bendixen G. Anti-adrenal, cellular hypersensitivity in Addison's disease. IV. In vivo and in vitro investigations on the mitochondrial fraction. *Clin Exp Immunol* 6:733-739 (1970).

Nerup J. Addison's disease-clinical studies. A report of 108 cases. *Acta Endocrinol (Copenh)* 76:127–141 (1974).

Neufeld M, MacLaren NK, Blizzard RM. Two types of autoimmune Addison's disease associated with different polyglandular autoimmune (PGA) syndromes. *Medicine (Baltimore)* 60: 355–362 (1981).

Nikoshkov A, Falorni A, Lajic S, *et al.* A conformation-dependent epitope in Addison's disease and other endocrinological autoimmune diseases maps to a carboxyl-terminal functional domain of human steroid 21-hydroxylase. *J Immunol* 162:2422–2426 (1999).

Nomura K, Depura H, Saruta T. Addison's disease in Japan: characteristics and changes revealed in a nationwide survey. *Intern Med* 33:602–606 (1994).

Novosad JA, Kalantaridou SN, Tong ZB, Nelson LM. Ovarian antibodies as detected by indirect immunofluorescence are unreliable in the diagnosis of autoimmune premature ovarian failure: a controlled evaluation. *BMC Womens Health* 3:2 (2003)

Oelkers W. Adrenal insufficiency. *N Engl J Med* 335:1206–1212 (1996)

Papadopoulos KI, Hallengren B. Polyglandular autoimmune syndrome type II in patients with idiopathic Addison's disease. *Acta Endocrinol (Copenh)* 122:472–478 (1990).

Park YS, Sanjeevi CB, Robles D *et al.* Additional association of intra-MHC genes, MICA and D6S273, with Addison's disease. *Tissue Antigens* 60:155-163 (2002).

Perniola R, Falorni A, Clemente MG, Forini F, Accogli E, Lobreglio G. Organ-specific and non-organ-specific autoantibodies in children and young adults with autoimmune polyendocrinopathy-candidiasis-ectodermal dystrophy (APECED). *Eur J Endocrinol* 143:497-503 (2000).

Petraglia F, Hartmann B, Luisi S, *et al.* Low levels of serum inhibin A and inhibin B in women with hypergonadotropic amenhorrea and evidence of high levels of activin A in women with hypothalamic amenhorrea. *Fertil Steril* 70:907-912 (1998).

Pitkänen J, Doucas V, Sternsdorf T *et al.* The autoimmune regulator protein has transcriptional transactivating properties and interacts with the common coactivator CREB-binding protein. *J Biol Chem* 275:16802–16809 (2000).

Pitkänen J, Vähämurto P, Krohn K *et al.* Subcellular localization of the autoimmune regulator protein. characterization of nuclear targeting and transcriptional activation domain. *J Biol Chem* 276:19597–19602 (2001).

Rabinowe SL, Jackson RA, Dluhy RG, Williams GH. Ia-positive T lymphocytes in recently diagnosed idiopathic Addison's disease. *Am J Med* 77:597–601 (1984).

Reith W, Mach B. The bare lymphocyte syndrome and the regulation of mhc expression. *Annu. Rev. Immunol.* 19:331-373 (2001).

Rotondi M, Falorni A, De Bellis A *et al.* Elevated serum interferon-γ-inducible chemokine-10/CXC chemokine ligand-10 in autoimmune primary adrenal insufficiency and *in vitro* expression in human adrenal cells primary cultures after stimulation with proinflammatory cytokines. *J Clin Endocrinol Metab* 90:2357–2363 (2005).

Rotondi M, Chiovato L, Romagnani S, Serio M, Romagnani P. Role of chemokines in endocrine autoimmune diseases. *Endocrine Rev* 28:492-520 (2007).

Ryan MM, Jones HR Jr. Myasthenia gravis and premature ovarian failure. *Muscle Nerve* 30:231-233 (2004).

Samy ET, Parker LA, Sharp CP, Tung KSK. Continuous control of autoimmune disease by antigen-dependent polyclonal CD4+CD25+ regulatory T cells in the regional lymph node. *J Exp Med* 202:771-781 (2005).

Samy ET, Setiady YY, Ohno K, Pramoonjago P, Sharp C, Tung KSK. The role of physiological self-antigen in the acquisition and maintenance of regulatory T-cell function. *Immunol Rev* 212:170-84 (2006).

Sedmak DD, Hart WR, Tubbs RR. Autoimmune oöphoritis: a histopathologic study involved ovaries with immunologic characterization of the mononuclear cell infiltrate. *Int J Gynecol Pathol* 6:73–81 (1987).

Skinningsrud B, Husebye ES, Gervin K *et al.* Mutation screening of PTPN22: association of the 1858T-allele with Addison's disease. *Eur J Hum Genet.* 16:977-982 (2008a).

Skinningsrud B, Husebye E, Pearce SH et al. Polymorphisms in CLEC16A and CIITA at 16p13 are associated with primary adrenal insufficiency. *J Clin Endocrinol Metab* 93:3310-3317 (2008b).

Sotsiou F, Bottazzo GF, Doniach D. Immunofluorescence studies on autoantibodies to steroid-producing cells, and to germline cells in endocrine disease and infertility. *Clin Exp Immunol* 39:97–111 (1980).

Stechmesser E, Scherbaum WA, Grossman T, Berg PA. An ELISA method for the detection of autoantibodies to adrenal cortex. *J Immunol Methods* 80:67–76 (1985).

Su MA, Giang K, Zumer K *et al.* Mechanisms of an autoimmune syndrome in mice caused by a dominant mutation in Aire. *J Clin Invest* 118:1712-1726 (2008).

Söderbergh A, Winqvist O, Norheim I, *et al.* Adrenal autoantibodies and organ-specific autoimmunity in Addison disease. *Clin Endocrinol (Oxf)* 45:453–460 (1996).

Tanaka H, Perez MS, Powell M *et al.* Steroid 21-hydroxylase autoantibodies: measurements with a new immunoprecipitation assay. *J Clin Endocrinol Metab* 82:1440–1446 (1997).

The Finnish-German APECED Consortium. An autoimmune disease, APECED, caused by mutations in a novel gene featuring two PHD-type zinc-finger domains. Autoimmune Polyendocrinopathy-Candidiasis-Ectodermal Dystrophy. *Nat Genet* 17:399–403 (1997).

Tonacchera M, Ferrarini E, Dimida A, *et al.* Gonadotrophin receptor blocking antibodies measured by the use of cell lines stably expressing human gonadotrophin receptors are not detectable in women with 46,XX premature ovarian failure. *Clin Endocrinol (Oxf)* 61:376-381 (2004).

Tsigkou A, Marzotti S, Borges L, et al. High serum inhibin concentration discriminates autoimmune oophoritis from other forms of primary ovarian insufficiency. *J.Clin.Endocrinol.Metab.* 93:1263-1269 (2008).

Welt CK, Falorni A, Taylor AE, Martin KA, Hall JE. Selective theca cell dysfunction in autoimmune oophoritis results in multifollicular development, decreased estradiol, and elevated inhibin B levels. *J Clin Endocrinol Metab* 90:3069-3076 (2005).

Wheatcroft NJ, Salt C, Milford-Ward A, Cooke ID, Weetman AP. Identification of ovarian antibodies by immunofluorescence, enzyme-linked immunosorbent assay or immunoblotting in premature ovarian failure. *Hum Reprod* 12:2617-2622 (1997)

Winqvist O, Karlsson FA, Kämpe O. 21-Hydroxylase, a major autoantigen in idiopathic Addison's disease. *Lancet* 339:1559–1562 (1992).

Winqvist O, Gustafsson J, Rorsman F, Karlsson FA, Kämpe O. Two different cytochrome P450 enzymes are the adrenal antigens in autoimmune polyendocrine syndrome type I and Addison's disease. *J Clin Invest* 92:2377–2385 (1993).

Wuepper KD, Weigienka LC, Hugh Fudenberg H. Immunologic aspect of adrenocortical insufficiency. *Am J Med* 46:206–216 (1969).

Yu L, Brewer KW, Gates S *et al.* DRB1*04 and DQ alleles: expression of 21-hydroxylase autoantibodies and risk of progression to Addison's disease. *J Clin Endocrinol Metab* 84:328-335 (1999).

Zelissen PM, Bast EJ, Croughs RJ. Associated autoimmunity in Addison's disease. *J Autoimmunity* 8:121–130 (1995).

16

Excretion of Steroid Hormones in Rodents: An Overview on Species Differences for New Biomedical Animal Research Models

Juan Manuel Busso[1,3] and Rubén Daniel Ruiz[2,3]
[1]Instituto de Ciencia y Tecnología de Alimentos, Facultad de Ciencias Exactas, Físicas y Naturales (FCEFyN) – Universidad Nacional de Córdoba (UNC)/ Consejo Nacional de Investigaciones Científicas y Técnicas (CONICET)
[2]Instituto de Fisiología, Facultad de Ciencias Médicas, UNC
[3] Established investigators from the CONICET
Argentina

1. Introduction

Living organisms have regular patterns and routines that involve obtaining food and carrying out life-history stages such as breeding, migrating, molting and hibernating. The acquisition, utilization, and storage of energy reserves (and other resources) are critical to lifetime reproductive success, and this reproductive process could be affected by predictable and unpredictable environmental changes (McEwen and Wingfield, 2003; Schneider, 2004). Allostasis is achieving physiological stability through change (see details in McEwen and Wingfield, 2003); the allostatic state refers to altered and sustained activity levels of the primary mediators, i.e., glucocorticosteroids that integrate physiology and associated behaviors in response to changing environments and challenges. Focused on these primary mediators, particularly in steroid hormones, it has been well accepted for a long time that variations (increases) of adrenal glucocorticoids are associated with stress responses. Moreover, measuring changes in glucocorticoid concentration (and also in levels of adrenaline and noradrenaline) has been the most frequently used strategy to monitor physiological responses to stress and distress challenges (Terlouw et al, 1997; Wielebnowski, 2003; Mormède et al, 2007; Sheriff et al., 2011). In terms of changes in steroid secretory patterns in response to a stressor, glucocorticoids are known to change over the course of minutes and those levels will subsequently (within hours to days) affect steroid reproductive hormones (such as testosterone, estradiol and progesterone) (Sapolsky et al., 2000).

While experiencing severe stress, animals, as humans, can succumb to disease or fail to reproduce or develop properly (Moberg, 2000). Therefore, animals have evolved a suite of physiological and behavioral strategies to cope with environmental changes as well as to survive in a particular given time and space (Buchanan, 2000; Romero, 2004). Therefore, "environmental endocrinology" has developed in response to the need to understand how hormones modulate and control physiological processes in animals exposed to the exigencies of their particular natural environment. This has only been possible through spectacular developments in hormone assay techniques, which now make feasible hormone measurements on microlitre volumes of body fluids (Bradshaw, 2007). Four biological samples have been employed up to the present: blood, saliva, excreta (feces and urine), and integumentary structures (hair and feathers), each of them having advantages and disadvantages for use with different species and research purposes (Sheriff et al., 2011).

Blood collection continues being an attractive and reliable technique for steroid analysis; several reports for different species are available in the literature, such as for Japanese quail (Arora, 1979) or chinchilla (Tappa et al, 1989); these *species-specific reports provide recommendations on safety, ease of collection and repeated collections*. However, in a study of endocrine dynamics this approach may be impractical because blood extraction is a powerful stressor and it is known that within minutes, glucocorticoid secretion is stimulated and gonadal steroid secretion declines. For example, blood samples collected only from birds reflect unstressed (baseline) glucocorticoid concentrations with a high degree of confidence within less than 2 minutes (Sapolsky et al., 2000; Romero and Reed, 2005). In addition, when experiments involve small animals it is usually difficult to obtain the necessary blood volume, and repeated blood sampling can interfere with subsequent hormone measurements, and it may even be harmful as it has been reported for chinchilla. In large-sized bird and mammalian species, such as Greater Rhea (Léche et al., 2009) and Clouded Leopard (Wielebnowsky et al., 2002), blood collection may be dangerous for the operator and certainly stressful for animals. Blood sample collection is always a critical procedure in the laboratory, and an impractical approach in nature without the aid of auxiliary techniques (such as anesthesia); therefore, these "Gold" microliters of plasma/serum are always appreciated by researchers.

Hormones secreted by adrenal and gonad glands go through the bloodstream to their target tissues and cells, where they initiate a change in cellular activity by attaching to a receptor protein. Thereafter, steroids are excreted into the bile to undergo metabolic changes in the intestinal tract due to the enzymatic activity of the intestinal microflora. Also, enterohepatic recirculation of steroid metabolites, with possible further metabolic changes in the liver, is known to occur in many species. The reabsorbed metabolites may be excreted in the bile again or pass into urine (Taylor, 1971). Evaluating steroid metabolite content and/or profiles in either urine or feces represents an alternative technical approach without perturbing individuals, populations or animal species. This experimental strategy has been applied to a wide range of research goals in captive and free-ranging wildlife, as well as domestic and laboratory species. Several reviews focusing on steroid metabolism and the validation of particularly fecal steroid assays have been published in the last years (Schwarzenberger et al., 1996; Brown and Wildt, 1997; Monfort, 2003; Palme et al., 2005; Schwarzenberger, 2007).

The obvious advantage of assessing urinary or fecal hormone concentrations is that adrenal and gonadal functions can be determined without even touching the animal: the waste is simply recovered from the adequately arranged ground or enclosure floor and analyzed in the laboratory. Resulting hormonal profiles are generally less "noisy" than those observed after analyzing blood because the excretory patterns represent a pool of metabolites rather than reflecting the often hour-to-hour fluctuating dynamism quantified in blood (Pukazhenthi and Wild, 2004). According to recent reviews, it seems that this approach, noninvasive monitoring, will be utilized more than ever when well-focused endocrine issues are addressed and some steroids are involved (Palme and Möstl, 2002; Pukazhenthi and Wildt, 2004; Palme, 2005; Schwarzenberger, 2007). In fact, international programs have trained science students, especially researches from Latin American PhD programs (Swanson and Brown, 2004), as it can found in the reports of Busso et al. (2005a, 2007), Ponzio et al. (2004) in Argentina, of Brousset Hernández-Jauregui et al. (2005) in Mexico, and of Moreira et al. (2007) in Brazil. Similarly, new studies fully developed in traditionally called developing countries are clear evidence of the usefulness of this non-invasive approach (Leche et al., 2009, 2011). Furthermore, national funds or grants in these developing countries are becoming available to develop this type of noninvasive hormone research; e.g., in Argentina, new doctoral fellowships are being granted to support these studies.

A particular disadvantage of fecal steroid analysis is the presence of a vast number of different fecal steroid metabolites even in closely related species. For the development of techniques for fecal steroid analysis, experiments on the metabolism of radioactively labeled steroids have provided a valuable insight into the metabolism and excretion of hormone metabolites via feces and urine (Schwarzenberger, 2007; see discussion below). By contrast, steroids voided into urine are not extremely degraded; however, the use of urine steroids has the particular disadvantage that urine collection in some animals requires restraint in a metabolic cage, surgical interference or rigorous surveillance to collect samples during urination (Peter et al., 1996; Monfort, 2003). In non-invasive monitoring of steroid activity, several aspects must be considered before undertaking a new study, and/or focusing on a new species, or applying a new immunoassay (Millspaugh and Washburn, 2004; Buchanan and Goldsmith, 2004; Palme, 2005; Touma and Palme, 2005; Wielebnowski and Watters, 2007; Hayward et al., 2010).

When we intend to measure steroid metabolites in excreta, firstly we need to obtain them, usually by an extraction technique that should be simple, safe and efficient. Secondly, we usually need an immunoassay to detect (accurately, precisely, and specifically) variation of steroid levels in the matrix of interest. All these laboratory and validation steps as well as interpretation of results are strongly affected by information about steroid metabolism and catabolism; animal biological characteristics must be also taken into account (individual development, reproductive stage, nutritional strategy, copying strategy, etc.) during result analysis. Although we have not focused our revision on these aspects, the reader must be aware of them and their importance in the application of non-invasive monitoring.

As we have addressed steroid excretion, we need to know some aspects about steroid excretion before employing some immunoassays to reveal steroid activity: 1) **route of excretion** of each hormone to be evaluated, 2) **time-course** of steroid secretion in blood-stream and its clearance into urine and feces, 3) **proportion of excreted metabolites during biological cycles**, 4) **identification of steroid metabolites in the matrix selected**. These variables may be determined by injecting the hormone, usually a radiolabeled steroid or, less frequently, a large amount of unlabeled steroid and tracking their metabolite excretion over time. For example, Wielebnowski and Watters (2007) indicate that the types of fecal steroid metabolites excreted, the main route of excretion, and the time it takes for metabolization and excretion to occur should be identified before selecting an antibody and assay system. Normative data on steroid excretion is essential for improving the application of non-invasive monitoring; in addition, this information would be an extraordinary source of knowledge to compare several aspects of animal environmental endocrinology.

Therefore, based on updated endocrine data from wild, laboratory and farmed rodents, we propose to develop a comparative endocrine survey of the routes of gonadal and adrenocortical steroid excretion. In our laboratory, chinchilla were subjected to radiometabolism studies of progesterone, corticosterone, testosterone and estradiol (Ponzio et al, 2004; Busso et al, 2005a, 2007). Since domesticated chinchilla still share some genomic characteristics with their counterparts in the wild, the analysis would serve as an adequate example of widely diverse interests (scientific, ecological, economic, cultural and emblematic values). Basically, our endocrinological studies contribute with some specific data from this particular large rodent to the existing data for other rodents. The information provided can be helpful for:

In situ studies: 1- assessment of ecological phenomena, focused on environmental endocrinology, i.e. by quantifying field concentrations of stress hormones in individual organisms; 2- identification of healthy individuals from endangered wild populations to develop reproductive *ex situ* programs.

Ex situ studies: 1- diagnosis of reproductive functions and dysfunctions of valuable farmed individuals 2- application of assisted reproductive techniques; 3- improvement of welfare of animal model for studying biomedical research; 4- development of new experimental biotypes for the study of hormonal disruptive effects of environmental pollute.

In general, reviews about those topics have apparently neglected information about rodents. These animals are not regarded as threatened mammals, and public appreciation about their biological importance is scarce and tends to overlook the ecological role and conservation problems of an order representing about 41% of mammalian species (Gippoliti and Amori, 1998; Amori and Gippoliti, 2001, 2003). However, the order Rodentia is a tremendous biodiversity example of life strategies, with more than 2000 species, which encompass a staggering diversity of form, behavior and physiology. Additionally, scientists have frequently employed several rodent species to conduct research, and have used rodents even as animal models for biomedical studies.

2. Excretion of steroid hormones

Nowadays, it is widely accepted that basic knowledge of the metabolism and excretion of glucocorticoids is necessary for the development of a non-invasive technique to monitor adrenocortical activity (Möstl and Palme, 2002). Similarly, information of sex steroid metabolism is essential to monitor steroidogenic activity of gonads (Brown et al, 1994). The first step in assay development is identifying the excretory routes for each hormone of interest; conducting an infusion study would be extremely valuable in domestic and nondomestic animals, if captive-held counterparts are available and the tests are feasible (Wielebnowski and Watters, 2007), such as the studies performed in domestic chinchilla to evaluate wild chinchilla (Busso et al, 2005a, 2007; see further details below). We also accept that, in practical terms, it is unnecessary to determine the specific molecular structure of the hormones being monitored in each species. However, it is critical to demonstrate that fluctuations in the hormone metabolites being measured provide physiologically relevant information (Monfort, 2003). Accordingly, it is well accepted that endocrine glands must be challenged to monitor their activation, e.g., by injecting ACTH or dexamethasone and measuring whether glucocorticoid levels in the tested matrix reflects the predicted changes in the blood. The use of a biological test or the so called "biologically relevant tests" (that expose an animal to a biological stressor to measure the glucocorticoids in samples) is also recommended; this ensures that the noninvasive monitoring will appropriately measure glucocorticoids in the field when animals are exposed to genuine stressors (Sheriff et al., 2011). Several reports may be useful to set up an experimental design for applying a non-invasive approach (Brown and Wildt, 1997; Wasser et al., 2000; Palme and Möstl, 2002;

Buchanan and Goldsmith, 2004; Millspaugh and Washburn, 2004; Palme, 2005; Goymann, 2005; Klasing, 2005; Palme et al., 2005; Wielebnowski and Watters, 2007).

Pharmacological and biological relevance tests are truly useful for validating non-invasive endocrine monitoring. Nevertheless, such validations should not miss the radiolabelling studies, since these allow us to discover, investigate and/or discuss the functional relevance of steroids. In fact, steroid receptors and the co-evolution of steroidogenic enzymes and steroid-inactivating enzymes had an important role in the evolution of complex regulatory networks in vertebrates, contributing to vertebrate survival and diversification in the last 500 million years (Baker, 1996, 2003).

Cholesterol is the precursor of the five major classes of steroid hormones. According to their number of carbon-atoms, these classes are: progestagens, glucocorticoids (and mineralcorticoids, C21); androgens (C19); and estrogens (C18). Because of their common precursor cholesterol, they are apparently all structurally related across birds and mammalian species; however, they show strong functional differences. Steroid hormones bind to intracellular proteins, termed receptors, which function as transcription factors. The receptors are specific for a given class of steroid. These receptors are members of the large superfamily of nuclear hormone receptors that include different hormones such as glucocorticoids, mineralocorticoids, vitamin A, thyroid and retinoids, as well as sex steroids (Brown, 1999). It is also well known that steroid hormones are synthesized in a number of endocrine tissues, mainly gonads, adrenals, and placenta.

Steroid hormones are dissociated from their receptors and metabolized by the target cell or the liver, which possess enzymes capable of altering the specific steroids and rendering them biologically inactive and water soluble. Typically, inactivation involves reduction or removal of side chain or attached groups or both, as well as the combination with other molecules (conjugation), such as glucose, to form a glucuronide or conjugation with sulfate. The relative emphasis on sulfate or glucuronide varies depending on the steroid and/or species (Norris, 2007). During this inactivation process, steroids are metabolized in the liver and excreted via the bile into the gut. Enterohepatic recirculation of steroid metabolites, with possible further metabolic changes in the liver, may facilitate steroid metabolite reabsorption; the reabsorbed metabolites would be excreted in the bile again or pass into urine. More than 40 years ago, Taylor (1971) revised studies on the excretion of steroid hormone metabolites in bile and feces. Regarding steroid metabolites, those of the less polar molecules tend to be excreted in bile to a greater extent than metabolites of polar steroids; e.g., progesterone metabolites are mainly present in bile (and feces). In contrast, hydrocorticortisone (cortisol) is almost completely excreted as urinary metabolites. On the basis of evidence reviewed, a hypothesis was postulated suggesting that the membrane of the bile canaliculi would have receptor sites specific for certain steroids metabolites (Taylor, 1971). The binding of these substances at the receptor sites is an obligatory step prior to active transfer of the substances across the canalicular membrane. In "primitive" mammals, such as rats and mice, the receptor sites have poor specificity and are therefore able to bind metabolites of most steroid hormones. In other species, evolution has resulted in a decrease in the number, specificity and binding capacity of these sites. Therefore, some steroid metabolites are partially bound and so excreted into bile (e.g., progesterone), whereas others are less firmly, or not, bound and therefore return to the blood by a passive or active transport. This hypothesis seems to go some way to explaining the difference in biliary excretion of steroid metabolites among species, and the excretion of different steroids by the same species. Radioinfusions have offered data as new evidence for increased caution in the inferences due to differences between species.

As pointed out above, it is possible to evaluate gut passage time using radiometabolism studies, in which radio-labeled steroids are usually injected and then clearance of radioactivity into urine and faecal compartments is monitored (Brown et al., 1994; Palme et al., 1996); this procedure reflects time delay quite precisely and therefore provides a rough estimate of the expected delay. The delay time between circulation of steroids in plasma and their appearance in urine samples is usually rather short (less than 5 h), but fecal steroid metabolites have an appreciable lag time (Palme et al., 1996; Schwarzenberger et al., 1996). For example, lag time or time course of fecal excretion may range from less than 30 minutes to more than one day, depending on the species, sometimes even within species, depending on the activity rhythms of animals (Palme and Möstl, 2002; Monfort, 2003; Palme, 2005). Recently, Touma et al. (2003) indicated that metabolism and excretion of corticosterone in urine and feces of mice are not only significantly affected by sex, but also by the time of day when the radioactive peak was observed (after administration). Several radiometabolism studies demonstrated that oestrogens in the form of estradiol and/or estrone are present in fecal samples; by contrast, testosterone, progesterone and, especially, cortisol/corticosterone are heavily metabolized and the original hormone is barely present in the feces (Schwarzenberger, 2007). Therefore, the route of excretion varies considerably among species, and among steroids within the same species.
This chapter focuses on the updated comparative endocrine analysis of the routes of excretion of gonadal and adrenocortical steroids, taking into account the published information on non-invasive analyses being used by a variety of scientists (e.g., conservation biologists, animal scientists) to examine glucocorticoid (i.e., stress hormone) and gonadal steroids (i.e. reproductive hormones) secretion in domestic and wild rodents. Also, radiolabeled procedures have also provided useful results for testing the efficiency of different protocols for extracting hormones from samples (Schwarzenberger et al, 1996).

3. Measurements of steroids in rodent excreta: Use of radiolobelled infusions for evaluation of corticosterone/cortisol, progesterone, testosterone and estradiol catabolism

Over 40% of mammal species belong to the order Rodentia. While rodents are often thought of as just mice and rats, more than 2000 species in this order encompass a staggering diversity of form, behavior and physiology. In fact, excluding the human species, the order Rodentia is the group of most prosperous modern mammals, occupying very different ecological niches in almost all the planet, mostly specialized in rapid reproduction that can be adjusted to different circumstances (Conaway, 1971; Young, 1985; Bronson, 1999). At present, based on rodent morphology of their lower jaw, living rodents are divided into two suborders: the Sciurognathi (squirrel and mouse-like forms) and the Hystriocognathi (cavy-like forms). Although this classification might still be a matter of debate as well as those based on the long-standing division of the insertion patterns of masseter muscles or the plane of incisor insertions (Mess et al., 2001; Huchon et al., 2002; Kay et al. 2008), these aspects are beyond the scope of present review. We currently support or choose the present classification of rodents as squirrel and mouse or cavy-like forms. It has been proposed that Rodentia is a monophyletic group; however, several molecular studies have suggested that the guinea pig and its relatives (such as Hystriocognathi or cavy-like forms) are closer to other orders of mammals than to families of rats and mice. For example, taking into account that insulin is a conservative molecule in mammals, as we might think of steroids,

Hystricognathi species represent an exception having a very divergent molecule with unusual physiological properties among rodents (Opazo et al, 2005).
In our laboratory, we have been studying aspects of reproductive biology in chinchilla (*Chinchilla lanigera*) for over 15 years (Ponce et al., 1998a, b; Carrascosa et al., 2002; Ponzio et al., 2004, 2007a, b, 2008; Busso et al., 2005a, b, c, 2007). This is an interesting taxon, since domesticated chinchilla used for the fur industry still share some genomic characteristics with their endangered (almost extinct) counterparts. Actually, *Chinchilla* spp. are critically endangered in South American wild populations according to the IUCN (IUCN/SSC Rodent Specialist Group):

Wild rodents
Chinchilla lanigera, a chinchillid from the Cordillera de la Costa and rocky Andean slopes of Chile (400-2500 m asl), which is threatened by the fur trade and habitat loss due to overgrazing, firewood collection, and mining. **Chinchilla brevicaudata**, another chincillid from the central Andean region of Peru, Bolivia, Argentina, and Chile. This species inhabits at higher altitudes (over 3,000 m asl), and is also threatened by the fur trade. Although its actual status is poorly known, it is already extinct in Argentina and Peru and probably is facing extinction in other parts of its range. The Convention on International Trade in Endangered Species of Wild Fauna and Flora (CITES), lists in Appendix I all South American populations of Chinchilla, but no other rodents. According to Lidicker (IUCN/SSC Rodent Specialist Group, 1989), these listings by IUCN and CITES do not mean for sure that the populations of most rodent species are in good health, but only that we know very little about them.

Box 1. a status in nature must be verified in CITES and IUCN before start a new radiolabelled steroid infusion

Back to steroid hormones, most of the knowledge about endocrine modulation of reproductive physiology in *Chinchilla* spp. has been derived from studies in females (Tam, 1971, 1972; Brookhyser and Aulerich, 1980; Gromadzka-Ostrowska and Sylarska-Gozdz, 1984; Gromadzka-Ostrowska et al., 1985). With respect to the male endocrine reproductive physiology, Cepeda et al. (2006) obtained a plasma testosterone profile during the annual reproductive cycle, showing that endocrine activity increased immediately before the breeding season. Other studies performed using blood sampling have also been reported in chinchilla (Brookhyser et al., 1977; Tappa et al., 1989); however, serial samples taken over time induced injury in some animals. Alternatively, we validated a tool for non-invasively assessing endocrine testicular and ovary activity as well as adrenocortical activity by detecting hormone changes in excreta (Ponzio et al., 2004; Busso et al., 2005a, 2007).
We subjected some males and females to radiometabolism studies of testosterone, and progesterone and estradiol, respectively; we also studied corticosterone excretion in males. Firstly, after assessing ^{14}C-testosterone metabolite excretion in male chinchilla (Busso et al., 2005a), several urinary and fecal androgen metabolites were separated by HPLC for their identification, but only fecal metabolites were associated with native testosterone. More than one metabolite derived from ^{14}C-testosterone showed immunoreactivity and further

biochemical and biological tests demonstrated that the employment of excreta would be useful to assess endocrine testicular function in this species. In female chinchillas, we also performed radiolabeled infusion of ^{3}H-estradiol and ^{14}C-progesterone, but in contrast to testosterone assessment, natural steroids were evaluated (were separated by HPLC-UV) in urinary and fecal extracts from pregnant individuals. This is a particular protocol to avoid the use of radioactive material in technical procedures, as normally expected at present. Chromatographic analyses demonstrated that most peaks were associated with the polar mobile phase in urine, whereas in feces, there were both polar and non-polar peaks. All HPLC fractions were individually analyzed by UV detector and by estradiol or progesterone immunoassays. These experiments suggest that chinchillas excrete native forms of progesterone and estradiol in low concentrations in urine and feces, whereas only progesterone-derived metabolites appear to be present in both excreta (Busso et al., 2007). Figure 1 depicts reproductive endocrine normative data with respect to route of steroid excretion in chinchilla (Hystricognathi rodent).

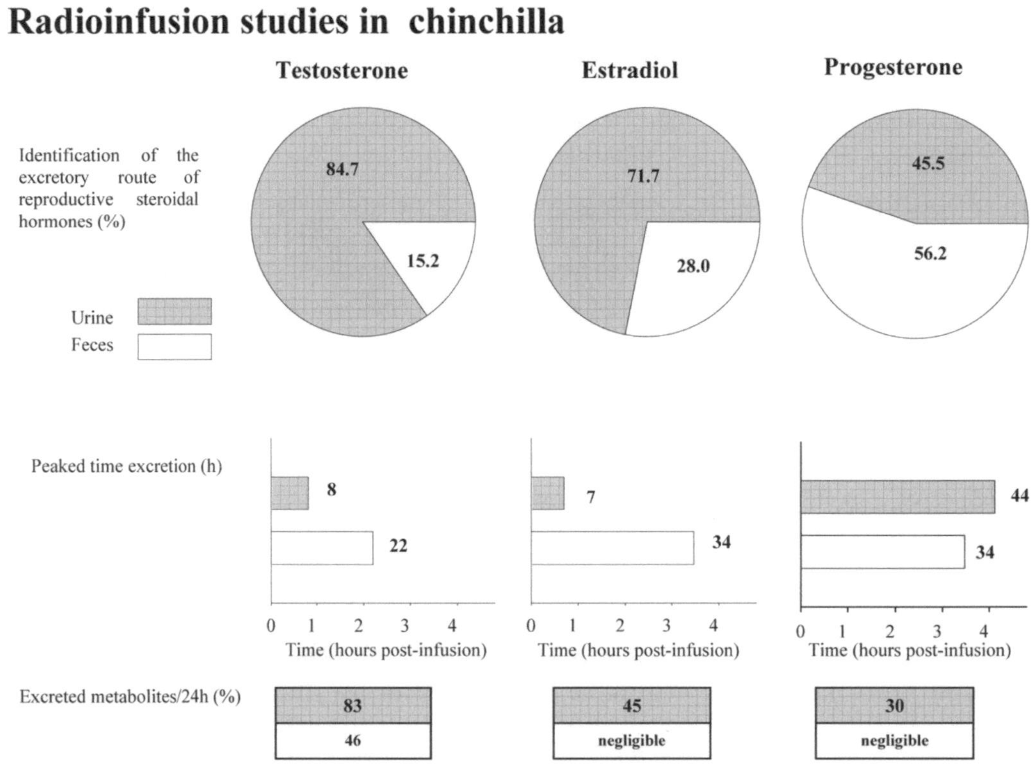

Fig. 1. Characterization of testosterone metabolite excretion in urine and feces after isotope administration (i.m.) in chinchilla males (n = 4; details in Busso et al. 2005a). Similarly, estradiol and progesterone metabolite excretion in excreta after isotope administration (i.p.) in chinchilla females (n = 4; details in Busso et al. 2007).

Furthermore, in the same experimental model, we also established that the urinary route of corticosterone excretion was predominant in male (Ponzio et al., 2004) and HPLC analysis revealed that most corticosteroids are excreted as readily hydrolysable steroid conjugates of

cortisol. Results shown together with data on corticosterone excretion in Figure 1 clearly demonstrate that urine is the main route, except for progesterone, where radioactive metabolites were almost equally found in urinary (45.5 ± 13.5%) and fecal extracts (56.2 ± 4.9%). As expected, radioactive peaks generally appeared earlier in urine than in feces. However, estradiol and progesterone radioactive metabolite time-courses showed great individual differences between 24-48 h post infusions, the highest percentages of excreted radioactive metabolites being detected during 48h post-infusion.
Interestingly, based on these results from our radiometabolism studies and those reported for other rodents subjected to radiolabeled infusion up to this moment, we considered that the route of steroid metabolite excretion varies depending on the rodentia suborder. Therefore, it was proposed that the urinary route is preferential in Hystrichomorpha (chinchilla and guinea pigs; currently considered cavy-like forms) while in the Sciurognathi (squirrel and mouse-like forms, formerly considered Sciumorpha or Myormorpha suborders), the primary excretory route is the feces (Busso et al., 2006, Ponzio et al., 2006).
To our best knowledge, Taylor (1971) provided the best compilation of radiometabolism studies in mammalian species reported in the literature up to the present. Two of Taylor's major conclusions are relevant for our purposes: a) different steroids are excreted to different extents in urine and feces; this is evident, for example, in our comparative endocrinological studies in chinchilla (see Figure 1); and b) the same steroid is excreted to different extents in urine and feces of different species; reports revised by Taylor in the 1970s and most of the reports published thereafter are included in Figure 2. In this illustration our compilation is arranged according to our hypothesis of preferential route of steroid metabolite excretion in Rodentia suborders (see details in legend). It can be useful to take into account certain physical-chemical natural characteristics of steroids; considering the physico-chemical characteristics of steroid polarity, steroids are firstly shown in Figure 2 according to their water solubility (considering that steroids are heavily metabolized and the original hormone is barely present, particularly in the feces). Anyway, according to recent revisions, taxonomic relatedness does still little to predict the precise nature of metabolites or their relative routes of excretion (urine versus feces; Palme et al. 2005; Schwanzenberger, 2007).

3.1 Hystricognathi (cavy-like forms)

Both Guinea pigs and chinchilla are commonly employed as animal models in biomedical investigations. These species belong to the hystricomorph group of rodents that are well represented in South America, and have remarkably long reproductive cycles compared to other rodents.
Few studies on the comparative aspects of steroid metabolism and excretion in cavy-like forms (chinchilla and guinea pig) are available; published data of most reproductive steroids indicate that they are excreted mainly by urine (except for progesterone in chinchilla, see above). Fewer studies are available for sex steroids in this group of rodents; Bogdan and Monfort (2001) evaluated fecal estrogen and progesterone profiles in breeding and non-breeding females of the North American porcupine (*Erethizon dorsatum; Erethizontoidae family*). For glucocorticoids, cortisol is the main adrenal steroid hormone present in guinea pig plasma (Malinowska and Nathanielsz, 1974). No studies applying radiolabeled glucocorticoids in guinea pig have been conducted according to our last search, but apparently cortisol metabolites are found in large quantities in urine (Fajer and Vogt, 1963).

Results of the application of a non-invasive technique in chinchilla indicate that glucocorticoids would present mainly in urine (Ponzio et al., 2004), and that cortisol would also be the main adrenal steroid. Cortisol was also detected in an experiment employing a cortisol RIA in blood samples of *Octodon degus* (*Octodontoidae family*); in addition, an ACTH positive effect on blood cortisol profile and cortisol fecal metabolite excretion was detected (Soto Gamboa et al., 2009). However, in the latter study it is difficult for us to establish a close correlation between results from different matrices because of sampling regimens.

3.2 Sciurognathi (squirrel and mouse-like forms)

Rats and mice are also widely used as animal models of human diseases in biomedical research. Other rodents such as those in the sciurid group, e.g., ground squirrel, have been extensively used as mammalian models of ecology, population regulation, and behavior. Nevertheless, Lepschy et al. (2007), as other authors, argued that the small body size of rodents and difficulties involved in blood sampling make it difficult to apply an invasive procedure. We should keep in mind that stress is a significant source of experimental errors and a major cause of stress in laboratory animals, and reducing stressful conditions in normal husbandry and in application of methods is essential to achieve an adequate level of reliability in the experimental results (Dahlin et al., 2009). Therefore, a non-invasive technique to monitor stress hormones in these animals is highly desirable (Siswanto et al., 2008; Touma et al., 2004; Thanos et al, 2009; Kalliokoski et al., 2010).

Likewise, Harper and Austad (2000) developed a noninvasive method for measuring adrenal activity in house mice, deer mice, and red-back voles (*members of Muridae and Cricetidae families*), as other authors did in old field mice (*Cricetidae family;* Good et al., 2003), in spiny mice (*Acomys cahirinus; Muridade family*) (Nováková et al., 2008; Frynta et al., 2009), in agouti and non-agouti deer mice (*Peromyscus maniculatus; Cricetidae family*) (Hayssen et al., 2002), and in Columbian ground squirrel (*Sciuridae family*) (Bosson et al, 2009). Similarly, although most of those authors did not perform a previous radioinfusion study, a noninvasive assessment proved to be useful also in different reproductive studies conducted in others small rodents (DeCantanzaro et al., 2003; Kuznetzov et al., 2004; Cavigelli et al., 2005; Chelini et al., 2005).

In mice, corticosterone and testosterone are excreted mainly by feces. Although several reports showed aspects of steroid metabolism in some rodents such as mice during the 1960s and 1970s, new studies have contributed to increase that limited information. Touma et al. (2003) injected mice i.p. with ^{3}H-corticosterone; although males excreted significantly more radioactive metabolites via the feces than females (72 vs 56%), this study demonstrated once again that most corticosterone metabolite excretion was via the feces in both sexes. Conversely, Kalliokoski et al. (2010) reported that corticosterone metabolite content is about 50% higher in urine than in feces; therefore, they recommended that future studies should analyze primarily the output in urine, although this matrix is volatile and difficult to collect. Billiti et al. (1998) employed 3 mice and 3 deer mice (3–24 months of age) to perform radiolabeled testosterone infusion (intraperitoneally), and found that the proportion of the injected testosterone excreted in feces was 62% for *Mus* spp. and 58% for *Peromyscus* spp. Noteworthy, it has been reported that in mice, the rate of excretion vs. time profile showed between two and three elimination phases in urine and feces (and more than 90% excreted testosterone metabolites were found during first 24 h). This information revealed that the first phase corresponded to radioactive testosterone that went directly to highly perfused tissues such as liver and kidney, and the second phase corresponded to a slower component in which hormone is sequestered in slowly perfused tissues such as adipose tissues; also, the route of administration, such as the intraperitoneal one, may favor the excretion of testosterone in one phase over another. All these are important considerations not only for future experiments but also for application in field studies.

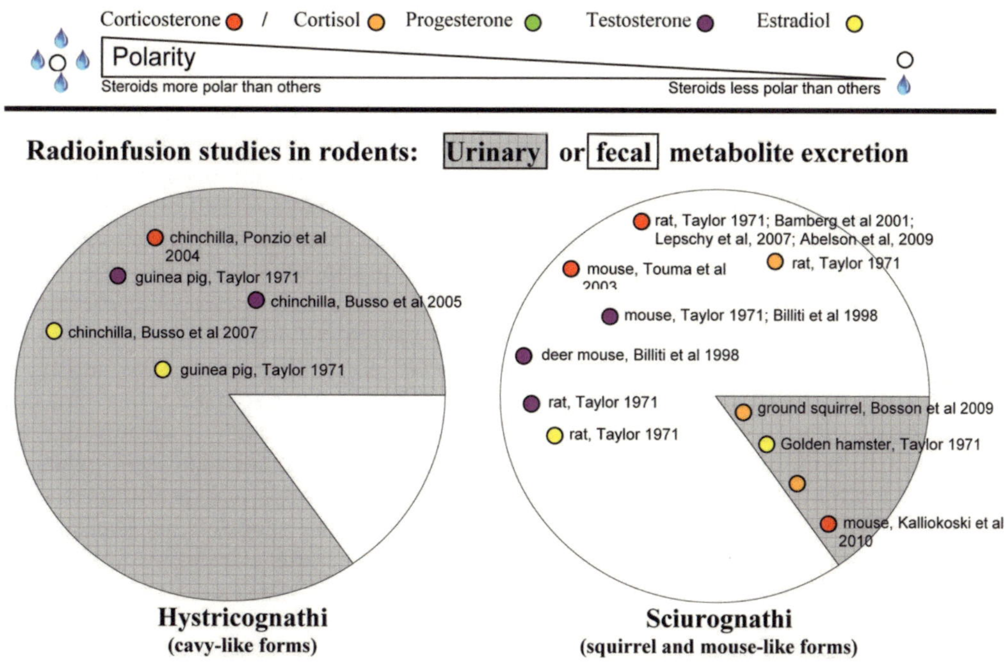

Fig. 2. Compilation of radiometabolism studies in rodent species reported in the literature. Firstly, adrenal and sex steroids are ordered according to solubility in aqueous phase in an "ideal" physical chemistry system in the laboratory. Pie charts are illustrated according to that hypothesis that postulates that in Hystricognathi rodents the urinary route (gray) is preferential, whereas in Sciurognathi, feces (white) is the primary excretory route (details in the text); the size of gray and white portions in both pie charts is only illustrative. Colors of circles are associated with steroids; in addition, circles as well as references were located according to the main route of excretion of each hormone of interest in the studied species, i.e. in Sicurognathi: feces: corticosterone in rat: similar results are revealed by different reports, e.g., Taylor, 1971; Bamberg et al., 2001; Lepschy et al., 2007 and Abelson et al., 2009.

Recently, cortisol radioinfusions were informed for squirrel species (Bosson et al., 2009; Dantzer et al., 2010) as well the application of noninvasive monitoring in Cape ground squirrel (Pettitt et al., 2007). In Columbian ground squirrel, this glucocorticoid is highly metabolized, with virtually none being excreted. The percentages of radioactive cortisol recovered were 31% and 6.5% in urine and feces, respectively; it can be argued that these values are low. The authors accepted this problem but, because of the characteristics of excreta collection, results were certain only for feces. Similar results were obtained by Dantzer et al. (2010), who injected radiolabeled cortisol in North American red squirrel; the hormone was entirely metabolized and excreted in both urine (70.3 ± 0.02%) and feces (29.7 ± 0.02%), with a lag time to peak excretion of 10.9 ± 2.3 h in feces. With respect to cortisol excretion in mouse-like forms, we found only one reference (for rat, Taylor, 1971); the main route was feces, as well as for corticosterone in other Sciurognathi rodents. Since squirrels belong to the Sciuridade family, which is closer to Lagomorpha than the Muridae family (rat and mouse, etc.), this genetic proximity would explain these results. Accordingly, low fecal excretion of glucocorticoid metabolites (about 8%) has also been found in European hares (*Lepus europaeus;* Teskey- Gerstl et al., 2000). In fact, Taylor (1971) informed (another species of Lagomorpha order) that only between 3-5% of testosterone or 4% of estradiol are excreted in rabbit feces.

Similarly to the studies analyzed above, different techniques have been applied in rats to monitor the route, time-course and proportions of excreted steroid metabolites. Bamberg et al. (2001) employed male Sprague-Dawley 8 week-old rats which were injected i.p. with ^{3}H-corticosterone (16 µCi) at 09:00. Meanwhile, Lepschy et al. (2007) started an experiment at the same time as the former study; however, each rat (both sexes were employed in this study; 12 week-old individuals) was intravenously injected with different doses of ^{3}H-corticosterone (62.1 µCi). Both studies showed that the main route of corticosterone excretion in the male was feces. It is quite difficult to compare both studies since a different sample collection technique was applied. Firstly, when employing only males, during the first day, urine or feces samples were collected at different time schedule. Lepschy et al. (2007) collected all voided excreta from both sexes during the first day (probably the most recommended). Both radioactive urinary peaks were detected earlier than feces peaks, but there was a great variability in urine: 1-6h and 4-10h, respectively. Technical differences in the study of the same steroid in the same species were further reported by Abelson et al. (2009), who studied male Sprague-Dawley rats after intravenous administration of a low dose (1µCi) of radioactive corticosterone. The amount of radioactivity detected in feces was highest and displayed a more pronounced peak 12h after injection when the substance was administered through a jugular vein catheter than through tail vein injection.

As expected, it is evident that there were great differences in the profiles of radioactive excretion among individuals in rodents, particularly in well studied species such rats and mice, as in others mammals (Brown et al, 1994; Palme et al, 1996), i.e., time course may change with the route and time of administration, even between sexes in some species (see detailed studies on rats: Touma et al., 2003; Eriksson et al., 2004; Abelson et al., 2009). Similarly, in chinchilla, Busso et al. (2005a, 2007) also indicated that radioactive urinary estradiol peaked between 24-48h, the radioactive peak being at 34h post-infusion. Several technical aspects, rather than biological ones, must be taken into account before deciding to undertake a new investigation; from molecular structure of interested hormone (free marked or conjugated steroid), through animal state and development, up to sample collection regimen, etc. Further studies are necessary to standardize how to obtain endocrinological information from animal "waste" as soon as possible.

A key advantage of measuring hormones in excreta is that this procedure integrates hormone levels over time, instead of measuring a single time point (as in snapshot) represented by hormone levels in blood. We consider that time peak excretion after radioinfusion or steroid hormone increase after gland has been stimulated is not a robust measure because there are too many sources of variation. Several variables, such as dietary preferences, gastrointestinal anatomy, digestive physiology, biochemical capabilities, and commensal microflora, called "nutritional strategy" by Klasing (2005) in birds, may affect retention time and consequently time course of excreted steroids among species and/or individuals of the same population. Besides, a different sample collection schedule also seriously affects interpretation of time course or hormonal profiles; collecting naturally all voided urine or feces is advisable, as it has been observed in many reports. Therefore, in attempting to collect all samples, some problems may arise, i.e., in the study of testosterone excretion in chinchilla, an "animal effect" associated with each hormonal profiles was found. This effect evoked a delayed excretion of testosterone metabolites in some males with respect to others; a constipation process was a probable source of variation that has previously been detected in other farmed animals (Palme et al., 1996; Busso et al., 2005a). It is advisable to use each animal as its own control, thereby minimizing the problems of individual differences in basal and peak levels (Touma and Palme, 2005).

Urinary and fecal excretion frequency may be affected by other factors, such as some stressors effects on different individuals. Nowadays, increasing evidence indicates considerable variation between individuals in the magnitude and pattern of their corticosterone responses (called "personalities"). Furthermore, regularity of food intake and resulting defecation frequency has not been investigated sufficiently and needs to be considered as a potential variable for steroid metabolite analyses. In addition, changes in defecation frequency and patterns due to seasonal variation, reproduction, or even stress may alter elimination rate and therefore systematically affect the amount of metabolites excreted per sample (Wielebnowski and Watters, 2007). Further experiments are necessary to enhance our understanding of kinetic parameters; these variables are still significant research topics or unresolved issues that will allow us to elucidate the relationship between physiological events and detection of changes in excreta.

Elimination of steroids via the urine is usually very rapid as maximal concentration is found within a few hours after administration of radioactive tracer and/or peak natural concentrations in the plasma; the first urinary samples collected usually exhibit most of the excreted metabolites. In feces, peak concentrations of radioactivity were observed after a certain lag time (usually after 24 h or up to 48h) (Monfort, 2003; Palme, 2005; Schwanzenberger, 2007). However, this is not a particularly useful or informative measure as it is highly dependent on the sampling regimen, and fails to account for differences in the general shape of the hormone excretion-time profile (Kalliokoski et al. 2010). Thus, we consider that proportion of total metabolites excreted per activity phase (such as dark/light cycle; endocrine cycles, etc.) would be more informative than the exact time of peak excretion; however, most importantly, hormone monitoring must be performed in repeated long-term studies.

The reviewed information is significantly useful because when monitoring stress and/or reproductive endocrine responses in a long-term study, competitive immunoassays will be used in different matrices (urine, feces, etc) to reveal adrenal and/or gonadal endocrine activities. Thus, depending on the species, the hormone, and the research question, it is relevant to "pick" the appropriate antibody and assay design that allows for detection of most, or at least a considerable amount, of the immunoreactive metabolites involved (Wielebnowski and Watters, 2007). Otherwise, some problems may arise when working with a matrix that exhibits lowest concentration of excreted metabolites. For example, an assay for testosterone fecal metabolites in guinea pig failed to clearly discriminate among intact males, castrated males, and females (Bauer et al., 2008). In addition, it was not possible to detect fecal progestagen changes throughout pregnancy, pre-partum and post-partum stages in chinchilla compared with results obtained from urine samples (Busso et al., 2007).

This does not mean that we do not recommend working with samples with low steroid concentrations. In fact, there are good examples like the report of Muir et al. (2001), involving urinary samples of female and male mice, since this mouse species excretes reproductive steroids mainly by feces. However, greatest efforts are needed when samples are collected from the less quantitative route of steroid excretion in a given species.

4. Remarkable issues for a precise assessment of steroid hormone excretion in rodents

Steroid hormones have demonstrated a major regulatory role in vertebrate physiology (affecting, for example, fetal and postnatal growth and development, and maintaining allostasis, particularly, progesterone or glucocorticoids, as other examples, which are important in female reproduction or are involved in the "fight or flight" response). The physiological changes mediated by adrenal and sex steroids receptors provided early vertebrates with an advantage in competing with the diverse organisms that evolved during the Cambrian explosion (Baker, 1997). Therefore, it is of great importance and interest to study how these hormonal modulators respond to different environmental conditions, such as the studies of chemical disruptors on endocrine activity with implications in normal neuroendocrine responses (Crews et al., 2000; Dickerson and Gore, 2007)

Let´s remember that rodents are eutherian mammals (Short, 1985) and that one obvious way of increasing or decreasing an animal's reproductive potential is by altering its gestation length. Three groups stand out with respect to gestation length/maternal weight ratio: hystricomorph rodents as well as primates have relatively long gestations, and whales with relatively short gestations. Hystricomorph rodents, here called cavy-like form, have evidently developed a different reproductive strategy than other rodents. By contrast, Sciurognathi species generally exhibit small body size, short lifespan, short gestation (21 days in mice and rats),numerous litters, and rapid rates of development, as well as short birth intervals (all these species called "r" strategist in ecology). All rodent species together amount to 2000 different taxa; however, information mostly comes from few species of two families (Muridae: Old World mice, rats, gerbils and relatives or Cricetidae: New World rat, mice, voles, hamsters and relatives). These families are genetically closely related and have been well studied: they display differences of degree but not of kind.

Contrarily, Hystricomorph rodents (about 170 species) appear to be more diversified in their patterns of reproduction than any other group of related mammals. The hystricomorph rodents, which are particularly well represented in South America, have colonized harsh environments at either high altitude or high latitudes. Under such conditions, it would be advantageous for a species like the chinchilla to prolong gestation (more than 100 days) so as to allow birth during clement weather. However, this environmental explanation cannot account for the long gestations of those hystricomorphs that live in subtropical forests, or those that live in underground burrows as the plains viscacha (Weir and Rowlands, 1973; Short, 1985; Bronson, 1999). Therefore, this group of mammals (rodents), excluding the human species, is the group of most prosperous modern mammals, occupying very different ecological niches almost worldwide, mostly specialized in different rhythms of reproduction that can be adjusted to different circumstances. This biodiversity offers several phenotypes or biotypes of animals to study general and comparative endocrinological aspects. Finally, how these animals have synchronized to cope with habitats and face environmental challenges up to present is one of our major research concerns.

Regarding our research work that focused on chinchilla, we considered only steroid excretion in rodents in this chapter. It was not our goal to thoroughly review the details of each species. We found out that few species of rodents were subjected to radiolabeled studies of steroid excretion. According to the latest publications, taxonomic relatedness does little to predict the precise nature of metabolites or their relative routes of excretion (urine versus feces; Palme et al. 2005; Schwanzenberger, 2007). The best way to clarify these questions is to perform radiometabolism experiments and a physiological and biological validation of the immunoassay, such as the work conducted in Columbian ground squirrel (Bosson et al., 2009). However, at present, radioinfusion as an experimental approach to the noninvasive study of adrenal and/or gonadal activity seems "old-fashioned". Accordingly, we did our best to include in the present revision as many reports of application of non-invasive hormone monitoring in rodents species as possible. We also know that it may not be possible to elucidate why different steroids are excreted in urine and feces to different extents; however, a better framework for rodents is now available with respect to differences among species in terms of the same steroid being excreted in urine and feces to different extents. In the assessment of adrenal and gonadal endocrine activities using non-invasive techniques, several extensive considerations should be taken into account (Buchanan and Goldsmith, 2004; Millspaugh and Washburn, 2004; Palme, 2005; Touma and Palme, 2005; Schwarzenberger, 2007; Wilebnowski and Watters, 2007); however, these aspects are beyond the scope of the present revision, but all of them may be affected by the ranking of the excretory routes.

Accordingly, multidisciplinary scientific efforts might be useful to increase our knowledge on comparative endocrinology in rodents, using different species as biotypes or new animal models for the studies. Some concerns about it have already been stated. Smale et al. (2005) pointed out that the study of neuroendocrinology in nontraditional mammals is an essential approach that complements methodologies (such as knock-out mouse) by taking advantage of allelic variation produced by natural selection. Obviously, the technical advantages of non-invasive hormonal monitoring with repeated measures in long-term studies have strongly encouraged biologists (and specialists such as ecologists, ethologists, etc.) as well as other professionals in human and veterinary medicine, zoological exhibition and/or animal production managers.

In summary, the application of noninvasive hormonal monitoring has proven very useful for the generation of normative data (for the species, reproductive cycles, stress responses, etc.) and particularly for the assessment of individual endocrine state. All the aspects shown in Box 2 must be addressed for a precise assessment of steroid hormone excretion.

Finally, one of the main advantages of measuring steroids in blood is the study of the dynamics of hormone secretion; however, great efforts must be made to meet the technical requirements for obtaining a blood sample for an accurate and reliable measurement (route of blood extraction, minimal obtained blood volume, extraction time to avoid stress interference in steroid profiles, etc.). Therefore, hormonal quantification in different biological matrices such urine and feces is an alternative approach. But also, this approach does not exclude technical disadvantages involved in sample collection, such as frequency of elimination of excreta, volume of excreta (which can affect the distribution of hormone metabolites, etc.). Therefore, both types of samples, blood and excreta, are seriously affected by the sampling protocol. Laboratories should continue reviewing (and possibly standardizing) this aspect. In addition, there are extra sources of variation affecting sampling protocol such as nutritional strategy, which also seriously alter the precise hormonal determination. Moreover the fact that an individual may be studied without being disturbed, another interesting aspect in the use of non-invasive hormone monitoring is that metabolite concentrations frequently are 2 to 4 times higher than plasma levels (Peter et al., 1996). However, this quantitative advantage is lost when the route of steroid excretion is unknown.

"Keys for a precise assessment of steroid hormone excretion"

- **Who?** ID of steroids of interest; particularly it is necessary to know species differences and to identify the main glucocorticoid by the adrenal gland in rodents (cortisol or corticosterone).
- **How much?** Percentage of hormone metabolite excretion into urine or feces; route of excretion may be determined by radiolabeled or unlabeled infusion of each hormone of interest.
- **When it happened?** Time course of steroid secretion in blood-stream and its clearance into urine and feces. The best approach is to collect all voided urine and excreted feces, because there is still no standardization with respect to sampling protocols. In the future, it seems that proportion of excreted metabolites during activity cycles (day/night; elimination phases) may be a better approach to understanding steroid excretion with respect to individual endocrine state.
- **Which matrix?** After choosing the biological matrix (urine or feces), identification of steroid metabolite in the matrix of interest is essential to obtain the best results in immunoassay performance. Each matrix has advantages and disadvantages.
- **How are results expressed?** To follow the endocrine gland activity in the best way possible, it would be useful to express hormone excretion rated by fixed period of time (i.e. hour of sample collection) and to inform total volume or weight/period of time of voided urine and excreted feces, respectively.
- **What else?** Sex, life stages (juvenile, adult, aging change), environmental characteristics (photoperiod, temperature, feeding strategy, coping strategy) must be taken into account to improve our knowledge.

ID: identification.

Box 2. Recycling information from excretes about animal stress and reproductive endocrine states in rodents.

5. Acknowledgements

J. M. Busso jmbusso@conicet.gov.ar and R. D. Ruiz are Established Investigators from CONICET, Argentina and their contributions were supported by CONICET, Agencia Córdoba Ciencia, SECyT-UNC and FONCyT, Argentina.

6. References

Abelson, KSP, Fard SS, Nyman J, Goldkuhl R, Hau J. (2009). Distribution of (^{3}H)-corticosterone in urine, feces and blood of male Sprague-Dawley rats after tail vein and jugular vein injection. In Vivo: 23: 381-386.

Amori G and Gippoliti S, (2003) A higher–taxon approach to rodent conservation priorities for the 21st century. Animal Biodiversity and Conservation, 26: 2: 1-18

Amori, G Gippoliti, S. (2001). Identifying priority ecoregions for rodent conservation at the genus level. Oryx 35, 158-165

Baker, ME. (1997). Steroid receptor phylogeny and vertebrate origins. Mol Cell Endocrinol, 135: 101-107.

Baker, ME. (2003). Evolution of adrenal and sex steroid action in vertebrates: a ligand-based mechanism for complexity. BioEssays, 25: 396-400.

Biddlecombe R.A. and Law B., (1996). Validation of an immunoassay. In Brian Law (ed): Immunoassay a practical guide. Taylor and Francis Ltd, London, pp 171-203.

Blanga-Kanfi S, Miranda H, Penn O, Pupko T, DeBry RW, Huchon D. (2009). Rodent phylogeny revised: analysis of six nuclear genes from all major rodents clades. BMC Evolutionary Biology 9:71, 2148-9-71.

Bosson CO, Palme R, Boonstra R. (2009). Assessment of the stress response in Columbian Ground Squirrels: laboratory and Field validation of an enzyme immunoassay for fecal cortisol metabolites. Physiol Biochem Zool 82: 291-301.

Bogdan D, Monfort SL. (2001). Faecal oestrogen and progesterone profiles in breeding and non-breeding female north American porcupine (*Erethizon dorsatum*). Mammalia 65, 73-82.

Bradshaw D. (2007). Enviromental endocrinology. Gen Comp Endocrinol, 152: 125–141.

Bronson FH. (1999). Rodentia. In Knobil E, Neill JD (eds): Encyclopedia of reproduction. Academic Press, New York, pp 282-289.

Brookhyser KM, Aulerich RJ, Vomachka AJ. (1977). Adaptation of the orbital sinus bleeding technique to the chinchilla (*Chinchilla laniger*). Lab. Anim. Sci. 27: 251-254.

Brousset Hernández-Jauregui DM, Galind Maldonado F, Valdez Pérez RA, Romano Pardo M, Schuneman de Aluja A. (2005). Cortisol in saliva, urine, and feces: non-invasive assessment of wild mammals. Vet Mex 36: 325-337.

Brown JL, Wildt DE. (1997). Assessing reproductive status in wild felids by noninvasive faecal steroid monitoring. Int. Zoo Yb. 35, 173-191.

Brown JL, Wasser SK, Wildt DE, Graham LH. (1994). Comparative aspects of steroid hormone metabolism and ovarian activity in felids, measured noninvasively in feces. Biol. Reprod. 51, 776-786.

Brown JL. Steroids hormones-Overview (1999): In Knobil E, Neill JD (eds): Encyclopedia of reproduction. Academic Press, New York, pp 282-289.

Buchanan KL (2000). Stress and the evolution of condition-dependent signals. TREE, 15: 156-160.

Buchanan K, Goldsmith A. (2004). Noninvasive endocrine data for behavioural studies: the importance of validation. Anim. Behav. 67: 183–185.

Busso JM, Ponzio MF, Dabbene V, Fiol de Cuneo M, Ruiz RD. (2005a) Assessment of urine and fecal testosterone metabolite excretion in *Chinchilla lanigera* males. Anim. Reprod. Sci. 86, 339-351.

Busso JM, Ponzio MF, Chiaraviglio M, Fiol de Cuneo M, Ruiz RD. (2005b). Elecroejaculation in the Chinchilla (*Chinchilla lanigera*): effects of anesthesia on seminal characteristics. Res. Vet. Sci. 78, 93-97.

Busso JM, Ponzio MF, Fiol de Cuneo M, Ruiz RD. (2005c). Year-round testicular volume and semen quality evaluations in captive *Chinchilla lanigera*. Anim. Reprod. Sci. 90, 127-134.

Busso JM. Estudio de la función reproductora y optimización de biotecnología para mejorar la eficacia reproductiva del género chinchillla. Fac Cs Ex, Fis y Nat-UNC, Córdoba-Argentina; Ph D Thesis 2006.

Busso JM, Ponzio MF, Fiol de Cuneo M, Ruiz RD,. (2007) Noninvasive monitoring of ovarian endocrine activity in the chinchilla (Chinchilla lanigera). Gen Comp Endocr; 150: 288-297.

Carrascosa RE, Martini AC, Ponzio MF, Busso JM, Ponce AA, Lacuara JL. (2001). Storage of *Chinchilla laniger* semen at 4°C for 24 or 72 h with two different cryoprotectants. Cryobiology 42, 301-306.

Cavigelli SA, Monfort SL, Whitney TK, Mechref YS, Novotny M, McClintock MK. (2005). Frequent serial fecal corticoid measures from rats reflect circadian and ovarian corticosterone rhytms. J. Endocrinol. 184, 153-163.

Chelini MOM, Souza NL, Rocha AM, Felippe ECG, Oliveira CA. (2005). Quantification of fecal estradiol and progesterone metabolites in Syrian hamsters (Mesocricetus auratus). Brazilian J of Medical and Biological Research, 38: 1711-1717.

Cepeda R, Adaro L, Peñailillo G. (2006) Morphometric Variations of Chinchilla laniger Prostate and Plasmatic Testosterone Concentration During its Annual Reproductive Cycle. Int J Morphol; 24: 89-97.

Conaway C.H. (1971). Ecological adaptation and mammalian reproduction. Biol. Reprod. 4, 239-247.

Crews D, Willingham E, Skipper JK. (2000). Endocrine disruptors: present issues, future directions. Q Rev Biol 75: 243-260.

Dahlin J, Lam J, Hau J, Astuti P, Siswanto H, Abelson KSP.(2009). Body weight and faecal corticosterone metabolite excretion in male Sprague-Dawley rats following short transportation and transfer from Group-housing to single-housing. Scand. J. Lab. Anim. Sci. 36: 205-213.

Dantzer B, McAdam AG, Palme R, Fletcher QE, Boutin S, Humphries MM, Boonstra R. (2010). Fecal cortisol metabolite levels in free-ranging North American red squirrels: Assay validation and the effects of reproductive condition. Gen Comp Endocrinol 167: 279–286

DeCantanzaro D, Muir C, Beaton EA, Jetha M. (2004). Non-invasive repeated measurement of urinary progesterone, 17 -estradiol, and testosterone in developing, cycling, pregnant, and postpartum female mice. Steroids 69, 687-696.

Dickerson SM, Gore AC. (2007). Estrogenic envrionmental endocrine-disrupting chemical effects on reproductive neuroendocrine function and dysfunction across the life cycle. Rev Endocr Metab Disord 8: 143-159.

Eriksson E, Royo F, Lyberg K, Carlsson H-E, Hau J. (2004). Effect of metabolic cage housing on immunoglobulin A and corticosterone excretion in faeces and urine of young male rats. Exp Physiol 89, pp 427-433

Fajer AB, Vogt M. (1963). Adrenocortical secretion in the Guinea-pig. J Physiol, 169: 373-385.

Frynta D, Nováková M, Kutalová H, Palme R, Sedlácek. (2009). Apparatus for collection of fecal samples from undisturbed Spiny mice (Acomys cahirinus)living in a complex social group. J Am Assoc Lab Anim Sci. 48: 196–201.

Gippoliti S, Amori G. (1998). Rodent conservation, zoos, and the importance of the "common species". Zoo Biol. 17, 263-265.

Good T, Khan MZ, Lynch WL. (2003). Biochemical and physiology validation of a corticosteroid radioimmunoassay for plasma and fecal samples in oldfield mice (Peromyscus polionotus). Physiol and Behav 80: 405- 411.

Goymann, W. (2005). Noninvasive monitoring of hormones in bird droppings. Physiological validation, sampling, extraction, sex differences, and the influence of diet on hormone metabolite levels. Ann NY Acad Sci 1046; 35-53.

Gromadzka-Osrttowska J, Zalewka B, Szylarska-Gozdz E. (1985). Peripheral plasma progesterone concentration and hematological indices during normal pregnancy of Chinchillas (*Chinchilla laniger*). Comp. Biochem. Physiol. 82 A, 661-665.

Gromadzka-Ostrowska, Zalewska B. (1984). Progesterone concentration and their seasonal changes during the estrus cycle of chinchilla. Acta. Theriogenology. 20: 251-258.

Harper JM, Austad SN. (2000). Fecal glucocorticoids: a noninvasive method of measuring adrenal activity in wild and captive rodents. Physiol. Biochem. Zool. 73, 12-22.

Hayssen V, Harper JM, DeFina R. (2002). Fecal corticosteroids in agouti and non-agouti deer mice (Peromyscus maniculatus). Comp. Biochem. Physiol., A, 132: 439- 446.

Hayward LS, Booth R, Wasser S. (2010). Eliminating the artificial effect of sample mass on avian fecal hormone metabolite concentration. Gen Comp Endocrinol, 169: 117-122

Homyack JA. (2010). Evaluating habitat quality of vertebrates using conservation physiology tools. Wildlife Res, 37: 332-342.

Huchon D, Madsen O, Sibbald MJJB, Ament K, Stanhope MJ, Catzeflis F, de Jong WW, Douzery EJP (2002). Rodent phylogeny and timescale for the evolution of glires: evidence from an extensive taxon sampling using three nuclear genes. Mol. Biol. Evol. 19: 1053–1065.

Kalliokoski O, Hua J, Jacobsen KR, Schumacher-Petersen C, Abelson KSP. (2010). Distribution and time course of corticosterone excretion in faces and urine of female mice with varying systemic concentrations. Gen Comp Endocrinol, 168: 450-454.

Kay EH, Hoekstra HE. (2008). Rodents. Current Biol, 18 R406-R410.

Klasing, KC (2005). Potential impact of nutritional strategy on noninvasive measurements of hormones in birds. Ann. N Y Acad. Sci. 1046: 5–16.

Kuznetsov VA, Tchabovsky AVT, Kolosova IE, Moshkin MP. (2004). Effect of habitat type and population density on the stress levels of Midday Gerbils (*Meriones meridianus Pall*) in free-living populations. Biol Bull Russ Acad Sci, 31: 628-632.

Arora KL. (1979). Blood sampling and intravenous injections in Japanese quail (*Coturnix coturnix japonica*). Lab Anim Sci. 29:114-118.

Lèche A, Busso JM, Navarro JL, Hansen C, Marín RH, Martella MB. (2011). Non-invasive monitoring of adrenocortical activity in Greater Rhea (*Rhea americana*) by measuring fecal glucocorticoid metabolites. Journal of Ornithology, in press.

Lèche A, Busso JM, Hansen C, Navarro JL, Marín RH, Martella MB (2009) Physiological stress in captive Greater rheas (*Rhea americana*): Highly sensitive plasma corticosterone response to an ACTH challenge. Gen Comp Endocrinol 162: 188-192

Malinowska KW, Nathanielsz PW. (1974). Plasma aldosterone, cortisol and corticosterone in the new-born guinea-pig. J. Physiol. 236: 83-93.

McEwen BS, Wingfield JC (2003). The concept of allostasis in biology and biomedicine. Horm and Behavior, 43: 2-15.

Mess A, Mohr B, Martin T. (2001). Evolutionary transformations of hystricognath rodentia and the climantic change in the Eocene to late Oligocene time interval. Zoossystmatics and Evol, 77: 193-206

Millspaugh J.J., Washburn B.E. (2004). Use of fecal glucocorticoid metabolite measures in conservation biology research: considerations for application and interpration. Gen. Comp. Endocrinol. 138, 189-199.

Moberg GP. (2000). Biological response to stress: implications for animal welfare. Chapter 1, in: Moberg GP, Mench JA (eds). The biology of animal stress. Basic principles and implications for animal welfare. CAB International, pp 1-22.

Monfort SL. (2003). Non-invasive endocrine measures of reproduction and stress in wild population. In Holt WV, Pickard AR, Rodger JC, Wild DE. (eds). Reproductive Science and integrated Conservation, Cambridge, London, pp 146-165.

Moreira N, Brown JL, Moraes W, Swanson WF, Monteiro-Filho EL. (2007). Effect of housing and environmental enrichment on adrenocortical activity, behavior and reproductive cyclicity in the female tigrina (Leopardus tigrinus) and margay (Leopardus wiedii). Zoo Biol, 26:441-60

Mormède P, Andanson S, Aupérin B, Beerda B, Guémené D, Malmkvist J, Manteca X, Manteuffel G, Prunet P, Van Reenen CG, Richard S, Veissier I. (2007). Exploration of the hypothalamic–pituitary–adrenal function as a tool to evaluate animal welfare. Physiol and Behav, 92: 317–339.

Möstl E., Palme R. (2002). Hormones as indicators of stress. Domest Anim Endocrinol 23: 67–74

Muir C, Spironello-Vella E, Pisani N, deCatanzaro D. (2001). Enzyme immunoassay of 17ß-Estradiol, estrone conjugates, and T in urinary and fecal samples from males and female mice. Horm. Metab. Res. 33,653-658.

Norris DO. (2007). Synthesis, Metabolism, and Actions of Bioregulators. In Vertebrate endocrinology, Fourth Edition. Elsevier Academic Press, pp 46-105.

Nováková M, Palme R, Kutalová H, Jansky L, Frynta D. (2008). The effects of sex, age and commensal way of life on levels of fecal glucocorticoid metabolites in spiny mice (Acomys cahirinus). Physiology and Behavior, 95: 187–193.

Opazo JC, Palma RE, Melo F, Lessa EP. (2005). Adaptative evolution of the insulin gene in Caviomorph Rodents. Mol. Biol. Evol. 22:1290–1298.

Pettitt BA, Wheaton CJ, Waterman JM. (2007). Effects of storage treatment on fecal steroid hormone concentrations of a rodent, the Cape ground squirrel (Xerus inauris). Gen Comp Endocrinol 150: 1-11.

Palme R, Fischer P, Schildorfer H, Ismail MN. (1996). Excretion of infused 14C-steroid hormones via faeces and urine in domestic livestock. Anim Reprod Sci, 43: 43-63.

Palme R., S. Rettenbacher, C. Touma, S.M. El-Bahr, and Möstl E. 2005. Stress hormones in mammals and birds: comparative aspects regarding metabolism, excretion, and noninvasive measurement in fecal samples. Ann N Y Acad Sci 1040:162–171.

Palme, R. (2005). Measuring fecal steroids: guidelines for practical application. Ann. N.Y. Acad. Sci. 1046: 75–80.

Peter, A. T., N. Kapustin, and J. K. Critser. (1996). Analysis of sex steroid metabolites excreted in the feces and urine of nondomesticated animals. *Compend Contin Educ Pract Vet* 18:781–789.

Ponce AA, Carrascosa RE, Aires VA, Fiol de Cuneo M, Ruiz RD, Ponzio MF Lacuara JL. (1998a) Activity of Chinchilla laniger spermatozoa collected by electroejaculation and cryopreserved. Theriogenology 50, 1239-1249.

Ponce AA, Aires VA, Carrascosa RE, Fiol de Cuneo M, Ruiz RD, Lacuara JL. (1998b). Functional activity of epididymal Chinchilla laniger spermatozoa cryopreserved in different extenders. Res. Vet. Sci. 64, 239-243.

Ponzio MF, Monfort SL, Busso JM, Dabbene VG, Ruiz RD, Fiol de Cuneo M. (2004). A non-invasive method for assessing adrenal activity in the chinchilla (Chinchilla lanigera). J. Exp. Zool. 3, 218-227.

Ponzio MF. "Detección de situaciones potencialmente estresantes y su repercusión sobre la fisiología reproductiva en un modelo animal (Chinchilla laniger)". Fac Cs Ex, Fis y Nat-UNC, Córdoba-Argentina; Ph D Thesis 2006.

Ponzio MF; Busso JM, Ruiz RD, Fiol de Cuneo, M. (2007) Time-related changes in functional activity and capacitation of chinchilla (Chinchilla lanigera) spermatozoa during in vitro incubation. Anim Reprod Sci; 102: 343-349.

Ponzio MF; Busso JM, Ruiz RD, Fiol de Cuneo, MF, Ponce, AA (2008). Functional activity of frozen thawed Chinchilla lanigera spermatozoa cryopreserved with glycerol or ethyleneglycol. Reprod Dom Anim; 43: 228-233.

Pukazhenthi BS, Wild DE. (2004). Which reproductive technologies are most relevant to studying, managing and conserving wildlife? Reprod Fert and Develp 16: 33-46.

Romero LM. (2004). Physiological stress in ecology: lessons from biomedial research. Trends in Ecol Evol, 19: 249-255.

Romero LM, Reed JM. (2005). Collecting baseline corticosterone samples in the field: is under 3 min good enough? Comp Biochem Physiol, Part A 140: 73- 79.

Sapolsky RM, Romero LM, Munck AU. (2000). How do glucocorticoids influence stress responses? Integrating permissive, suppressive, stimulatory, and preparative actions. Endocr. Rev. 21:55-89.

Schneider JE. (2004). Energy balance and reproduction. Physiol and Behav, 81: 289-317.

Schwarzenberger F, Möstl E, Palme R, Bamberg E. (1996). Faecal steroid analysis for on-invasive monitoring of reproductive status in farm, wild and zoo animals. l, Anim Reprod Sci 42: 515-526.

Schwarzenberger F. (2007) The many uses of non-invasive faecal steroid monitoring in zoo and wildlife species. Inter Zoo Yearbook; 41: 52 - 74

Sheriff MJ, Dantzer B, Delehanty B, Palme R, Boonstra R. (2011). Measuring stress in wildlife: techniques for quantifying glucocorticoids. Oecologia Feb 23. [Epub ahead of print]

Short, RV. Species differences in reproductive mechanisms. (1985). In Austin CR, and Short RV (eds): chapter 2, Reproduction in mammals. Cambridge University Press, pp 62-101.

Siswanto H, Hau J, Carlsson H-E, Goldkuhl R, Abelson KSP. (2008). Corticosterone concentration in blood and excretion in faces after ACTH administration in male Sprague-Dawley rats. In Vivo (International Journal of Experimental and Clinical Pathophysiology and Drug Research), 22:435-440.

Soto Gamboa M, Gonzalez S. (2009). Validation of a radioimmunoassay for measuring fecal cortisol metabolites in the hystricomorph rodent, *Octodon degus*. J Exp Zool, 311A:496–503.

Smale L, Heideman PD, French JA. (2005). Behavioral neuroendocrinology in nontraditional species of mammals: things the 'knockout' mouse CAN'T tell us. Horm Behav, 48: 474–483.

Swanson WF, Brown JL. (2004). Internation training programs in reproductive sciences for conservation of Latin American felids. Anim Reprod Sci, 82-83: 21-34.

Tam W.H. (1971). The production of hormonal steroids by ovarian tissues of the chinchilla (*Chinchilla lanigera*). J. Endocr. 50, 267-279.

Tam WH (1972). Steroid metabolic pathways in the ovary of the chinchilla (Chinchilla laniger). J Endocr; 52: 37-50.

Tappa B, Amao H, Takahashi KW (1989). A simple method for intravenous injection and blood collection in the chinchilla (Chinchilla laniger). Lab Anim 23: 73-75.

Taylor W., (1971). The excretion of steroid hormone metabolites in bile and feces. Vitam. Horm. N.Y. 29, 201-285.

Thanos PK, Cavigelli SA, Michaelides M, Olvet DM, Patel U, Diep MN, Volkow. (2009). A non-invasive method for detecting the metabolite stress response in rodents: characterization and disruption of the circadian corticosterone rhythm. Physiol Res 58: 219-228.

Terlouw EMC. Schouten WGP, Ladewig J. Physiology (1997). In: Appleby MC, Hughes Bo (eds), chapter 10 Animal Welfare. CABI International, pp 143-158.

Teskey-Gerstl A, Bamberg E, Steineck T, Palme R. (2000). Excretion of corticosteroids in urine and faeces of hares (*Lepus europaeus*). J. Comp. Physiol. B. 170, 163-168.

Touma C., Sachser N., Mostl E., and Palme R., (2003). Effects of sex and time of day on metabolism and excretion of corticosterone in urine and feces of mice. Gen. Comp. Endocrinol. 130, 267-278.

Touma C, Palme R. (2005). Measuring fecal glucocorticoid metabolites in mammals and birds: the importance of validation. Ann N Y Acad Sci 1046:54–74.

Touma C, Palme R, Sachser N. (2005). Analyzing corticosterone metabolites in fecal samples of mice: a noninvasive technique to monitor stress hormone. Horm and Behav, 45: 10– 22.

Wasser SK, Kathleen EH, Brown JL, Cooper K, Crockett CM, Bechert U, Millspaugh JJ, Larson S, Monfort SL. (2000). A generalized fecal glucocorticoid assay for use in a diverse array of nondomestic mammalian and avian species. Gen. Comp. Endocr. 120, 260-275.

Weir BJ, Rowland IW. (1973). Reproductive strategies of mammals. Annu Rev Ecol Syst 4: 139-163.

Wielebnowski N. (2003). Stress and distress: evaluating their impact for the well-being of zoo animals. J. Am. Vet. Med. Assoc. 223, 973-977.

Wielebnowski NC, Fletchall N, Carlstead K, Busso JM, Brown JL. (2002). Noninvasive assessment of adrenal activity associated with husbandry and behavioral factors in the North American clouded leopard population. Zoo Biol. 21, 77-98.

Wielebnowski N, Watters J. (2007). Applying fecal endocrine monitoring to conservation and behavior studies of wild mammals: important considerations and preliminary tests. Israel J Ecology and Evolution, 53: 439-460.

Young JZ. (1985). Roedores y lagomorfos. En: La vida de los vertebrados. Ediciones Omega, Barcelona, pp 533-542.

Part 5

Metabolic Bone Disease

17

New Trends in Calcium and Phosphorus Metabolism Disorders – Hypoparathyroidism

Gonzalo Díaz-Soto[1] and Manuel Puig-Domingo[2]
[1]*Servicio de Endocrinología y Nutrición, Hospital Clínico de Valladolid. Centro de Investigación de Endocrinología y Nutrición Clínica (IEN). Facultad de Medicina de Valladolid*
[2]*Servei de Endocrinologia i Nutrició. Hospital Germans Trias i Pujol. Badalona Universitat Autònoma de Barcelona. Spain*

1. Introduction

Numerous physiological functions are regulated by calcium. In fact, ionized intracellular calcium (Ca2+) is the most common signal transduction element, a universal cofactor for various enzymes and a crucial participant in different physiologically relevant pathways at the cell membrane level. Thus, ensuring a stable level of extracellular Ca2+ is a priority for preserving many cell functions as automatism of nerve and muscle activity, contraction of cardiac, skeletal and smooth muscle, release of neurotransmitters and secretion of endocrine and exocrine hormones, among others.

The levels of extracellular Ca2+ and phosphorus (P) are tightly regulated by complex mechanisms that have evolved from a phylogenetic perspective, in order to maintain their extracellular concentrations within relatively narrow limits. Among key participants in the regulation of Ca2+, parathyroid hormone (PTH), calcitonin and 1-25 dihydroxyvitamin D are major hormones involved in mineral ion homeostasis, through their effects on parathyroid glands, bone, kidney and intestine.

Although, injury or removal of the parathyroid glands during neck surgery is by far the most common cause of acute and chronic hypoparathyroidism, there are other no so common causes as parathyroid hormones or vitamin D related disorders that may contribute to an impaired parathyroid function.

Conventional treatment of chronic hypocalcemia, particularly hypoparathyroidism, is based on calcium salts, vitamin D (mainly calcitriol), and drugs that increase renal tubular reabsorption of calcium as thiazides. Recently, new treatments have been developed, increasing the therapeutic armamentarium for hypocalcemic disorders, as synthetic recombinant human parathyroid hormone (rhPTH) 1–34 administered once or twice daily in patients with hypoparathyroidism. This treatment modality has proved to reduce urinary calcium excretion compared with calcitriol therapy and to maintain serum calcium in the normal range, thus avoiding chronic hypercalciuria that may lead to renal function impairment, nephrocalcinosis and renal insufficiency in the long term. What is more, new rhPTH release formulations are currently under investigation, opening a new field to explore for the treatment of hypoparathyroidism.

In this chapter, we will discuss the regulation of the metabolism of calcium and phosphorus and their integrated pathways to maintain their levels within physiological limits with special focus on hypocalcemic disorders and new treatment approaches.

2. Physiological regulation of calcium and phosphorus metabolism

Extracellular Ca2+ participates in the regulation of numerous physiological functions, as automatism of nerve and muscle activity, contraction of cardiac, skeletal and smooth muscle, release of neurotransmitters and secretion of endocrine and exocrine hormones among others; thus, physiological concentrations of extracellular ionized Ca2+ remain virtually constant at 1.2 mM (5 mg/dL) (Brown, 1991). For these reason, different physiological mechanisms are involved for maintaining extracellular Ca2+ level whiting these narrow limits that includes parathyroid hormone (PTH), calcitonin and 1-25 dihydroxyvitamin D as major hormones participating in mineral ion homeostasis, through their effects on parathyroid glands, bone, kidney and intestine.

2.1 General Homeostasis of calcium and phosphorus metabolism

The bone acts as a true storehouse of Ca2+ and P, containing nearly the total Ca2+ and P of the body in its mineral structure. Only 1% of Ca2+ from the bone is in constant exchange with extracellular Ca2+ and under tight regulation as this quantitatively minor amounts play a crucial physiological role (Kronenberg et al, 2007).

Extracellular Ca2+ not bound to proteins (albumin and globulins mainly), called as ionized Ca2+, acts as the biological active fraction. Its physiological concentration remains virtually constant at 1.2 mM tightly controlled by hormonal mechanisms.

In contrast, resting cytosollic calcium concentration is about 100 nM but fluctuations allow increases up to 1 microM (100 folders) through cellular activation by releasing Ca2+ from intracellular stores (endoplasmic reticulum, mitochondria) and through activated channels thanks to a very large chemical gradient (10,000:1). Intracellular Ca2+ acts as a key intracellular messenger and cofactor for various enzymes and biological functions (Valero et al, 2008).

On the other hand, organic P is a main constituent and coenzyme for numerous physiological processes as replication, differentiation, development, energy expenditure and storage. Any alteration on P homeostasis cause severe disorders that affect global organ functions (Figure 1).

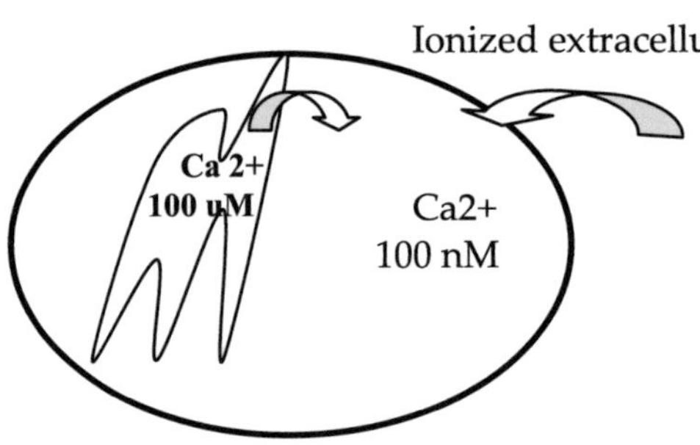

Fig. 1. Calcium concentration in the cell, plasma and intracellular stores and main fluxes (endoplasmic reticulum).

The levels of extracellular Ca2+ and P are tightly regulated by complex mechanisms in a coordinated way that has evolved from a phylogenetic perspective in order to maintain their extracellular concentrations within relatively narrow limits.

2.2 Parathyroid hormone

The parathyroid cell is a prototypical extracellular Ca2+ sensing cell (Brown, 1998). This characteristic allows the constant monitoring of extracellular ionized Ca2+ levels, thus, increasing extracellular Ca2+ is sensed by plasma membrane receptor of parathyroid glands cells (the calcium sensing receptor -CaSR-) that mediates the reduction of PTH hormone secretion (Figure 2) (Riccardi & Gamba, 1999).

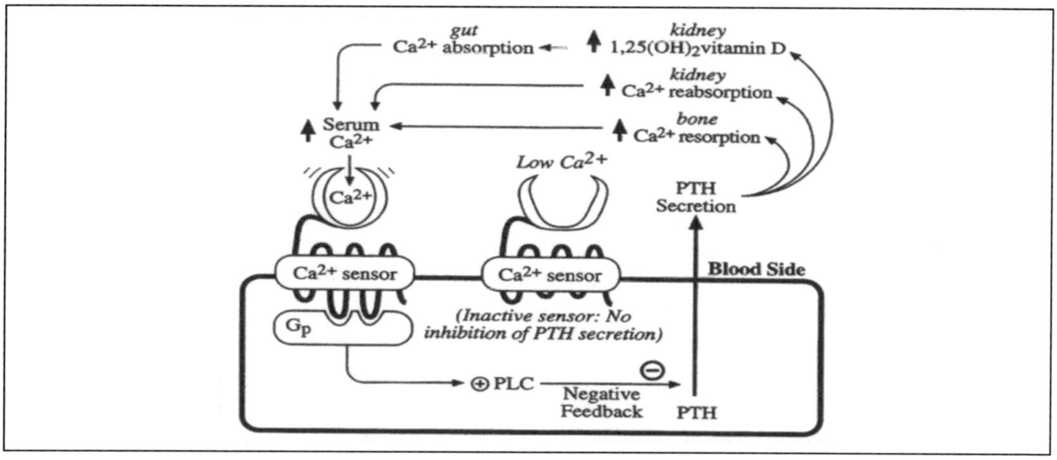

Fig. 2. PTH regulation on parathyroid gland by extracellular Ca2+ levels through CaSR http://chemistry.gravitywaves.com/CHE452/20_Calcium%20Homeostasis16.htm March 15 2011. Dr Noel Sturm

In last years, inherited diseases caused by mutations of the CaSR have been studied (Health et al, 1996). Loss-of-function mutations induce a loose of sensitivity to extracellular Ca2+ levels and a disruption of the downregulation mechanism of PTH secretion as in familiar hypocalciuric hypercalcemia and neonatal severe hyperparathyroidism. These inherited diseases are characterized by mild or severe hypercalcemia. Gain of function mutations have been described in recent years, and in these conditions the hypersensitivity to Ca2+ levels cause hypocalcemia due to a premature inhibition of PTH secretion by the parathyroid gland as in autosomal dominant hypoparathyroidism (Polak et al, 1994).

Parathyroid hormone (PTH) is secreted by parathyroid glands regulated by ionized extracellular Ca2+ through CaSR. PTH is a 84 amino acids peptide hormone synthesized as a large pre-prohormone that exerts its biological effects on its intact configuration or by different amino terminal fragments. A continuous PTH high level as seen in hyperparathyroidism induces stimulation of bone resorption and the release of Ca2+ and P to plasma, and consequently leads to a decrease of bone mineral density. On the other hand, intermittent administration of PTH has the opposite effect and it is the basis of its use in the treatment of severe osteoporosis. In the kidney, PTH acts stimulating Ca2+ reabsorption and P urinary excretion. Indirectly, PTH provides active vitamin D by hydroxylation of 25(OH)D3 in position 1 (1,25(OH)2D3) which increases calcium absorption at the gut level.

In summary, PTH acts as a Ca2+ rising hormone and a major regulatory of Ca2+ metabolism; conversely, increasing levels of Ca2+ exert a downregulation feed back effect on PTH secretion (Shoback, 2008).

2.3 Calcitonin

Calcitonin is a 32 amino acid peptide hormone secreted by parafollicular cells (C cells) of the thyroid gland. Despite of its important role in few vertebrae animals, in humans its role on Ca2+ and P metabolism is less important. However, it is used in the treatment of hypercalcemia due to its decreasing Ca2+ renal reabsorption effect and its inhibition Ca2+ bone resorption; thus, calcitonin has a net hypocalcemic effect on plasma Ca2+ levels in hypercalcemic disorders. Its regulation is mediated by Ca2+ ionized extracellular levels in part through the CaSR as in parathyroid glands, although other hormone and vitamin factors could also play an important role. Finally, calcitonin is also secreted by different neuroendocrine tumours, as medullary thyroid carcinoma, and it used as tumour marker (Kudo et al, 2011).

2.4 Vitamin D

Vitamin D acts as a real hormone. Its synthesis and tissue concentration is more dependent of seasonal and sun exposure factors rather than oral intake. Endogenous inactive vitamin D (colecalciferol-Vitamin D3) is synthesized by ultraviolet radiation, although nutritional alternative sources (supplemented dairy products, fat fish and liver) could eventually provide sufficient quantities for covering daily needs. Vitamin D3 activation requires hydroxylation of the 25th and 1st positions to get full biological activity (1,25(OH)2D3); this process takes place in the liver and kidney where hydroxylation is successively performed and at the kidney level activation of 1-hydroxilase is partially dependent of PTH. Vitamin D can also be hydroxilated at position 24 which renders inactive the molecule.

The main effect of vitamin D on Ca2+ and P metabolism is to stimulate calcium absorption in the bowel by means of the binding of its active form 1,25(OH)2D3 to the vitamin D nuclear receptor (VDR) (Shiohara et al, 2005). A less pronounced but also an important effect of vitamin D is to promote Ca2+ and P apposition in the bone and to stimulate calcium excretion in the kidney. The VDR is a ubiquitous receptor which is expressed in most tissues and cell lines and in fact vitamin D has been implicated in numerous biological actions as activation of the immune system, autoimmune diseases, cardiovascular risk, proliferation and differentiation of cancer cell lines among others (Fernandez et al, 2009; Mathieu & Adorini, 2002; Nagpal et al, 2005).

Calcium and vitamin D intake is currently though to be under normal requirements, especially in old populations due to loss of efficiency of vitamin D synthesis and age-related down regulation of 1alpha kidney hydroxylation in relation with kidney function, as well as insufficient sun exposure in aged people. At the moment, a worldwide high prevalence of vitamin D deficiency has been described (Rosen, 2011).

2.5 Integrated homeostasis of calcium metabolism

The levels of extracellular Ca2+ and P are tightly regulated by complex interrelation of PTH, calcitonin and 1-25 dihydroxyvitamin D through their balanced effects on parathyroid glands, bone, kidney and intestine target organs (Figure 3).

PTH secretion is regulated by extracellular Ca2+ levels and activation of 25(OH)D3 to 1,25(OH)2D3 is regulated by PTH action on kidney. 1,25(OH)2D3 enhances calcium absorption on gut. On the same way, calcitonin regulation is mediated by Ca2+ ionized extracellular level. These complex mechanisms work in concert to keep Ca2+ and P+ in a constant concentration for maintaining under optimal conditions some critical physiological functions as automatism of nerve and muscle activity, contraction of cardiac, skeletal and smooth muscle, release of neurotransmitters and secretion of endocrine and exocrine hormones among others.

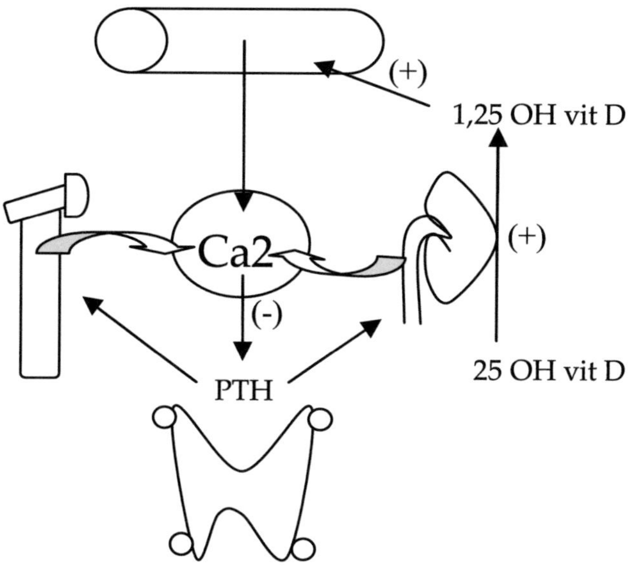

Fig. 3. Integrated physiological homeostasis of calcium metabolism.

Calcium and vitamin D insufficiency leads to an increase in calcium intestinal absorption, renal uptake and calcium bone reabsorption. The first step to reach the new equilibrium is initiated by the low extracellular calcium concentration which is sensed by CaSR and triggers PTH secretion by the parathyroid glands. The increment of PTH level increases the synthesis of the activated form of vitamin D and stimulates absorption of tubular calcium on kidney. On the other hand, 1,25 OH vitamin D acts on the nuclear pathways of the entherocytes to increase absorption of dietary calcium, which is quantitatively the most important response to calcium and vitamin D insufficiency. To summarize, chronic calcium and vitamin D insufficiency provoques a continuous compensatory hyperparathyroidism aimed to maintain Ca2+ and P+ into the physiological levels; this chronic hyperactivation of the parathyroid glands may have deleterious consequences at the long term.

3. Hypocalcemic disorders

Any alteration of this close balance between the hormones involved in calcium metabolism could originate disorders characterized by the presence hypocalcemia.
Although, injury or removal of the parathyroid glands during neck surgery is the most common cause of acute and chronic hypoparathyroidism, other not so common causes should be evaluated and ruled out, mainly caused by alteration in intestinal absorption (vitamin D related) or by decrease reabsorption at the bone and kidney levels (parathyroid hormones related).

3.1 Parathyroid hormones related disorders

Parathyroid hormones related hypocalcaemia could be differentiated from other causes by a low or inappropriately normal PTH level in the presence of low calcium levels, mild hyperphosphatemia and low 1,25(OH)2D3.

PTH related causes of hypocalcemia include:

3.1.1 Parathyroid glands destruction

Injury or removal of the parathyroid glands during neck surgery is the most common cause of acute and chronic hypoparathyroidism. Its incidence rate is usually related to surgeon's experience, the type of pathology and the surgical technique performed (Sthepen, 2000). Although postsurgical hypoparathyroidism is usually a transitory problem, occasionally, it persists in 0.4%-33% of cases depending on the series (Page & Strunsky 2007; Torregrosa et al, 2005). It may be caused by vascular interruption or involuntary removal during surgery and it uses to be permanent if there is no remission after 6-9 months after surgery.

After hyperparathyroidism adenoma removal, a transient suppressive hypoparathyroidism can occur in the first 48 hours after surgery of functional nature. In these cases, hungry bone syndrome should be ruled out and could be identified as hypophosphatemia is virtually always an associated feature after surgery of a severe and of long duration hyperpathyroidism.

However, any infiltrative or autoimmune disease that affects all parathyroid glands could cause hypoparathyroidism. Wilson disease, hemochromatosis, metastic disease can infiltrate parathyroid glands causing their dysfunction (Angelopoulos et al, 2006). Autosomal recessive autoimmunity hypoparathyroidism can be part of autoimmunity polyglandular syndrome type 1, in which Addison disease and mucocutaneous candidiasis are found together with hypocalcemia (Husebye et al, 2009). This syndrome has been related to the autoimmunity regulatory gene AIRE. Autoimmunity antibodies against parathyroid glands and CaSR can support this diagnosis (Dittmar & Kahaly, 2003).

3.1.2 Congenital/inherited parathyroid disorders

Transient neonatal hypocalcaemia is a quite frequent disorder that is usually resolved during the first days after birth. Hyperparathyroidism and diabetes of the mother are the most common causes. However, hypocalcemia disorders that are not resolved during first 4 weeks or life require a more extended diagnosis work-up. Inactivating mutations of some transcription factors as glial cell missing factor (GCM) and SOX3 have been related to neonatal hypoparathyroidism.

In some cases, hypoparathyroidism is part of more complex malformative syndromes arising during the embryonic development, as Di George's syndrome. Di George's syndrome or velo-cardio-facial syndrome is the most frequent severe malformation (1/3000) and it is caused by embryonic disorder of third, fourth and fifth branchial pouches, resulting in the absence of parathyroid glands associated with cardiac malformations, abnormal facies, thymus hypoplasia, and cleft palate. It is caused by deletions in 22q11, and less frequently in 10p (Kobrynski & Sullivan, 2007). Other not so common causes of neonatal/inherited hypoparathyroidism are Kenny-Caffey syndrome and Barakat syndrome among others.

Gain of function mutations of CaSR amino-terminal domain have been published in recent years; in these cases, hypersensitive sensing to Ca2+ levels cause hypocalcemia by premature inhibition of PTH secretion by the parathyroid glands expressed as an autosomal dominant hypoparathyroidism (Pollak et al, 1994). In these patients hypocalcemia is found together with hypercalciuria and normal PTH. In such a situation, treatment with vitamin D results in the development of hypercalcemia which may lead to nephrocalcinosis and renal failure; thus, treatment is aimed to avoid symptoms of hypocalcemia and not to achieve normocalcemia (Pearce et al, 1996).

3.1.3 Pseudohypoparathyroidism

Pseudohypoparathyroidism is characterized by peripheral PTH resistance despite of elevated PTH levels, and hypocalcaemia plus hiperphophatemia plasma levels similar to what is found in hypoparathyroidism after having ruled out magnesium deficiency and renal failure. It may be associated to a characteristic morphotype called Albright´s hereditary osteodysthophy. Its genetic bases and clinical features will be described in detail in another chapter.

3.2 Vitamin D related hypocalcemia

Hypocalcemia syndrome due to vitamin D related disorders is mainly caused by alterations in intestinal absorption of dietary calcium. Hypocalcemic disorders in the context of vitamin D deficiency are characterized by elevated PTH plasma levels and hypophosphatemia with an increased renal phosphate clearance (Figure 4). Increased PTH is of compensatory nature aimed to maintain Ca2+ and P+ within the physiological levels by calcium mobilization from skeleton, increased renal reabsorption of calcium and increased renal 1alpha hydroxylation.

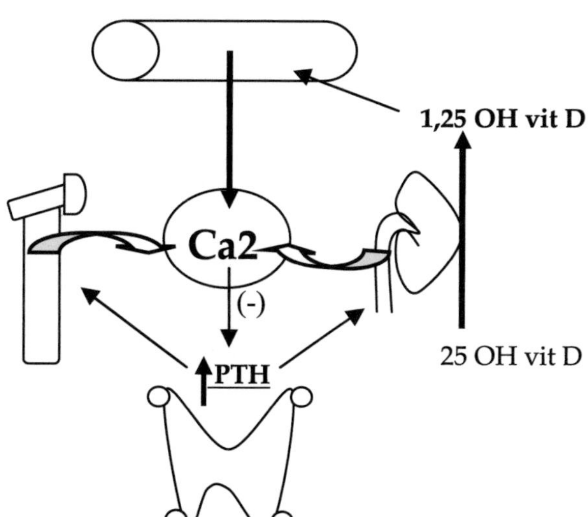

Fig. 4. Adaptation to vitamin D and calcium insufficiency (adaptation pathways on bold type).

Vitamin D related hypocalcaemia could be caused by:

3.2.1 Vitamin D absorption/synthesis deficiency

Vitamin D deficiency is mostly seen in old people, although younger populations may also suffer from this condition. As vitamin D could be sourced by skin synthesis under

ultraviolet irradiation and/or dietary intake, any deficiency on dietary intake or reduction on intestinal fat-soluble vitamin D absorption (gastrectomy, intestinal illness, chronic hepatic insufficiency) and any decrease in skin synthesis due to insufficient solar irradiation or used of high solar protective factor sun blocks, could cause a vitamin D deficiency. It also causes a compensatory hyperparathyroidism and has been correlated with seasonal psychiatric and immune disorders in northern countries (Rosen, 2011).
Modern food industry has supplemented dairy products with vitamin D although it has not been correlated with improvements in general population vitamin D levels.

3.2.2 Impaired 1 or 25 alpha hydroxilation of Vitamin D

Any alteration on hepatic or kidney functions could lead on deficient hydroxylation of vitamin D, as in renal or liver failure. This would cause an intestinal calcium absorption and a compensatory increase in circulating PTH.
It is a common clinical entity especially in chronic renal failure under dialysis. The failure of 1alpha hydroxilation at the kidney level causes a decrease in plasma calcium by malabsorption of dietary calcium intake and a compensatory elevation of PTH (secondary hyperparathyroidism) without an increased phosphate clearance because of kidney failure. Treatment of compensatory hyperparathyroidism is based on the administration of the active form of vitamin D (1-25(OH)2 Vit D) to cover 1alpha hydroxilase deficit, an increase in calcium intake and phosphate binders (Messa et al, 2010). Regulation of PTH secretion with non hypercalcemic Vitamin D analogs and calcimimetics (parathyroid CaSR sensitizers) has been a revolution in the treatment of secondary hyperparathyroidism associated to renal failure (Borstand et al, 2010).

3.2.3 Impaired entero-hepatic circulation of vitamin D

Vitamin D is a fat-soluble vitamin, so it is under entero-hepatic circulation and adiposity and hepatic deposit. Any alteration on entero-hepatic circulation or accelerated hepatic metabolism and its nature is mainly drug-induced: anticonvulsants, tuberculostatic treatment, and bile acid sequestrants; any of these could cause an accelerated loss of vitamin D.

3.2.4 Calcitriol resistance-Hereditary vitamin D resistant rickets

Some inherited disorders have been described to be associated with vitamin D resistance; their frequency is very low. They are characterized by a biochemical profile concordant with vitamin D deficiency and compensatory hyperparathyroidism with normal or even elevated levels of vitamin D that indicates a resistance vitamin D status. Most mutations described in vitamin D resistant rickets involve intranuclear vitamin D receptor (VDR) at the DNA binding domain and it affects the regulation of gene expression (Mallory et al, 2004).
Clinical features are variable but it uses to appear during childhood with hypocalcaemia and hypophosphatemia, associated with alopecia, bone deformations and short stature. Treatment with high doses of calcitriol do not use to be successful, although it depends on the specific mutations on VDR. Vitamin D analogues have opened new therapeutic possibilities on this rare illness. Treatment with sequestrant compounds could cause an accelerated loss of vitamin D.

3.3 Other causes

Other hypocalcaemia causes include: bone apposition in osteoblastic metastasis; sequestration by intravascular drugs or by acute hyperphosphatemic states (rhabdomyolysis, chemotherapy); treatment or ion alterations and vitamin D insufficiency in HIV infected patients; critical illness as acute pancreatitis.

4. Acute hypocalcaemia treatment

Acute hypocalcaemia is a medical emergency that requires a quick diagnosis and treatment. However, chronic hypocalcaemia is frequently asymptomatic and treatment must be aiming to normalization of calcium levels without increasing complications (Cooper & Gottoes, 2008).

Acute hypocalcaemia can be diagnosed by measuring total calcium levels using protein correction to calculate free extracellular calcium (a decrease in calcium of 0.8 mg/dl for every 1 g/dL decrease in albumin) or by direct monitoring of ionized Ca2+ (Kronenberg et al, 2007).

Symptoms are correlated with acute instauration and magnitude of the deficiency, especially in relation to neuromuscular excitability as carpopedal spasm. In acute and severe cases of hypocalcemia general tetany, broncospasm and serious cardiac arrhythmias have been described, thus serum calcium levels must be measured frequently in this period, and electrocardiographic monitoring must be done during initial replacement therapy.

Acute hypocalcemia treatment requires prompt normalisation of calcium plasma levels using intravenous calcium infusion; other ions alterations are particularly important, i.e. the correction of hypomagnesaemia that causes impaired secretion of PTH from parathyroid glands and precludes the correction of hypocalcemia.

5. Chronic hypocalcemia treatment

The conventional treatment of chronic hypocalcemia and hypoparathyroidism is based on calcium salts, vitamin D (mainly calcitriol), and drugs that increase renal tubular reabsorption of calcium as thiazides. However, over the past few years, the administration of synthetic recombinant human parathyroid hormone (rhPTH) 1-34 once or twice daily, even with more physiological releasing devices in patients with hypoparathyroidism has proved to reduce urinary calcium excretion compared with calcitriol therapy, and to maintain serum calcium in the normal range, thus avoiding chronic hypercalciuria that may lead to renal function impairment, nephrocalcinosis and renal insufficiency in the long term. On the other hand, new vitamin D analogues have been investigated to maintain calcium levels on normal range without hypercalciuria complications.

In this section we will describe conventional and new treatment approaches of chronic hypocalcemia mainly focused on post surgical hypoparathyroidism, due to the important innovations appeared in last years.

5.1 Conventional treatments

The conventional treatment of chronic hypocalcaemia and hypoparathyroidism is based on calcium salts, vitamin D (mainly calcitriol), and drugs that increase renal tubular reabsorption of calcium as thiazides.

Treatment objectives are to maintain free ionized calcium levels within the normal interval or plasma calcium in the lower half or slightly below the normal range (8.0-8.5 mg/dL), and to avoid hypercalciuria (< 250 mg urine calcium/24 hours) and other treatment complications. It should be directed at the underlying disorder (Shoback, 2008).

5.2 Calcium salts

Long-term treatment of patients with chronic hypocalcemia is warranty with 1 to 3 g of elementary calcium per day in the various forms of salts available (table 1) because of the increased excretion of calcium. Interrupting the supplement can rapidly lower an elevated calcium value. It should be must be scheduled in 3-4 doses with meals to facilitates its absorption. Calcium carbonate is by far the most used calcium salts due to its low cost, despite of gastrointestinal adverse effects and that it requires gastric acidification to assure its absorption; thus achlorhydric patients or under proton-pump inhibitors treatment should be avoid unlike citrate calcium and should be taken with food or citrus drinks to promote maximal absortion. Besides, calcium citrate is preferable because it increases urinary citrate thus helping calcium to stay in solution (Harvey et al, 1988). Of the calcium preparations available, only the carbonate and citrate salts contain sufficient elemental calcium (per tablet) for the efficient treatment of most patients with hypoparathyroidism. Other preparations may be used in patients who cannot tolerate citrate and carbonate salts. The percentage of elemental calcium is lower in these other preparations, and do not adds any benefit (Maeda et al, 2006; Shoback, 2008).

Calcium Salts	Ca element content	Milligrams of salt needed 1 g preparation elementary calcium
Calcium Carbonate	40%	2500
Calcium Phospathe	38%	2631
Calcium Chloride	27%	3700
Calcium Citrate	21%	4762
Calcium Lactate	13%	7700
Calcium Gluconate	9%	11100

Table 1. Calcium salts available. Calcium carbonate: constipation is a common side effect; calcium carbonate is best absorbed with meals and with acid present in the stomach. Calcium citrated: Recommended in patients who have achlorhydria or who are taking a proton-pump inhibitor, in order to achieve sufficient absorption of calcium (Maeda et al, 2006).

5.3 Vitamin D

All patients with hypoparathyroidism must be treated with vitamin D or analogues in addition to calcium. Vitamin D chosen must be selected depending on the underlying disorder, thus impaired renal 1alpha hydroxylation should be treated with 1alpha hydroxilated analogues, but vitamin D insufficiency could be treated with non hydroxilated vitamin D metabolites (Cooper & Gittoes, 2008).

Compared to PTH, replacement with calciferol steroids leads to a higher urinary excretion of Ca with an increased risk of nephrocalcinosis. Vitamin D toxicity is an important concern and may occur at any time. Manifestations may include altered mental status, fatigue, thirst, dehydration, reduced renal function, nephrolithiasis, and constipation. Treatment involves discontinuation of the vitamin D preparation and the calcium salt intake. Depending on the severity, and especially if the toxic effects are related to treatment with vitamin D metabolites with long half-lives, intravenous saline infusion and possibly oral glucocorticoids may quickly antagonize vitamin D action and restore normocalcemia in a short period of time. Levels of 25-hydroxyvitamin D must be monitored, even in patients receiving calcitrol and alfacalcidiol to assess vitamin D dosage adequacy. The target 25-hydroxyvitamin D level is 30 ng/ml.

The current most used drugs are dihydrotachysterol (average half-time 7 days), alphacalcidol (average half life-2 days) and calcitriol (average half life-1 day) depending on underlying pathology (table 2). Not all drugs are available in all countries and short half-life compound are more recommendable due to its higher security. Theorically, for patients with labile calcemia, dihydrotachysterol may be preferable because it provides better stability but a higher risk of intoxication. When an additional rapid effect is needed or security is the priority short-acting drugs can be added. (Maeda et al, 2006).

On hypoparathyroidism, calcitriol is preferred over vitamin D2/D3 because of its potency, rapid onset and offset of action. The vast majority of patients require calcitriol in dosages of 0.25 μg, taken twice daily, and extremely rare cases up to 0.5 μg four times daily. However, vitamin D and calcium dosage show a remarkable variability so straight monitoring and titration is warranted at the beginning of the treatment.

Vitamin D metabolites	25/1a hydroxilation required	Dosage per day	Onset of action	Offset of action
Vitamin D2 (ergocalciferol)/ Vitamin D3 (cholecalciferol)	+/+	25,000-100,000 UI once daily	10-14 days	14-25 days
1, 25 OH Vitamin D (Calcitriol)	-/-	0.25-1 ug twice daily	1-2 days	2-3 days
1a hydroxivitamin D (alfacalcidiol)	+/-	0.5-3.0 ug daily	1-2 days	5-7 days
Dihydrotachysterol	-/-	0.2-1.0 mg once daily	4-7 days	7-21 days
25 (OH) vitamin D (Calcidiol)	-/+	0.625-5 mg	4-8 weeks	6-12 weeks

Table 2: Vitamin D metabolites and actions (Maeda et al, 2006; Shoback, 2008).

5.4 Enhanced calcium renal tubular reabsorption: Thiazides

Hypoparathyroidism causes increased excretion of urinary calcium in relation to serum calcium and chronic vitamin D treatment predisposes to hypercalciuria, nephrolithiasis, and nephrocalcinosis. The use of drugs that increase renal tubular reabsorption of calcium as thiazides could be useful in hypocalcemia as complementary treatment and may help to control hypercalciuria (Porter et al, 1978). In fact, patients should be evaluated annually to rule out complications of vitamin D chronic treatment as nephrocalcinosis by imaging techniques and cataracts with an ophthalmic revision (Levine , 2001), besides high water intake is recommended, at least 1.5-2.5 L/day.

5.5 New treatment approaches

Treatment of hypoparathyroidism/hypocalcemia with vitamin D metabolites and calcium salts are usually well tolerated. However, quality of life studies suggest that despite optimization or normalization of biochemical values, patients with treated hypoparathyroidism show scores of depression, anxiety and somatisation higher than matched controls (Arlt et al, 2002). What is more, vitamin D and calcium salts are not an absolutely safe treatment. In fact, treatment is aimed to target low-normal calcium levels in order to prevent hypercalciuria and deterioration of renal function at long term.

In last years, the administration of synthetic human PTH 1-34 once or twice-daily in patients having hypoparathyroidism has proved to reduce the level of urinary calcium excretion compared with calcitriol therapy as well as maintaining serum calcium in the normal range, avoiding chronic hypercalciuria that may lead to impairment of renal function, nephrocalcinosis and renal insufficiency. Cost and inconvenience of injection treatment in the case of rPTH are the reasons why currently classic treatment with vitamin D plus calcium is preferred, despite the risk of hypercalciuria and long term impairment of renal function. However, in recent years, successful rhPTH treatment has been reported in cases of hypocalcemia and hypoparathyroidism not controlled by conventional therapy, thus indicating its usefulness is such a resistant cases (Angelopolulos et al, 2007; Mahajan et al, 2009; Puig-Domingo et al, 2008, Sanda et al, 2008, Shiohara et al, 2006; Winer et al, 2008).

On the other hand, research on calcium sensing receptor and vitamin D analogues have opened new and promising investigation in future treatments. In fact, in last years clinical availability of cinacalcet, the agonist of Calcium Sensing Receptor has proved to be effective for the treatment of hyperparathyroidism (Marcocci et al, 2009). Research on antagonists of calcium sensing receptor (calcilytic agents) may be used to promote inactivation of the receptor in the parathyroid glands and increase PTH secretion, specially in those hypocalcemic patients with activated CaSR mutations (Nemeth et al, 2001; Leth et al, 2010).

5.6 Recombinant human PTH

Hypoparathyroidism is one of the few endocrine diseases for which hormone-replacement therapy is not the treatment approach. Over the last 10 years, some clinical assays using synthetic recombinant human parathyroid hormone 1–34 (rhPTH) administered once or twice daily in adults and children with hypoparathyroidism, have proved to maintain serum calcium in the normal range as well as reducing urinary calcium excretion compared with conventional treatment with vitamin D (Winer et al, 1993, 1996, 1998, 2003, 2008, 2010). This treatment modality may prevent renal function impairment, nephrocalcinosis and renal insufficiency in the long term as it avoids the chronic hypercalciuric state associated to vitamin D administration. On the other hand, many studies have shown that rhPTH treatment in adult subjects with osteoporosis produces a rapid rise in bone mineralization, which may contribute to a faster recovery of lost bone mineral content of these patients (Farocki et al, 2007).

Despite these advantages, rhPTH has not become the treatment of choice for hypoparathyroidism, because conventional treatment with vitamin D and calcium salts is usually well tolerated, and rhPTH injection is more expensive. However, in recent years, successful rhPTH treatment has been reported in cases of hypocalcaemia and hypoparathyroidism not controlled by conventional therapy as an off-label treatment.

Only a few small, randomized trials have assessed the use of injectable PTH (1-34) and supplemental calcium in patients with this condition in a relative short period of follow-up of 3 years. In those trials, rhPTH has proved to maintain calcium levels between normal or slightly below normal range but with a significantly reduction of urinary calcium excretion. Twice-daily rhPTH versus once allowed a marked reduction in the total daily PTH 1–34 dose, with less fluctuations in serum calcium, normalization of urine calcium and significantly improved metabolic control both in adults and children. Also, rhPTH efficacy has been extensively published in case reports dealing with hypocalcemic disorders not controlled under conventional treatment, some of them trying to mimic more physiological delivery as using multipulse subcutaneous pump PTH delivery (Puig-Domingo et al, 2008). Major concerns of rhPTH use are related to safety; those data have been obtained mainly from osteoporosis treatment studies. Animal toxicity studies have raised concerns regarding dose-dependent PTH effects on the bone (Sato et al, 2002). Long-term, supraphysiological doses of recombinant human PTH 1–34 (rhPTH), given under continuous delivery rather than in a pulsatile way to rats with normal functioning parathyroid glands, was associated to an increased risc of osteosarcoma development. However, this higher risk has been associated to a particular effect on rat bones and does not seem relevant to PTH-deficient patients receiving physiological replacement doses. In fact, post commercialisation follow-up has not detected an increase in human osteosarcoma diagnosis until now (Harper et al, 2007). Anyway, more physiological release of PTH as using subcutaneous pumps delivery or patch could be even a safer alternative (Horwitz & Stewart, 2008).

5.7 Calcium sensing receptor antagonists

PTH secretion is regulated by a cell surface receptor that detects small changes in the level of plasma calcium, the calcium sensing receptor (figure 2). This receptor provides a particularly interesting and new molecular target for drugs useful for treating calcium and bone disorders. At the moment, a calcimimetic (compounds that mimic or potentiate the effects of extracellular calcium at the CaSR) is commercialized as cinacalcet (Mimpara ®) and it is approved and used in non surgical or tertiary hyperparathyroidism (Marcocci et al, 2009).

In the same way, molecules that blocked CaSR activity will stimulate PTH secretion. Although, there is no calcilytic compound available yet for therapeutic human use, some of them are under research with promising preliminary results, especially for the treatment of patients with CaSR activating mutations whose treatment with vitamin D and calcium does not correct the underlying pathophysiological defect, and they often worsen hypercalciuria and accelerate kidney stone formation or nephrocalcinosis resulting in impaired renal function under conventional treatment (Letz et al, 2010).

6. Conclusion

Numerous physiological functions are regulated by calcium metabolism, thus, ensuring a stable level of extracellular Ca2+ is a priority for preserving normal homeostasis. In this respect, levels of extracellular Ca2+ and phosphorus are tightly regulated by complex mechanisms in which key participants are parathyroid hormone, calcitonin and 1-25 dihydroxyvitamin D through their effects over parathyroid glands, bone, kidney and intestine. Any alteration of this close balance between the hormones involved in calcium metabolism could originate hypocalcemia.

Although post surgical hypoparathyroidism is the most common cause, diagnosis and treatment of hypocalcemic disorders require a detailed study and infrequent causes should also be evaluated and ruled out. Hypoparathyroidism could be classified into two main groups: vitamin D related causes and parathyroid hormone related causes. Although, conventional treatment of chronic hypocalcaemia and hypoparathyroidism is based on calcium salts, vitamin D (mainly calcitriol) and drugs that enhance renal tubular reabsorption of calcium, the administration of synthetic recombinant human parathyroid hormone (rhPTH) 1-34 and research in calcium sensing receptor have opened new promising fields in the last few years.

7. References

Angelopoulos NG, Goula A, Rombopoulos G, Kaltzidou V, Katounda E, Kaltsas D, Tolis G. (2006) Hypoparathyroidism in transfusion-dependent patients with beta-thalassemia. J Bone Miner Metab.24(2):138-45.

Angelopoulos NG, Goula A, Tolis G. 2007 Sporadic hypoparathyroidism treated with teriparatide: a case report and literature review. Exp Clin Endocrinol Diabetes. Jan;115(1):50-4..

Arlt W, Fremerey C, Callies FReincke M, Schneider P, Timmermann W, Allolio B. (2002) Well-being, mood and calcium homeostasis in patients with hypoparathyroidism receiving standard treatment with calcium and vitamin D. Eur J Endocrinol 146:215-22.

Borstnar S, Erzen B, Gmeiner Stopar T, Kocjan T, Arnol M, Kandus A, Kovac D. (2010) Treatment of hyperparathyroidism with cinacalcet in kidney transplant recipients. Transplant Proc. Dec;42(10):4078-82.

Brown, EM. (1991) Extracellular Ca2+ sensing, regulation of parathyroid cell function, and role of Ca2+ and other ions as extracellular (first) messengers. Physiological Review. 71: 371-411

Brown EM, Pollak M, Hebert SC (1998) The extracellular calcium-sensing receptor: its role in health and disease. Annu Rev Med.;49:15-29..

Cooper MS, Gittoes NJ.(2008) Diagnosis and management of hypocalcaemia. BMJ Jun 7;336(7656):1298-302.

Dittmar M, Kahaly GJ. (2003) Polyglandular autoimmune syndromes: immunogenetics and long-term follow-up. J Clin Endocrinol Metab. Jul;88(7):2983-92.

Harvey JA, Zobitz MM, Pak CY (1998) Dose dependency of calcium absorption: a comparison of calcium carbonate and calcium citrate. J Bone Miner Res. Jun;3(3):253-8.

Heath H 3rd, Odelberg S, Jackson CE, Teh BT, Hayward N, Larsson C, Buist NR, Krapcho KJ, Hung BC, Capuano IV, Garrett JE, Leppert MF. (1996) Clustered inactivating mutations and benign polymorphisms of the calcium receptor gene in familial benign hypocalciuric hypercalcemia suggest receptor functional domains.J Clin Endocrinol Metab. Apr;81(4):1312-7.

Horwitz MJ, Stewart AF. (2008) Hypoparathyroidism: is it time for replacement therapy? J Clin Endocrinol Metab. Sep;93(9):3307-9.

Husebye ES, Perheentupa J, Rautemaa R, Kämpe O. (2009) Clinical manifestations and management of patients with autoimmune polyendocrine syndrome type I. J Intern Med. May;265(5):514-29.

Kobrynski LJ, Sullivan KE.(2007) Velocardiofacial syndrome, DiGeorge syndrome: the chromosome 22q11.2 deletion syndromes. Lancet.Oct 20;370(9596):1443-52.

Kronenberg HM, Melme S, Polonsky KS. Larsen, PR. Williams Textbook Of Endocrinology. Elsevier Saunders pp 1202-1204

Kudo T, Miyauchi A, Ito Y, Yabuta T, Inoue H, Higashiyama T, Tomoda C, Hirokawa M, Amino N. (2011) Serum calcitonin levels with calcium loading tests before and after total thyroidectomy in patients with thyroid diseases other than medullary thyroid carcinoma. Endocr J. 2011 Feb 24

Farooki A, Fornier M & Girotra M. 2007 Anabolic therapies for osteoporosis. New England Journal of Medicine 357 2410–2411.

Fernández CA, Puig-Domingo M, Lomeña F, Estorch M, Camacho Martí V, Bittini AL, Marazuela M, Santamaría J, Castro J, Martínez de Icaya P, Moraga I, Martín T, Megía A, Porta M, Mauricio D, Halperin I. Effectiveness of retinoic acid treatment for redifferentiation of thyroid cancer in relation to recovery of radioiodine uptake. J Endocrinol Invest. 32(3):228-33.

Harper KD, Krege JH, Marcus R, Mitlak BH. 2007 Osteosarcoma and teriparatide? J Bone Miner Res. Feb;22(2):334.

Letz S, Rus R, Haag C, Dörr HG, Schnabel D, Möhlig M, Schulze E, Frank-Raue K, Raue F, Mayr B, Schöfl C. (2010) Novel activating mutations of the calcium-sensing receptor: the calcilytic NPS-2143 mitigates excessive signal transduction of mutant receptors. J Clin Endocrinol Metab. Oct;95(10):E229-33.

Levine M. 2001 Hypoparathyroidism and pseudohypoparathyroidism. In: DeGroot LJ, Jameson JL. Endocrinology, 4th ed. Philadelphia: WB Saunders. pp. 1133-53.

Maeda SS, Fortes EM, Oliveira UM, Borba VC, Lazaretti-Castro M. (2006) Hypoparathyroidism and pseudohypoparathyroidism. Arq Bras Endocrinol Metabol. 2006 Aug;50(4):664-73.

Mahajan A, Narayanan M, Jaffers G, Concepcion L. 2009 Hypoparathyroidism associated with severe mineral bone disease postrenal transplantation, treated successfully with recombinant PTH. Hemodial Int. Oct;13(4):547-50.

Malloy PJ, Xu R, Peng L, Peleg S, Al-Ashwal A, Feldman D. 2004. Hereditary 1,25-dihydroxyvitamin D resistant rickets due to a mutation causing multiple defects in vitamin D receptor function. Endocrinology. 45(11):5106-14.

Marcocci C, Chanson P, Shoback D, Bilezikian J, Fernandez-Cruz L, Orgiazzi J, Henzen C, Cheng S, Sterling LR, Lu J, Peacock M. (2009) Cinacalcet reduces serum calcium concentrations in patients with intractable primary hyperparathyroidism. J Clin Endocrinol Metab. 2009 Aug;94(8):2766-72.

Mathieu C, Adorini L. 2002. The coming of age of 1,25-dihydroxyvitamin D(3) analogs as immunomodulatory agents. Trends Mol Med.8(4):174-9.

Messa P, Cafforio C, Alfieri C. (2010) Calcium and phosphate changes after renal transplantation. J Nephrol. Nov-Dec;23 Suppl 16:S175-81.

Nagpal S, Na S, Rathnachalam R. 2005 Noncalcemic actions of vitamin D receptor ligands. Endocr Rev.26(5):662-87.

Nemeth EF, Delmar EG, Heaton WL, Miller MA, Lambert LD, Conklin RL, Gowen M, Gleason JG, Bhatnagar PK, Fox J. (2001) Calcilytic compounds: potent and selective Ca2+ receptor antagonists that stimulate secretion of parathyroid hormone. J Pharmacol Exp Ther. Oct;299(1):323-31.

Page C, Strunski V. 2007 Parathyroid risk in total thyroidectomy for bilateral, benign, multinodular goitre: report of 351 surgical cases. J Laryngol Otol.;121(3):237-41.

Pearce SH, Williamson C, Kifor O, Bai M, Coulthard MG, Davies M, Lewis-Barned N, McCredie D, Powell H, Kendall-Taylor P, Brown EM, Thakker RV. (1996) A familial syndrome of hypocalcemia with hypercalciuria due to mutations in the calcium-sensing receptor. N Engl J Med. Oct 10;335(15):1115-22.

Pollak MR, Brown EM, Estep HL, McLaine PN, Kifor O, Park J, Hebert SC, Seidman CE, Seidman JG. (1994) Autosomal dominant hypocalcaemia caused by a Ca(2+)-sensing receptor gene mutation. Nat Genet. Nov;8(3):303-7.

Porter RH, Cox BG, Heaney D, Hostetter TH, Stinebaugh BJ, Suki WN. (1978) Treatment of hypoparathyroid patients with chlorthalidone. N Engl J Med. Mar 16;298(11):577-81.

Puig-Domingo M, Díaz G, Nicolau J, Fernández C, Rueda S, Halperin I. (2008) Successful treatment of vitamin D unresponsive hypoparathyroidism with multipulse subcutaneous infusion of teriparatide. Eur J Endocrinol. Nov;159(5):653-7.

Riccardi D, Gamba G. (1999) The many roles of the calcium-sensing receptor in health and disease. Arch Med Res. Nov-Dec;30(6):436-48.

Rosen CJ. 2011 Clinical practice. Vitamin D insufficiency. N Engl J Med. 20;364(3):248-

Sanda S, Schlingmann KP, Newfield RS. 2008 Autosomal dominant hypoparathyroidism with severe hypomagnesemia and hypocalcemia, successfully treated with recombinant PTH and continuous subcutaneous magnesium infusion. J Pediatr Endocrinol Metab. Apr;21(4):385-91.

Sato M, Ma YL, Hock JM, Westmore MS, Vahle J, Villanueva A , Turner CH. 2002 Skeletal efficacy with parathyroid hormone in rats was not entirely beneficial with long-term treatment. Journal of Pharmacological and Experimental Therapeutics 302 304–313.

Shiohara M, Shiozawa R, Kurata K, Matsuura H, Arai F, Yasuda T, Koike K. Effect of parathyroid hormone administration in a patient with severe hypoparathyroidism caused by gain-of-function mutation of calcium-sensing receptor. Endocr J.53(6):797-802.

Shoback D. (2008) Clinical practice. Hypoparathyroidism.N Engl J Med. Jul 24;359(4):391-403.

Sthephen J. 2000 Hyperparathyroid and hypoparathyroid disorders. N Engl J Med. 343(25):1863-75.

Torregrosa NM, Rodríguez JM, Llorente S, Balsalobre MD, Rios A, Jimeno L, Parrilla P. 2005 Definitive treatment for persistent hypoparathyroidism in a kidney transplant patient: parathyroid allotransplantation. Thyroid. 15(11):1299-302.

Valero RA, Senovilla L, Núñez L, Villalobos C. The role of mitochondrial potential in control of calcium signals involved in cell proliferation. Cell Calcium. Vol. 44, nº 3 (September 2008) pp 259-69.

Winer KK, Yanovski JA, Cutler GB Jr. (1996) Synthetic human parathyroid hormone 1-34 vs calcitriol and calcium in the treatment of hypoparathyroidism. JAMA. Aug 276(8):631-6.

Winer KK, Yanovski JA, Sarani B, Cutler GB Jr.(1998) A randomized, cross-over trial of once-daily versus twice-daily parathyroid hormone 1-34 in treatment of hypoparathyroidism. J Clin Endocrinol Metab. 1998 Oct;83(10):3480-6.

Winer KK, Ko CW, Reynolds JC, Dowdy K, Keil M, Peterson D, Gerber LH, McGarvey C, Cutler GB Jr. (2003) Long-term treatment of hypoparathyroidism: a randomized controlled study comparing parathyroid hormone-(1-34) versus calcitriol and calcium. J Clin Endocrinol Metab. 2003 Sep;88(9):4214-20

Winer KK, Sinaii N, Peterson D, Sainz B Jr, Cutler GB Jr. 2008 Effects of once versus twice-daily parathyroid hormone 1-34 therapy in children with hypoparathyroidism. J Clin Endocrinol Metab. Sep;93(9):3389-95.

Winer KK, Sinaii N, Reynolds J, Peterson D, Dowdy K, Cutler GB Jr.(2010) Long-term treatment of 12 children with chronic hypoparathyroidism: a randomized trial comparing synthetic human parathyroid hormone 1-34 versus calcitriol and calcium. J Clin Endocrinol Metab. 2010 Jun;95(6):2680-8.

18

Monogenic Phosphate Balance Disorders

Helge Raeder, Silje Rafaelsen and Robert Bjerknes
Department of Clinical Medicine, University of Bergen, Norway

1. Introduction

The last decade has seen that several of the dominant and recessive forms of hypo- and hyperphosphatemic bone disease have received their molecular explanation. This has led to new insight into the pathophysiology of hypo- and hyperphosphatemic bone disease, as well as the understanding of a bone-kidney axis which operates integrated and in parallel with the classical parathyroid-kidney axis in the regulation of phosphorus content in the body. In addition, it has led to the recognition of a Janus face of some of the involved genes, showing both hyper- and hypofunction, dependent on the nature of the mutation. In this book chapter, we will present an update on the emerging insight of monogenic hypo- and hyperphosphatemic disorders.

2. Genetic mechanisms and pathophysiology

Hypophosphatemia may lead to bone or dental disease resulting from decreased mineralization (calcification) of bone or dental matrix or osteoid. The simultaneous blood calcium levels will also influence the degree of mineralization. Hypophosphatemia leads to rickets in children or to osteomalacia in adults. In many of the hypophosphatemic conditions, there is also an impairment of renal activation of vitamin D, further aggravating disease. The mineralization of teeth can also be affected, and there are clinical forms where bone affection is minimal and the dental disorders dominate.

Hyperphosphatemia may lead to increased mineralization of both bone and non-bone tissues (ectopic calcification) due to an increase in the body content of phosphorus. This results in tumoral calcinosis with calcification of muscles, skin and vessels. The monogenic forms affect the renal handling of phosphorus by various mechanisms resulting from inactivation or activation of the involved genes.

With the advancement of genetic insight and the subsequent possibility to study subjects with mutations and a wide range of phenotypes, a broader phenotypic pattern is recognized. Consequently, we suggest the more appropriate terms of monogenic hypophosphatemia and monogenic hyperphosphatemia for these disorders, and that the specific disorders should be classified according to the affected gene, e.g. *PHEX*-hypophosphatemia and *FGF23*-hyperphosphatemia (Table 1).

We will now provide an overview of the genes directly implicated in monogenic phosphate balance disorders. Please refer to textbooks for a discussion of genes indirectly affecting phosphate balance (i.e. genes leading to defective parathyroid gland development or disrupted PTH receptor function).

Gene	Classical disease name	Suggested new name
PHEX	X-linked dominant hypophosphatemic rickets	*PHEX*-hypophosphatemia
DMP1	AR hypophosphatemic rickets	*DMP1*-hypophosphatemia
GALNT3	Familial hyperphosphatemic tumoral calcinosis	*GALNT3*-hyperphosphatemia
FGF23	AD hypophosphatemic rickets	*FGF23*- hypophosphatemia
	Familial hyperphosphatemic tumoral calcinosis	*FGF23*- hyperphosphatemia
FGFR1	Osteogophonic dysplasia with hypophosphatemia	*FGFR1*- hypophosphatemia
KL	Hypophosphatemic rickets and hyperparathyroidism	*KL*-hypophosphatemia
	Hyperphosphatemic tumoral calcinosis	*KL*-hyperphosphatemia
SLC34A1	Hypophosphatemic nefrolithiasis/ osteoporosis	*SLC34A1*-hypophosphatemia
SLC34A3	HHRH	*SLC34A1*-hypophosphatemia
SLC9A3R1	Hypophosphatemic nephrolithiasis/ osteoporosis	*SLC9A3R1*-hypophosphatemia
ENPP1	AR hypophosphatemic rickets, type 2	*ENPP1*-hypophosphatemia

Table 1. Overview of genes directly implicated in monogenic phosphate balance disorders AR, autosomal recessive; AD autosomal dominant, HHRH, Hereditary hypophosphatemic rickets with hypercalciuria.

2.1 PHEX

The *PHEX* (Phosphate-regulating endopeptidase homolog, XB; MIM* 300550) gene consists of 22 exons (Sabbagh, Boileau et al. 2003) and was positionally cloned in 1995 (HYP Consortium 1995). This gene is encoding a transmembrane protein and belongs to the type II integral membrane zinc-dependent endopeptidase family. The gene is expressed in a wide variety of tissues including the kidney with a higher expression in mature osteoblasts and odontoblasts. The substrate for the gene product is not known, but the pathogenesis seems to involve phosphate regulating humoral factors, phosphatonins, where the fibroblast growth factor-23 (FGFR-23) is central (Jonsson, Zahradnik et al. 2003; Juppner 2007; Bastepe and Juppner 2008). (See section 2.11 for a discussion on the physiological and pathophysiological mechanisms involved.) The protein is also believed to be involved in bone and dentin mineralization. Both the whole-body and bone-specific (osteocalcin-promoted inactivation) knockout mouse model of PHEX as well as the spontaneous Hyp mouse model display increased bone production, increased levels of serum FGF23, decreased kidney membrane NPT2 and osteomalacia (Yuan, Takaiwa et al. 2008). Cell studies indicate mechanistic defects both during protein processing in the endoplasmic reticulum and cell membrane (Sabbagh, Boileau et al. 2001) and as abrogated catalytic activity (Sabbagh, Boileau et al. 2003).

There are several mutations associated with PHEX-hypophosphatemia (see the PHEX mutation database: http://www.phexdb.mcgill.ca/) and most of the mutations are located in the region encoding the extracellular domain, but there are also examples of pathological mutations in the 5'UTR (Dixon, Christie et al. 1998) and 3'UTR (Ichikawa, Traxler et al. 2008) of the gene.

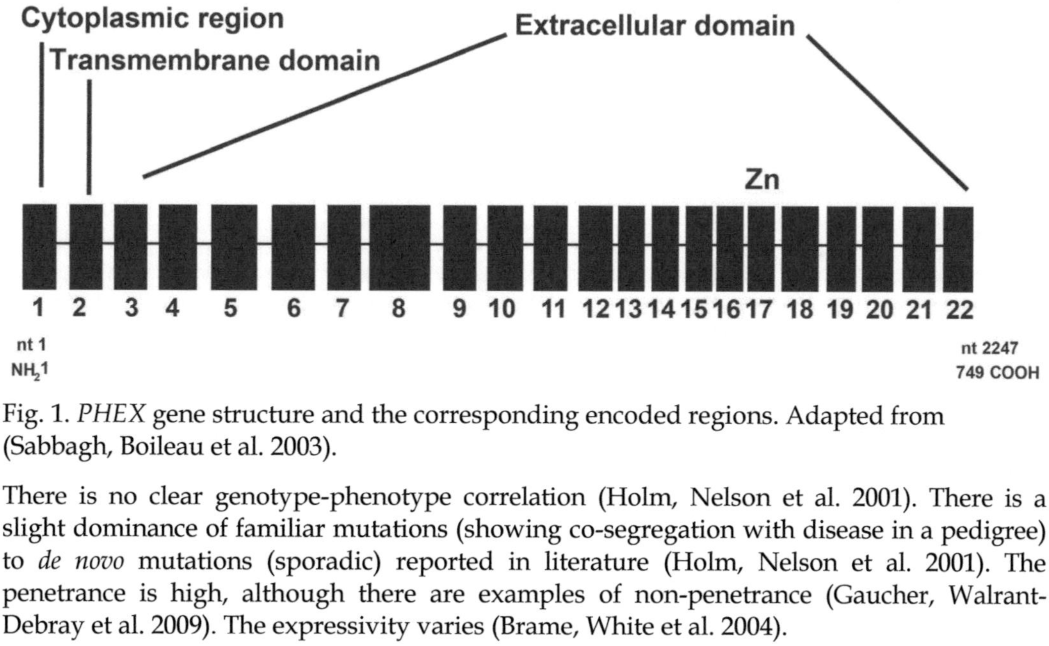

Fig. 1. *PHEX* gene structure and the corresponding encoded regions. Adapted from (Sabbagh, Boileau et al. 2003).

There is no clear genotype-phenotype correlation (Holm, Nelson et al. 2001). There is a slight dominance of familiar mutations (showing co-segregation with disease in a pedigree) to *de novo* mutations (sporadic) reported in literature (Holm, Nelson et al. 2001). The penetrance is high, although there are examples of non-penetrance (Gaucher, Walrant-Debray et al. 2009). The expressivity varies (Brame, White et al. 2004).

2.2 DMP1

The *DMP1* gene (dentin matrix acidic phosphoprotein 1; MIM* 600980) gene consists of 6 exons on chromosome 4q21, and was first implicated in a phosphate balance disorder in 2006 Lorenz-Depiereux, Bastepe et al. 2006). *DMP1* is highly expressed in osteocytes, and is a member of the 'SIBLING' (small integrin binding ligand n-linked glycoprotein) family of non-collagenous extracellular matrix proteins involved in bone mineralization (Huq, Cross et al. 2005). The *DMP1* knockout model displays rickets and osteomalacia with isolated renal phosphate wasting associated with elevated FGF23 levels and normocalciuria (Feng, Ward et al. 2006). In humans, homozygous or compound heterozygous mutations in *DMP1* leads to hypophosphatemic rickets with elevated FGF23, isolated phosphate wasting, and no evidence of hypercalciuria. The exact relation between DMP1 and FGF23 levels is not known, but in vitro studies have shown that vitamin D increases the expression of both (Farrow, Davis et al. 2009).

There are only a few reported mutations in the literature (Feng, Ward et al. 2006; Lorenz-Depiereux, Bastepe et al. 2006; Farrow, Davis et al. 2009; Koshida, Yamaguchi et al. 2010; Makitie, Pereira et al. 2010; Turan, Aydin et al. 2010), making *DMP1* mutations a rare cause of hypophosphatemic rickets (Gaucher, Walrant-Debray et al. 2009).

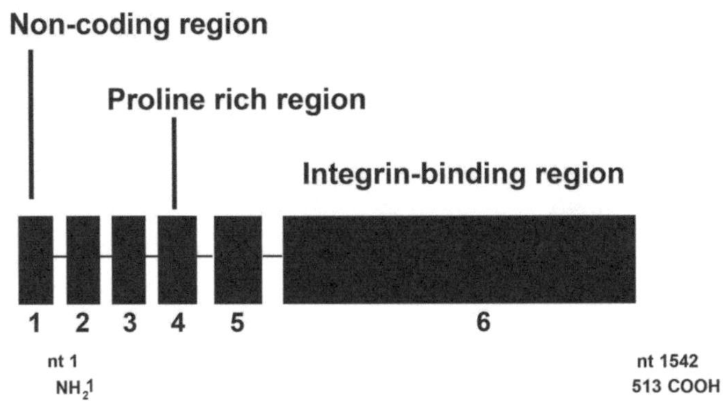

Fig. 2. *DMP1* gene structure and the corresponding encoded regions. Based on (Huq, Cross et al. 2005).

2.3 GALNT3

The O-glycosylation of serine and threonine residues on many glycoproteins depend on enzymatic catalyzation of the reaction UDP-GalNAc + polypeptide-(Ser/Thr)-OH to GalNAc-alpha-O-Ser/Thr-polypeptide + UDP. GalNAcT3 is one of 24 members in the UDP-GalNAc:polypeptide N-acetylgalactosaminyltransferase protein family involved in this process.

GalNAcT3 is encoded by the *GALNT3* gene (MIM *601756) on chromosome 2q24-q31, which contains 10 exons. GalNAcT3 is thought to protect FGF23 from proteolysis (Kato, Jeanneau et al. 2006) by *O*-glycosylation, and a deactivating mutation in *GALNT3* will thus lead to increased breakdown of FGF23. Mutations in *GALNT3* were the first to be associated with familial tumoral calcinosis (FTC) (Topaz, Shurman et al. 2004), and are also seen in the closely related disease, the hyperphosphatemic hyperostosis syndrome (HHS). These are the only diseases known to be caused by mutations in the family of UDP-GalNAc:polypeptide N-acetylgalactosaminyltransferases. Although the process of O-glycosylation is important in many tissues, mutations in *GALNT3* lead to a very restricted phenotype with hyperphosphatemia, periarticular calcifications and hyperostosis. This is thought to be explained by functional redundancy of this protein family. In addition to the effects on bone and renal phosphate handling caused by altered FGF23 metabolism, mutations in *GALNT3* are also thought to have direct effect in the process of ectopic calcification in extraosseous tissues (Chefetz and Sprecher 2009).

2.4 FGF23

The *FGF23* gene (MIM*605380) on chromosome 12 is composed of 3 exons, and encodes a member of the fibroblast growth factor family. The protein product, FGF23, acts via its receptor FGFR1 (fibroblast growth factor receptor 1, see 2.5), but is also dependent on the co-receptor Klotho (α-Klotho) to exert its functions (see below). Furthermore, FGF23 belongs to the FGF19 family where the two other family members, FGF19 and FGF21, (also binding to FGFR1) are dependent on ß -Klotho to exert their functions, illustrating the role of a co-receptor to ensure tissue specificity and function (Kurosu, Choi et al. 2007). FGF23 exerts its physiological effects on the kidney by the downregulation of the *CYP27B1* gene leading to a loss of compensatory increase in 1,25(OH)$_2$vitamin D levels, and by the endocytosis of the type IIa and IIc Na/phosphate (Pi) cotransporters (Npt2a and Npt2c) from the renal proximal tubular brush border membrane.

Heterozygous activating mutations in the cleavage site RXXR motif of exon 3 of *FGF23*, leads to stabilization and decreased degradation of the FGF23. The clinical phenotype is autosomal dominant hypophosphatemic rickets (Econs, McEnery et al. 1997; 2000).

Homozygous inactivating missense mutations in *FGF23* lead to hyperphosphatemic familial tumoral calcinosis, due to decreased renal excretion of phosphate and increased renal α-hydroxylation of vitamin D (Benet-Pages, Orlik et al. 2005; Ichikawa, Baujat et al. 2010).

2.5 FGFR1

The Fibroblast growth factor receptor 1 gene *FGFR1* (MIM*136315) located on chromosome 8p11 encodes a protein member of the FGFR (1-4) family, where the members are all receptor tyrosine kinases. FGFR1-3 are implicated in skeletal development, and various mutations in the corresponding genes are responsible for a number of skeletal dysplastic syndromes (Passos-Bueno, Wilcox et al. 1999). There are several subclasses of FGFRs, depending on the number of immunoglobulin-like loops and splicing differences in the third loop. FGFR1C combines with Klotho (*KL*) to become the functional receptor for FGF23 (Urakawa, Yamazaki et al. 2006).

Mutations in the *FGFR1C* lead to constitutive activation of the receptor and subsequent downregulation of the expression of the sodium-phosphate co-transporters NaPiIIa and NaPiIIc, as well as the downregulation of the *CYP27B1* gene leading to a loss of compensatory increase in 1,25(OH)$_2$vitamin D levels (Shimada, Hasegawa et al. 2004).

2.6 *KL*

Klotho (*KL*) (MIM*604824) is located to chromosome 13q12, comprises 5 exons, and encodes the protein Klotho (also known as α-Klotho), which in mice is considered a hormone with anti-aging properties (Kurosu, Yamamoto et al. 2005). *KL* knockout mice will go through a rapid aging process, and have decreased insulin secretion and increased insulin sensitivity (Kuro-o, Matsumura et al. 1997), while overexpression of *KL* leads to a prolonged life span in mice (Kurosu, Yamamoto et al. 2005). In addition, Klotho has been associated with disturbances of phosphate metabolism, as it is an obligate co-receptor for the binding of FGF23 to FGFR1C. In humans, there are two *KL* transcripts; one encoding a membrane bound protein and one encoding a secreted protein. Human *KL* is expressed mainly in the kidney, and the secreted variant seems to dominate (Matsumura, Aizawa et al. 1998). Recent findings from mouse studies suggest that Klotho has endocrine, paracrine and autocrine effects independent of FGF23 (Hu, Shi et al. 2010).

Inactivating mutations will lead to familial hyperphosphatemic tumoral calcinosis, similar to the phenotypes seen in *GALNT3*-hyperphosphatemia and *FGF23*-hyperphosphatemia (Ichikawa, Imel et al. 2007).
There is also one report of an activating translocation of the *KL* gene, leading to hypophosphatemic rickets with a phenotype similar to *PHEX*-hypophosphatemia but with additional distinctive dysmorphic features of the head (Brownstein, Adler et al. 2008).

2.7 SLC34A1

The solute carrier 34 (*SLC34*) gene family includes the three genes *SLC34A1*, *SLC34A2* and *SLC34A3*, all encoding sodium/phosphate cotransporters. *SLC34A2* encodes the intestinal NaPi-IIb, and will not be further discussed. *SLC34A1* and *SLC34A3* encode the two renal sodium/phosphate cotransporters, and the latter is described in 2.8 section.
The *SLC34A1* (MIM*182309) gene is expressed in the renal proximal tubule, and encodes the type IIa Na/Pi cotransporter (NaPi-IIa), which plays a central role in renal phosphate handling in various animal models. The expression of NaPi-IIa in the brush border membrane is regulated at the post translational level, by endocytosis and lysosomal degradation or microtubular recruitment (Tenenhouse 2005). Both PTH and FGF23 lead to increased endocytosis of NAPi-IIa, and thus decreased reabsorption of Pi from filtered urine, whereas hypophosphatemia and 1,25 dihydroxyvitamin D stimulate phosphate reabsorption (Tenenhouse 2005). There also seems to be a directly regulating effect of dietary Pi on Na/Pi cotransport in proximal tubules, and the existence of an intestinal-renal axis for phosphate regulation has been proposed [review: (Biber, Hernando et al. 2009)]. NaPi-IIa double knockout mice have hypophosphatemia, phosphaturia, elevated 1,25 dihydroxyvitamin D with resulting hypercalcemia, hypercalcuria and nephrocalcinosis/nephrolithiasis (Beck, Karaplis et al. 1998). This phenotype resembles hereditary hypophosphatemic rickets with hypercalcuria (HHRH) seen in humans, which interestingly is not caused by mutations in *SLCA34A1*, but rather by mutations in *SLC34A3* (NaPi-IIc) (see 2.8).
In man, a few cases have been described of heterozygous mutations in *SLC34A1*, leading to a syndrome of hypophosphatemia, osteoporosis and nephrolithiasis (Prie, Huart et al. 2002).

2.8 SLC34A3

The human *SLC34A3* (MIM*609826) gene, consists of 13 exons on chromosome 9q34, and homozygous mutations in this gene lead to hereditary hypophosphatemic rickets with hypercalciuria (HHRH) (Bergwitz, Roslin et al. 2006; Lorenz-Depiereux, Benet-Pages et al. 2006). The phenotype of HHRH resembles that of NaPi-IIa knockout mice, but the patients also display rickets or osteomalacia. In animal models the type IIc Na/Pi cotransporter (NaPi-IIc) has been shown to play a more minor role in proximal tubular phosphate resorption than NaPi-IIa. The opposite might be the case in man (Amatschek, Haller et al. 2010).

2.9 SLC9A3R1

The *SLC9A3R1* (MIM*604990) gene on chromosome 17 encodes the protein NHERF1 (sodium/hydrogen exchanger regulatory factor 1), which plays a part in maintaining the cytoskeleton in polarized cells with microvilli, such as renal tubular cells. Three different mutations in *SLC9A3R1* have recently been identified in 7 subjects with hypophosphatemia due to phosphaturia, nephrolithiasis and osteoporosis (Karim, Gerard et al. 2008).

2.10 ENPP1

The *ENPP1* (ectonucleotide pyrophosphatase/phosphodiesterase 1) (MIM*173335) gene on chromosome 6q22-q23 comprises 23 exones and encodes a type II transmembrane glycoprotein ectoenzyme responsible for the generation of inorganic pyrophosphate (PPi). PPi is an inhibitor of hydroxyapatite crystal growth, and also suppress chondrogenesis. In mice, *ENPP1* is expressed in plasma cells, on hepatocytes, renal tubules, salivary duct epithelium, epididymis, capillary endothelium in the brain, and chondrocytes (Harahap and Goding 1988). In man it has been shown that *ENPP1* is expressed in liver, cartilage and bone, and is thought to regulate physiological mineralization processes and pathological chondrocalcinosis (Huang, Rosenbach et al. 1994).

Homozygous mutations in *ENPP1* are known to cause generalized arterial calcifications of infancy (GACI) (Rutsch, Vaingankar et al. 2001; Rutsch, Ruf et al. 2003). Recently, homozygous mutations in *ENPP1* have been shown to cause autosomal recessive hypophosphataemic rickets (Levy-Litan, Hershkovitz et al. 2010). In some families, identical mutations cause GACI in some family members and hypophosphatemic rickets in other family members (Lorenz-Depiereux, Schnabel et al. 2010). Prolonged survival in GACI has been observed in subjects who have simultaneously displayed renal phosphate loss (Rutsch, Boyer et al. 2008).

Mutations in *ENPP1* have also been associated with susceptibility to insulin resistance and obesity (Goldfine, Maddux et al. 2008).

2.11 An integrated model for the physiological and pathophysiological mechanisms in the renal phosphate regulation

Figure 3 shows the integrated physiological and pathophysiological mechanisms in the renal phosphate regulation. The parathyroid-renal axis has been the traditional model explaining how PTH stimulates the renal tubular cells to phosphaturia as a negative feedback loop response to elevated phosphate levels (Figure 3A). In this model PTH acts via its receptor to block the sodium-phosphate co-transporters NaPiIIa and NaPiIIc encoded by the *SLC34A1* and *SLC34A3* genes, respectively. In addition, PTH stimulates the *CYP27B1* gene leading to a compensatory increase in 1,25(OH)$_2$vitamin D levels as a negative feedback loop to reduced serum levels of 1,25(OH)$_2$vitamin D and calcium. There is, however, also a PTH-independent pathway where hormonal substances from bone, phosphatonins, stimulate the renal tubular cells to phosphaturia in a negative feedback response to elevated serum phosphate and 1,25(OH)$_2$vitamin D levels. Recent emerging insight has laid the foundation for this model of a bone-kidney axis (Quarles 2003), where fibroblast growth factor 23 (FGF23) seems to be the central phosphatonin inhibiting phosphate reabsorption and hence inducing phosphaturia (Figure 3B). In contrast to PTH, FGF23 inhibits *CYP27B1* gene leading to an absent compensatory increase in 1,25(OH)$_2$vitamin D levels, recognized by clinicians as inappropriate normal 1,25(OH)$_2$vitamin D levels. In the normal state *PHEX* and *DMP1* gene products seem to inhibit FGF23 production, whereas the *GALNT3* gene product seems to stimulate FGF23 production. By interfering with the bone-kidney axis, increased FGF23 levels seem to play a central role in the pathogenesis of *PHEX*-hypophosphatemia (Jonsson, Zahradnik et al. 2003) (Figure 3C) and potentially also *DMP1*-hypophosphatemia (Lorenz-Depiereux, Bastepe et al. 2006; Turan, Aydin et al. 2010) and *FGF23*- hypophosphatemia (Imel, Hui et al. 2007), but the mechanisms are still poorly known (Strom and Juppner 2008). It is also poorly known how increased FGF23 levels in *FGF23*- hyperphosphatemia and *GALNT3*-

hyperphosphatemia explain the opposite condition of hyperphosphatemia (Topaz, Shurman et al. 2004; Benet-Pages, Orlik et al. 2005). A current model postulates that mutations in *PHEX* lead to increased FGF23 production by cancelled *PHEX*-mediated inhibition of FGF23 production (Figure 3 C).

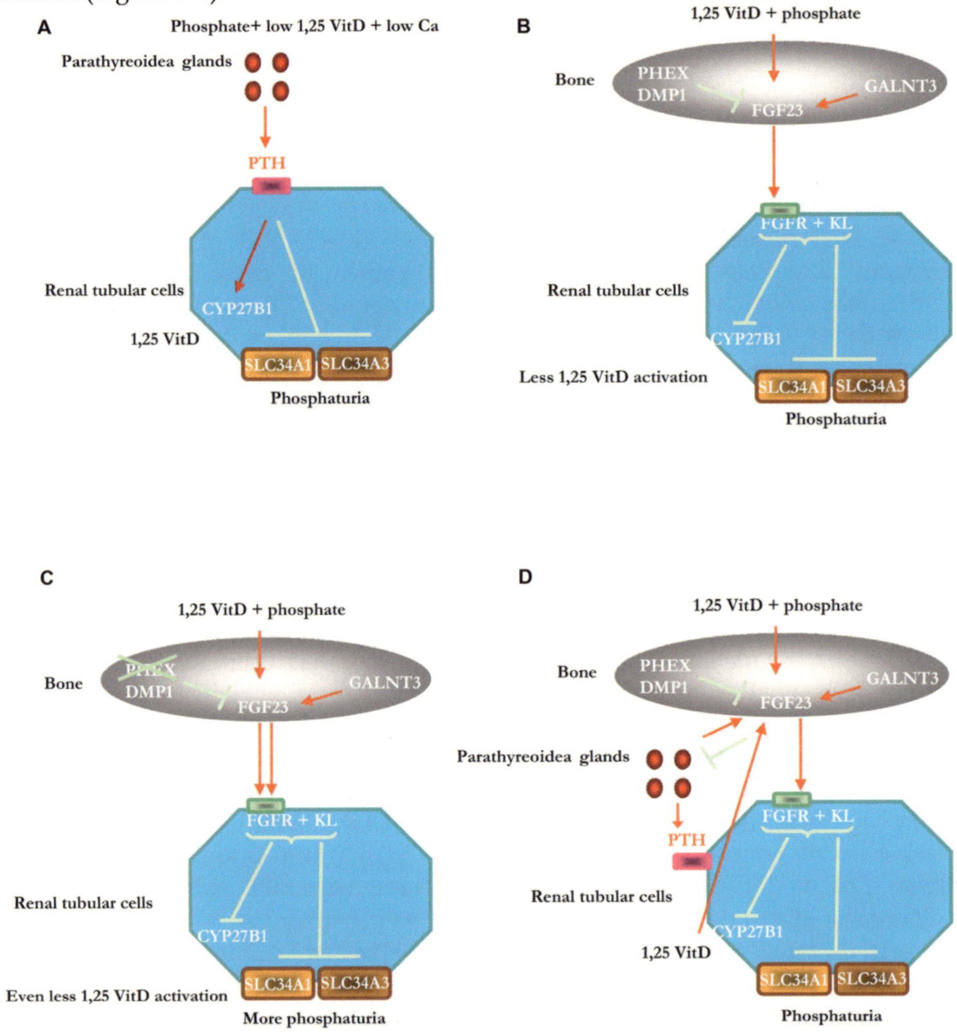

Fig. 3. Physiological and pathophysiological conditions in the phosphate regulation. For sake of clarity, only gene names are depicted and not the corresponding gene products. Adapted from (Bastepe and Juppner 2008; Strom and Juppner 2008).

Both the parathyroid-renal axis and the bone-kidney axis seem to be negative feedback loops where increased serum phosphate levels compared to a biological set value leads to phosphaturia. These two axes are different with respect to $1,25(OH)_2$vitamin D: Whereas low $1,25(OH)_2$vitamin D levels stimulating $1,25(OH)_2$vitamin D activation is the major regulation in the parathyroid-renal axis, high $1,25(OH)_2$vitamin D levels inhibiting $1,25(OH)_2$vitamin D activation is the major regulation in the bone-kidney axis. Recent work also points to interactions between these feedback loops where FGF23 inhibits PTH, whereas PTH possibly stimulates FGF23 (Figure 3D). Mutations in genes encoding the sodium-phosphate co-transporters such as *SLC34A1*, *SLC34A3* and *SLC9A3R1* lead to increased phosphaturia but since the 1,25(OH)$_2$vitamin D activation is unaffected, there is a normal compensatory increase in 1,25(OH)$_2$vitamin D levels. Whether gene mutations lead to hypophosphatemia or hyperphosphatemia is dependent on the location of the gene product in the pathways outlined above and whether the mutation is activating or inactivating the affected gene.

3. Diagnostic considerations

The diagnosis of monogenic hypo- or hyperphosphatemia requires the demonstration of affected phosphate balance in patients in which acquired causes of phosphate disturbance have been excluded. A family history of rickets, kidney stones, soft tissue calcification, bone deformities or recurrent fractures, as well as an indication of monogenic inheritance pattern is usually found, unless the patient seems to represent a sporadic case. In the case of hypophosphatemia, there is typically low plasma phosphate, low renal tubular reabsorption of phosphate (% TRP) and tubular threshold maximum for phosphate for glomerular filtration rate (TmP/GFR), raised alkaline phosphatase, normal PTH, and inappropriate and normal 25(OH) and 1,25(OH)$_2$ vitamin D levels. Moreover, the urinary calcium excretion is normal, whereas X-ray changes may demonstrate rickets or osteomalacia. FGF23 levels are typically high, either due to overproduction or under-catabolism, and in children with rickets, the combined evaluation of FGF23 and PTH leads differential diagnosis in the direction of impaired phosphate homeostasis (high FGF23 and normal PTH) or altered metabolism of vitamin D, calcium or magnesium (low FGF23 and high PTH) (Alon 2010). In the case of hyperphosphatemia, there is usually high plasma phosphate, an inappropriate normal % TRP and TmP/GFR, a low or normal PTH and normal renal function. In some cases, the clinical picture and inheritance pattern will suggest a specific genetic diagnosis, and, in addition, the blood FGF23 levels and hypercalciuria may differentiate between different genetic disorders of phosphate balance, although the clinical role of blood FGF23 levels is at present not fully elucidated.

3.1 PHEX

PHEX-hypophosphatemia (X-linked dominant) is usually a progressive disorder with a typical onset at the age when the child starts to walk. The most common clinical manifestations include genu varus, radiological rickets, short stature, bone pain, dental abscesses and calcification of tendons, ligaments and joint capsules with boys being more severely affected than girls and a wide variation between families (Econs, Samsa et al. 1994; Carpenter 1997; Bastepe and Juppner 2008). Some patients may even have craniosynosteosis and spinal stenosis. Many patients suffer from long lasting dental problems, particularly tooth decay and recurrent spontaneous dental abscesses that occur in the absence of a history of trauma or dental decay. Histological findings include high pulp horns, globular dentin, and defects of dentin and enamel. The primary teeth are most commonly affected, as the mineralization process starts in utero. Permanent teeth develop after birth, and adequate treatment improve development in some cases (Batra, Tejani et al. 2006). In children with rickets, a low serum phosphorus level, combined with high serum alkaline phosphatase and normal serum calcium is typical (Carpenter 1997). Urinary leakage of phosphate is demonstrated by low % TRP and TmP/GFR, whereas urinary calcium is normal. The PTH levels are usually normal or slightly elevated, even before the onset of therapy. The 25(OH)vitamin D is normal, and there is no compensatory increase in 1,25(OH)$_2$vitamin D levels due to defective renal activation of vitamin D, and, hence, no hypercalciuria. The FGF23 levels are increased (Jonsson, Zahradnik et al. 2003), and since the lower extremities are more severely affected than the other parts of the skeleton, radiographs of the knees and ankles will demonstrate the extent of rickets. The diagnosis of *PHEX*-hypophosphatemia is confirmed by genetic analysis.

3.2 DMP1

DMP1-hypophosphatemia (autosomal recessive) is usually a progressive disorder with a typical onset at the age when the child starts to walk. The condition is rarer than *PHEX*-hypophosphatemia, but is phenotypically quite similar to *PHEX*- and *FGF23*-hypophosphatemie. There is no compensatory increase in 1,25(OH)$_2$vitamin D levels due to defective renal activation of vitamin D and hence no hypercalciuria. The circulation levels of FGF23 are increased (Feng, Ward et al. 2006). The degree of skeletal abnormalities varies between families (Makitie, Pereira et al. 2010). Some patients also have dental affection, with hypomineralization, enlarged pulp chambers, and decrease in the dentin and enamel layers, which can cause dental abscesses and loss of teeth (Koshida, Yamaguchi et al. 2010; Turan, Aydin et al. 2010).

3.3 GALNT3

GALNT3-hyperphosphatemia is the result of biallelic mutation in the *GALNT3*-gene, and leads to typical tumoral calcinosis (TC) (Topaz, Shurman et al. 2004) or hyperostosis-hyperphosphatemia syndrome (HHS). There are several mutations in the *GALNT3* gene, and the same mutation can lead to TC in some patients and HHS in other (Ichikawa, Baujat et al. 2010). TC is characterized by ectopic calcifications in soft tissues and around large joints, recognized clinically as palpable masses and/or on radiography. Calcifications may also be found in the retina, in blood vessels, as testicular microlithiasis, and there might be dental abnormalities. HHC is characterized by hyperostosis of long bones, seen radiographically as cortical hyperostosis, diaphysitis and periosteal apposition. The biochemical findings in TC and HHC are similar, with elevated serum phosphate levels, increased or normal 1,25(OH)$_2$vitamin D levels. The levels of serum calcium and parathyroid hormone are normal. Some authors suggest that TC and HHS are clinical variants of the same disease (Ichikawa, Baujat et al. 2010).

3.4 FGF23

FGF23-hypophosphatemia (autosomal dominant) shows a variable age at onset of disease.

The expression of disease varies, and some children may have fracture tendency without skeletal deformities, whereas other children may have only temporary renal phosphate loss (Econs and McEnery 1997). Tooth abscesses and loss also occurs (Imel, Hui et al. 2007).

FGF23-hyperphosphatemia (autosomal recessive) shows typical tumoral calcinosis , or more rarely the hyperostosis-hyperphosphatemia syndrome (Benet-Pages, Orlik et al. 2005).

3.5 FGFR1

FGFR1R-hypophosphatemia is characterized by osteoglophonic dysplasia and can be associated with hypophosphatemia (Farrow, Davis et al. 2006). Clinical features are skeletal abnormalities leading to dwarfism and facial abnormalities similar to achondroplasia. There is often failure of tooth eruption, and mandibular malformations. Patients may also have various degrees of craniosynostosis (White, Cabral et al. 2005).

3.6 *KL*

To date only one case of *KL*-hypophosphatemia has been described in the literature (Brownstein, Adler et al. 2008). A 1-year old girl suffered from poor linear growth and increasing head size. She had clinical and radiological signs of rickets, hypophosphatemia, renal phosphate wasting and elevated levels of parathyroid hormone and alkaline phosphatase. A balanced translocation between chromosomes 9 and 13 was detected (t(9,13)(q21.13;q13.1)). This translocation had led to upregulation of *KL*-transcription. After a few years she demonstrated dysmorphic features of the face, and also an Arnold-Chiari 1 malformation (Brownstein, Adler et al. 2008). Dental affection has not been described.

KL-hyperphosphatemia has also been described in only one report (Ichikawa, Imel et al. 2007). A 13 year old girl presented with severe calcifications in soft tissues and in the vasculature, including the dura and the carotid arteries. In addition to hyperphosphatemia and hypercalcemia, she presented with hyperparathyroidism and elevated levels of FGF23. She had no signs of premature aging, which is seen in *KL* knockout mice. Dental affection has not been described.

3.7 SLC34A1 and SLC34A3

In *SLC34A1*- and *SLC34A3*-hypophosphatemia, there is hypophosphatemic rickets with hypercalciuria without other tubular defects (Tieder, Modai et al. 1985). The inheritance pattern is autosomal recessive. Since there is normal renal activation of vitamin D (in contrast to *PHEX*-hypophosphatemia and *DMP1*-hypophosphatemia), hypophosphatemia leads to a normal compensatory increase in 1,25$(OH)_2$vitamin D levels and increased absorption of calcium and phosphate from the gut.

3.8 SLC9A3R1

A total of 7 cases of SLC9A3R1-hypophosphatemia (hypophosphatemia, nephrolithiasis/osteoporosis) have been described to date (Karim, Gerard et al. 2008). All patients were adults, and had either nephrolithiasis and/or bone demineralization combined with hypophosphatemia and hyperphosphaturia. 1,25 (OH)2 vitamin D levels were either elevated or in the upper normal range. Dental affection has not been described.

3.9 ENPP1

ENPP1-hypophosphatemia (autosomal recessive) has a variable age at onset and a variable phenotype including Generalized Arterial Calcification of Infancy (GACI). Also there seems to be phenotypic variation within the same family among affected subjects carrying the same mutation. Whereas the classic presentation is that of severe arterial calcification leading to death in infancy, some patients have renal phosphate wasting and hypophosphatemia. This phosphate loss seems to attenuate the tendency of arterial calcifications, and is associated with prolonged survival (Lorenz-Depiereux, Schnabel et al. 2010).

4. Management principles

4.1 Hypophosphatemia

Hypophosphatemic rickets is in childhood usually treated with elementary phosphorus at doses preferentially between 30 and 60 (100) mg/kg bodyweight and 24 hours, usually divided by 4-6 doses, whereas the deficient 1,25(OH)$_2$vitamin D production is treated with active vitamin D, e.g. alphacalcidol or calcitriol in doses of 20 to 70 ng/kg bodyweight and 24 hours, usually divided by 2 doses. It should, however, be emphasized that the dosage ranges for both phosphate and active vitamin D are wide, dependent on the severity of the disease, the compliance and the occurrence of complications. In *SLC34A1*- and *SLC34A3*-hypophosphatemia, activation of vitamin D is normal, and, consequently, there is no need for treatment with vitamin D.

It is important to adjust the drug doses individually and bear in mind that insufficient doses of elementary phosphorus and vitamin D may fail to prevent or correct skeletal deformities (rickets, osteomalacia) and can lead to growth retardation. On the other hand, excessive doses may lead to nephrocalcinosis (high phosphate doses), as well as hypercalciuria and hypercalcemia (high vitamin D levels). Secondary (and even tertiary) hyperparathyroidism is seen in patients with insufficient doses of vitamin D or excessive doses of phosphorus. We recommend aiming at normal levels of PTH, which in severe cases may be obtained by adding the calcimimetic drug cinacalcet to the treatment (Raeder, Bjerknes et al. 2008).

Close monitoring is necessary to balance the effects of phosphorus supplement and active vitamin D. Growth, serum calcium, phosphorus, alkaline phosphatase, PTH, as well as urinary calcium/creatinine ratio should be determined every 3-6 months, and X-rays of ankles, knees and wrist should be taken yearly. Renal ultrasound should be obtained yearly to assess nephrocalcinosis.

Supplementary treatment with growth hormone is currently not recommended for the growth retardation caused by hypophosphatemia (Huiming and Chaomin 2005), but may be warranted in selected cases. Corrective osteotomies are seldom necessary in childhood, and it should always be deferred until the rickets has healed. Future therapeutic possibilities may include direct targeting of blood FGF23 levels.

4.2 Hyperphosphatemia

Patients with hyperphosphatemia due to monogenic phosphate balance disorders, i.e. *GALNT3*-hyperphosphatemia, *FGF23*-hyperphosphatemia and *KL*-hyperphosphatemia, develop ectopic and vascular calcifications. Combined use of intestinal phosphate binders and the carbonic anhydrase inhibitor acetazolamide has been reported to lower serum phosphorus levels and reduce tumoral masses in some patients (Garringer, Fisher et al. 2006). However, other reports suggest that neither medical nor surgical treatment seems to be effective in controlling ectopic calcifications in these conditions (Carmichael, Bynum et al. 2009). Future therapeutic possibilities may include direct targeting of blood FGF23 levels.

4.3 Genetic diagnostics and predictive testing

Identification of a specific mutation has important therapeutic and prognostic implications and tailored follow-up as outlined above. Distinction between *PHEX*-hypophosphatemia and *DMP1*-hypophosphatemia can be done clinically based on the inheritance pattern, but in some cases there is an ambiguous inheritance pattern (Figure 4) and a genetic test will resolve this ambiguity.

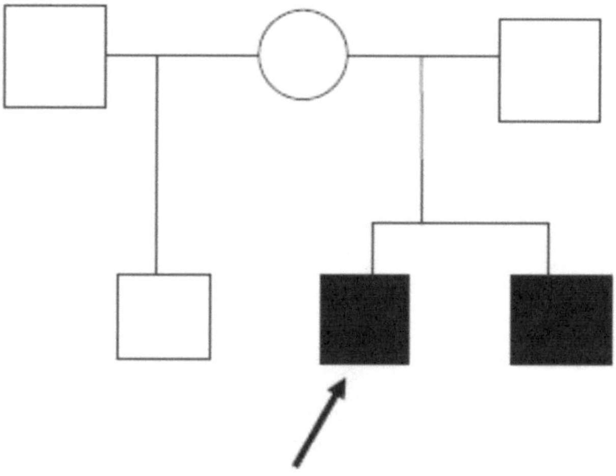

Fig. 4. An example of ambiguous inheritance pattern. Note that in this case, the pattern is compatible both with an X-linked disorder (i.e. *PHEX*-hypophosphatemia) and an AR disorder (i.e. *DMP1*-hypophosphatemia).

Monogenic phosphate balance disorders warrant genetic counseling, because of the known inheritance pattern and the high penetrance. This is also the case for novel gene variants where it is necessary to establish evidence for causality based on co-segregation studies and prediction tools (such as Polyphen http://genetics.bwh.harvard.edu/pph/)). Predictive genetic testing is less straightforward, and the legal regulations vary in different countries. Communicating genetic information can be difficult and it is important to take into account how well the individual understands both genetics in general and the disorder itself and the consequences of potentially diagnosing other family subjects. The basic fact that there is a 25% or 50% probability for a child to carry the family's mutation should be conveyed to the parents. In addition, the probability for the development of the disorder in the presence of a mutation (i.e. the penetrance) is not always 100%. The variable and in some cases unpredictable age of onset of some of the disorders should also be discussed. By increasing knowledge of the clinical spectrum of mutations, novel expected manifestations need to be discussed with the patient. A system for follow-up is required for children without a phenotype but with affected family members and where parents still request that their child be tested. This follow-up may include periodic testing for hypophosphatemia, with a frequency dependent on age and the suspected condition.

5. Research perspectives

We have established a national database of patients with hypophospahtemic bone disorder in order to study phenotype-genotype correlation in this disease and to be able to explore novel pathophysiologic pathways based on insight obtained from studies of families with no previously known genetic cause of monogenic hypophosphatemic bone disorder. We believe that a new classification of disease based on genetic etiology instead of clinical criteria may facilitate the finding of new phenotypes since it will facilitate the study of unobserved phenotypes, both in the patients and in their presumably unaffected relatives carrying mutations. In addition, it is possible that emerging new treatment options may vary based on the genetic diagnosis which warrants studies of associations between gene variants and therapeutic effects. Future studies of monogenic phosphate balance disorders will probably continue to include genomewide studies of families with genetically unexplained phosphate balance disorders. Animal and cell studies will probably also continue to contribute to the understanding of disease mechanism, and, in particular, the use of induced pluripotent stem cells (iPS) seems to be a promising new tool in the mechanistic and therapeutic studies (Rosenzweig 2010) as well as the use of small molecule screens in the search for new therapeutic options in monogenic disease (Shaw, Blodgett et al. 2011) .

6. Conclusion

As we have discussed in this book chapter, several of the dominant and recessive forms of hypo- and hyperphosphatemic bone disease have received their molecular explanation leading to new insight into the pathophysiology of hypo- and hyperphosphatemic bone disease. The major advancement in pathophysiological understanding has come from the understanding of a bone-kidney axis where the central bone phosphatonin FGF23 acts on FGFR1-receptors in the kidneys to promote phosphaturia and from the understanding of all the factors converging on this axis. In fact, this axis ties together the known monogenic forms of renal phosphate disorders. In addition, the understanding of the genetics and pathophysiology of these disorders has led to the recognition of the two faces of some of the involved genes, showing both hyper- and hypofunction, dependent on the nature of the mutation, which is in particular the case for mutations affecting the *KL* and *FGF23* genes.

We recommend the use of a genetic-oriented classification instead of the traditional disease-oriented classification since we believe that this will facilitate a broader understanding of the phenotype of monogenic phosphate balance disorders. Whereas increased molecular understanding has led to a more precise diagnosis, it has not yet led to new established treatment. We believe, however, that the molecular understanding will indeed facilitate the development of new treatment options with the use of the powerful tools including iPS cells and small molecular screens.

7. References

ADHR Consortium (2000). "Autosomal dominant hypophosphataemic rickets is associated with mutations in FGF23." Nat Genet 26(3): 345-348.

Alon, U. S. (2010). "Clinical practice : Fibroblast growth factor (FGF)23: a new hormone." European journal of pediatrics.

Amatschek, S., M. Haller, et al. (2010). "Renal phosphate handling in human--what can we learn from hereditary hypophosphataemias?" Eur J Clin Invest 40(6): 552-560.

Bastepe, M. and H. Juppner (2008). "Inherited hypophosphatemic disorders in children and the evolving mechanisms of phosphate regulation." Rev Endocr Metab Disord 9(2): 171-180.

Batra, P., Z. Tejani, et al. (2006). "X-linked hypophosphatemia: dental and histologic findings." J Can Dent Assoc 72(1): 69-72.

Beck, L., A. C. Karaplis, et al. (1998). "Targeted inactivation of Npt2 in mice leads to severe renal phosphate wasting, hypercalciuria, and skeletal abnormalities." Proc Natl Acad Sci U S A 95(9): 5372-5377.

Benet-Pages, A., P. Orlik, et al. (2005). "An FGF23 missense mutation causes familial tumoral calcinosis with hyperphosphatemia." Hum Mol Genet 14(3): 385-390.

Bergwitz, C., N. M. Roslin, et al. (2006). "SLC34A3 mutations in patients with hereditary hypophosphatemic rickets with hypercalciuria predict a key role for the sodium-phosphate cotransporter NaPi-IIc in maintaining phosphate homeostasis." Am J Hum Genet 78(2): 179-192.

Biber, J., N. Hernando, et al. (2009). "Regulation of phosphate transport in proximal tubules." Pflugers Arch 458(1): 39-52.

Brame, L. A., K. E. White, et al. (2004). "Renal phosphate wasting disorders: clinical features and pathogenesis." Seminars in nephrology 24(1): 39-47.

Brownstein, C. A., F. Adler, et al. (2008). "A translocation causing increased alpha-klotho level results in hypophosphatemic rickets and hyperparathyroidism." Proc Natl Acad Sci U S A 105(9): 3455-3460.

Carmichael, K. D., J. A. Bynum, et al. (2009). "Familial tumoral calcinosis: a forty-year follow-up on one family." The Journal of bone and joint surgery. American volume 91(3): 664-671.

Carpenter, T. O. (1997). "New perspectives on the biology and treatment of X-linked hypophosphatemic rickets." Pediatric clinics of North America 44(2): 443-466.

Chefetz, I. and E. Sprecher (2009). "Familial tumoral calcinosis and the role of O-glycosylation in the maintenance of phosphate homeostasis." Biochim Biophys Acta 1792(9): 847-852.

Dixon, P. H., P. T. Christie, et al. (1998). "Mutational analysis of PHEX gene in X-linked hypophosphatemia." J Clin Endocrinol Metab 83(10): 3615-3623.

Econs, M. J. and P. T. McEnery (1997). "Autosomal dominant hypophosphatemic rickets/osteomalacia: clinical characterization of a novel renal phosphate-wasting disorder." The Journal of clinical endocrinology and metabolism 82(2): 674-681.

Econs, M. J., P. T. McEnery, et al. (1997). "Autosomal dominant hypophosphatemic rickets is linked to chromosome 12p13." J Clin Invest 100(11): 2653-2657.

Econs, M. J., G. P. Samsa, et al. (1994). "X-Linked hypophosphatemic rickets: a disease often unknown to affected patients." Bone and mineral 24(1): 17-24.

Farrow, E. G., S. I. Davis, et al. (2006). "Extended mutational analyses of FGFR1 in osteoglophonic dysplasia." American journal of medical genetics. Part A 140(5): 537-539.

Farrow, E. G., S. I. Davis, et al. (2009). "Molecular analysis of DMP1 mutants causing autosomal recessive hypophosphatemic rickets." Bone 44(2): 287-294.

Feng, J. Q., L. M. Ward, et al. (2006). "Loss of DMP1 causes rickets and osteomalacia and identifies a role for osteocytes in mineral metabolism." Nat Genet 38(11): 1310-1315.

Garringer, H. J., C. Fisher, et al. (2006). "The role of mutant UDP-N-acetyl-alpha-D-galactosamine-polypeptide N-acetylgalactosaminyltransferase 3 in regulating serum intact fibroblast growth factor 23 and matrix extracellular phosphoglycoprotein in heritable tumoral calcinosis." The Journal of clinical endocrinology and metabolism 91(10): 4037-4042.

Gaucher, C., O. Walrant-Debray, et al. (2009). "PHEX analysis in 118 pedigrees reveals new genetic clues in hypophosphatemic rickets." Hum Genet 125(4): 401-411.

Gaucher, C., O. Walrant-Debray, et al. (2009). "PHEX analysis in 118 pedigrees reveals new genetic clues in hypophosphatemic rickets." Human genetics 125(4): 401-411.

Goldfine, I. D., B. A. Maddux, et al. (2008). "The role of membrane glycoprotein plasma cell antigen 1/ectonucleotide pyrophosphatase phosphodiesterase 1 in the pathogenesis of insulin resistance and related abnormalities." Endocr Rev 29(1): 62-75.

Harahap, A. R. and J. W. Goding (1988). "Distribution of the murine plasma cell antigen PC-1 in non-lymphoid tissues." J Immunol 141(7): 2317-2320.

Holm, I. A., A. E. Nelson, et al. (2001). "Mutational analysis and genotype-phenotype correlation of the PHEX gene in X-linked hypophosphatemic rickets." The Journal of clinical endocrinology and metabolism 86(8): 3889-3899.

Hu, M. C., M. Shi, et al. (2010). "Klotho: a novel phosphaturic substance acting as an autocrine enzyme in the renal proximal tubule." FASEB J 24(9): 3438-3450.

Huang, R., M. Rosenbach, et al. (1994). "Expression of the murine plasma cell nucleotide pyrophosphohydrolase PC-1 is shared by human liver, bone, and cartilage cells. Regulation of PC-1 expression in osteosarcoma cells by transforming growth factor-beta." J Clin Invest 94(2): 560-567.

Huiming, Y. and W. Chaomin (2005). "Recombinant growth hormone therapy for X-linked hypophosphatemia in children." Cochrane database of systematic reviews(1): CD004447.

Huq, N. L., K. J. Cross, et al. (2005). "A review of protein structure and gene organisation for proteins associated with mineralised tissue and calcium phosphate stabilisation encoded on human chromosome 4." Archives of oral biology 50(7): 599-609.

HYP Consortium. A gene (PEX) with homologies to endopeptidases is mutated in patients with X-linked hypophosphatemic rickets. Nature Genetics 1995;11:130-6

Ichikawa, S., G. Baujat, et al. (2010). "Clinical variability of familial tumoral calcinosis caused by novel GALNT3 mutations." Am J Med Genet A 152A(4): 896-903.

Ichikawa, S., E. A. Imel, et al. (2007). "A homozygous missense mutation in human KLOTHO causes severe tumoral calcinosis." J Clin Invest 117(9): 2684-2691.

Ichikawa, S., E. A. Imel, et al. (2007). "A homozygous missense mutation in human KLOTHO causes severe tumoral calcinosis." J Musculoskelet Neuronal Interact 7(4): 318-319.

Ichikawa, S., E. A. Traxler, et al. (2008). "Mutational survey of the PHEX gene in patients with X-linked hypophosphatemic rickets." Bone 43(4): 663-666.

Imel, E. A., S. L. Hui, et al. (2007). "FGF23 concentrations vary with disease status in autosomal dominant hypophosphatemic rickets." J Bone Miner Res 22(4): 520-526.

Jonsson, K. B., R. Zahradnik, et al. (2003). "Fibroblast growth factor 23 in oncogenic osteomalacia and X-linked hypophosphatemia." N Engl J Med 348(17): 1656-1663.

Juppner, H. (2007). "Novel regulators of phosphate homeostasis and bone metabolism." Therapeutic apheresis and dialysis : official peer-reviewed journal of the International Society for Apheresis, the Japanese Society for Apheresis, the Japanese Society for Dialysis Therapy 11 Suppl 1: S3-22.

Karim, Z., B. Gerard, et al. (2008). "NHERF1 mutations and responsiveness of renal parathyroid hormone." N Engl J Med 359(11): 1128-1135.

Kato, K., C. Jeanneau, et al. (2006). "Polypeptide GalNAc-transferase T3 and familial tumoral calcinosis. Secretion of fibroblast growth factor 23 requires O-glycosylation." The Journal of biological chemistry 281(27): 18370-18377.

Koshida, R., H. Yamaguchi, et al. (2010). "A novel nonsense mutation in the DMP1 gene in a Japanese family with autosomal recessive hypophosphatemic rickets." J Bone Miner Metab 28(5): 585-590.

Kuro-o, M., Y. Matsumura, et al. (1997). "Mutation of the mouse klotho gene leads to a syndrome resembling ageing." Nature 390(6655): 45-51.

Kurosu, H., M. Choi, et al. (2007). "Tissue-specific expression of betaKlotho and fibroblast growth factor (FGF) receptor isoforms determines metabolic activity of FGF19 and FGF21." The Journal of biological chemistry 282(37): 26687-26695.

Kurosu, H., M. Yamamoto, et al. (2005). "Suppression of aging in mice by the hormone Klotho." Science 309(5742): 1829-1833.

Levy-Litan, V., E. Hershkovitz, et al. (2010). "Autosomal-recessive hypophosphatemic rickets is associated with an inactivation mutation in the ENPP1 gene." Am J Hum Genet 86(2): 273-278.

Lorenz-Depiereux, B., M. Bastepe, et al. (2006). "DMP1 mutations in autosomal recessive hypophosphatemia implicate a bone matrix protein in the regulation of phosphate homeostasis." Nat Genet 38(11): 1248-1250.

Lorenz-Depiereux, B., A. Benet-Pages, et al. (2006). "Hereditary hypophosphatemic rickets with hypercalciuria is caused by mutations in the sodium-phosphate cotransporter gene SLC34A3." Am J Hum Genet 78(2): 193-201.

Lorenz-Depiereux, B., D. Schnabel, et al. (2010). "Loss-of-function ENPP1 mutations cause both generalized arterial calcification of infancy and autosomal-recessive hypophosphatemic rickets." Am J Hum Genet 86(2): 267-272.

Makitie, O., R. C. Pereira, et al. (2010). "Long-term clinical outcome and carrier phenotype in autosomal recessive hypophosphatemia caused by a novel DMP1 mutation." J Bone Miner Res 25(10): 2165-2174.

Matsumura, Y., H. Aizawa, et al. (1998). "Identification of the human klotho gene and its two transcripts encoding membrane and secreted klotho protein." Biochem Biophys Res Commun 242(3): 626-630.

Passos-Bueno, M. R., W. R. Wilcox, et al. (1999). "Clinical spectrum of fibroblast growth factor receptor mutations." Hum Mutat 14(2): 115-125.

Prie, D., V. Huart, et al. (2002). "Nephrolithiasis and osteoporosis associated with hypophosphatemia caused by mutations in the type 2a sodium-phosphate cotransporter." N Engl J Med 347(13): 983-991.

Quarles, L. D. (2003). "Evidence for a bone-kidney axis regulating phosphate homeostasis." J Clin Invest 112(5): 642-646.

Raeder, H., N. Shaw, et al. (2008). "A case of X-linked hypophosphatemic rickets (XLH): complications and the therapeutic use of cinacalcet." Eur J Endocrinol. 159 (Suppl. 1):101-105.

Rosenzweig, A. (2010). "Illuminating the potential of pluripotent stem cells." The New England journal of medicine 363(15): 1471-1472.

Rutsch, F., P. Boyer, et al. (2008). "Hypophosphatemia, hyperphosphaturia, and bisphosphonate treatment are associated with survival beyond infancy in generalized arterial calcification of infancy." Circ Cardiovasc Genet 1(2): 133-140.

Rutsch, F., N. Ruf, et al. (2003). "Mutations in ENPP1 are associated with 'idiopathic' infantile arterial calcification." Nat Genet 34(4): 379-381.

Rutsch, F., S. Vainganka r, et al. (2001). "PC-1 nucleoside triphosphate pyrophosphohydrolase deficiency in idiopathic infantile arterial calcification." Am J Pathol 158(2): 543-554.

Sabbagh, Y., G. Boileau, et al. (2003). "Structure and function of disease-causing missense mutations in the PHEX gene." The Journal of clinical endocrinology and metabolism 88(5): 2213-2222.

Sabbagh, Y., G. Boileau, et al. (2001). "Disease-causing missense mutations in the PHEX gene interfere with membrane targeting of the recombinant protein." Human molecular genetics 10(15): 1539-1546.

Shaw, S. Y., D. M. Blodgett, et al. (2011). "Disease allele-dependent small-molecule sensitivities in blood cells from monogenic diabetes." Proceedings of the National Academy of Sciences of the United States of America 108(2): 492-497.

Shimada, T., H. Hasegawa, et al. (2004). "FGF-23 is a potent regulator of vitamin D metabolism and phosphate homeostasis." J Bone Miner Res 19(3): 429-435.

Strom, T. M. and H. Juppner (2008). "PHEX, FGF23, DMP1 and beyond." Curr Opin Nephrol Hypertens 17(4): 357-362.

Tenenhouse, H. S. (2005). "Regulation of phosphorus homeostasis by the type iia na/phosphate cotransporter." Annu Rev Nutr 25: 197-214.

Tieder, M., D. Modai, et al. (1985). "Hereditary hypophosphatemic rickets with hypercalciuria." The New England journal of medicine 312(10): 611-617.

Topaz, O., D. L. Shurman, et al. (2004). "Mutations in GALNT3, encoding a protein involved in O-linked glycosylation, cause familial tumoral calcinosis." Nat Genet 36(6): 579-581.

Turan, S., C. Aydin, et al. (2010). "Identification of a novel dentin matrix protein-1 (DMP-1) mutation and dental anomalies in a kindred with autosomal recessive hypophosphatemia." Bone 46(2): 402-409.

Urakawa, I., Y. Yamazaki, et al. (2006). "Klotho converts canonical FGF receptor into a specific receptor for FGF23." Nature 444(7120): 770-774.

White, K. E., J. M. Cabral, et al. (2005). "Mutations that cause osteoglophonic dysplasia define novel roles for FGFR1 in bone elongation." Am J Hum Genet 76(2): 361-367.

Yuan, B., M. Takaiwa, et al. (2008). "Aberrant Phex function in osteoblasts and osteocytes alone underlies murine X-linked hypophosphatemia." The Journal of clinical investigation 118(2): 722-734.

19

Pseudohypoparathyroidism in Children

Benjamin U. Nwosu
University of Massachusetts Medical School
Worcester, Massachusetts,
USA

1. Introduction

Albright hereditary osteodystrophy (AHO) is a genetic syndrome characterized by a distinctive set of developmental and skeletal defects that may easily be misdiagnosed as exogenous obesity in children. There are very few publications detailing the comprehensive management of children and adolescents with this disorder. This chapter provides a comprehensive discussion of the various aspects of this disorder. At the end, the reader should be able to: (1) List the clinical features of Albright hereditary osteodystrophy, (2) Identify the genetic and molecular abnormalities of AHO, (3) List the clinical features of pseudohypoparathyroidism type 1a (PHP 1a), (4) Describe the management of children and adolescents with PHP 1a.

2. Genetics of Albright hereditary osteodystrophy

The molecular basis for AHO is a heterozygous mutation of the gene that encodes the G-stimulatory subunit ($G_s\alpha$) of guanine nucleotide-binding protein—the *GNAS* gene—that is located at chromosome 20q13.2. This type of mutation leads to a loss of expression or function of the $G_s\alpha$ which impairs the transmission of stimulatory signals to adenylate cyclase, limiting cyclic AMP generation necessary for hormone action(Lietman, 2008).

The *GNAS* gene is subject to imprinting. Patients with AHO who have *GNAS* mutations on maternally inherited alleles manifest resistance to multiple hormones, such as parathyroid hormone (PTH), thyroid stimulating hormone (TSH), gonadotropins, growth-hormone-releasing hormone (GHRH), and glucagon(Brickman, 1986; Weinstein, 2004). These defects lead to PHP 1a. On the other hand, patients with AHO who have *GNAS* mutations on paternally inherited alleles have only the phenotypic features of AHO without hormonal resistance, a condition termed pseudopseudohypoparathyroidism (PPHP) (Lietman, 2008). PHP 1b is an autosomal dominant disorder that is associated with the presence of hormone resistance that is limited to PTH target organs, normal $G_s\alpha$ activity, and the absence of features of AHO(Levine, 1983). PHP 1c is associated with features of AHO, resistance to multiple hormones, and normal GNAS activity while PHP type 2 is associated with renal resistance to PTH action and the absence of AHO phenotype(Levine, 2000).

More than 50 different loss-of-function mutations of *GNAS* have been reported in more than 70 affected individuals. Pohlenz *et al.*(Pohlenz, 2003) have reported a missense mutation, which results in the amino-acid substitution (Lys338Asn) in codon 338 of exon 12 of the *GNAS* gene associated with congenital hypothyroidism in AHO, though they did not state the precise mechanism by which this mutation leads to hypothyroidism. A Q35X mutation in exon 1 has been associated with growth-hormone deficiency(Germain-Lee, 2003), whereas a *de novo*, missense mutation, W281R in exon 11, has been linked to progressive osseous heteroplasia, a rare, autosomal-dominant condition that presents in childhood as dermal ossification that progresses to involve deep skeletal muscles(Chan, 2004). Germain-Lee *et al.*(Germain-Lee, 2003) identified a patient with a Q29X mutation, and Nwosu *et al.* (Nwosu, 2009) reported the association of Q29X mutation with a phenotype that includes Albright hereditary osteodystrophy, morbid obesity, acanthosis nigricans, insulin resistance, growth-hormone deficiency, hypothyroidism, and subcutaneous calcification.

3. Clinical features

3.1 General appearance

The developmental and skeletal defects that characterize AHO include short stocky physique (Figure 1a), round face, mental deficiency, heterotopic ossification, and brachymetaphalangism(Weinstein, 1993) (Figure 1 b, c). AHO is present in types 1a and 1c and PPHP. Hormonal resistance is seen in PHP 1a, PHP 1c and PHP type 2.

3.2 Stature

The prevalence of short adult height in PHP 1a is reported to be as high as 80%(Nagant de Deuschaisnes, 2007). Although height during childhood may be normal, adult height is often subnormal. The reason for the short stature in PHP 1a is multifactorial and includes GHRH resistance and chondrocytic dysfunction as explained below in section 3.8.

3.3 Mental deficiency

Learning disabilities and psychomotor retardation have been described in PHP 1a(Chen, 2005). The mechanism of this mental deficiency is unknown and early institution of thyroid hormone replacement does not seem to prevent the development of mental deficiency(Weisman, 1985). There appears to be a correlation with reduced $G_s\alpha$ since patients with PHP 1b do not present with mental deficiency in spite of equivalent serum calcium and phosphate abnormalities(Wilson, 1994). This mental deficiency is generally mild, but ranges from moderately severe delay to normal educational ability.

3.4 Ectopic calcification

In patients with PHP 1a, soft-tissue calcification has been reported in various body parts, especially in the subcutaneous tissues, and rarely in the brain and cardiac septum(Schuster, 1992). Persistent hyperparathyroidism is believed to have some causative role in this abnormal calcification. This situation is distinct from progressive osseous heteroplasia (Chan, 2004), a rare condition that causes dermal ossification.

3.5 Brachymetaphalangism

The hand abnormalities in the PHP and PPHP forms of AHO are indistinguishable (Poznanski, 1977). The malformations involve both the phalanges and metacarpals and are often symmetrical(Wilson, 1994) (Figure 1b). Shortening of the distal phalanx of the thumb is estimated to occur in 75% of AHO patients(Poznanski, 1977). Similar shortening occur in the metacarpals. Metacarpal shortening often involves the fourth and the fifth metacarpals(Poznanski, 1977; Steinbach, 1965). Shortening of the metatarsals (Figure 1c), especially the third and fourth, is seen in about 70% of persons with AHO(Steinbach, 1966).

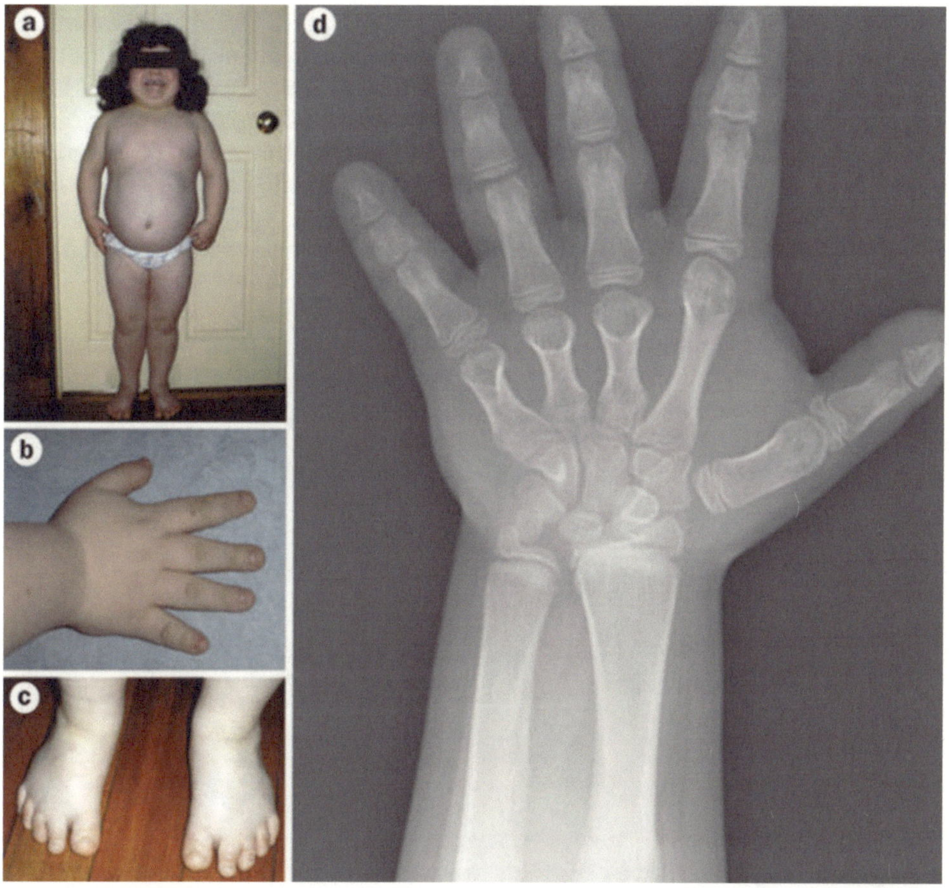

Fig. 1. a, b, c, d. Features suggestive of Albright hereditary osteodystrophy(Nwosu, 2009) Figure 1 | Features suggestive of Albright hereditary osteodystrophy in the patient. a | Photo of a patient at 5 years of age showing an obese phenotype, round face, broad chest, short neck and digits consistent with pseudohypoparathyroidism type 1a. b | Photo of the patient's hand at 5 years of age showing brachyphalangism of the fingers, especially the third through fifth digits. c | Photo of the patient's feet at 5 years of age showing brachyphalangism of the toes. d | Bone age radiograph of the patient at 7 years of age showing premature fusion of the epiphyses of the distal phalanges of the thumb, midphalanges of both the second and fifth fingers, and shortening of the third through fifth metacarpals. Her bone age was read as 13 years at a chronological age of 7 years and 8 months.

3.6 Obesity and insulin resistance

Insulin resistance has not been described in patients with PHP 1a, and acanthosis nigricans is not a typical finding in AHO. Germain-Lee et al(Germain-Lee, 2003) reported a patient with acanthosis nigricans in a cohort of 13 patients with PHP 1a who had normal

hemoglobin A1c and fasting insulin levels. Nwosu et al(Nwosu, 2009) described a child with PHP 1a with acanthosis nigricans and insulin resistance (Figure 2).
A patient with Albright hereditary osteodystrophy-like syndrome with a normal *GNAS* gene that was complicated by type 2 diabetes mellitus with severe insulin resistance, growth-hormone deficiency and diabetes insipidus has been described(Sakaguchi, 1998). Long *et al.*(Long, 2007) reported that obesity is a more prominent feature of PHP 1a than of PPHP, and that severe obesity is characteristic of PHP 1a. They postulated that paternal imprinting of $G_s\alpha$ occurs in the hypothalamus such that maternal, but not paternal, $G_s\alpha$ mutations lead to loss of the melanocortin signaling cascade, which is important for signaling satiety. This loss of satiety signaling then leads to greater alteration in energy balance and notably greater insulin resistance in individuals with PHP 1a (as shown in Figure 2) than in those with PPHP.

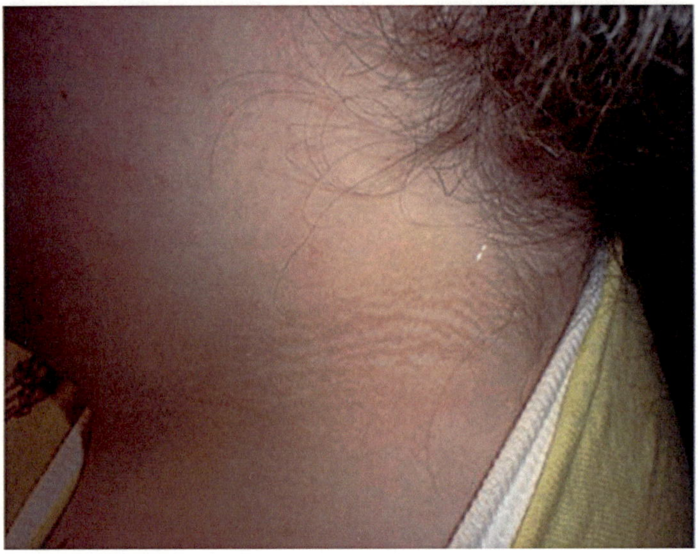

Fig. 2. Acanthosis nigricans of the neck folds in a patient with Albright Hereditary Osteodystrophy(Nwosu, 2009)

The insulin receptor belongs to a large class of tyrosine kinase receptors, and is structurally distinct from the heptahelical G_s receptors. The development of insulin resistance in the patient shown in Figure 2 most probably resulted from the combined effects of obesity, growth-hormone treatment, a family history of type 2 diabetes mellitus, and abnormal melanocortin signaling, as noted above. Obesity is the most common cause of insulin resistance in children(Caprio, 2002). It is postulated to represent a subclinical inflammatory state that promotes the production of proinflammatory factors, such as interleukin 6 and tumor necrosis factor, which are involved in the pathogenesis of insulin resistance(Bastard, 2006). Growth hormone antagonizes insulin's effects on glucose metabolism by inhibiting insulin-induced glucose uptake through the inhibition of insulin receptor substrate-2-associated phosphatidylinositol-3-kinase activity, without affecting glucose transporter 4 translocation(Sasaka-Suzuki N, 2009). A family history of type 2 diabetes mellitus conveys not only heritable genetic information, but also reveals familial behaviors and social norms that may exacerbate the individual's risk for insulin resistance and frank diabetes(Meigs, 2008).

3.7 Biochemical profile

The biochemical profile in patients with PHP 1a shows evidence of PTH resistance, with elevated serum concentrations of PTH and phosphate, and low or normal serum levels of ionized calcium. Serum TSH concentrations are elevated from infancy indicating TSH resistance at the receptor-complex level. Subnormal peak growth-hormone levels of <7.5 μg/l are commonly found when growth-hormone stimulation tests are carried out(Scott, 1995). Serum gonadotropins are either normal or slightly elevated in women with AHO despite their hypoestrogenic status(Namnoum, 1998). This is believed to be due to partial resistance to gonadotropins in the granulosa and theca cells of the ovary(Namnoum, 1998).

3.8 Bone age and other skeletal and radiologic features

The bone ages of children with PHP 1a are more advanced than would be expected for their stage of sexual maturation. Premature epiphyseal fusion occurs selectively in the hands and feet of affected patients(de Wijn, 1982; Steinbach, 1966). Furthermore, the phalanges of patients either lack epiphyses or have epiphyses that are partially fused when they first develop, which makes accurate assessments of bone age very difficult(Steinbach, 1966). This abnormal epiphyseal fusion is postulated to result from the loss of $G_s\alpha$, which induces resistance to parathyroid-hormone-related protein which, in turn, promotes premature differentiation of proliferating chondrocytes into hypertrophic chondrocytes(Kobayashi, 2002; Tavella, 2004; van der Eerden, 2000). This series of events leads to early closure of the growth plate and limb-reduction defects. Despite early fusion of the epiphyses in the phalanges, the epiphyses of long bones may remain open, thus an increase in height with growth-hormone therapy is still possible.

Other radiological features of PHP 1a in children include rickets which results from low levels of 1,25-dihydroxyvitamin D as a result of PTH resistance(Wilson, 1994). Generalized osteoporosis and osteitis fibrosa cystica(Burnstein, 1985; Steinbach, 1966) can be seen, and these pathologies are suggestive of some preservation of the skeletal remodeling response to the raised levels of circulating PTH(Kerr, 1987). Some of the skeletal abnormalities associated with AHO include shortened ulna, radial and tibial bowing, coxa vara, coxa valga and caudal narrowing of interpedicular distance(Wilson, 1994).

3.9 Hormonal defects and manifestations

In addition to the AHO phenotype, biochemical and hormonal derangements in PHP 1a lead to characteristic patterns of presentation. PHP 1a is associated with resistance to multiple hormones, such as PTH, TSH, gonadotropins, growth-hormone-releasing hormone, and glucagon(Brickman, 1986; Weinstein, 2004).

PHP 1a accompanied by growth-hormone deficiency was first described in 1995(Scott, 1995). The short stature of patients with PHP 1a results from a combination of several factors, such as epiphyseal defects and resistance to GHRH(Scott, 1995). This hormone resistance results in the inability of GHRH to stimulate pituitary somatotropes to produce growth hormone. Many patients with PHP 1a present with subclinical hypothyroidism in infancy (Pohlenz, 2003; Scott, 1995), as a result of resistance to TSH action. Resistance to PTH action could lead to hypocalcemia which could be complicated by hypocalcemic seizures, and/or muscle spasms. Resistance to the actions of the gonadotropins results in hypogonadism or menstrual irregularities in women with PHP 1a. The mechanism of this reproductive dysfunction is believed to be due to a partial resistance of the theca and granulosa cells of the ovary to gonadotropins due to deficient $G_s\alpha$ activity (Namnoum, 1998).

Whereas resistance to PTH, TSH, growth-hormone-releasing hormone, follicle-stimulating hormone, and luteinizing hormone may lead to clinical manifestations, the blunted cyclic AMP response to glucagon documented by Brickman *et al.*(Brickman, 1986) in patients with PHP 1a is apparently subclinical, as the glucose response is intact.

4. Differential diagnosis

The differential diagnoses of a child with this AHO phenotype include exogenous obesity, Cushing syndrome, severe hypoparathyroidism, Prader–Willi syndrome, and Laurence–Moon–Biedl–Bardet syndrome.

The generalized metacarpal and phalangeal shortening characteristics of acrodysostosis has been observed in cases of AHO(Ablow, 1977). Acrodysostosis presents with similar features as AHO including short stature, brachymetaphalangism, advanced bone age, mental deficiency and other radiologic features. However, cutaneous ossification does not occur in acrodysostosis, and pronounced nasal hypoplasia is a distinguishing feature of acrodysostosis, but has been described in PHP 1a(Ablow, 1977).

Turner syndrome and multiple familial exostoses are associated with short stature and metacarpal shortening but are easily distinguished from AHO(Wilson, 1994).

A diagnosis is usually reached by reviewing patient's family history, establishing the components of the AHO phenotype, such as short fourth metacarpals, and connecting these findings to the existing hormonal defects such as a history of subclinical hypothyroidism or parathyroid hormone resistance.

5. Treatment and management

The defect in PHP 1a leads to resistance to multiple hormones that mediate their actions through cyclic AMP(Spiegel, 1982). These include PTH, TSH, growth-hormone-releasing hormone, gonadotropins, glucagon, and possibly TSH-releasing hormone(Balavoine, 2008). Patients with $G_s\alpha$ deficiency could, therefore, develop hypothyroidism, hypogonadism, growth-hormone deficiency, and pseudohypoparathyroidism, depending on the degree of $G_s\alpha$ activity in specific tissues(Scott, 1995).

5.1 Hypoparathyroidism

The initial medical management of all patients with severe, symptomatic hypocalcemia should be with intravenous calcium. The recommended initial dose for newborn babies , infants and children is 0.5–1.0 ml/kg of 10% calcium gluconate administered over 5 min. Administration of oral calcium and 1α-hydroxylated vitamin D metabolites, such as calcitriol, is recommended for patients with symptomatic hypocalcemia. The goals of therapy are to maintain serum total and ionized calcium levels within the reference range and to reduce PTH levels to near normal. This normalization is important because elevated PTH levels in patients with PHP 1a could cause increased bone remodeling and lead to secondary hyperparathyroid bone disease(Abraham, 2007).

5.2 Growth-hormone deficiency

Some children with PHP 1a have hypothalamic growth-hormone deficiency and may benefit from therapy with recombinant human growth hormone to achieve optimal adult height. In those patients in whom defective growth-hormone secretion is suspected, the epiphyseal defects, commonly mischaracterized as bone-age advancement, should not disqualify these children from being considered for growth-hormone therapy. In addition to its effect on statural growth, growth-hormone therapy also seems to improve body composition in patients with PHP 1a(Nwosu, 2009).

5.3 Hypothyroidism

Most patients with PHP 1a present with subclinical hypothyroidism before the onset of hypocalcemia. Hypothyroidism is treated with thyroid hormone replacement using levothyroxine at age-appropriate and weight-appropriate doses. The aim of management is to normalize serum concentrations of TSH and free T_4.

5.4 Hypogonadism

Common reproductive dysfunctions in persons with PHP 1a include delayed puberty, oligomenorrhea and infertility(Abraham, 2007). Each condition requires age-appropriate therapy; for example, low-dose estrogenic formulations are used to induce puberty in adolescent girls with delayed puberty.

5.5 Obesity and insulin resistance

Patients with PHP 1a who also have a family history of type 2 diabetes mellitus may have familial risk factors for development of insulin resistance, prediabetes and type 2 diabetes mellitus. Growth-hormone therapy improves body composition, but may worsen insulin resistance. Lifestyle modifications should be incorporated in the management of patients with PHP 1a phenotype who may be at risk of metabolic syndrome. Early introduction of oral insulin-sensitizing agents, such as metformin, may be necessary when lifestyle modification is ineffective, especially in patients with prediabetes.

6. Conclusion

Accurate understanding of the features of AHO will prevent its misdiagnosis as exogenous obesity. Children diagnosed with PHP 1a should be further evaluated for associated endocrinopathies, such as resistance to growth-hormone-releasing hormone, which may lead to growth-hormone deficiency. Preliminary data suggest that the short stature in patients with PHP 1a may be ameliorated with growth-hormone therapy in some cases(Scott, 1995). The advanced bone age seen in PHP 1a is due to a chondrocytic signaling defect, and not due to excess production of sex hormones; therefore, bone-age advancement should not preclude affected children from being considered for growth-hormone therapy. However, a combination of growth-hormone therapy, family history of type 2 diabetes mellitus, and obesity in these children might lead to metabolic complications, such as insulin resistance, prediabetes and type 2 diabetes mellitus.

7. Future directions

A comprehensive management of a child with PHP 1a must address the controversies surrounding authorization of growth hormone therapy for these patients. This is because most health insurance carriers decline authorization for GH therapy in these patients because of the apparent bone age advancement that affects the digital bones but not the long bones.

It is equally important to address increasing weight gain in these patients as they are at risk for obesity and its co-morbidities. Even though insulin resistance is not part of the syndrome, there are increasing reports of worsening insulin resistance in these patients which predisposes them to frank diabetes mellitus. This is due to the synergistic effects of prevalent obesity and the pre-existing AHO phenotype.

The presence of delayed puberty may indicate LH and FSH resistance in these patients. There is no clear protocol for initiating sex hormone therapy in these patients. Most pediatric endocrinologists address this problem by adopting similar therapeutic modalities for the induction of the development of secondary sexual characteristics as in patients with Turner syndrome.

Most patients with PHP 1a have variable levels of mental deficiency. It is important to address this problem very early in life by recommending additional classroom supervision, and in severe cases, instituting an individualized educational plan.

In summary, a comprehensive management of a patient with PHP 1a includes a thorough assessment for associated hormonal defects, the obese phenotype and its comorbidities, and the degree of intellectual deficiency.

8. Acknowledgement

We thank Ms. Jessica Kowaleski for her clerical assistance. This work was supported in part by a grant to Dr Nwosu by the Faculty Scholars Diversity Program, University of Massachusetts Medical School.

9. References

Ablow, R. C., Hsia, Y. E., & Brandt, I. K. (1977). Acrodysostosis coinciding with pseudohypoparathyroidism and pseudo-pseudohypoparathyroidism. *AJR Am J Roentgenol, 128*(1), 95-99.

Abraham, M. R., & Khadori, R. K. (2007). Pseudohypoparathyroidism. *eMedicine, http://www.emedicine.com/med/TOPIC1940.HTM.*

Balavoine, A. S., Ladsous, M., Velayoudom, F. L., Vlaeminck, V., Cardot-Bauters, C., d'Herbomez, M., & Wemeau, J. L. (2008). Hypothyroidism in patients with pseudohypoparathyroidism type ia: Clinical evidence of resistance to tsh and trh. *Eur J Endocrinol, 159*(4), 431-437.

Bastard, J. P., Maachi, M., Lagathu, C., Kim, M. J., Caron, M., Vidal, H., Capeau, J., & Feve, B. (2006). Recent advances in the relationship between obesity, inflammation, and insulin resistance. *Eur Cytokine Netw, 17*(1), 4-12.

Brickman, A. S., Carlson, H. E., & Levin, S. R. (1986). Responses to glucagon infusion in pseudohypoparathyroidism. *J Clin Endocrinol Metab, 63*(6), 1354-1360.

Burnstein, M. I., Kottamasu, S. R., Pettifor, J. M., Sochett, E., Ellis, B. I., & Frame, B. (1985). Metabolic bone disease in pseudohypoparathyroidism: Radiologic features. *Radiology, 155*(2), 351-356.

Caprio, S. (2002). Insulin resistance in childhood obesity. *J Pediatr Endocrinol Metab, 15 Suppl 1*, 487-492.

Chan, I., Hamada, T., Hardman, C., McGrath, J. A., & Child, F. J. (2004). Progressive osseous heteroplasia resulting from a new mutation in the gnas1 gene. *Clin Exp Dermatol, 29*(1), 77-80.

Chen, Y. J., Shu, S. G., & Chi, C. S. (2005). Pseudohypoparathyroidism: Report of seven cases. *Acta Paediatr Taiwan, 46*(6), 374-380.

de Wijn, E. M., & Steendijk, R. (1982). Growth and maturation in pseudo-hypoparathyroidism: A longitudinal study in 5 patients. *Acta Endocrinol (Copenh), 101*(2), 223-226.

Germain-Lee, E. L., Groman, J., Crane, J. L., Jan de Beur, S. M., & Levine, M. A. (2003). Growth hormone deficiency in pseudohypoparathyroidism type 1a: Another manifestation of multihormone resistance. *J Clin Endocrinol Metab, 88*(9), 4059-4069.

Kerr, D., & Hosking, D. J. (1987). Pseudohypoparathyroidism: Clinical expression of pth resistance. *Q J Med, 65*(247), 889-894.

Kobayashi, T., Chung, U. I., Schipani, E., Starbuck, M., Karsenty, G., Katagiri, T., Goad, D. L., Lanske, B., & Kronenberg, H. M. (2002). Pthrp and indian hedgehog control differentiation of growth plate chondrocytes at multiple steps. *Development, 129*(12), 2977-2986.

Levine, M. A. (2000). Clinical spectrum and pathogenesis of pseudohypoparathyroidism. *Rev Endocr Metab Disord, 1*(4), 265-274.

Levine, M. A., Downs, R. W., Jr., Moses, A. M., Breslau, N. A., Marx, S. J., Lasker, R. D., Rizzoli, R. E., Aurbach, G. D., & Spiegel, A. M. (1983). Resistance to multiple hormones in patients with pseudohypoparathyroidism. Association with deficient activity of guanine nucleotide regulatory protein. *Am J Med, 74*(4), 545-556.

Lietman, S. A., Goldfarb, J., Desai, N., & Levine, M. A. (2008). Preimplantation genetic diagnosis for severe albright hereditary osteodystrophy. *J Clin Endocrinol Metab, 93*(3), 901-904.

Long, D. N., McGuire, S., Levine, M. A., Weinstein, L. S., & Germain-Lee, E. L. (2007). Body mass index differences in pseudohypoparathyroidism type 1a versus pseudopseudohypoparathyroidism may implicate paternal imprinting of galpha(s) in the development of human obesity. *J Clin Endocrinol Metab, 92*(3), 1073-1079.

Meigs, J. B., Shrader, P., Sullivan, L. M., McAteer, J. B., Fox, C. S., Dupuis, J., Manning, A. K., Florez, J. C., Wilson, P. W., D'Agostino, R. B., Sr., & Cupples, L. A. (2008). Genotype score in addition to common risk factors for prediction of type 2 diabetes. *N Engl J Med, 359*(21), 2208-2219.

Nagant de Deuschaisnes, C., Krane, SM. (2007). *Hypoparathyroidism* (3rd ed.). San Diego: Academic Press.

Namnoum, A. B., Merriam, G. R., Moses, A. M., & Levine, M. A. (1998). Reproductive dysfunction in women with albright's hereditary osteodystrophy. *J Clin Endocrinol Metab, 83*(3), 824-829.

Nwosu, B. U., & Lee, M. M. (2009). Pseudohypoparathyroidism type 1a and insulin resistance in a child. *Nat Rev Endocrinol, 5*(6), 345-350.

Pohlenz, J., Ahrens, W., & Hiort, O. (2003). A new heterozygous mutation (l338n) in the human gsalpha (gnas1) gene as a cause for congenital hypothyroidism in albright's hereditary osteodystrophy. *Eur J Endocrinol, 148*(4), 463-468.

Poznanski, A. K., Werder, E. A., Giedion, A., Martin, A., & Shaw, H. (1977). The pattern of shortening of the bones of the hand in php and pphp--a comparison with brachydactyly e, turner syndrome, and acrodysostosis. *Radiology, 123*(3), 707-718.

Sakaguchi, H., Sanke, T., Ohagi, S., Iiri, T., & Nanjo, K. (1998). A case of albright's hereditary osteodystrophy-like syndrome complicated by several endocrinopathies: Normal gs alpha gene and chromosome 2q37. *J Clin Endocrinol Metab, 83*(5), 1563-1565.

Sasaka-Suzuki N, A. K., Ogata T, Kasahara K. (2009). Gh inhibition of glucose uptake in adipocytes occurs without affecting glut-4 translocation thorugh an irs-2pi 3-kinase-dependent pathway. *J. Biol. Chem.*

Schuster, V., & Sandhage, K. (1992). Intracardiac calcifications in a case of pseudohypoparathyroidism type ia (php-ia). *Pediatr Cardiol, 13*(4), 237-239.

Scott, D. C., & Hung, W. (1995). Pseudohypoparathyroidism type ia and growth hormone deficiency in two siblings. *J Pediatr Endocrinol Metab, 8*(3), 205-207.

Spiegel, A. M., Levine, M. A., Aurbach, G. D., Downs, R. W., Jr., Marx, S. J., Lasker, R. D., Moses, A. M., & Breslau, N. A. (1982). Deficiency of hormone receptor-adenylate cyclase coupling protein: Basis for hormone resistance in pseudohypoparathyroidism. *Am J Physiol, 243*(1), E37-42.

Steinbach, H. L., Rudhe, U., Jonsson, M., & Young, D. A. (1965). Evolution of skeletal lesions in pseudohypoparathyroidism. *Radiology, 85*(4), 670-676.

Steinbach, H. L., & Young, D. A. (1966). The roentgen appearance of pseudohypoparathyroidism (ph) and pseudo-pseudohypoparathyroidism (pph). Differentiation from other syndromes associated with short metacarpals, metatarsals, and phalanges. *Am J Roentgenol Radium Ther Nucl Med, 97*(1), 49-66.

Tavella, S., Biticchi, R., Schito, A., Minina, E., Di Martino, D., Pagano, A., Vortkamp, A., Horton, W. A., Cancedda, R., & Garofalo, S. (2004). Targeted expression of shh affects chondrocyte differentiation, growth plate organization, and sox9 expression. *J Bone Miner Res, 19*(10), 1678-1688.

van der Eerden, B. C., Karperien, M., Gevers, E. F., Lowik, C. W., & Wit, J. M. (2000). Expression of indian hedgehog, parathyroid hormone-related protein, and their receptors in the postnatal growth plate of the rat: Evidence for a locally acting growth restraining feedback loop after birth. *J Bone Miner Res, 15*(6), 1045-1055.

Weinstein, L. S., Liu, J., Sakamoto, A., Xie, T., & Chen, M. (2004). Minireview: Gnas: Normal and abnormal functions. *Endocrinology, 145*(12), 5459-5464.

Weinstein, L. S., & Shenker, A. (1993). G protein mutations in human disease. *Clin Biochem, 26*(5), 333-338.

Weisman, Y., Golander, A., Spirer, Z., & Farfel, Z. (1985). Pseudohypoparathyroidism type 1a presenting as congenital hypothyroidism. *J Pediatr, 107*(3), 413-415.

Wilson, L. C., & Trembath, R. C. (1994). Albright's hereditary osteodystrophy. *J Med Genet, 31*(10), 779-784.

20

Retinoids and Bone

H. Herschel Conaway[1] and Ulf H. Lerner[2,3]
[1]*Department of Physiology and Biophysics, University of Arkansas for Medical Sciences,*
[2]*Department of Molecular Periodontology, Umeå University*
[3]*Center for Bone and Arthritis Research at Institute of Medicine, Sahlgrenska Academy at University of Gothenburg,*
[1]*USA*
[2,3]*Sweden*

1. Introduction

Vitamin A (retinol) can be produced in the body by hydrolysis of retinyl esters or reduction of retinal. Liver and eggs, which are good animal sources of vitamin A, contain retinyl esters. Plant sources such as carrots and spinach contain pro-vitamin A carotenoids, which can be cleaved to retinal. Retinal, also called retinaldehyde, is interconvertible with retinol (Fig. 1). Retinal also serves as an intermediate in the irreversible production of all-trans-retinoic acid (ATRA), which is considered the major biologically active derivative of vitamin A [Moise *et al.* 2007, Chambon 1996]. Another important derivative of vitamin A is the visual chromophore 11-cis-retinal [Wald 1968]. Binding of 11-cis-retinal to proteins called opsins is the chemical basis of vision. Vitamin A formed from retinyl esters or carotinoids in the normal diet, or ingested in fortified foods or dietary supplements, is stored in the liver and transported to tissues as a complex bound to retinol binding protein [Moise *et al.* 2007].

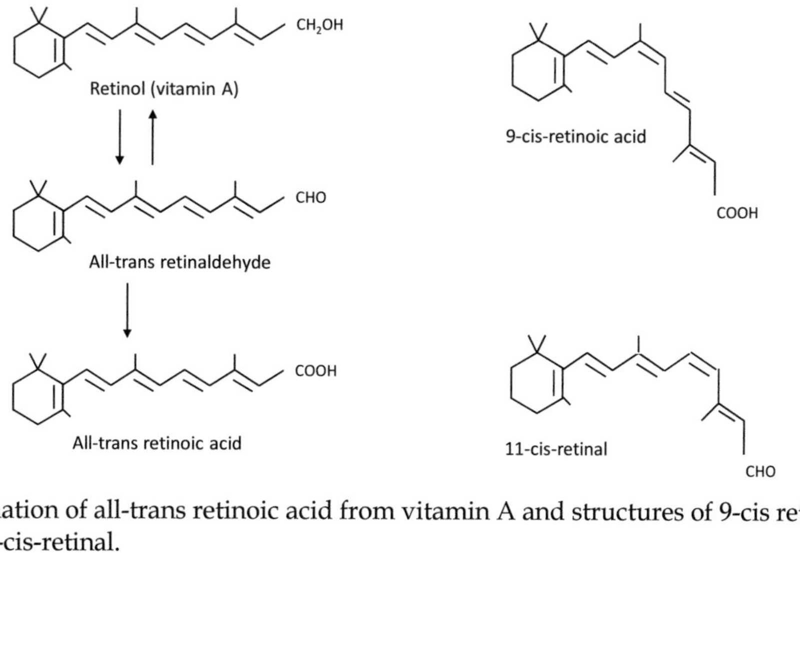

Fig. 1. Formation of all-trans retinoic acid from vitamin A and structures of 9-cis retinoic acid and 11-cis-retinal.

Effects of retinoids are mediated primarily by two families of nuclear hormone receptors, retinoic acid receptors (RARs) and the retinoid X receptors (RXRs) [Bastein *et al.* 2004]. Each receptor family is made up of three isoforms (α, β and γ), produced by separate genes. RARs can be activated by ATRA and the isomer 9-*cis* retinoic acid (9-cis RA), while RXRs are activated by 9-*cis* RA. RARs form heterodimers with RXRs and these heterodimers and RXR homodimers function as transcription factors, activating RAREs in the promoter regions of target genes. Most retinol signaling in cells is thought to be mediated by ATRA binding RAR in RAR/RXR heterodimers [Mic *et al.* 2003]. It is still not clear if 9-*cis* RA is formed physiologically in cells and what role this isomer may play as a specific ligand for RXR [Mic *et al.* 2003]. Activated retinoid receptors function as transcription factors, activating specific RA response elements (RAREs) for transcriptional regulation of target genes [Bastein *et al.* 2004, Mic *et al.* 2003].

Peroxisome proliferator-activated receptors (PPARs), α, β/δ, and γ, represent another group of nuclear hormone receptors that forms heterodimers with RXR. PPAR/RXR heterodimers also function as transcription factors, activating specific response elements of target genes [Mangelsdorf and Evans 1995, Bocher *et al.* 2002, Wilson *et al.* 2000]. Recent studies have indicated that ATRA not only can bind RARs, but can serve as a ligand for PPAR β/δ as well [Berry *et al.* 2007]. Channelling of ATRA to RARs or PPAR β/δ is suggested to depend on the intracellular binding proteins, RA binding protein II or keratinocyte fatty acid binding protein 5, which deliver ATRA to either RAR or PPAR β/δ, respectively [Schug *et al.* 2007].

Vitamin A plays an essential role in numerous biological processes, including vision, cellular proliferation, differentiation, and apoptosis, organ development and function, and immunity [Moise *et al.* 2007, Mark *et al.* 2006, Mark *et al.* 2009]. Numerous malformations and impaired vision, growth, organ function, and reproduction have been noted with vitamin A deficiency. Vitamin A is used in developing countries to help correct vitamin A deficiency [Moise *et al.* 2007]. Supplementation with vitamin A has had an enormous worldwide impact, saving countless lives, at minimal costs per patient. There is also widespread use of vitamin A derivatives (retinoids) for treatment of various skin conditions, such as acne [Peck *et al.* 1979], and for different cancers, including acute promyelocytic leukemia (APL), Kaposi's sarcoma, head and neck squamous cell carcinoma, ovarian carcinoma, and neuroblastoma [Siddikuzzaman *et al.* 2010]. Use of retinoids has proved particularly useful for treatment of APL [Siddikuzzaman *et al.* 2010]. Pharmacological concentrations (10^{-7} - 10^{-6}M) of ATRA block repression by a PML- RARα fusion protein that interferes with normal RARα transcriptional regulation in APL.

Besides serving as an intermediate in retinoic acid formation, recent studies have shown that retinal (retinaldehyde) is present at biologically active concentrations in fat tissue, where it antagonizes PPAR-γ activity, inhibits adipogenesis, and improves insulin sensitivity [Ziouzenkova *et al.* 2007]. These observations suggest that retinal may be an additional vitamin A derivative that plays an important role as a mediator of biological processes.

Hypervitaminosis A in experimental animals has been linked to increased bone resorption, decreased bone mass, and increased fractures [Frankel *et al.* 1986, Hough *et al.* 1988, Johansson *et al.* 2002]. There are also case studies in humans showing that significantly increased intake of vitamin A increases bone resorption, causes hypercalcemia, and induces skeletal pain [Frame *et al.* 1974]. Supplementation of the diet with vitamins is a common occurrence in developed countries and there is presently debate over whether more modest increases in vitamin A might promote skeletal abnormalities. Some studies have shown that increased vitamin A intake or elevated serum retinol levels [Michaelsson *et al.* 2003] are associated with an increased incidence of hip fracture or decreased bone mass [Melhaus *et al.* 1998, Feskanich *et al.* 2002, Promislow *et al.* 2002]; however, other studies have shown no deleterious effect on bone mass or fracture risk, and, in some instances, protection from bone loss because of increased vitamin A has been reported [Ribaya-Mercado and Blumberg 2007, Caire-Juvera *et al.* 2009]. In studies where vitamin A analogues have been evaluated, decreases in bone mass have been reported following isotretinoin and acitretin usage in some instances, but a recent, large scale, case-control study has found no increased risk of fracture with these agents [Vestergaard *et al.* 2010].

2. Bone tissue

Skeletal tissue is comprised primarily of either cortical (compact) or trabecular (cancellous) bone. In the adult, approximately 80% of skeletal mass is cortical bone and 20% trabecular bone. Cortical bone is found in the shafts of long bones and the outer surfaces of all other bones in the body. It is organized around blood vessels into cylinders of consolidated bone called osteons, or Haversian systems. Unlike trabecular bone, cortical bone does not contain bone marrow. Trabecular bone is characterized as a network of thin spicules of bone ("spongy bone"), which is found in the interior of vertebrae, flat bones in the skull, the pelvis and sacrum, and the distal and proximal parts of long bones. Both cortical and trabecular bone are important for bone strength. In the adult skeleton, both types of bone are remodelled and modelled [Martin and Seeman 2008]. Modelling of bone is a process that changes the size and shape of bone either by bone resorption without subsequent bone formation, or bone formation without prior bone resorption. Remodelling of bone is the process by which old bone is replaced by new bone. It is initiated by bone resorption to remove damaged bone, followed by new bone formation in the area resorbed. Remodelling does not change the size or shape of the bones. Remodelling is more frequent in trabecular bone than in cortical bone, one of the reasons why a metabolic bone disease like postmenopausal osteoporosis affects primarily bones with proportionally increased amounts of trabecular bone, e.g. vertebrae, distal radius, and proximal femur. Remodelling is believed to be initiated by microcracks in the mineralized bone extracellular matrix and subsequent osteocytic apoptosis, which triggers osteoclast formation and resorption of the micro-damaged area [Martin and Seeman 2008]. The process causes release of "coupling factors" which attract and activate osteoblasts to form new bone under a canopy of bone lining cells [Martin and Sims 2005, Boyce *et al.* 2009, Martin *et al.* 2009]. When osteoblasts fill the resorption lacunae made by osteoclasts with new bone in the bone multicellular unit (BMU), remodelling is in balance and bone mass remains constant. This equilibrium involves bidirectional interactions between osteoclasts and osteoblasts to fine tune the balance between bone formation and bone resorption.

The skeleton is a support structure that serves as a reservoir for calcium, phosphate, and numerous other minerals, protects vital organs such as brain, heart, lung, and bone marrow, and recently has been implicated in glucose- and energy metabolism [Confavreux *et al.* 2009]. Three systemic hormones that play primary roles in calcium homeostasis and bone formation and resorption are parathyroid hormone (PTH), 1,25(OH)$_2$-vitamin D$_3$, and calcitonin. PTH and 1,25(OH)$_2$-vitamin D$_3$ stimulate bone resorption when serum calcium decreases, whereas calcitonin inhibits bone resorption when serum calcium is increased. Sex hormones also play important roles, with increased bone resorption and decreased bone formation occurring when levels of either estrogen or testosterone are decreased. Other agents known to play significant roles in bone turnover are the thyroid hormones, glucocorticoids, follicle stimulating hormone, and the retinoids. Interestingly, there is also a great deal of cross talk between bone cells and the immune system. This occurs during both normal physiological remodelling and in pathological inflammatory conditions involving bone, like rheumatoid arthritis and peridontitis [Takayanagi 2009].

3. Osteoclast differentiation

Osteoclasts are multinucleated giant cells found on bone surfaces that stain for tartrate resistant acid phosphatise (TRAP). They are formed by fusion of mononucleated progenitor cells derived from hematopoetic myeloid stem cells, which also give rise to macrophages and dendritic cells. For fusion of osteoclast precursors to occur, they must be differentiated specifically along the osteoclastic lineage [Lorenzo and Horowitz 2008, Edwards and Mundy 2011]. Formation of osteoclasts is controlled by osteoblasts at the bone surface. Thus, osteoblasts are responsible for not only bone formation, but regulate bone resorption as well. In addition to hematopoetic cells, bone marrow also contains pluripotent mesenchymal cells which are able to support differentiation of osteoclasts [Askmyr *et al.* 2009]; however, mature osteoclasts do not form within bone marrow, but enter the circulation as mononucleated osteoclast progenitors and home to periosteal and endosteal tissues. The details of this attraction are not known at present, but stomal cell-derived factor-1 (SDF-1 or CXCL12) produced by osteoblasts and CXCR4 expressed by osteoclast progenitors may play important roles [Kollet *et al.* 2006]. To what extent the circulating osteoclast progenitor cells are primed in the bone marrow, or to what extent priming occurs in the periosteum and endosteum is also not known at present. Nor is it known if osteoclast formation in trabecular bone in the close vicinity of bone marrow is different from osteoclast formation in periosteal tissues, which are always some distance from bone marrow. Recently, one group has presented evidence for the existence of a unique periosteal macrophage - osteomac which not only can form osteoclasts, but is also able to control bone formation [Chang *et al.* 2008]. Increasing evidence indicates that osteoclast formation does not follow a common pathway and that osteoclasts are different in different parts of the skeleton [Everts *et al.* 2009, Henriksen *et al.* 2011].

Crude bone marrow cultures, or co-cultures of periosteal osteoblasts and purified osteoclast progenitors from either bone marrow or spleens, have shown that osteoclast formation requires close physical contact of progenitor cells with either stromal cells in the bone marrow or osteoblasts. Molecularly, it has been found that macrophage colony-stimulating factor (M-CSF) and receptor activator of nuclear factor κB ligand (RANKL) are two products of stromal cells/osteoblasts that play key roles in regulating osteoclast formation. M-CSF supports progenitor cell proliferation and survival, and RANKL is responsible for progenitor differentiation to osteoclasts, rather than to macrophages or dendritic cells [Takayanagi 2009, Lorenzo and Horowitz 2008, Nakashima and Takayanagi 2009]. RANKL, which is a member of the TNF superfamily, functions by binding to RANK on osteoclast progenitor cells. Osteoprotegerin (OPG), a soluble protein released from stromal cells/osteoblasts, is another key factor regulating osteoclastogenesis. OPG functions as a decoy receptor for RANKL, blocking interaction between RANKL and RANK. The expression of RANKL is thought to be restricted to a relatively small number of cells: bone marrow stromal cells, osteoblasts, periodontal ligament cells, synovial fibroblasts, T-, B- and NK-cells, while OPG appears to be ubiquitously expressed. It is the relative expression of RANKL and OPG which determines whether osteoclast formation will take place. Enhancement of the RANKL/OPG ratio in stromal cells or osteoblasts by hormones and cytokines causes stimulation of bone resorption.

Following RANKL binding to trimeric RANK, association of the cytoplasmic tail of RANK with TNF receptor-associated factor 6 (TRAF 6) leads to activation of several kinases, including IKKβ, MAPKs such as p38 and JNK, and PI3K (Fig. 2). Subsequently, transcription factors such as NF-κB, AP-1, MITF, NFATc1 and Akt are activated. Within the NF-κB family of transcription factors, p50 and p52 seem to be the most important subunits [Boyce *et al.* 2010]. RANK signaling leads to induction and activation of c-fos, which functions as a component of the transcription factor, activator protein-1 (AP-1). Mice with double knockouts of p50/p52 or with deletion of the c-Fos gene lack osteoclasts and exhibit osteopetrosis. The induction of the master transcription factor for osteoclastogenesis, NFATc1, is dependent on NF-κB and c-fos signaling by RANK [Negishi-Koga and Takayanagi 2009]. In cooperation with RANK, immunoglobulin-like receptors associated with adaptor proteins harboring the immunoreceptor tyrosine-based activation motif (ITAM) activate phospholipase Cγ, calcium signaling, and the formation of calcineurin required for activation of NFATc1 [Nemeth *et al.* 2011]. The activation of specific genes necessary for osteoclastogenesis and osteoclast function is regulated by NFATc1 cooperating with other transcription factors, such as AP-1, CREB, PU.1, and MITF. Important osteoclast genes include those encoding calcitonin receptor and TRAP, which serve as osteoclast markers, cathepsin K, which is involved in breakdown of bone matrix collagen, Atp6i and chloride chanel-7, involved in acidification and dissolution of bone mineral crystals, and the integrins α_v and β_3, which are important for attachments of osteoclasts to bone surfaces.

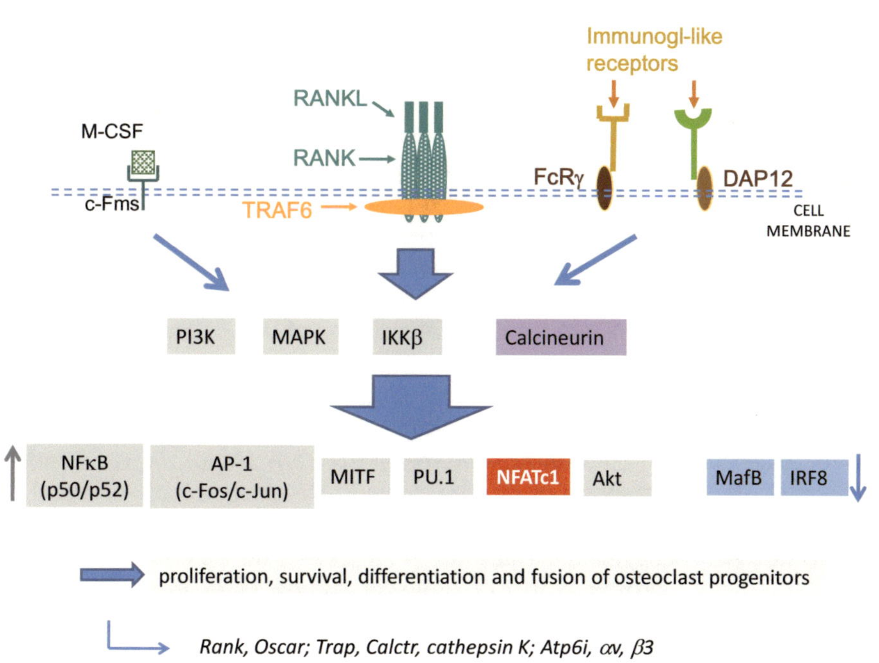

Fig. 2. Osteoclastogenic pathways, transcription factors, and genes stimulated by M-CSF and RANKL.

4. Retinoids and bone resorption in vitro

The effect of vitamin A on bone resorption has been studied the most thoroughly in rodent models. It has been known since the 1920´s that excess vitamin A has effects on the skeleton. In classical experiments in 1952 employing cultured fetal mouse limb bones, Dame Honor Fell showed that hypervitaminosis A stimulated osteoclast formation and bone resorption [Fell and Mellanby 1952]. Thirteen years later, Larry Raisz showed that vitamin A could stimulate bone resorption in organ cultures of fetal rat long bones [Raisz 1965]. Since those early experimental reports, there have been additional studies in organ cultures of fetal rat long bones [Scheven and Hamilton 1990], fetal rat calvariae [Delaissé *et al.* 1988] and calvarial bones from both fetal [Delaissé *et al.* 1988] and newborn [Raisz *et al.* 1977, Togari *et al.* 1991, Kindmark *et al.* 95, Conaway *et al.* 1997] mice confirming the osteoclastogenic effects of vitamin A and derivatives. An investigation indicating that ATRA increases mRNA expression of *RANKL* in primary human osteoblast-like cultures and decreases mRNA expression and protein formation of OPG in human MG-63 osteosarcoma cells [Jacobson *et al.* 2004] led to the suggestion that bone resorption stimulated by the retinoid is due to an increased RANKL/OPG ratio; however, until recently, there had been no data from bone or bone culture systems showing how vitamin A or derivatives stimulated bone resorption. In a recent investigation, we have reported that stimulation of osteoclastogenesis and bone resorption by retinoids in neonatal mouse calvarial bone is due to increased RANKL mRNA and protein expression. Supporting evidence for the role of RANKL was the observation that exogenous OPG administration blocked retinoid induced calvarial bone resorption [Henning *et al.* 2011].

Resorption in the bone organ culture systems depends on increased osteoclast formation and/or enhanced osteoclast activity. Attempts to elucidate effects of vitamin A on mature osteoclasts have generated conflicting results. It has been reported that bone resorbing activity of rabbit osteoclasts incubated on dentine slices is enhanced by ATRA [Saneshige *et al.* 1995]. Additionally, the vitamin A derivative isotretinonin has been observed to increase activity of rat osteoclasts incubated on cortical bone slices [Lakkakorpi and Väänänen 1991]. In contrast, bone resorbing activity of embryonic chicken osteoclasts on either bovine cortical bone or sperm whale dentine has been reported to be decreased by ATRA [O´Neill *et al.* 1992]. Furthermore, degradation of bone particles incubated with chicken osteoclasts is said to be enhanced by retinol and ATRA [Oreffo *et al.* 1988], which differs from experiments using osteoclast-like cell lines from human giant cell bone tumors, where Colucci *et al.* have found that ATRA inhibits degradation of bone matrix in rat bone particles [Colucci *et al.* 1996].

Evaluations of the effects of vitamin A on osteoclast formation have also generated conflicting data. In human bone marrow cultures, ATRA has been reported to stimulate formation of osteoclast-like multinucleated cells that are incapable of resorbing bone [Thavarajah *et al.* 1991]. Formation of multinucleated osteoclasts unable to resorb bone has also been reported following ATRA treatment of bone marrow cultures from egg laying hens [Chiba *et al.* 1996]. Scheven and Hamilton [1990] found no effect of ATRA on osteoclast formation in rat bone marrow cultures; however, when Hata *et al.* [1992] stimulated osteoclast formation in rat bone marrow cultures with $1{,}25(OH)_2$-vitamin D_3, they found inhibition with ATRA. Using an acyclic retinoid, geranylgeranoic acid, Wang *et al.* [2002] also found that osteoclast formation in mouse bone marrow cultures stimulated by $1{,}25(OH)_2$-vitamin D_3 was inhibited. Inhibition by the retinoid was most likely due to inhibition of osteoclast progenitor cells, since inhibition of osteoclast formation by geranylgeranoic acid was also observed in mouse bone marrow macrophage (BMM) cultures stimulated by RANKL. In agreement with these latter observations, we have recently shown that ATRA, as well as 9-cis retinoic acid, inhibit osteoclast formation in mouse bone marrow cell cultures stimulated with either 1,25$(OH)_2$-vitamin D_3 or PTH [Conaway *et al.* 2009], an effect associated with decreased expression of the osteoclast genes *Calcr, Acp5,* and *Catsk,* which code for the calcitonin receptor, TRAP, and cathepsin K, respectively. ATRA did not affect 1, 25$(OH)_2$-vitamin D_3 stimulated mRNA expression of *Rankl,* nor did the retinoid affect the decrease of *Opg* expression induced by 1,25$(OH)_2$-vitamin D_3, suggesting that the inhibitory effect was at the level of osteoclast progenitors rather than stromal cells. Osteoclast formation in both crude bone marrow cultures and spleen cell cultures stimulated by RANKL was also inhibited by ATRA and 9-cis retinoic acid. Moreover, osteoclast formation stimulated by RANKL in highly purified mouse BMM cultures was inhibited by ATRA and 9-cis retinoic acid, providing good evidence that the retinoids inhibited osteoclastogenesis by directly affecting osteoclast progenitor cells.

Inhibition of osteoclast progenitor cell differentiation by ATRA was due to inhibition of AP-1 and Nfatc1 pathways, but did not involve the NF-κB pathway [Conaway *et al.* 2009]. ATRA inhibited mRNA and protein expression of the transcription factors c-Fos and Nfatc1 induced by RANKL. RANKL also enhanced the mRNA expression of *Fra-1, Fra-2* and *JunB* in mouse BMM, but ATRA inhibited only *Fra-2*. The decrease of the macrophage transcription factor MafB caused by RANKL during osteoclastogenesis was blunted by ATRA, suggesting that ATRA arrested precursor cells at the macrophage stage. In agreement with these observations, it has been observed that ATRA inhibits Nfatc1 expression, translocation, and DNA-binding in RAW264.7 cells and mouse BMM [Balkan *et al.* 2011].

Mouse BMM express RARα and RARβ, but little RARγ. By use of different agonists and antagonists, it was demonstrated that ATRA induced inhibition of RANKL stimulated osteoclast formation in BMM was mediated by RARα [Conaway *et al.* 2009]. As discussed above, ATRA can also serve as a ligand for PPARβ/δ. However, ligands specific for this receptor did not mimic the inhibitory effect of ATRA.

Effects of retinoids on osteoclast formation have also been studied using osteoclast progenitor cells isolated from peripheral blood. Woods *et al.* [1995] found that monocytes from chicken peripheral blood spontaneously formed giant cells with osteoclast like features and that this process was inhibited by ATRA. Recently, it was shown that ATRA inhibited osteoclast formation in RANKL stimulated cultures of human $CD14^+$ monocytes from peripheral blood [Hu *et al.* 2010]. In agreement with observations in RANKL stimulated mouse BMM, inhibition of osteoclast formation in human $CD14^+$ cells was associated with decreased mRNA expression of osteoclastic genes such as *ACP5* and *CATSK,* and the transcription factor *NFATc1,* indicating that retinoids inhibit osteoclast formation by inhibiting osteoclast differentiation rather than fusion of differentiated progenitor cells. The authors attributed the inhibition to decreased expression of RANK mRNA and protein; however, it remains to be shown if this is the primary event.

5. Retinoids and bone resorption in vivo

In short term *in vivo* studies where rodents were treated with increased concentrations of retinoids (ATRA or Ro 13-6298), it has been reported that thinning of cortical bone due to significant stimulation of periosteal resorption occurs at the same time that cancellous bone resorption is inhibited [Kneissel *et al.* 2005]. Furthermore, in a recent one week study where rats were fed increased vitamin A, increased cortical osteoclasts and cortical bone thinning were also observed; however, in these animals, endosteal osteoclasts disappeared because of impaired endosteal/marrow blood flow, which resulted in hypoxia and pathological endosteal mineralization [Lind *et al.* 2011]. This resulted in thinner, more brittle bones with little apparent affect on bone mass. Vitamin A and retinoids stimulate resorption in cultured fetal mouse and rat limb bones [Fell and Mellanby 1952, Raisz 1965, Scheven *et al.* 1990], but these studies are normally based on calcium release to medium and do not distinguish between cortical and cancellous bone breakdown. On the other hand, calvarial bone is considered to be a good model for periosteal resorption of cortical bone and it is established that vitamin A and ATRA are effective stimulators of osteoclastogenesis and bone resorption in calvarial bone [Raisz *et al.* 1977, Togari *et al.* 1991, Kindmark *et al.* 1995, Conaway *et al.* 1997]. As stated previously, retinoids are also good inhibitors of osteoclastogenesis in mouse bone marrow cell and BMM cultures. Thus, when comparing results of *in vitro* and *in vivo* experimental studies attempting to access the effects of increased vitamin A, it appears there may be good agreement regarding cortical osteoclast formation and function stimulated by vitamin A. In contrast, it seems a continuum of effects may occur in the endosteum, with increased vitamin A inhibiting endosteal osteoclast formation and function, and impaired blood flow and hypoxia promoting osteoclast death.

6. Conclusion

In developed countries, the diet is often supplemented with vitamin A and there is presently controversy over whether increased intake of vitamin A might promote skeletal fragility [Michaelsson *et al.* 2003, Melhaus *et al.* 1998, Feskanich *et al.* 2002, Promislow *et al.* 2002, Ribaya-Mercado and Blumberg 2007, Caire-Juvera *et al.* 2009]. If cortical bone thinning and suppression of osteoclastogenesis in cancellous bone play prominent roles in fracture incidence in humans following increased intake of vitamin A, this would be substantially different from conditions such as postmenopausal osteoporosis and glucocorticoid excess, where the increased incidence of fracture is due primarily to cancellous bone loss. These different paradigms for bone fragility may help explain some of the differing outcomes in studies evaluating vitamin A intake and fracture risk. It also seems possible that a duality of retinoid action on osteoclast precursors in cortical and cancellous bone might be manifest as different degrees of cortical resorption and cancellous inhibition, depending on other systemic and environmental factors. This would also affect bone mass and fracture risk, as would the development of hypoxia and death of endosteal osteoclasts. Our improving understanding of vitamin A action in bone cells is not only promising to be extremely valuable for future experimentation, but appears to warrant new evaluations of bone mass and fracture risk in patients with increased intake of vitamin A as well.

7. Acknowledgements

Studies performed in the author´s laboratories were supported by grants from the Swedish Research Council, Swedish Dental Society, the Royal 80 Year Fund of King Gustav V, the Swedish Rheumatism Association, Medical Faculty at Umeå University, Combine, ALF/LUA grants from the Sahlgrenska University Hospital and the County Council of Västerbotten.

8. References

Askmyr M, Sims NA, Martin TJ, Purton LE. (2009) What is the true nature of the osteoblastic hematopoetic stem cell niche? *Trends Endocrinol Metab* 20:303-309

Balkan W, Rodríguez-Gonzales M, Pang M, Fernandez I, Troen BR. (2011) Retinoic acid inhibits Nfatc1 expression and osteoclast differentiation. *J Bone Miner Metab* Epub ahead of print 2011

Bastien, J., and Rochette-Egly, C. (2004) Nuclear retinoid receptors and the transcription of retinoid-target genes. *Gene* 328, 1–16

Berry, D.C., and Noy, N. (2007) Is PPARβ/δ a retinoid receptor? *PPAR. Res.* 73256:1-5

Bocher, V., Pineda-Torra, I., Fruchart, J.C., and Staels, B. (2002) PPARs: transcription factors controlling lipid and lipoprotein metabolism. *Ann. N. Y. Acad. Sci.* 967:7-18

Boyce BF, Yao Z, Xing L. (2009) Osteoclasts have multiple roles in bone in addition to bone resorption. Crit Rev *Eukaryot Gene Expr* 19:171-180

Boyce BF, Yao Z, Xing L. (2010) Functions of nuclear factor κB in bone. *Ann NY Acad Sci* 1192:367-375

Caire-Juvera, G., Ritenbaugh, C., Wactawski-Wende, J., Snetselaar, L., G. and Chen, Z. (2009) Vitamin A and retinol intakes and the risks of fractures among participants of the Women's Health Observational Study. *Am. J. Clin. Nutr.* 89: 323-330

Chambon, P.(1996) A decade of molecular biology of retinoic acid receptors *FASEB J* 10, 940-954

Chang MK, Raggatt LJ, Alexander KA, Kuliwaba JS, Fazzalari NL, Schroder K, Maylin ER, Ripoll VM, Hume DA, Pettit AR. (2008) Osteal tissue macrophages are intercalated throughout human and mouse bone lining tissues and regulate osteoblast function in vitro and in vivo. *J Immunol* 181:1232-44

Chiba M, Teitelbaum SL, Cao X, Ross FP. (1996) Retinoic acid stimulates expression of the functional osteoclast integrin $\alpha_v\beta_3$: transcriptional activation of the β_3 but not the α_v gene. *J Cell Biochem* 62:467-475

Colucci S, Grano M, Mori G, Scotlandi K, Mastrogiacomo M, Mori C, Zambonin Zallone A. (1996) Retinoic acid induces cell proliferation and modulated gelatinases activity in human osteoclast-like cell lines. *Biochem Biophys Res Commun* 227:47-52

Conaway HH, Grigorie D, Lerner UH. (1997) Differential effects of glucocorticoids on bone resorption in neonatal mouse calvariae stimulated by peptide and steroid-like hormones. *J Endocrinol* 155:513-521

Conaway HH, Persson E, Halén M, Granholm S, Svensson O, Pettersson U, Lie A, Lerner UH. (2009) Retinoids inhibit differentiation of hematopoetic osteoclast progenitors. *FASEB J* 23:3526-3538

Confavreux CB, Levine RL, Karsenty G. (2009) A paradigm of integrative physiology, the crosstalk between bone and energy metabolism. *Mol Cell Endocrinol* 310:21-29

Delaissé JM, Eeckhout Y, Vaes G. (1988) Bone-resorbing agents affect the production and distribution of procollagenase as well as the activity of collagenase in bone tissue. *Endocrinology* 123:264-276

Edwards JR, Mundy GR. (2011) Advances in osteoclast biology: old findings and new insights from mouse models. *Nat Rev* Rheumatol EPUB ahead of print

Everts V, de Vries TJ, Helfrich MH. (2009) Osteoclast heterogeneity: lessons from osteopetrosis and inflammatory conditions. *Biochim Biophys Acta* 1792:757-765

Fell HB, Mellanby E. (1952) The effect of hypervitaminosis A on embryonic limb-bones cultivated in vitro. *J Physiol* 116:320-349

Feskanich, D., Singh, V., Willett, W.C. and Colditz, G.A. (2002) Vitamin A intake and hip fractures among postmenopausal women. *JAMA* 287:47-54

Frame, B., Jackson, C.E., Reynolds, W. A. and Umphrey, J. E. (1974) Hypercalcemia and skeletal effects in chronic hypervitaminous A. *Annals of Internal Medicine* 80:44-48

Frankel, T.L., Seshadri, M.S., McDowall, D.B., and Cornish, C.J. (1986) Hypervitaminosis A and calcium-regulating hormones in the rat. *J. Nutr.* 116:578-587

Hata K, Kukita T, Akamine A, Kukita A, Kurisu K. (1992) Trypsinized osteoclast-like multinucleated cells formed in rat bone marrow cultures efficiently form resorption lacunae on dentine. *Bone* 13:139-146

Henning P, Pirhayati A, Pettersson U, Svensson O, Conaway HH, Lerner UH. (2011) Stimulation of mouse calvarial periosteal resorption and inhibition of osteoclast formation in human peripheral $CD14^+$ cells by vitamin A. Abstract at 3rd Joint Meeting European Calcified Tissue Society and International Bone and Mineral Society, Athens May 7-11, 2011.

Henriksen K, Bollerslev J, Everts V, Karsdal MA. (2011) Osteoclast activity and subtypes as a function of physiology and pathology - implications for future treatments of osteoporosis. *Endocr Rev* 32:31-63

Hough, S., Avioli, L.V., Muir, H., Gelderblom, D., Jenkins, G., Kurasi, H., Slatopolsky, E., Bergfeld, M.A. and Teitelbaum, S. L. (1988) Effects of hypervitaminosis A on the bone and mineral metabolism of the rat. *Endocrinology* 122:2933-2939

Hu L, Lind T, Sundqvist A, Jacobson A, Melhus H. (2010) Retinoic acid increases proliferation of human osteoclast progenitors and inhibits RANKL-stimulated osteoclast differentiation by suppressing RANK. *PLoS One* 5:e13305

Jacobson A, Johansson S, Branting M, Melhus H. (2004) Vitamin A differentially regulates RANKL and OPG expression in human osteoblasts. *Biochem Biophys Res Commun* 322:162-167

Johansson, S., Lind, P.M., Håkansson, H., Oxlund, H., Orberg, J., and Melhus, H. (2002) Subclinical hypervitaminosis A causes fragile bones in rats. *Bone* 31:685-689

Kindmark A, Melhus H, Ljunghall S, Ljunggren Ö. (1995) Inhibitory effects of 9-cis and all-trans retinoic acid on $1,25(OH)_2$ vitamin D_3-induced bone resorption. *Calcif Tissue Int* 57:242-244

Kollet O, Dar A, Shivtiel S, Kalinkovich A, Lapid K, Sztainberg Y, Tesio M, Samstein RM, Goichberg P, Spiegel A, Elson A, Lapidot T. (2006) Osteoclasts degrade endosteal components and promote mobilization of hematopoetic progenitor cells. *Nat Med* 12:657-664

Kneissel, M., Studer, A. and Cortesi, M. S. (2005) Retinoid-induced bone thinning by subperiosteal osteoclast activity in adult rodents. *Bone* 36, 202-214

Lakkakorpi PT, Väänänen HK. (1991) Kinetics of the osteoclast cytoskeleton during the resorption cycle in vitro. *J Bone Miner Res* 6:817-826

Lind, T., Lind, P.M., Jacobson, A., Hu, L., Sundqvist, A., Risteli, J., Yebra-Rodriguez, A., Rodriguez-Navarro, A., Andersson, G. and Melhaus, H. (2011) High dietary intake of retinol leads to bone marrow hypoxia and diaphyseal endosteal mineralization in rats. *Bone* 48, 496-506

Lorenzo J, Horowitz M, Choi Y. (2008) Osteoimmunology: interactions of the bone and immune system. *Endocr Rev* 29: 403-440

Mangelsdorf, D.J., and Evans, R.M. (1995) The RXR heterodimers and orphan receptors. *Cell* 83:841-850

Mark, M., Ghyselinck, N.B., and Chambon, P. (2006) Function of retinoid nuclear receptors: lessons from genetic and pharmacological dissections of the retinoic acid signaling pathway during mouse embryogenesis. *Annu. Rev. Pharmacol. Toxicol.* 46: 451-480

Mark, M., Ghyselinck, N.B., and Chambon, P. (2009) Function of retinoic acid receptors during embryonic development. *Nuclear Receptor Signaling* 7, e002

Martin TJ, Seeman E. (2008) Bone remodeling: its local regulation and the emergence of bone fragility. Best Pract Res *Clin Endocrinol Metab* 22:701-722

Martin TJ, Sims NA. (2005) Osteoclast-derived activity in the coupling of bone formation to resorption. *Trends Mol Med* 11:76-81

Martin TJ, Gooi JH, Sims NA. (2009) Molecular mechanisms in coupling of bone formation to resorption. *Crit Rev Eukaryot Gene Expr* 19:73-88

Melhus, H., Michaelsson, K., Kindmark, A., Bergstrom, R., Holmberg, L., Mallmin, H., Wolk, A. and Ljunghall, S. (1998) Excessive dietary intake of vitamin A is associated with reduced bone mineral density and increased risk of hip fracture. *Ann. Intern. Med.* 129:770-778

Mic, F. A., Molotkov, A., Benbrook, D. M., and Duester, G. (2003) Retinoid activation of retinoid acid receptor but not retinoid X receptor is sufficient to rescue lethal defect in retinoic acid synthesis. *Proc. Natl. Acad. Sci. U. S. A.* 100, 7125–7140

Michaelsson, K., Lithell, H., Vessby, B. and Melhus, H. (2003) Serum retinol levels and the risk of fracture. *N. Engl. J. Med.* 348:287-294

Moise, A.R., Noy, N., Palcqewski, K., and Blaner, W.S. (2007) Delivery of retinoid-based therapies to target tissues. *Biochemistry* 46, 4449- 4458

Nakashima T, Takayanagi H. (2009) Osteoclasts and the immune system. *J Bone Miner Metab* 27:519-529

Negishi-Koga T, Takayanagi H. (2009) Ca^{2+}-NFATc1 signalling is an essential axis of osteoclast differentiation. *Immunol Rev* 231:241-256

Nemeth K, Schoppet M, Al-Fakhri N, Helas S, Jessberger R, Hofbauer LC, Goettsch C. (2011) The role of osteoclast-associated receptor in osteoimmunology. *J Immunol* 186:13-18

O´Neill RPJ, Jones JS, Boyde A, Taylor ML, Arnett TR. (1992) Effect of retinoic acid on the resorptive activity of chick osteoclasts in vitro. *Bone* 13:23-27

Oreffo RO, Teti A, Triffitt JT, Francis MJ, Carano A, Zallone AZ. (1988) Effect of vitamin A on bone resorption: evidence for direct stimulation of isolated chicken osteoclasts by retinol and retinoic acid. *J Bone Miner Res* 3:203-210

Peck, G.L.,Olsen, T.G., Yoder, F.W., Peck GL, Olsen TG, Yoder FW, Strauss JS, Downing DT, Pandya M, Butkus D, Arnaud-Battandier J.(1979) Prolonged remissions of cystic and conglobate acne with 13-cis-r retinoic acid . *N. Engl. J. Med.* 300: 329-333

Promislow, J.H.E., Goodman-Gruen, D., Slymen, D.J. and Barrett-Connor, E. (2002) Retinol intake and bone mineral density in the elderly: The Rancho Bernardo study. *J. Bone Miner. Res.* 17:1349-1358

Raisz LG. (1965) Bone resorption in tissue culture. Factors influencing the response to parathyroid hormone. *J Clin Invest* 44:103-116

Raisz LG, Simmons HA, Gworek SC, Eilon G. (1977) Studies on congenital osteopetrosis in microphthalmic mice using organ cultures: impairment of bone resorption in response to physiologic stimulators. *J Exp Med* 145:857-865

Ribaya-Mercado, J. D. and Blumberg, J. B. (2007) Vitamin A: Is it a risk factor for osteoporosis and bone fracture? *Nutr. Rev.* 65: 425-438

Saneshige S, Mano H, Tezuka K, Kakudo S, Mori Y, Honda Y, Itabashi A, Yamada T, Miyata K, Hakeda Y, Ishi J, Kumegawa M. (1995) Retinoic acid directly stimulates osteoclastic bone resorption and gene expression of cathepsin K/OC-2. *Biochem J* 309:721-724

Schug, T.T., Berry, D.C., Shaw, N.S., Travis, S.N. and Noy, N. (2007) Opposing effects of retinoic acid on cell growth result from alternate activation of two different nuclear receptors. *Cell* 129:723-733

Siddikuzzaman, Guruvayoorappan, C. and Berlin Grace, V., M. (2010) All trans retinoic acid and cancer. *Immunopharmacol. and Immunotoxicol.* EPUB ahead of print 1-9

Scheven BAA, Hamilton NJ. (1990) Retinoic acid and 1,25$(OH)_2$-vitamin D_3 stimulate osteoclast formation by different mechanisms. *Bone* 11:53-59

Takayanagi H. (2009) Osteoimmunology and the effects of the immune system on bone. Nat Rev Rheumatol 5:667-676

Thavarajah M, Evans DB, Kanis JA. (1991) 1,25$(OH)_2D_3$ induces differentiation of osteoclast-like cells from human bone marrow cultures. *Biochem Biophys Res Commun* 176:1189-1195

Togari A, Kondo M, Arai M, Matsumoto S. (1991) Effects of retinoic acid on bone formation and resorption in cultured mouse calvaria. *Gen Pharmacol* 22:287-292

Vestergaard, P., Rejnmark, L. and Mosekilde,L. (2010) High-dose treatment with vitamin A analogues and risk of fractures. *Arch. Dermatol.* 146:478-482.

Wald, G. (1968) Molecular basis of visual excitation. *Science* 162, 230-239

Wang X, Wu J, Shidoji Y, Muto Y, Ohishi N, Yagi K, Ikegami S, Shinki T, Udagawa N, Suda T, Ishimi Y. (2002) Effects of geranylgeranoic acid in bone: induction of osteoblast differentiation and inhibition of osteoclast formation. *J Bone Miner Res* 17:91-100

Wilson, T.M., Brown, P.J., Sternbach, D.D., and Henke, B.R. (2000) The PPARs: from orphan receptors to drug discovery. *J. Med. Chem.* 43:527-550

Woods C, Domenget C, Solari F, Gandrillon O, Lazarides E, Jurdic P. (1995) Antagonistic role of vitaminD3 and retinoic acid on the differentiation of chicken hematopoetic macrophages into osteoclast precursor cells. *Endocrinology* 136:85-95

Ziouzenkova, O., Orasanu, G., Sharlach, M., Adiyama T. E., Berger, J.P., Viereck, J., Hamilton, J. A., Tang, G., Dolnikowski, G. G., Vogel, S., Duester, G. and Plutzky, J. (2007) Retinaldehyde represses adipogenesis and diet-induced obesity. *Nature Med.* 13: 695-702

21

Environmental Endocrinology: Endocrine Disruptors and Endocrinopathies

Eleni Palioura, Eleni Kandaraki and Evanthia Diamanti-Kandarakis
Medical School University of Athens, Greece

1. Introduction

An endocrine disruptor (ED) is defined by the US- Environmental Protection Agency as "an exogenous agent that interferes with the production, release, transport, metabolism, binding, action, or elimination of natural hormones in the body responsible for the maintenance of homeostasis, reproduction, development, and/or behavior" (U.S. EPA., 1997). This definition encompasses a rather heterogeneous group of molecules from naturally occurring substances (e.g., phytoestrogens) to biochemically manufactured compounds such as plasticizers, pesticides, industrial solvents, pharmaceutical agents (diethylstilbestrol) and heavy metals.

Endocrine disruptors were originally considered to exert their biological action through nuclear steroid receptors by mimicking or antagonizing natural hormone's action (Waring & Harris, 2005) with the majority of them acting as pseudoestrogens and less possessing anti-androgenic or anti-estrogenic properties (McLachlan et al., 2006). Today, basic scientific research shows that the mechanisms are much broader than originally recognized and include interaction with transcriptional factors, non-nuclear steroid hormone receptors, gene regulation or even transgenerational effects by targeting germ cell lines (Anway & Skinner, 2006, 2008; Tabb & Blumberg, 2006).

In addition, targets for endocrine disruption extend beyond the traditional estrogen/androgen -mediated reproductive system. Within the last few years, scientists also have expressed concern about the potential role of EDs in increasing trends in obesity and diabetes, the major life-threatening diseases of modern word. At present, all hormone-sensitive physiological systems seem to be vulnerable to EDs, including brain and hypothalamic neuroendocrine systems; pituitary; thyroid; cardiovascular system; mammary gland; adipose tissue; pancreas; ovary and uterus in females; and testes and prostate in males (Diamanti-Kandarakis et al., 2009).

Undoubtedly, the issue of endocrine disruption has attracted considerable scientific attention with the weight of data obtained from wildlife populations, animal models and epidemiological studies growing extensively during the last years. After all, the unprecedented increase in the production and use of industrial and agricultural chemicals during last decades makes human exposure inevitable through multiple sources. Adults are exposed mainly through the ingestion of contaminated drinking water, food and breathing polluted air. Infants are exposed to EDs through breast milk, baby products, and polluted air while fetuses are exposed through the placenta and are more vulnerable to harmful, irreversible, pathological changes in adult life. People occupationally exposed to pesticides, fungicides and industrial chemicals are considered to be at highest risk for developing an endocrine abnormality as well as humans acutely exposed to an accidental release of an endocrine disrupting chemical.

This chapter reviews the evidence linking endocrine disrupting chemicals to a broad spectrum of clinical perturbations from reproduction and thyroid to metabolic regulation.A summarized review of literature focused on the strongest experimental data and human epidemiological studies targets to elucidate the underlying interactions between endocrine disruptors and endocrine abnormalities.

2. Reproductive function and endocrine disruptors

Reproductive health is traditionally considered as one of the well-studied fields in endocrine disruption. The effects of EDs on reproduction are amply documented in both wildlife and laboratory populations while interfering with human reproductive function is highly plausible. Establishing causality between human reproductive health and exposure to a certain environmental contaminant is challenging as several confounders need to be taken into account.

A critical concern is the potential lag between exposure to EDs and the manifestation of a reproductive disorder as in humans this period may be years or decades after initial exposure. The timing of exposure is key to human disease as the developmental periods from periconception and during pregnancy, infancy, childhood, and puberty are considered as critical and sensitive windows of susceptibility to environmental insults .Furthermore, chronic exposure to low amounts of mixtures of EDs than acute exposure to a single compound, as in many animal models, is the most possible scenario when studying human reproduction. In addition, as in other systems in the organism, EDs effects on human reproduction could be varied by individual differences in metabolism, body composition and susceptibility due to genetic polymorphisms (Diamanti-Kandarakis et al., 2009).

In the human female, the first evidence of endocrine disruption was provided almost four decades ago by diethylstilbestrol (DES), a synthetic oestrogen prescribed therapeutically in a large scale in the mid-20th century in order to prevent miscarriage in pregnant women. The observation of an uncommon gynecologic neoplasm, vaginal adenocarcinoma, in daughters born 15–22 yr earlier to women treated with this potent synthetic estrogen during pregnancy was the first clinical evidence of DES disruption on reproductive system (Herbst et al., 1971). Posterior studies have identified additional adverse effects in female off springs including increased risk for structural reproductive tract anomalies with a characteristic T-shaped uterus, infertility, menstrual irregularity and poor pregnancy outcomes manifested as spontaneous abortion, ectopic pregnancy, and preterm delivery (Kaufman et al., 1982, 2000; Palmer et al., 2001). Furthermore, DES grand-daughters born to mothers prenatally exposed to diethylstilbestrol exhibit irregular menstrual cycles and possible infertility (Titus-Ernstoff et al., 2006) .These robust clinical observations together with experimental data support the causal role of DES in female reproductive disorders.

Increasing data from wildlife and laboratory studies support a role of EDs in the pathogenesis of several other female reproductive disorders during a broad developmental spectrum from puberty onset to menopause (Diamanti-Kandarakis et al., 2010; McLachlan et al., 2006; Woodruff et al., 2008). The catalogue of reproductive aberrations possible related to

ED exposure is extending to include early/delayed puberty, polycystic ovarian syndrome (PCOS), impaired fertility and fecundity, premature ovarian failure, endometriosis, uterine fibroids, aneuploidy, pregnancy complications as well as breast and endometrial tumors (Caserta et al., 2008; Diamanti-Kandarakis et al., 2009).

To give few examples, earlier menarche onset has been observed in girls exposed to polychlorinated biphenyls(PCBs), polybrominated biphenyls (PBBs), phthalate esters and DDT while there are other data that link phthalates to premature thelarche and increased risk of endometriosis (Woodruff et al., 2008). With regard to human puberty, scientific interest is focused on the potential effect of environmental factors on puberty timing. This is based on the observation that since the 19th century there have been significant modifications in puberty timing with earlier age of thelarche and menarche in girls (Euling et al., 2008a).This puberty timing alteration has been associated, apart from apparent improvements in general health and nutrition, with a potential impact of endocrine-disrupting chemicals, particularly the estrogen mimics and antiandrogens (Euling et al., 2008b, Jacobson-Dickman & Lee, 2009).

Adult female reproductive functions are also disrupted by environmental chemicals with the strongest evidence incriminating heavy metals and especially lead exposure. Most modifiable risk appears to be associated with exposures in unique populations (contaminated fish consumers) or occupational groups (farmworkers) (Mendola et al., 2008). Furthermore, recent evidence imply a potential role of Bisphenol A (BPA) in the PCOS pathophysiology given that in women with PCOS, BPA levels were found to be higher compared to BMI-matched healthy women and also to be positively and strongly associated with androgen levels (Kandaraki et al., 2010). Serum BPA concentrations are significantly higher in men than in women (Takeuchi et al., 2002) and in women with ovulatory dysfunction compared to regularly ovulating women (Takeuchi et al., 2004). As PCOS pathogenesis remains partly unraveled, the role of environmental factors and in particular BPA could also been proposed in PCOS development.

With regard to male reproductive system, research has been mainly focused on three major health endpoints; impaired semen quality and infertility, urogenital tract abnormalities-cryptorchidism and hypospadias- and testicular germ cell cancer. This is probably related to the epidemiologic evidence that suggest a decline in human semen quality over the last 50 years (Carlsen et al., 1992) and temporal increasing trends in the prevalence of urogenital tract malformations such as cryptorchidism and hypospadias (Toppari et al., 2001). Interestingly, it is hypothesized that the above-mentioned abnormalities share a common embryogenic origin as parts of a pathogenic entity coined as "testicular dysgenesis syndrome" (TDS). This hypothesis proposes that a prenatal, synergistic, interaction between environmental, genetic and maternal factors lead to abnormal testis development (dysgenesis)(Skakkebæk et al., 2001) and secondarily to impaired androgen production and germ cell development due to Sertoli and Leydig cells' dysfunction (Sharpe & Skakkebæk, 2003). The existence of TDS as a distinct clinical entity and of possible associations with EDs is an area of active research.

Some substances that have been incriminated to have an aggravating impact on sperm parameters include polychlorinated biphenyls (Dallinga et al., 2002; Hauser et al., 2003), phthalates (Duty et al., 2003; Hauser et al., 2006) and non-persistent pesticides (Juhler et al., 1999; Padungtod et al., 2000).Epidemiologic evidence for EDC exposure and cryptorchidism or hypospadias are limited. Concerning ED exposure and cryptorchidism and/or hypospadias, the strongest epidemiological data are those suggesting an association between residency in agricultural areas and/or measures of direct parental exposure to non-organochlorine pesticides (Diamanti-Kandarakis et al., 2009).

Overall, the epidemiologic data on the environmental EDs suggest that there may be associations between exposure and adverse health outcomes in men. However, the limited human data highlight the need for further research on these chemicals. Future longitudinal epidemiology studies with appropriately designed exposure assessments are needed to determine potential causal relationships, to identify the most important time windows of exposure, and to define individual susceptibility factors for adverse effects on men's health in response to exposure.

3. Thyroid and endocrine disruptors

Thyroid hormones have been evolutionarily preserved as important regulators of development, tissue growth and metabolism among all vertebrates and in some invertebrate species (Heyland and Moroz, 2005). Given their importance for normal physiological processes, considerable concern has aroused regarding the clinical impact of environmental factors on thyroid function to the extent that human could be affected. This interaction is biologically plausible as a variety of heterogeneous synthetic chemicals has been recognized to interfere with thyroid homeostasis by acting on different points of regulation of thyroid hormone synthesis, release, transport through the blood, metabolism and clearance (Howdeshell, 2002) or directly at the receptor level (Zoeller, 2007).

Polychlorinated biphenyls (PCBs), Polybrominated diphenyl ethers (PBDEs), Bisphenol-A, dioxin, Perchlorate and furans have been incriminated as potential disruptors of thyroid homeostasis through their ability to affect the hypothalamic- pituitary- thyroid axis (Boas et al., 2006; Zoeller, 2010). Correlations between levels of these compounds in the body and circulating thyroid hormone levels, thyrotropin levels, thyroid volume and prevalence of thyroid antibodies have been reported by several researchers, however, inconsistency exists across studies (Hagmar et al., 2001; Langer et al., 2008; Meeker et al., 2007).

Literature on thyroid disrupting chemicals includes human epidemiological studies that indicate a potential association between exposure to endocrine disruptors and disturbance of thyroid function (Persky et al., 2001; Steinmaus et al., 2007; Takser et al., 2005) with most data pointing towards subtle alterations of the thyroid axis within normal ranges which may, in turn, be harmful especially for human fetus (Boas et al., 2006). Fetus' growth and brain development are very sensitive to modifications of thyroid homeostasis with a significant risk of neurological and cognitive deficiencies.

Overall, the literature on thyroid-disrupting effects of individual chemicals is rapidly increasing, as animal exposure studies and in vitro tests reveal a multitude of potential mechanisms of action. Quick and robust tools should be developed to identify potential thyroid disrupting chemicals and their multiple mechanisms of action. Furthermore, a better understanding of the mechanisms underlying disruption of the thyroid function may lead to changes in public policy in order to limit adverse outcomes for future generations.

4. Obesity epidemic and endocrine disruptors

A potential role of environmental contaminants on the escalating rates of human obesity has been hypothesized as an exogenous factor that may impair body's natural weight-control mechanisms (Baillie-Hamilton, 2002). As the current epidemic in obesity cannot be solely explained by alterations in food intake, physical activity and/or genetic predispotion, the contribution of environmental factors becomes suspicious.

Research on this field has been mainly focused on the identification of environmental "obesogens", molecules that inappropriately regulate lipid metabolism and adipogenesis and also on the molecular mechanisms underlying these metabolic alterations (Grün et al., 2006; Tabb & Blumberg, 2006). After all, recent epidemiology studies indicate that exposure to EDs during development is associated with overweight and obesity later in life. In a cross-sectional analysis of six urinal phthalates metabolites in a total sample of 4369 participants, positive correlations were observed between body mass index (BMI) and waist circumference and most of the metabolites in adult males (Hatch et al., 2008). High serum Polychlorinated Bisphenyls levels have been associated with high levels of total serum lipids and BMI in a Native American cohort (Goncharov et al., 2008) and prenatal and early life PCB exposures were associated with increased weight in boys and girls at puberty (Gladen et al., 2000).

So far, several experimental data have pointed to the effect of endocrine disrupting chemicals on lipid metabolism suggesting that adipocyte *per se* may represent a cell vulnerable to disruption. A characteristic example of such interaction is provided by the organotin tributyltin (TBT) that has been shown to modulate adipocyte differentiation by acting as an agonist for retinoid X receptor (RXR) and peroxisome proliferators-activated receptor γ (PPAR γ), the nuclear receptors that play important roles in lipid homeostasis and adipogenesis (Grün & Blumberg, 2006; Kanayama et al., 2005). Therefore, as it is speculated by Tabb & Blumberg, chronic life-time or developmental exposure to TBT could activate RXR and/or RXR:PPAR-γ signalling leading to long-term alterations of the total adipocyte number and/or a lipid haemostasis (Tabb & Blumberg, 2006).

Another chemical showed to display "obesogenic" properties *in vivo* is diethylstilbestrol. Female mice neonatally exposed to both low and high doses of this estrogenic compound exhibited increased body weight in adulthood. The low dose did not affect body weight during treatment but was associated with a significant increase in body weight in the adult animal by 4 to 6 months of age while the highest dose resulted in a significant decrease in mice weight during treatment followed by a "catch-up" before puberty and consecutively elevated body weight during adulthood (Newbold et al., 2008). Further studies indicated that the increase in body weight in DES-exposed mice was associated with an increase in the percent of body fat as determined by mouse densitometry (Newbold et al., 2007).

Bisphenol A is also postulated to play a role in the development of obesity by interacting with lipid homeostasis and body weight control mechanisms through pleiotropic modes of action. Micromolar concentrations of BPA were shown to enhance adipocyte differentiation and lipid accumulation in target cells in a dose-dependent manner (Masuno et al., 2002, 2005; Wada et al., 2007). From a molecular perspective, these effects are liked with up-regulation of gene expressions involved in lipid metabolism and adipogenic transcription factors (Phrakonkham et al., 2008; Wada et al., 2007). *In vivo* studies confirm the above observations. Perinatal exposure to low doses of BPA increases adipose storage in rodents in adult life (Rubin et al, 2001; Somm et al, 2009). A similar effect is observed when exposure takes place during gestation (Nikaido et al., 2004).

Many other environmental chemicals are suspected to be candidate obesogens including pesticides; for example, organochlorines such as DDT, endrin, lindane, and hexachlorobenzene; organophosphates; carbamates; polychlorinated biphenyls; other plastic components such as phthalates; perfluoroctanoic acid (PFOA); heavy metals such as cadmium, lead, and arsenic; and solvents (Newbold, 2010). Although the epidemiological link between specific obesogen exposure and obesity is highly suggestive, causality and overall significance currently remain ambiguous. New detailed longitudinal studies are merited as a high-priority investigative goal to establish the magnitude of the contributing risk by individual obesogens.

5. Metabolic disorders and endocrine disruptors

The issue of potential ED interference with metabolic imbalances is very timely especially in light of a recent cross-sectional study in the general adult population of the United States that reported an association between higher urinary BPA concentrations with diabetes, cardiovascular diagnoses and clinically abnormal concentrations of the liver enzymes γ-glutamyltransferase (Lang et al., 2008). An analysis of the posterior data from the US National Health and Nutrition Survey (NHANES) conducted by Melzer et al. confirmed the association between urinary BPA levels with coronary heart disease (Melzer et al., 2010).

These adverse effects of BPA on humans' metabolism appear to be confirmative of previously reported actions in animal models. Indeed, a series of studies by Alonso-Magdalena et al. have illustrated the potency of this estrogenic compound to directly affect pancreatic cells' function and to favor metabolic disorders (Alonso-Magdalena et al., 2005, 2006, 2010). Low doses of BPA acutely induced a change in glycemic balance characterized by a decrease in glycose levels that correlated with a rise of plasma insulin in adult male mice (Alonso-Magdalena et al., 2006). Furthermore, long term administration of BPA in β-cells from these rodents resulted to an increase in the insulin content and insulin secretion of the islets of Langerhans while BPA-treated mice appeared to be insulin resistant (Alonso-Magdalena et al., 2006). Pancreatic a-cells have also been implied as potential targets for endocrine disruption given that low doses of Bisphenol A were shown to impair the molecular signaling that leads to secretion of glycagon by suppressing intracellular calcium ion oscillations in α-cells in response to low blood glucose levels (Alonso-Magdalena et al., 2005).

Interestingly, gestational exposure to BPA has been recently linked to impaired glucose tolerance and reduced insulin sensitivity in adult mice' life when compared with non-exposed male offspring. Pregnant mothers were also affected as indicated by the aggravated insulin resistance during pregnancy and post-partum in this population in comparison to non-treated mothers (Alonso-Magdalena et al., 2010). As demonstrated in these rodent studies, BPA may contribute to metabolic disorders relevant to glucose homeostasis and, therefore, this altered blood glucose homeostasis may subsequently enhance the development of type 2 diabetes. Interestingly, human studies have also implied BPA to favor metabolic syndrome development through an inhibitory effect on adiponectin release from adipose depots of patients with morbidity obesity undergoing gastric bypass surgery (Hugo et al., 2008).

Other compounds that have been correlated with alterations in blood glucose homeostasis in humans are dioxins (Bertazzi et al., 2001; Henriksen et al., 1997) and arsenic (Lai et al., 1994; Meliker et al., 2007).

In conclusion, accumulating data are pointing to the potential role of endocrine disrupting chemicals either directly or indirectly in the pathogenesis of adipogenesis and diabetes ,the major epidemics of modern world.

6. Conclusion

Accumulative evidence from experimental and human studies imply that exposure to endocrine disruptors may have significant impact to all hormone-sensitive endocrine systems. The catalogue of endocrinopathies possible related to EDs is expanding to include a broad spectrum of disorders from reproductive function to metabolic regulation (see Table 1).

Human exposure to EDs is well-documented to occur through multiple sources, however, several parameters considerably complicate the assessment of EDs' interaction with human health. For instance, it is important to keep in mind that humans are continuously exposed to a multitude of pollutants which can act together, and lead to effects that are different from those of the individual pollutants that are usually studied in the laboratory. Furthermore,

the multiplicity of targets and the fact that many targets can be disrupted at the same time within an organism make difficult to truly evaluate the affect of an endocrine disrupting chemical to many endocrine systems. In addition, humans are not usually exposed to a single compound but to a mixture of EDs and as these chemicals may interact additively or antagonistically, the final clinical outcome may be variable. After all, human disorders are more likely the additive result of chronic exposure to low amounts of mixtures of EDs.

Another important parameter is timing of exposure as the biological effects of a compound vary depending not only on the nature of the chemical and dose, but on the susceptibility of the individual to this. The timing of exposure appears as a determining factor in the developmental programming hypothesis, which proposes that exposure of the developing tissues/organs to an adverse stimulus or insult during critical or sensitive times of development can permanently reprogram normal physiological responses leading to hormonal disorders later in life (Gluckman et al., 2005). In other words, when estimating the effect of a compound on human health the time of exposure may determine the clinical outcome. Importantly, the consequences of an exposure may not be apparent at the actual time of exposure, but may manifest later in life. Indeed, the potential lag between exposure to EDs and the manifestation of an endocrine disorder in humans may be years or decades after initial exposure.

Although direct causal links between exposures to EDs and disease states in humans are difficult to draw, results from basic research and epidemiological studies make it clear that more screening for exposures and targeting at-risk groups is a high priority. Innovative technologies designed to improve the assessment of human exposure and reproductive and endocrine health endpoints should be applied. Furthermore, scientific community should adopt a united approach with collaboration between different professional groups and government policy to prompt precautionary actions against excess exposure. After all, endocrine disruption is on the agenda of many experts' groups, steering committees and panels of governmental organizations, industry, and academia throughout the world.

Endocrine systems	Endocrine Disorders Possibly Related To Endocrine Disruptors' Exposure
Male reproductive system	Testicular Dysgenesis Syndrome Altered semen quality Hypospadias/ cryptorchidism Testicular cancer Prostate cancer
Female reproductive system	Precocious/delayed puberty Impaired fertility/fecundity Reproductive tract anomalies Endometriosis Menstrual and Ovarian dysfunction Pregnancy complication (Preterm delivery/Pregnancy lost) Premature menopause Impaired mammary gland differentiation / Breast cancer
Thyroid	Altered thyroid hormones
Adipose tissue	Promote adipogenesis Altered body weight Disturbed adipokine secretion
Pancreas	Diabetes mellitus Disturbed insulin secretion Disturbed glycagon secretion

Table 1. Endocrine system as a target for disruption: The potential impact of endocrine disruptors on endocrine system based on experimental and human data.

7. References

Alonso-Magdalena, P.; Vieira, E.; Soriano, S.; Menes, L.; Burks, D.; Quesada, I. & Nadal A. (2010). Bisphenol A exposure during pregnancy disrupts glucose homeostasis in mothers and adult male offspring. *Environ Health Perspect.,* Vol.118, No. 9, pp.1243-50

Alonso-Magdalena, P.; Laribi, O.; Ropero, AB.; Fuentes, E.; Ripoll, C.; Soria, B. & Nadal A. (2005). Low Doses of Bisphenol A and Diethylstilbestrol Impair Ca2+ Signals in Pancreatic α-Cells through a Nonclassical Membrane Estrogen Receptor within Intact Islets of Langerhans. *Environ Health Perspect,* Vol.113, No. 8, pp.969-77

Alonso-Magdalena, P.; Morimoto, S.; Ripoll, C.; Fuentes, E. & Nadal, A. (2006). The Estrogenic Effect of Bisphenol -A Disrupts Pancreatic β-Cell Function In Vivo and Induces Insulin Resistance. *Environ Health Perspect,* Vol.114, No. 1, pp.106-12

Anway, MD. & Skinner, MK. (2006). Epigenetic Transgenerational Actions of Endocrine Disruptors. *Endocrinology,* Vol.147, No.6, pp43-49

Anway, MD. & Skinner, MK. (2008). Transgenerational effects of the endocrine disruptor vinclozolin on the prostate transcriptome and adult onset disease. *Prostate* 2008; Vol.68, No.5, pp.517-529

Baillie-Hamilton, PF. (2002). Chemical toxins: a hypothesis to explain the global obesity epidemic. *J Altern Complement Med.,* Vol.8, No.2, pp.185-92

Bertazzi, PA.; Consonni, D.; Bachetti, S.; Rubagotti, M.; Baccarelli, A.; Zocchetti, C. & Pesatori, AC. (2001). Health Effects of Dioxin Exposure: A 20-Year Mortality Study. *Am J Epidemiol,* Vol.153, No.11, pp.1031–44

Boas, M.; Feldt-Rasmussen, U.; Skakkebæk, NE. & Main KM. (2006). Environmental chemicals and thyroid function. *Eur J Endocrinol.,* Vol.154, No.5,pp.599–611

Carlsen, E.; Giwercman, A.; Keiding, N. & Skakkebaek, NE.(1992). Evidence for decreasing quality of semen during past 50 years. *BMJ,* Vol.305, No.6854, pp.609-13

Caserta, D.; Maranghi, L.; Mantovani, A.; Marci, R.; Maranghi ,F. & Moscarini M. (2008). Impact of endocrine disruptor chemicals in gynaecology. *Hum Reprod Update,* Vol.14, No.1, pp.59–72

Dallinga, JW.; Moonen, EJ.; Dumoulin, JC.; Evers, JL.; Geraedts, JP. & Kleinjans JC. (2002). Decreased human semen quality and organochlorine compounds in blood. *Hum Reproduction,* Vol.17, No.8, pp.1973-9

Diamanti-Kandarakis, E., Bourguignon, JP., Giudice, LC., Hauser, R., Prins, GS., Soto, AM., Zoeller, RT. & Gore AC. Endocrine-disrupting chemicals: an Endocrine Society scientific statement. Endocr Rev. 2009;30(4):293-342.

Diamanti-Kandarakis, E.; Palioura, E.; Kandarakis, SA. & Koutsilieris, M. (2010) The impact of endocrine disruptors on endocrine targets. *Horm Metab Res.,* Vol.42, No.8, pp.543-52

Duty, SM.; Silva, MJ.; Barr, DB.; Brock, JW.; Ryan, L.; Chen, Z.; Herrick, RF.; Christiani, DC. & Hauser, R. (2003). Phthalate exposure and human semen parameters. *Epidemiology,* Vol.14, No.3, pp.269-77

Euling, SY.; Herman-Giddens, ME.; Lee, PA.; Selevan, SG.; Juu,l A.; Sørensen, TI.; Dunkel, L.; Himes, JH; Teilmann, G. & Swan, SH. (2008)a. Examination of US puberty-timing data from 1940 to 1994 for secular trends: panel findings. *Pediatrics.,* Vol.121, No.3, pp.172-91

Euling, SY.; Selevan, SG.; Pescovitz, OH. & Skakkebaek NE. (2008)b. Role of environmental factors in the timing of puberty. *Pediatrics.,* Vol.12, No.3, pp.167-71

Gladen, BC.; Ragan, NB. & Rogan, WJ. (2000). Pubertal growth and development and prenatal and lactational exposure to polychlorinated biphenyls and dichlorodiphenyl dichloroethene. *J Pediatr,* Vol.136, No.4, pp.490-496

Gluckman, PD.; Hanson, MA. & Pinal C. (2005). The developmental origins of adult disease. *Matern Child Nutr.,* Vol. 1, No.3, pp.130-141

Goncharov, A.; Haase, RF.; Santiago-Rivera, A.; Morse, G.; Akwesasne Task Force on the Environment; McCaffrey, RJ.; Rej, R. & Carpenter DO. (2008). High serum PCBs are associated with elevation of serum lipids and cardiovascular disease in a Native American population. *Environ Res,* Vol.106, No.2, pp.226-239

Grün, F. & Blumberg, B. (2006). Environmental obesogens: organotins and endocrine disruption via nuclear receptor signaling. *Endocrinology,* Vol. 147, No. 6, pp.50-5

Grün, F.; Watanabe, H.; Zamanian, Z.; Maeda, L.; Arima, K.; Cubacha, R.; Gardiner, DM.; Kanno, J.; Iguchi, T. & Blumberg, B. (2006). Endocrine-Disrupting Organotin Compounds Are Potent Inducers of Adipogenesis in Vertebrates. *Mol Endocrinol.,* Vol.20, No.9, pp.2141-55

Hagmar, L.; Bjork, J.; Sjodin, A.; Bergman, A. & Erfurth, EM. (2001). Plasma levels of persistent organohalogens and hormone levels in adult male humans. *Arch Environ Health,* Vol. 56, No.2, pp.138-143

Hatch, EE.; Nelson, JW.; Qureshi, MM.; Weinberg, J.; Moore, LL.; Singer M. & Webster TF. (2008). Association of urinary phthalate metabolite concentrations with body mass index and waist circumference: a cross-sectional study of NHANES data, 1999-2002. *Environ Health.*, Vol.7, pp.27

Hauser, R.; Chen, Z.; Pothier, L.; Ryan, L. & Altshul, L. (2003).The relationship between human semen parameters and environmental exposure to polychlorinated biphenyls and p,p'-DDE. *Environ Health Perspect,* Vol.111, No.12, pp.1505-11

Hauser, R.; Meeker, JD.; Duty, S.; Silva, MJ. & Calafat, AM. (2006). Altered semen quality in relation to urinary concentrations of phthalate monoester and oxidative metabolites. *Epidemiology,* Vol.17, No.6, pp. 682-91

Henriksen, GL.; Ketchum, NS.; Michalek, JE. & Swaby, JA. (1997). Serum dioxin and diabetes mellitus in veterans of Operation Ranch Hand. *Epidemiology,* Vol.8, No.3, pp.252-8

Herbst, AL.; Ulfelder, H. & Poskanzer DC. (1971). Adenocarcinoma of the vagina. Association of maternal stilbestrol therapy with tumor appearance in young women. *N Engl J Med,* Vol.284, No.15, pp.878-881

Heyland, A & Moroz, LL. (2005). Cross-kingdom hormonal signaling: an insight from thyroid hormone functions in marine larvae. *J Exp Biol.,* Vol.208, No.23, pp.4355-61

Howdeshell, KL. (2002). A model of the development of the brain as a construct of the thyroid system. *Environ Health Perspect,* Vol.110, No.3, pp.337-348

Hugo, ER.; Brandebourg, TD.; Woo, JG.; Loftus, J.; Alexander, JW. & Ben-Jonathan, N. (2008). Bisphenol A at environmentally relevant doses inhibits adiponectin release from human adipose tissue explants and adipocytes. *Environ Health Perspect.,* Vol.116, No.12, pp.1642-7

Jacobson-Dickman, E. & Lee, MM. (2009). The influence of endocrine disruptors on pubertal timing . *Curr Opin Endocrinol Diabetes Obes,* Vol.16, No.1, pp.25–30

Juhler, RK.; Larsen, SB.; Meyer, O.; Jensen, ND.; Spanò, M.; Giwercman, A. & Bonde JP. (1999). Human semen quality in relation to dietary pesticide exposure and organic diet. *Arch Environ Contam Toxicol,* Vol.37, No.3, pp.415-23

Kanayama, T.; Kobayashi, N.; Mamiya, S.; Nakanishi, T. & Nishikawa J. (2005). Organotin Compounds Promote Adipocyte Differentiation as Agonists of the Peroxisome Proliferator-Activated Receptor -γ /Retinoid X Receptor Pathway. *Mol Pharmacol.,* Vol. 67, No.3, pp.766-74

Kandaraki, E.; Chatzigeorgiou, A.; Livadas, S.; Palioura, E.; Economou, F.; Koutsilieris, M.; Palimeri, S.; Panidis, D. & Diamanti-Kandarakis E. Endocrine Disruptors and Polycystic Ovary Syndrome (PCOS): Elevated Serum Levels of Bisphenol A in Women with PCOS. *J Clin Endocrinol Metab.* 2010 Dec 30. [Epub ahead of print]

Kaufman, RH. (1982). Structural changes of the genital tract associated with in utero exposure to diethylstilbestrol. *Obstet Gynecol Annu.,* Vol.11, pp.187-202

Kaufman, RH.; Adam, E.; Hatch, EE.; Noller, K.; Herbst, AL.; Palmer, JR. & Hoover, RN. (2000). Continued follow-up of pregnancy outcomes in diethylstilbestrol-exposed offspring. *Obstet Gynecol,* Vol.96, No.4, pp.483-9

Lai, MS.; Hsueh, YM.; Chen, CJ.; Shyu, MP.; Chen, SY.; Kuo. TL.; Wu, MM. & Tai TY. (1994). Ingested inorganic arsenic and prevalence of diabetes mellitus. *Am J Epidemiol.,* Vol.139, No.5, pp.484-92

Lang, IA.; Galloway, TS.; Scarlett, A.; Henley, WE.; Depledge, M.; Wallace, RB. & Melzer D. (2008). Association of Urinary Bisphenol A Concentration With Medical Disorders and Laboratory Abnormalities in Adults. *JAMA.,* Vol.300, No.11, pp.1303-10

Langer, P.; Koban, A.; Tajtakovα, M.; Koška, J.; Radikovα, Z.; Kšinantovα, L.; Imrich, R.; Hucková, M.; Drobná, B.; Gasperíková, D.; Seböková, E. & Klimes, I. (2008). Increased thyroid volume, prevalence of thyroid antibodies and impaired fastingand impaired fasting glucose in young adults from organochlorine cocktail polluted area: Outcome of transgenerational transmission? *Chemosphere,* Vol.73, No.3, pp.1145-1150

Masuno, H.; Iwanami, J.; Kidani, T.; Sakayama, K. & Honda K. (2005). Bisphenol a accelerates terminal differentiation of 3T3-L1 cells into adipocytes through the phosphatidylinositol 3-kinase pathway. *Toxicol Sci.,* Vol.84, No.2, pp.319-27

Masuno, H.; Kidani, T.; Sekiya, K.; Sakayama, K.; Shiosaka, T.; Yamamoto, H. & Honda K.(2002). Bisphenol A in combination with insulin can accelerate the conversion of 3T3-L1 fibroblasts to adipocytes. *J Lipid Res.,* Vol.43, No.5, pp.676-84.

McLachlan, JA.; Simpson, E. & Martin, M. (2006). Endocrine disrupters and female reproductive health. *Best Pract Res Clin Endocrinol Metab,* Vol.20, No.1, pp.63–75

Meeker, JD.; Altshul, L. & Hauser R. (2007). Serum PCBs, *p,p'*-DDE and HCB predict Thyroid Hormone Levels in Men. *Environ Res.,*Vol. 104, No.2, pp.296–304

Meliker, JR.; Wahl, RL.; Cameron, LL. & Nriag, JO. (2007). Arsenic in drinking water and cerebrovascular disease, diabetes mellitus, and kidney disease in Michigan: a standardized mortality ratio analysis. *Environmental Health,* Vol.6, pp.4

Melzer, D.; Rice, NE.; Lewis, C.; Henley, WE, & Galloway TS. (2010). Association of Urinary Bisphenol A Concentration with Heart Disease: Evidence from NHANES 2003/06. *PLoS One.,* Vol.5, No. 1, e.8673

Mendola, P.; Messer LC. & Rappazzo K. (2008). Science linking environmental contaminant exposures with fertility and reproductive health impacts in the adult female. *Fertil Steril.,* Vol.89, No.2, pp.81-94

Newbold RR. (2010). Impact of environmental endocrine disrupting chemicals on the development of obesity. *Hormones (Athens),* Vol.9, No.3, pp.206-17

Newbold, RR.; Padilla-Banks, E.; Jefferson, WN. & Heindel JJ. (2008). Effects of endocrine disruptors on obesity. *Int J Androl,* Vol.31, No.2, pp.201-208, ISSN 0105-6263

Newbold, RR.; Padilla-Banks, E.; Snyder, RJ.; Phillips, TM. & Jefferson WN. (2007). Developmental exposure to endocrine disruptors and the obesity epidemic. *Reprod Toxicol,* Vol.23, No.3, pp.290-296

Nikaido, Y.; Yoshizawa, K.; Danbara, N.; Tsujita-Kyutoku, M.; Yuri, T.; Uehara, N. & Tsubura, A. (2004). Effects of maternal xenoestrogen exposure on development of the reproductive tract and mammary gland in female CD-1 mouse offspring. *Reprod. Toxicol,* Vol.18, No.6, pp.803–811

Palmer, JR.; Hatch, EE.; Rao, RS.; Kaufman, RH.; Herbst, AL.; Noller, KL.; Titus-Ernstoff, L. & Hoover RN. (2001). Infertility among women exposed prenatally to diethylstilbestrol. *Am J Epidemiol,* Vol.154, No.4, pp.316–21

Persky, V.; Turyk, M.; Anderson, HA.; Hanrahan, LP.; Falk, C.; Steenport, DN.; Chatterton, R Jr. & Freels, S.; Great Lakes Consortium. (2001). The effects of PCB exposure and fish consumption on endogenous hormones. *Environ Health Perspect.,* Vol.109, No.12, pp.1275-83

Phrakonkham, P.; Viengchareun, S.; Belloir, C.; Lombes, M.; Artur, Y. & Canivenc-Lavier MC. (2008). Dietary xenoestrogens differentially impair 3T3-L1 preadipocyte differentiation and persistently affect leptin synthesis. *J. Steroid Biochem. Molec. Biol,* Vol.110, No.1-2, pp.95–103

Rubin, BS.; Murray, MK.; Damassa, DA.; King, JC. & Soto, AM. (2001). Perinatal exposure to low doses of bisphenol-A affects body weight, patterns of estrous cyclicity and plasma LH levels. *Environ Health Perspect.,* Vol.109, No.7, pp.675–680

Skakkebæk, NE.; Rajpert-De Meyts, E. & Main KM. (2001). Testicular dysgenesis syndrome: an increasingly common developmental disorder with environmental aspects. *Hum Reprod Update,* Vol.16, No.5, pp. 972-978

Sharpe, RM. & Skakkebæk NE. (2003). Male reproductive disorders and the role of endocrine disruption: advances in understanding and identification of areas for future research. *Pure Appl Chem,* Vol.75, pp.2023-2038

Somm, E.; Schwitzgebel, VM.; Toulotte, A.; Cederroth, CR.; Combescure, C.; Nef, S.; Aubert, ML. & Hüppi PS. (2009). Perinatal Exposure to Bisphenol A Alters Early Adipogenesis in the Rat. *Environ Health Perspect,* Vol.117, No. 10, pp.1549–1555.

Steinmaus, C.; Miller, MD. & Howd, R. (2007). Impact of smoking and thiocyanate on perchlorate and thyroid hormone associations in the 2001-2002 national health and nutrition examination survey. *Environ Health Perspect.,* Vol.115, No.9, pp.1333–1338

Tabb, MM., & Blumberg, B. (2006). New Modes of Action for Endocrine-Disrupting Chemicals. *Mol Endocrinol.,* Vol.20, No.3, pp.475–482

Takeuchi, T. & Tsutsumi, O. (2002). Serum Bisphenol A Concentrations Showed Gender Differences, Possibly Linked to Androgen Levels. *Biochem Biophys Res Commun.,* Vol.291, No.1, pp.76–78

Takeuchi, T.; Tsutsumi, O.; Ikezuki, Y.; Takai, Y. & Taketani Y. (2004). Positive relationship between androgen and the endocrine disruptor, bisphenol A, in normal women and women with ovarian dysfunction. *Endocr J.,* Vol.51, No.2, pp.165-9

Takser, L.; Mergler, D.; Baldwin, M.; de Grosbois, S.; Smargiassi ,A. & Lafond, J. (2005). Thyroid hormones in pregnancy in relation to environmental exposure to organochlorine compounds and mercury. *Environ Health Perspect.,* Vol. 113, No.8, pp.1039-45

Titus-Ernstoff, L.; Troisi, R.; Hatch, EE.; Wise, LA.; Palmer, J.; Hyer, M.; Kaufman, R.; Adam, E.; Strohsnitter, W.; Noller, K.; Herbst, AL.; Gibson-Chambers, J.; Hartge, P. & Hoover RN. (2006). Menstrual and reproductive characteristics of women whose mothers were exposed in utero to diethylstilbestrol (DES). *Int J Epidemiol,* Vol.35, No.4, pp.862-868

Toppari, J.; Kaleva, M. & Virtanen HE.(2001). Trends in the incidence of cryptorchidism and hypospadias, and method0logical limitations of registry-based data. *Hum Reprod Update* Vol.7, No.3, pp.282-6

U.S. EPA. (1997). Special report on Environmental Endocrine Disruption: An Effects Assessment and Analysis. Office of Research and Development, 1997, EPA/630/R-96/012, Washington D.C.

Wada, K.; Sakamoto, H.; Nishikawa, K.; Sakuma, S.; Nakajima, A.; Fujimoto, Y. & Kamisaki Y. (2007). Life style-related diseases of the digestive system: endocrine disruptors stimulate lipid accumulation in target cells related to metabolic syndrome. *J Pharmacol Sci.,* Vol.105, No.2, pp.133-7

Waring, RH. & Harris RM. (2005). Endocrine disrupters: A human risk? *Mol Cell Endocrinol.,* Vol.244, No.1-2, pp.2-9

Woodruff, TJ.; Carlson, A.; Schwartz, JM. & Giudice, LC. (2008). Proceedings of the Summit on Environmental Challenges to Reproductive Health and Fertility: Executive Summary. *Fertil Steril,* Vol. 89, No.2, pp.281–300

Zoeller, RT. (2007). Environmental chemicals impacting the thyroid: targets and consequences. *Thyroid,* Vol.17, No.9, pp.811-817

Zoeller, TR. (2010). Environmental chemicals targeting thyroid. *Hormones (Athens).,* Vol.9, No.1,pp. 28-40